Pabulo H. Rampelotto (Ed.)

Enzymes and Their Biotechnological Applications

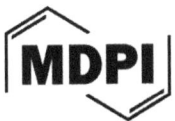

MDPI

This book is a reprint of the special issue that appeared in the online open access journal *Biomolecules* (ISSN 2218-273X) in 2013 (available at: http://www.mdpi.com/journal/biomolecules/special_issues/biotechnological_applications).

Guest Editor
Pabulo H. Rampelotto
Federal University of Rio Grande do Sul
Brazil

Editorial Office
MDPI AG
Klybeckstrasse 64
Basel, Switzerland

Publisher
Shu-Kun Lin

Assistant Editor
Rongrong Leng

1. Edition 2015

MDPI • Basel • Beijing • Wuhan

ISBN 978-3-03842-147-4 (PDF)
ISBN 978-3-03842-148-1 (Hbk)

Table of Contents

IV

List of Contributors

Jose L. Adrio: Neol Biosolutions SA, BIC Granada, Granada 18016, Spain.

Sergio D. Aguirre: Department of Biochemistry and Biomedical Sciences, McMaster University, 1280 Main St. W., Hamilton, ON L8S 4K1, Canada.

Birgitte K. Ahring: Section for Sustainable Biotechnology, Aalborg University Copenhagen, A C Meyers Vaenge 15, 2450 Copenhagen SV, Denmark; Bioproducts, Sciences & Engineering Laboratory, Washington State University, 2710 Crimson Way, Richland, WA 99354, USA.

M. Monsur Ali: Department of Biochemistry and Biomedical Sciences, McMaster University, 1280 Main St. W., Hamilton, ON L8S 4K1, Canada.

Manuela Avi: LONZA AG, Rottenstrasse 6, Visp 3930, Switzerland.

Christopher D. Boone: Biochemistry & Molecular Biology, University of Florida, P.O. Box 100245, Gainesville, FL 32610, USA.

Elisabetta De Angelis: Flavia 110, Trieste 34147, Italy.

Rubén de Regil: Unidad de Biotecnología Industrial, CIATEJ, A.C. Av. Normalistas 800, Col. Colinas de la Normal, Guadalajara, Jal, C.P. 44270, Mexico.

Arnold L. Demain: Research Institute for Scientists Emeriti (R.I.S.E.), Drew University, Madison, NJ 07940, USA.

Cynthia Ebert: Dipartimento di Scienze Chimiche e Farmaceutiche, Università degli Studi di Trieste, Piazzale Europa 1, Trieste 34127, Italy.

Mohammad S. Eram: Department of Biology, University of Waterloo, 200 University Avenue West, Waterloo, Ontario N2L 3G1, Canada; Current address: Structural Genomics Consortium, University of Toronto, Toronto, Ontario M5G 1L7, Canada.

Valerio Ferrario: Dipartimento di Scienze Chimiche e Farmaceutiche, Università degli Studi di Trieste, Piazzale Europa 1, Trieste 34127, Italy.

Lucia Gardossi: Dipartimento di Scienze Chimiche e Farmaceutiche, Università degli Studi di Trieste, Piazzale Europa 1, Trieste 34127, Italy.

Gianfranco Gilardi: Department of Life Sciences and Systems Biology, University of Torino, via Accademia Albertina 13, Torino 10123, Italy.

Sonika Gill: Biochemistry & Molecular Biology, University of Florida, P.O. Box 100245, Gainesville, FL 32610, USA.

Andrew Habibzadegan: Biochemistry & Molecular Biology, University of Florida, P.O. Box 100245, Gainesville, FL 32610, USA.

Dietmar Haltrich: Food Biotechnology Laboratory, BOKU–University of Natural Resources and Life Sciences Vienna, Muthgasse 11, Vienna 1190, Austria.

Yi Jiang: Department of Polymer Chemistry, Zernike Institute for Advanced Materials, University of Groningen, Nijenborgh 4, 9747 AG Groningen, The Netherlands; Dutch Polymer Institute (DPI), P.O. Box 902, 5600 AX Eindhoven, The Netherlands.

Jun-ichi Kadokawa: Graduate School of Science and Engineering, Kagoshima University, 1-21-40 Korimoto, Kagoshima 890-0065, Japan; Research Center for Environmentally Friendly Materials Engineering, Muroran Institute of Technology, 27-1 Mizumoto-cho, Muroran, Hokkaido 050-8585, Japan.

Balázs Krámos: Department of Inorganic and Analytical Chemistry, Budapest University of Technology and Economics, Gellért tér 4, Budapest H-1111, Hungary.

Iris Krondorfer: Food Biotechnology Laboratory, BOKU–University of Natural Resources and Life Sciences Vienna, Muthgasse 11, Vienna 1190, Austria.

Kouichi Kuroda: Division of Applied Life Sciences, Graduate School of Agriculture, Kyoto University, Sakyo-ku, Kyoto 606-8502, Japan.

Wan Chi Lam: School of Energy and Environment, City University of Hong Kong, Tat Chee Avenue, Kowloon, Hong Kong, China.

Sanford Leuba: Program in Molecular Biophysics and Structural Biology, Hillman Cancer Center, University of Pittsburgh, 5117 Centre Ave., Pittsburgh, PA 15213, USA; Department of Cell Biology, Hillman Cancer Center, University of Pittsburgh, 5117 Centre Ave., Pittsburgh, PA 15213, USA.

Yingfu Li: Department of Biochemistry and Biomedical Sciences, McMaster University, 1280 Main St. W., Hamilton, ON L8S 4K1, Canada; Department of Chemistry and Chemical Biology, McMaster University, 1280 Main St. W., Hamilton, ON L8S 4K1, Canada; Michael G. DeGroote Institute for Infectious Disease Research, McMaster University, 1280 Main St. W., Hamilton, ON L8S 4K1, Canada.

Carol Sze Ki Lin: School of Energy and Environment, City University of Hong Kong, Tat Chee Avenue, Kowloon, Hong Kong, China.

Katja Loos: Department of Polymer Chemistry, Zernike Institute for Advanced Materials, University of Groningen, Nijenborgh 4, 9747 AG Groningen, The Netherlands; Dutch Polymer Institute (DPI), P.O. Box 902, 5600 AX Eindhoven, The Netherlands.

Mette Lübeck: Section for Sustainable Biotechnology, Aalborg University Copenhagen, A C Meyers Vaenge 15, 2450 Copenhagen SV, Denmark.

Peter S. Lübeck: Section for Sustainable Biotechnology, Aalborg University Copenhagen, A C Meyers Vaenge 15, 2450 Copenhagen SV, Denmark.

Kesen Ma: Department of Biology, University of Waterloo, 200 University Avenue West, Waterloo, Ontario N2L 3G1, Canada.

Robert McKenna: Biochemistry & Molecular Biology, University of Florida, P.O. Box 100245, Gainesville, FL 32610, USA.

János András Mótyán: Department of Biochemistry and Molecular Biology, Faculty of Medicine, Medical and Health Science Center, University of Debrecen, POB 6, Debrecen H-4012, Hungary.

Kamila Napora-Wijata: ACIB (Austrian Centre of Industrial Biotechnology) GmbH, Petersgasse 14/III, Graz 8010, Austria.

Gábor Náray-Szabó: Laboratory of Structural Chemistry and Biology and HAS-ELTE Protein Modeling Group, Eötvös Loránd University, Pázmány Péter St. 1A, Budapest H-1117, Hungary.

Luciano Navarini: Flavia 110, Trieste 34147, Italy.

Poonam Singh Nigam: Biomedical Science Research Institute, University of Ulster, Coleraine BT52 1SA, UK.

Julianna Oláh: Department of Inorganic and Analytical Chemistry, Budapest University of Technology and Economics, Gellért tér 4, Budapest H-1111, Hungary.

Ramesh N. Patel: SLRP Associates Consultation in Biotechnology, 572 Cabot Hill Road, Bridgewater, NJ 08807, USA.

Joelle N. Pelletier: Chimie, Université de Montréal, 2900 Boulevard Edouard-Montpetit, Montréal, Québec, H3T 1J4, Canada; CGCC, the Center in Green Chemistry and Catalysis, Montréal, H3A 0B8, Canada; PROTEO, the Québec Network for Protein Function, Structure and Engineering, Québec, G1V 0A6, Canada; Biochimie, Université de Montréal, 2900 Boulevard Edouard-Montpetit, Montréal, Québec, H3T 1J4, Canada.

Clemens K. Peterbauer: Food Biotechnology Laboratory, BOKU–University of Natural Resources and Life Sciences Vienna, Muthgasse 11, Vienna 1190, Austria.

Daniel Pleissner: School of Energy and Environment, City University of Hong Kong, Tat Chee Avenue, Kowloon, Hong Kong, China.

Natalie M. Rachel: Chimie, Université de Montréal, 2900 Boulevard Edouard-Montpetit, Montréal, Québec, H3T 1J4, Canada; CGCC, the Center in Green Chemistry and Catalysis, Montréal, H3A 0B8, Canada; PROTEO, the Québec Network for Protein Function, Structure and Engineering, Québec, G1V 0A6, Canada.

Karen Robins: LONZA AG, Rottenstrasse 6, Visp 3930, Switzerland.

Bruno J. Salena: Dvision of Gastroenterology, Department of Medicine, McMaster University, 1280 Main St. W., Hamilton, ON L8S 4K1, Canada.

Georgina Sandoval: Unidad de Biotecnología Industrial, CIATEJ, A.C. Av. Normalistas 800, Col. Colinas de la Normal, Guadalajara, Jal, C.P. 44270, Mexico.

Grant Schauer: Program in Molecular Biophysics and Structural Biology, Hillman Cancer Center, University of Pittsburgh, 5117 Centre Ave., Pittsburgh, PA 15213, USA; Department of Cell Biology, Hillman Cancer Center, University of Pittsburgh, 5117 Centre Ave., Pittsburgh, PA 15213, USA.

Nicolas Sluis-Cremer: Department of Medicine, Division of Infectious Diseases, 3550 Terrace St., Pittsburgh, PA 15261, USA.

Manoj N. Sonavane: ACIB (Austrian Centre of Industrial Biotechnology) GmbH, Petersgasse 14/III, Graz 8010, Austria.

Annette Sørensen: Section for Sustainable Biotechnology, Aalborg University Copenhagen, A C Meyers Vaenge 15, 2450 Copenhagen SV, Denmark; Bioproducts, Sciences & Engineering Laboratory, Washington State University, 2710 Crimson Way, Richland, WA 99354, USA.

Petra Staudigl: Food Biotechnology Laboratory, BOKU–University of Natural Resources and Life Sciences Vienna, Muthgasse 11, Vienna 1190, Austria.

Gernot A. Strohmeier: ACIB (Austrian Centre of Industrial Biotechnology) GmbH, Petersgasse 14/III, Graz 8010, Austria; Institute of Organic Chemistry, TU Graz, Stremayrgasse 9, Graz 8010, Austria.

X

Ferenc Tóth: Department of Biochemistry and Molecular Biology, Faculty of Medicine, Medical and Health Science Center, University of Debrecen, POB 6, Debrecen H-4012, Hungary.

József Tőzsér: Department of Biochemistry and Molecular Biology, Faculty of Medicine, Medical and Health Science Center, University of Debrecen, POB 6, Debrecen H-4012, Hungary.

Antonio Trincone: Institute of Biomolecular Chemistry, National Research Council, Via Campi Flegrei, 34, Pozzuoli 80078, Naples, Italy.

Mitsuyoshi Ueda: Division of Applied Life Sciences, Graduate School of Agriculture, Kyoto University, Sakyo-ku, Kyoto 606-8502, Japan.

Francesca Valetti: Department of Life Sciences and Systems Biology, University of Torino, via Accademia Albertina 13, Torino 10123, Italy.

Gert O.R. Alberda van Ekenstein: Department of Polymer Chemistry, Zernike Institute for Advanced Materials, University of Groningen, Nijenborgh 4, 9747 AG Groningen, The Netherlands.

Harumi Veny: Department of Chemical Engineering, Faculty of Engineering, University of Malaya, Malaysia.

Margit Winkler: ACIB (Austrian Centre of Industrial Biotechnology) GmbH, Petersgasse 14/III, Graz 8010, Austria.

Albert J.J. Woortman: Department of Polymer Chemistry, Zernike Institute for Advanced Materials, University of Groningen, Nijenborgh 4, 9747 AG Groningen, The Netherlands.

About the Guest Editor

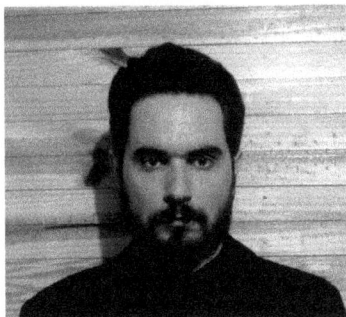

Pabulo Henrique Rampelotto is a molecular biologist currently developing his research at the Federal University of Rio Grande do Sul (Brazil). Prof. Rampelotto is the founder and Editor-in-Chief of the Springer Book Series **Grand Challenges in Biology and Biotechnology**. In addition, he serves as Editor-in-Chief of **Current Biotechnology** as well as Associate Editor, Guest Editor and member of the editorial board of several scientific journals in the field of Life Sciences and Biotechnology. Prof. Rampelotto is also a member of four scientific advisory boards (Astrobiology/SETI Board, Biotech/Medical Board, Policy Board, and Space Settlement Board) of the Lifeboat Foundation, alongside several Nobel Laureates and other distinguished scientists, philosophers, educators, engineers, and economists. Some of the most distinguished team leaders in the field have published their work, ideas, and findings in his books and special issues.

Preface

The development of new enzymes is one of the most thriving branches of biotechnology. Although the applications of enzymes are already well established in some areas, recent advances in modern biotechnology have revolutionized the development of new enzymes. The use of genetic engineering has further improved manufacturing processes and enabled the commercialization of enzymes that could previously not be produced. Protein engineering and the possibility of introducing small changes to proteins brings ever more powerful means of analysis to the study of enzyme structure and its biochemical and biophysical properties, which have led to the rational modification of enzymes to match specific requirements and also the design of new enzymes with novel properties. The developments in bioinformatics and the availability of sequence data have significantly increased the efficiency of identifying genes with biotech potential from nature. Complementary to chemical synthesis, biosynthesis of drug metabolites with mammalian or microbial bioreactors offers certain advantages, and sometimes is the only practical route to the desired metabolite. At the same time, new technological developments are stimulating the chemical and pharmaceutical industry to embrace enzyme technology. Altogether, these advances have made it possible to provide tailor-made enzymes, displaying new activities and adapted to new process conditions, enabling a further expansion of their use in several branches of biotechnology. This Special Issue focuses on the discovery and development of new enzymes and their application in different areas of biotechnology. The Special Issue contains a collection of papers written by authors who are leading experts in the field, including selected papers from the 4th International Symposium on Enzymes & Biocatalysis (SEB-2013) and will influence future trends in one of the fastest growing fields of research.

Pabulo H. Rampelotto
Guest Editor

Angling for Uniqueness in Enzymatic Preparation of Glycosides

Antonio Trincone

Abstract: In the early days of biocatalysis, limitations of an enzyme modeled the enzymatic applications; nowadays the enzyme can be engineered to be suitable for the process requirements. This is a general bird's-eye view and as such cannot be specific for articulated situations found in different classes of enzymes or for selected enzymatic processes. As far as the enzymatic preparation of glycosides is concerned, recent scientific literature is awash with examples of uniqueness related to the features of the biocatalyst (yield, substrate specificity, regioselectivity, and resistance to a particular reaction condition). The invention of glycosynthases is just one of the aspects that has thrust forward the research in this field. Protein engineering, metagenomics and reaction engineering have led to the discovery of an expanding number of novel enzymes and to the setting up of new bio-based processes for the preparation of glycosides. In this review, new examples from the last decade are compiled with attention both to cases in which naturally present, as well as genetically inserted, characteristics of the catalysts make them attractive for biocatalysis.

Reprinted from *Biomolecules*. Cite as: Trincone, A. Angling for Uniqueness in Enzymatic Preparation of Glycosides. *Biomolecules* **2013**, *3*, 334-350.

1. Introduction

In a brilliant, recently published analysis of the research-guided development in the field of biocatalysis during the last century, different authors recognized three historical waves of innovations that totally changed the field of biocatalysis to the present industrially accomplished level [1]. In a nutshell, while in the past limitations of an enzyme modeled the enzymatic process, today the enzyme can be engineered to be suitable for the process requirements. However this general bird's-eye view cannot be specific for articulated contexts in which each single class of enzyme or selected enzymatic process is at the present state. In another similar general bird's-eye analysis, Riva identified a long wave of successes still far from reaching the end in biocatalysis [2], due to the difficulties encountered in the shift from "classical" processes to biobased ones. It is clear that exploiting natural catalysts to obtain selective transformations of non-natural substrates is far from being fully explored; among many others, the cases represented by the new concept of "third generation biorefineries" [2] (producing chemicals from biomasses), or by the new glycoside hydrolases and other enzymes found in marine environments [3] have re-fostered new research trends in the field. As a matter of example, although investigation into hemicellulases as biorefining enzymes has been slow, as reported in a recent analysis [4], xylan-related biocatalysis has continued to make steady progress in many areas, including the discovery and characterization of a wide range of hemicellulases. Talking more specifically about biobased glycosynthesis, these studies are opening new prospects for the use of pentose sugars as building blocks for engineered pentosides as non-ionic surfactants or prebiotic food/feed ingredients.

Carbohydrates are involved in a broad range of functions in cell living systems. Structural roles and energy storage as functions were recognized during the first half of the last century while attainments in glycobiology and glycochemistry, during the last twenty years, have further revealed that carbohydrate parts of biomolecules (glycoproteins, glycolipids, *etc.*) are involved in important biological functions mainly related to cell recognition events [5–7]. It should not be neglected that carbohydrates are important molecules also in the technological domain. Synthetic carbohydrate-containing polymers have a wide range of applications in medical biotechnology [8]. A number of novel dietary carbohydrates produced by enzymatic syntheses have been introduced into food technology during the last decade [9]. In innovative fine chemical manufacturing solutions, straightforward synthesis of products is of interest (e.g., chromophoric oligosaccharides of strictly defined structure as valuable tools for the kinetic analysis of hydrolytic activities and for characterization of new exo- or endo-glycosidases). Finally, in cosmetics, prodrug action of enzymatically glycosylated natural lipophilic antioxidants is currently under consideration.

In general glycosylation is considered to be an important and quite special method for the structural modification of a compound. It allows the conversion of a lipophilic compound into a hydrophilic one changing pharmacokinetic properties or creating drug delivery systems. It could also be generalized that in a glycoside, the type of aglycon determines the application: long alkyl chains allow glycosides to possess useful properties as surfactants and emulsifiers; aglycon based on unsaturated alkyl chains are said to be valuable, as glycosides, for fungal infections or as antimicrobial agents; glycosides of peptides and steroids are used in antitumor formulations and cardiac-related drugs, respectively; and glycosides of flavors and fragrances are used as "controlled release" compounds [10,11].

Sugar units have more than one site through which the chains are extended. Each of these sites frequently shows very similar reactivity, thus the masking of reactive centers by protecting groups is essential in order to direct coupling through the right position. For this reason protection and deprotection steps of functional groups are in use extensively in the arsenal of the synthetic carbohydrate chemist; moreover ensuring the correct stereochemistry of the glycosidic linkage formed entails additional difficulty. Carbohydrate related synthetic chemistry can still be considered one of the well-explored branches of organic chemistry and very rich in significant and spectacular successes, although important alternative biomethodologies for assembling glycosidic linkages are presently known and acknowledged. It is worth noting that in comparison with chemical methods, enzymatic glycosylation is particularly useful for the modification of complex biologically active substances, when generally harsh conditions or use of toxic (heavy metals) catalysts are undesirable. Enzymes may represent an imperative choice in fields such as agriculture and food or cosmetics where chemical strategies are not acceptable [12]. In a very recent report detailing different examples of enzymatic glycosylation of small molecules, the authors concluded that challenging substrates require tailored catalysts, and the progress in the field of enzyme engineering and screening of new catalytic activities are both expected to result in new applications of biocatalytic glycosylations in various industrial sectors [13].

The enzymes responsible for the synthesis of glycosidic linkage have been recognized as transglycosylases and named glycosyltransferases, specifying the glycosyl donor and the reaction product. These enzymes transfer sugar moieties from activated donors to specific acceptors, forming stereochemically specific glycosidic bonds, and are responsible *in vivo* for the synthesis of most cell-surface glycoconjugates, using eight common sugar nucleotides as activated donors (Leloir pathway). Sugar phosphates act as donors for other glycosyltransferases (non-Leloir pathway). Another widespread group of enzymes, named glycoside hydrolases (glycosidases), exists; they are involved in the carbohydrate metabolism being responsible for the hydrolysis of glycosidic linkages; they can act as exo- or endo-glycosidases and are involved in a series of important biological events such as energy uptake, in processes inherent cell wall metabolism, in glycan processing during *in vivo* glycoprotein synthesis, *etc*. Based on historical grounds, glycoside hydrolases were implicated in most experimental observations during the early studies into the biological synthesis of glycosidic linkages at the beginning of the last century. Hence, the concepts of enzymatically promoted synthesis by both hydrolysis-reversal and glycosyl transfer soon appeared [14]. By the end of the 1980s, several research projects [15] testified the importance of different and interesting glycoside hydrolases, especially from the marine environment; their main application was centered on the structural identification efforts that faced the complexity of oligosaccharide structures before the instrumental exploit of 2D NMR and MS spectroscopy.

Different wild-type glycosidases and their modified versions are enzymes deserving new expectations in research and development today. Significant progress has been made in recent years for the application of these enzymes: even while the major breakthrough was the invention of glycosynthases, protein engineering, metagenomics and reaction engineering led to the discovery of an expanding number of novel enzymes and to the setting up of new bio-based processes for the preparation of important glycosides. This review will compile different examples where glycoside hydrolases are the key enzymes in the process.

2. Natural Enzymes for the Synthesis of Glycosidic Linkages

In chemical terms, considering both hydrolytic or synthetic aspects of esterases, glycosidases, phosphatases, transglycosidases and peptidases, the enzymatic mechanisms are based on displacement reactions and could be grouped together. This line of thought proved to be highly productive in historical terms, allowing the collection and rationalization of the amount of mechanistic data especially for glycosidases and transglycosylases. The stereochemistry of the mechanisms of glycoside hydrolases was analyzed by Koshland [16] more than 60 years ago and allowed the classification of inverting and retaining enzymes according to the anomeric configuration found in the product with respect to that in the starting substrate. Very recently, it has become clear that other mechanisms have evolved, such as the one based on elimination [17]. In 2010, in an interesting review on diversity of catalytic base nucleophile of glycoside hydrolases, it was reported that a variety of systems are used to replace this function, including substrate-assisted catalysis, a network of several residues, and the use of non-carboxylate residues or exogenous nucleophiles [18].

Glycosyltransferases-mediated reactions are thought to proceed via an oxocarbenium-ion-like transition state as proposed for glycosidase reactions on the basis of solid structural, mechanistic and *ab initio* molecular orbital calculations data [19]. Glycosyltransferases are catalysts for natural glycosylation reactions, known as "Leloir" glycosyl transferases (GT). Glycoside phosphorylases (GP), requiring glycosyl phosphates and transglycosidases (TG), employing non-activated carbohydrates (e.g., sucrose), are additional examples of synthetic enzymes. However glycoside hydrolases (GH) can also be used for synthetic purposes under either kinetic (transglycosylation) or thermodynamic (reverse hydrolysis) control.

In this paragraph new examples related to the transfer of glycosyl residues between two oxygen nucleophiles are compiled with attention to those cases in which the natural characteristics of the catalyst make it attractive for biocatalysis (importance of molecular skeleton of substrates, yield, regioselectivity, resistance to particular reaction condition, *etc.*).

2.1. Interesting Transfer of Glycosyl Residues in Natural Enzymes for the Synthesis of Glycosidic Linkages

Hyaluronic acid, synthesized by hyaluronan synthases, is a biopolymer abundant in extracellular matrices that is degraded by hyaluronidases. Biocompatibility and biodegradability of this polymer and of related small derivatives are of great interest in pharmaceutics in a number of molecular devices for drug delivery. Bovine testicular hyaluronidase (BTH) is a commercially available hyaluronidase preparation that has long been considered a prototype of mammalian hyaluronidases. Presumably all mammalian hyaluronidases can catalyze hydrolysis as well as transglycosylation reactions of hyaluronic acid fragments (Figure 1). In the case of BTH, the hydrolysis is favored at acidic pH values, while transglycosylation occurs preferentially at neutral pH and at low NaCl concentrations. The availability of recombinant expression systems for the production of purified human hyaluronidases PH-20 and Hyal-1 has facilitated the first detailed analysis of the enzymatic reaction products for these two enzymes. HA hexasaccharide, which is generally accepted as being the minimum substrate of BTH, is not a substrate of recombinant human PH-20 and Hyal-1 as recently demonstrated [20] although BTH and PH-20 belong to the same type of hyaluronidase. Interestingly, HA octasaccharide can be used as the substrate of Hyal-1 at pH 3.5. The substrate was converted quickly at concentration between 25 µM to 1 mM; above 1 mM weak substrate inhibition was observed. The study of transfer reactions, selectivities and yields are all features of interest for a possible use of these enzymes in biocatalytic steps for the manipulation of important biomolecules [21].

Additional new examples of this enzyme can be derived from other environments: the venoms of two classes of fish, freshwater stingray (members of the genus Potamotrygon) and stonefish (members of the genus Synanceia), contain, along with proteinaceous toxins, also hyaluronidases. These proteins are considered as spreading factors that facilitate the tissue diffusion of toxins by degrading hyaluronan; owing to this quick action it can possess very interesting features for biocatalysis [22].

Figure 1. Tetrasaccharidic moiety of a hyaluronic acid chain and point of attach of hyaluronase for the hydrolysis and transglycosylation reactions.

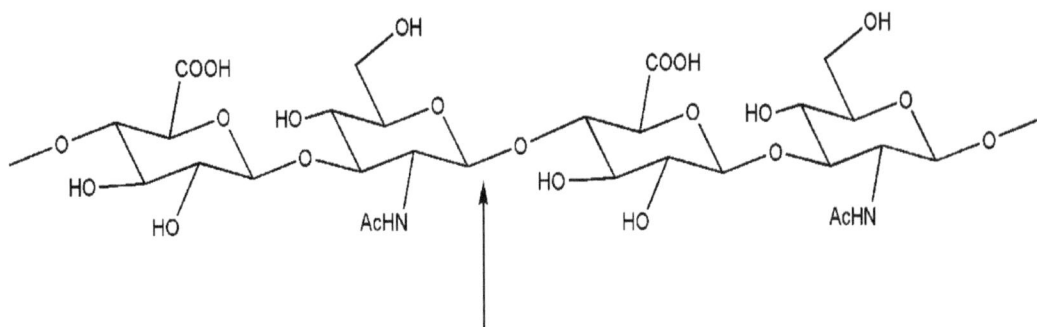

Sensitive and reliable enzymatic tools for the analysis of glycan chains are needed. The O-linked glycans are attached to serine or threonine through the GalNAc residue at the reducing end. The hydrolysis of the *O*-glycosidic α-linkage between GalNAc of the disaccharide Gal-β-1,3-GalNAc- and threonine or serine, is catalyzed by endo-α-N-acetylgalactosaminidase (EC 3.2.1.97). Most of the enzymes of this type are strictly specific for the disaccharidic structure and have no action on substrates with longer or different glycosyl chains. Using the protein sequence of a known endo-α-GalNAcase from *B. longum*, four potential sequences were found from BLAST (Basic Local Alignment Search Tool) search. Cloned and expressed proteins were purified and characterized [23]. Substrate specificity was investigated on aryl substrates as indicated in Figure 2 or by using natural glycoproteins. All three new enzymes are active on Core 1 substrate (Gal-β-1,3-GalNAc) while only two of them (EngEF and EngPA) were active after 24 h on Core 3 disaccharide (Glc-β-1,3-GalNAc). Interestingly, these enzymes acted also as transglycosylating agents; when reacted with simple alkanols (from methanol to nonanol) as acceptors, Core 1 and Core 3 acted as donor disaccharides in test reactions. Although the yields as judged by TLC analysis were low (at 0.8–1.6 mM donor and 13% v/v alkanols), positive reactions were observed up to 4–5 alkanol carbon atoms. As stated by the authors in the concluding remarks, the action of EngEF and EngPA enzymes acting on Core 3 in addition to Core 1 *O*-glycans could make these enzymes powerful tools for the release of *O*-glycan sugars from glycoproteins. More importantly they can also be used as templates in future protein engineering experiments for a possible creation of endo-α-GalNAcases capable of acting on O-linked glycans, regardless of their sugar composition.

One of the last outstanding results in transglycosylation reactions in the last decade is, without any doubt, the recognition that endo-β-*N*-acetylglucosaminidase can transglycosylate a large oligosaccharide onto various glycosyl acceptors. In 2001, the Shoda group reported on the synthesis of a novel disaccharide possessing a 1,2-oxazoline moiety and tested it with a series of enzymes for transglycosylation activity. Typical oxazoline substrate 1, as depicted in Figure 3, reacted with Endo-M or Endo-A from *Mucor hiemalis* or *A. protophormiae*, respectively and the acceptor GlcNAc-β-1-*O*-pNP for the synthesis of a trisaccharidic derivative in high yield [24]. These interesting biocatalysts (Endo-M or Endo-A), which belong to GH family 85 were inactive when they have to use acceptors capped with an α-1,6-fucose (1,6-fucosyl-GlcNAc derivative as acceptors for transglycosylation). But more recently, the Huang group, screening various endo-β-N-acetylglucosaminidases using appropriate synthetic oxazoline donors and compound 2, Figure 3, as acceptor substrate, found that endo-β-N-acetylglucosaminidases from *Flavobacterium meningosepticum* (including Endo-F2 and Endo-F3), were able to glycosylate α-1,6-fucosylated GlcNAc derivative to provide natural, core-fucosylated complex type N-glycopeptides [25]. The product(s) were isolated in high yield by HPLC and this efficiency of transglycosylation is quite impressive, given the fact that only two-fold of the donor substrate was used.

Figure 2. Substrates and percentages of products liberated at the link indicated by each single enzyme.

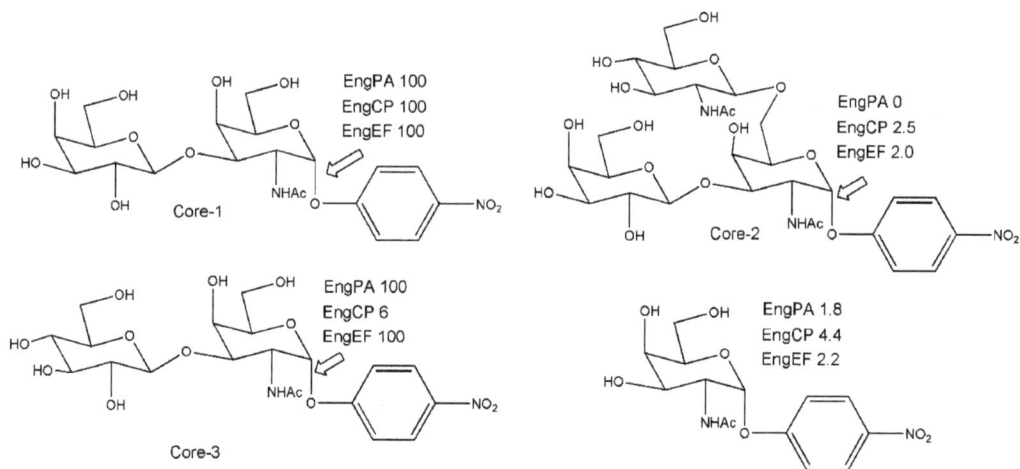

Starting from the known consideration that extracellular glycosidases from fungi, (used to access low molecular weight sugars by their hydrolytic action on polymeric substrates), must possess high flexibility in substrate specificity, the group of Kren recently investigated new enzymes in which the 4-hydroxy moiety of the pyranose ring of the substrate is not essential for binding to the enzyme active site. In their report they emphasize also the transglycosylation activity of β-N-acetylhexosaminidase from *Talaromyces flavus*. The results reported on the production of three novel 4'-deoxy-disaccharides prepared in high yields (52% total disaccharide fraction) starting with phenyl 2-acetamido-2,4-dideoxy-substrate. The conditions of the transglycosylation reaction were first optimized on an analytical scale by varying the concentrations and ratios of the reaction components and identifiying the following reaction conditions as the most efficient: 75 mM donor, 300 mM acceptor, incubation for 5–6 h at 35 °C [26].

Figure 3. Typical oxazoline substrate 1 reacting with Endo-M or Endo-A and capped α-1,6-fucose (1,6-fucosyl-GlcNAc derivative) used as acceptors for transglycosylation by Endo-F2 and Endo-F3 [25].

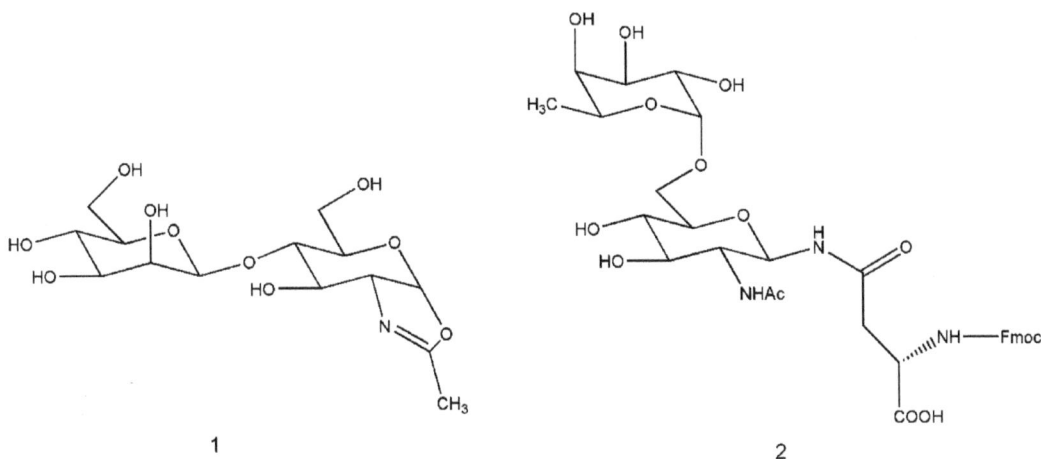

1   2

The enzymatic formation of β-D-fucosides is hardly described in the scientific literature. An extraordinarily broad substrate specificity for both hydrolysis and transglycosylation was exhibited by a glycosidase isolated from the China white jade snail. Acceptor specificity for monosaccharides and transfer efficiency have both been investigated for this promising enzyme [27] and from the results obtained, the authors indicated a very high transfucosylation efficiency using p-nitrophenyl derivative of β-D-fucose at 10 mM and acceptors (at 20–100 mM) such as glucose (88% yield) and xylose (93% yield); the interglycosidic linkage formed with glucose is β-1,6 thus they proposed this biocatalyst as a useful candidate for disaccharide synthesis. The Fuc-β-Xyl disaccharide formed in other reactions is a building block for the synthesis of asterosaponins of marine origin, although in natural compound the interglycosidic linkage is different (Fuc-β-(1-2)-Xyl) [28].

In screening a suitable biocatalyst for galactosylation of nucleosides, Ye *et al.* very recently found that β-galactosidases from *Kluyveromyces lactis* (Sigma, USA) and a crude glycosidase extract of apple seeds, had high hydrolytic activities toward oNPGal, but could not catalyze transglycosylation reactions between oNPGal and 2β-deoxynucleosides [29]. Indeed, only very few reports have appeared in the literature in the last 10 years leading with successful glycosidase-mediated nucleoside glycosylation: (i) after low-yielding results using β-galactosidase from *Aspergillus oryzae* [30], the first successful approach, which appeared in 2007; was (ii) the convenient synthesis of β-galactosyl derivatives of antiviral and anticancer nucleosides, utilizing the purified β-galactosidase activity from the hepatopancreas of *Aplysia fasciata* [31] and the second valid method is (iii) the regioselective galactosylation of floxuridine (FUdR) catalyzed by a commercial β-galactosidase from bovine liver with a high yield (75%) and an excellent 5-β-regioselectivity (>99%) [32] using o-nitrophenyl β-D-galactoside as glycosyl donor. Such desirable products were synthesized with satisfactory yields (41%–68%) and moderate to high 5β-regioselectivities (87%–100%), also by using the crude enzyme extract.

In the hepatopancreas and visceral mass of the mollusc *Aplysia fasciata* a wide range of glycoside hydrolases (α-glucosidase, β-galactosidase, β-glucosidase, β-mannosidase and others) were found and successfully used for the hydrolysis and synthesis of glycosidic bonds. The formation of α-D-oligoglucosides from maltose (up to tetra- and pentasaccharides) was studied in detail [33] and it was also demonstrated that the enzyme was able to form mono- and di- and poly-glucosides of different externally added acceptors [3 and references cited therein]. This activity has been applied in the very recent chemoenzymatic synthesis of α-6-sulfoquinovosyl-1,2-*O*-diacylglycerols, a class of natural lipids that have attracted biomedical attention as possible antitumors, antivirals, and immunomodulators. This synthesis started with the enzymatically controlled transfer of glucose from maltose (10:1 molar ratio) to (*rac*)-1,2-*O*-isopropylidene glycerol. The 1,2 glycerol acetonide conversion of 59% in 29 h was obtained and reaction products were exclusively 3-α-glycosyl derivatives of 1,2-*O*-isopropylidene glycerol. In particular 3-α-glucosyl-1,2-*O*-isopropylidene glycerol was produced as the major component (30% yield) together with a mixture of di- and tri-saccharide analogues (23% and 6% yields, respectively). Under similar conditions the transglycosidase of *Aspergillus niger* and the α-glucosidase of *Bacillus stearothermophilus* gave 3-α-glucosyl-1,2-*O*-isopropylidene glycerol with yields below 2%. This comparison suggests that marine enzymes may offer a viable option for the synthesis of different types of glycolipids [34].

There are other glycoside hydrolase activities that are hardly used in synthesis. A thermostable α-L-arabinofuranosidase was reported in 2002 for its ability to perform transarabinosylation reactions for the synthesis of different α-L-arabinofuranosides of various alcohols. The same enzyme was later reported as a useful biocatalyst for the synthesis of p-nitrophenyl α-L-arabinofuranosyl-(1-2)-α-L-arabinofuranoside, p-nitrophenyl β-D-xylopyranosyl-(1-2) -β-D-xylopyranoside, p-nitrophenyl β-D-xylopyranosyl-(1-3)-β-D-xylopyranoside and benzyl α-L-arabinofuranosyl-(1-2)- α-D-xylopyranoside. Such a disaccharidic motif could be used as the reference compound for the analysis of hemicellulase action and for raising antibodies to well-defined motifs for immunochemical-based analyses of plant cell walls [35]. The same group reported also the synthesis of galactofuranosides using the above catalyst [36]. β-D-galactofuranose is a cell wall constituent in several pathogenic species including *Mycobacterium tuberculosis* and *leprae*, agents of tuberculosis and leprosy, respectively. The synthesis of galactofuranose analogues acting as inhibitors of the biosynthetic enzymes (UDP-galactopyranose mutase and galactofuranosyl transferases) or the synthesis of galactofuranosides that could be used for the elaboration of vaccines, is important for this aspect. Authors reported also on the chemical synthesis of p-nitrophenyl galactofuranoside used as donor and the low yield obtained (16%) could act as an additional center of interest for the synthetic aspect of this kind of enzyme.

An interesting case of the effect of solvents in transglycosylation reactions has been studied recently for the synthesis of *N*-acetyl-D-lactosamine, Gal-β-1,4-GlcNAc (LacNAc), catalyzed by the β-galactosidase from *Thermus thermophilus* (TTP0042). The authors studied the percentages of all products formed (self-condensation products, hydrolytic originating galactose and transfer regioisomers). The low yield (about 20%) of LAcNAc when the reaction is performed in buffer is increased by up to 91% when the process takes place in the presence of glycerol based solvents.

According to conformational studies of the enzyme structure by circular dichroism and fluorescence, the authors concluded that in the presence of these solvents the enzyme modifies secondary and tertiary structure and this may also be the cause of some additional regioselectivity changes observed [37]. Unfortunately no molecular details were furnished, indeed no clear relationship between the very different solvent structures used and the regioselectivity change was envisaged.

A new and interesting fungal diglycosidase was isolated from *Acremonium* sp. It has an α-rhamnosyl-β-glucosidase activity with transglycosylation potential of the entire disaccharide (rutinose) moiety from natural products to different acceptors. This enzyme allowed the synthesis of the diglycoconjugated fluorogenic substrate 4-methylumbelliferyl-rutinoside. The synthesis was performed in one step from the corresponding aglycone, 4-methylumbelliferone, and hesperidin as rutinose donor with a 16% yield regarding the sugar acceptor [38]. Despite the low yield, the fluorogenic substrate formed, 4-methylumbelliferyl rutinoside (Figure 4), which is not commercially available, is important for the study of diglycosidases since it allows the detection of enzymes specific for rutinose mobilization. Although the activity of this enzyme could seem quite specific for a broad interest, we must bear in mind its potential use for industrial processing of plant-based foods and the ability to transglycosylate rutinosyl units from abundant and inexpensive by-products of citrus industry.

Figure 4. Transrutinosylation performed by diglycosidase isolated from Acremonium sp.

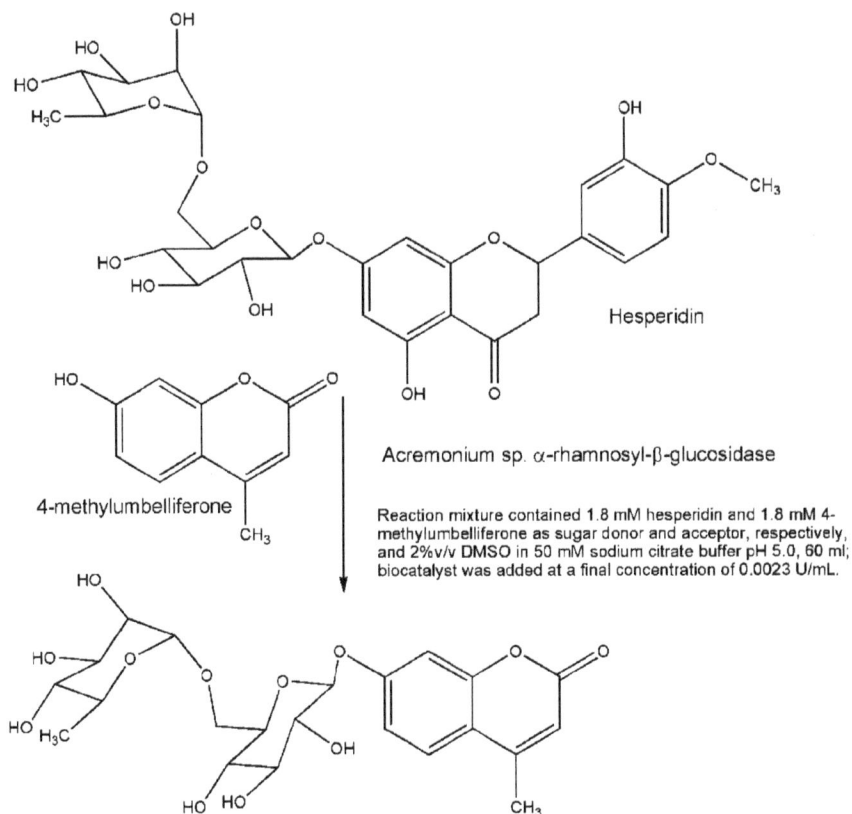

Reaction mixture contained 1.8 mM hesperidin and 1.8 mM 4-methylumbelliferone as sugar donor and acceptor, respectively, and 2%v/v DMSO in 50 mM sodium citrate buffer pH 5.0, 60 ml; biocatalyst was added at a final concentration of 0.0023 U/mL.

3. Engineered Enzymes

From 2004 to 2013 PubMed indexed 78 hits having the words glycosynthase(s) in the title, including review articles that accounted for *ca.* 20%. Similar figures can be found in Scopus and in Web of Knowledge. Using data published up to the mid-term of 2003, Perugino *et al.* compiled a review [39] accounting for 11 different glycoside hydrolases from bacteria, eukarya and archaea, that were modified as efficient glycosynthases. In 2012, in an update report from the same lab [40] a quadrupled value was found. Although these lists were declared not exhaustive, a similar number is also reported in the review of 2011 from Wong labs [41]. Indeed a number of excellent reviews periodically survey the most recent achievements in the field of glycosynthases from different perspectives, such as their production and application to the synthesis of glycoconjugates. The obvious success is due to quantitative yields that can be reached in reactions using these active-site modified glycoside hydrolases. The glycosynthase approach is certainly of great help while keeping molecular diversity offered by different natural glycoside hydrolases, including features such as resistance to temperature, organic solvent, *etc.,* making this aspect very interesting for the exploitation of these enzymes in biocatalysis. A survey of all these examples will not be repeated here, where instead just one case of a spectacular glycosphingolipids synthesis is reported below.

The focus in the remaining part of this paragraph, dedicated to engineered enzymes, is on those cases where genetic modifications could help in different manner than increasing yield by glycosynthase philosophy.

3.1. Preparative Glycosphingolipids Synthesis Operated by Glycosynthase

Pharmacological interest for glycosphingolipids, a class of glycolipids based on the aminodiol sphingosine, is high since these compounds have numerous biological functions in processes of human physiology [42]. Gangliosides are a subclass of glycosphingolipids containing also sialic acid in the oligosaccharide moiety, composed of different sugars. Certain gangliosides are involved in viral infections mechanisms. Commercial sources for glycosphingolipids rely on isolation of compounds from natural sources, such as bovine brain and canine blood. This is impractical for large-scale preparation, as well as posing risks for contamination and requiring great effort for extensive purification. A spectacular example of application of glycosynthase technology for high yield production of different gangliosides has been recently reported [43]. The work is based on the transformation of a natural hydrolytic enzyme, the endoglycoceramidase II (EGC II) from *Rhodococcus* strain M-777, in a glycosynthase. This glycosynthase version of the enzyme with Ala, Ser or Gly as substituents of active site nucleophile, is not capable of performing hydrolysis, but it can react in synthetic mode using α-anomer of different oligosaccharidic fluorides (di- to pentasaccharides) in the presence of acceptors such as D-erythro-sphingosine or sphingosine analogues (Figure 5). Yields from 70% to 100% were obtained for the lyso product on 300 mg scale.

Figure 5. Reaction yields for EGCII glycosynthase with various glycosyl fluoride.

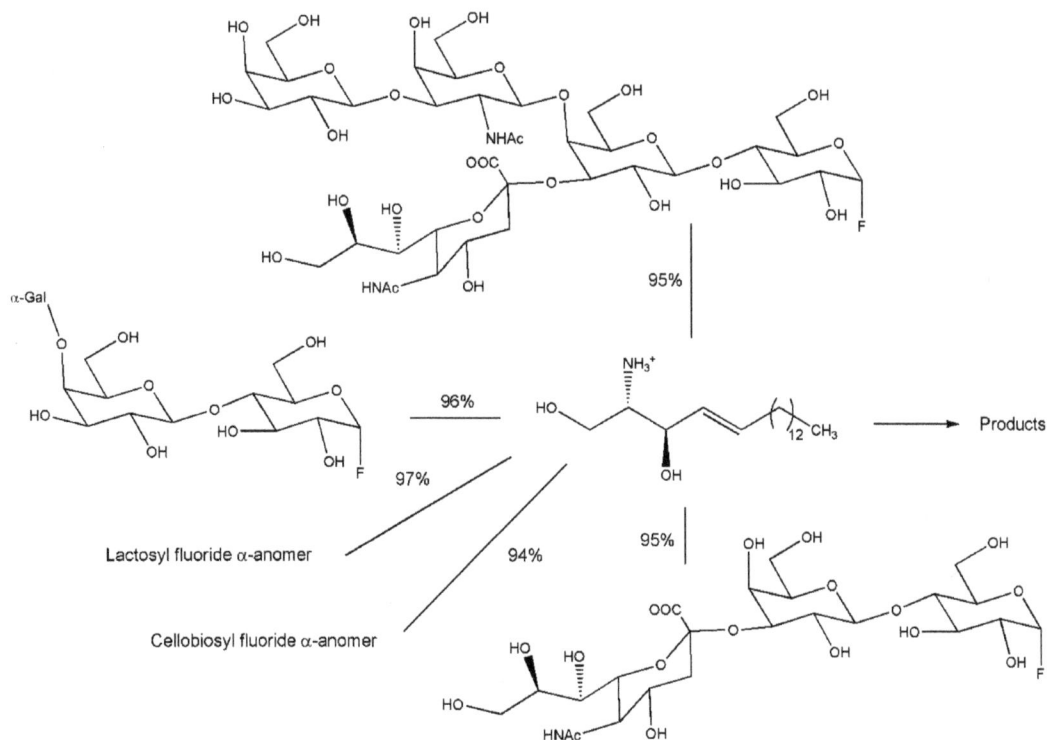

Reactants so structurally different could pose problems, but the solubility of the hydrochloride salt of the sphingosine in aqueous buffer (25 mM after sonication at 37 °C) is considered by the authors a benefit for possible molecular diversity that can be obtained with successive acylation steps with structurally diverse acyl chains. In fact, N-acyl substituents in ceramides affects biological activity of these compounds to some extent, and the acyl substituent has also been identified as a convenient position for conjugation of non-lipid substituents, including fluorescent tags [44].

3.2. Engineering Glycoside Hydrolases not at the Active Site

Engineering the active-site environs is a technique that has been used to enhance the transglycosylation activity of glycosidases and to modify other features of interest in biocatalysis. When structural architecture of the active site is not known, a site-specific "randomization" approach could be used in which an amino acid residue near the catalytic site can be replaced by each of all other amino acids to screen mutant enzyme(s) of interest. This strategy was used to obtain α-glucosidase variant(s) for increasing the production of theanderose, a trisaccharide obtained from sucrose by α-glucosylation to the C6 of glucose. An amino acid residue (Gly273 or Thr272) near the putative catalytic site (Glu271) of this *Bacillus* α-glucosidase was replaced by all other naturally-occurring amino acids thus increasing the transglucosylation activity. The highest specificity for theanderose formation (*i.e.*, the highest content of theanderose in the reaction product) was obtained with the isoleucine containing mutant (T272I), which showed 1.74 times higher productivity (per sucrose-hydrolyzing unit) of theanderose than that of the wild-type enzyme. The authors concluded, however, that elucidation of three-dimensional structures should help to understand the details of the mechanism eliciting the specificity obtained [45]. More recently, the transglycosylation/hydrolysis ratio was shown to be 3- and 8-fold increased with two mutants of a different enzyme, the *Thermotoga neapolitana* β-glucosidase. The asparagine mutant (N291T) of this enzyme showed also altered regioselectivity. In particular TLC analysis of the transglycosylation products indicated that while the mutant retained its β-1,3 regioselectivity, β-1,4 and β-1,6 selectivities were lost when pNPG and arbutin were used as a donor and acceptor, respectively [46]. In another case, Feng *et al.* in 2005 described directed evolution applied to the β-glycosidase of *Thermus thermophilus* to increase the ability of this enzyme in transglycosylation reaction. The most efficient mutations of phenylalanine and asparagine (F401S and N282T), were located just in front of the acceptor subsite and the authors suggested that repositioning of the glycone in its subsite together with a better fit of the acceptor in the acceptor subsite, might favor the attack of a glycosyl acceptor in the mutant at the expense of water; this conclusion was based on molecular modeling techniques. They also concluded that their results suggest that directed evolution of the glycosidases in transglycosidases could be an alternative to the glycosynthase strategy; in fact, for certain mutants, synthesis by self-condensation of nitrophenyl glycosides became nearly quantitative [47]. However when the asparagine (N282T) mutant was analyzed with external added acceptor pNPGlcNAc using oNPGal as donor, the NMR study of kinetic formation of transglycosylation products showed that those due to self-condensation (Galβ1-3Gal-oNP and Galβ1-6Gal-oNP) are kinetically favored over the condensation product Galβ1-4GlcNAc-pNP, suggesting that oNPGal is a better acceptor than pNPGlcNAc; competition between self-condensation and condensation could be responsible for the moderate yield of the desired product Gal β1-4GlcNAc-pNP. Based on the analysis of catalytic context, the authors studied *in silico* the complex alanine mutant-acceptor (A221W)/pNPGlcNAc establishing that the docking of the acceptor is not perturbed by the mutation, compared to the WT case. Donor docking was also studied with A221W mutant complexed with oNPGal to analyze precisely the perturbation as compared with WT. In WT enzyme there is enough room for oNPGal in the acceptor sites allowing the self-condensation reaction. In the A221W mutant, a drastic steric conflict occurs between the galactose ring and the tryptophan substituting alanine and this effect was seen by the authors as the most promising for preventing the self-condensation reaction. The mutation A221W was thus introduced by directed mutagenesis. The analysis of products and relative yields of this double mutant N282T/A221W shows that these results are consistent with the MM calculations. The authors proposed their approach as convenient in that relatively stable activated sugars can be used [48]. While this work shows the value of a rational approach to eliminate the side effects of transglycosylation reactions, a thermophilic glycosynthase from *Sulfolobus solfataricus* was indeed shown to act in presence of external formate on stable activated sugars such as oNP-glyco donors [49].

A random mutagenic approach coupled to a screening procedure was applied in another thermophilic case in nature. The screening was based on the reduction of the hydrolysis of a potential transglycosylation product (lactosucrose, β-D-galactopyranosyl-(1-4)-D-sucrose) formed in presence of sucrose, thus providing mutant enzymes possessing improved synthetic properties for the transglycosylation [50]. The application of thermostable β-galactosidases such as the β-galactosidase BgaB from *Geobacillus stearothermophilus* is of interest for transgalactosylation because at higher temperatures higher lactose concentration can be used to favor the synthesis.

A complete change of product profile of the reaction was observed for one of the mutants obtained by site directed mutagenesis of α-amylase of *Bacillus amyloliquefaciens*. The Val289 residue substituted with tyrosine showed less than 15% activity compared to the wild-type, but it acquired transglycosylation activity, producing longer oligosaccharides. The analysis of all mutants produced led to the conclusion that changes in the hydrolytic property of α-amylase may be due to factors like the geometry and electrostatics of the environment around the active site [51].

It could be of interest in this paragraph to mention the development of methodologies for the screening of large libraries of mutant enzymes. In a paper of 2009 Konè *et al.* reported on digital screening methodology as a system dedicated to the screening for sugar-transfer activity [52], which gave great impetus to the study of glycosidases with efficient transglycosidases activity as an alternative to glycosyltransferases or glycosynthases. Recently, from genomic and metagenomic program results, protein sequences with unknown functions are increasing, thus effective screening methodologies have become an important aspect of this research. In the field of polysaccharide degrading enzymes, a profiling method reported in 2012 by the Helbert group is worth noting. Polysaccharidases are important enzymes that are used as specific tools to improve conversion of lignocellulosic biomass into sugar monomers prior to ethanol production, for: degradation of microbial polysaccharides, obtaining bioactive materials, for structural determination of unknown complex polysaccharides structures, *etc.* The profiling strategy is based on a series of filtrations necessary to eliminate any reducing sugars not directly generated by enzyme degradation. After enzymatic action, filtrates are assayed with a ferricyanide solution to reveal the reducing sugars produced by glycoside hydrolases or polysaccharide lyases; however matrix-assisted laser desorption ionization mass spectrometry (MALDI-MS), presenting several unique advantages for the structural characterization of degradation products of carbohydrates, is also considered as providing an effective methodology [53,54].

4. Conclusions

Although not exhaustively catalogued in this review, the scientific literature of the last decade, with regard to the process of enzymatic preparation of glycosides, enables the reader to conclude that research for uniqueness, in terms of enzymatic features, is still active. This is in contrast with the tempting generalization about enzymes as plastic biomolecules fully receptive to be engineered by appropriate changes, although this plasticity has been successfully demonstrated in some examples [1]. The list of naturally "unique" enzymes cited in this review includes examples found among the most promising subjects of biocatalytic applications: (i) hyaluronidases for producing and/or transferring hyaluronic oligosaccharides of pharmaceutical interest or (ii) disaccharidases such as endo-α-*N*-acetylgalactosaminidase (for the analysis of glycan chains) and (iii) the fungal rutinosidase used in the synthesis of related fluorogenic derivative of 4-methylumbelliferone, are of specific interest. Among engineered enzymes, even though glycosynthases have to be seen as the most successful approach to reach quantitative transfer yields in transglycosylations, engineered enzymes examples with mutations only in the active-site environ (and not at active site aminoacids), demonstrated that biocatalytic features are well manipulated also in this way, thus enlarging competence to regioselectivity and or specificity for heteroacceptors and not only to reaction yield as devised for glycosynthases.

This overview should increase the interest from biocatalyst practitioners towards both naturally unique enzymes and for infrequent mutations capable of inducing biocatalytically interesting features.

Acknowledgments

The support for bibliographic search facilities is provided by Consiglio Nazionale delle Ricerche.

References

1. Bornscheuer, U.T.; Huisman, G.W.; Kazlausaks, R.J.; Lutz, S.; Moore, J.C.; Robins, K. Engineering the third wave of biocatalysis. *Nature* **2012**, *485*, 185–194.
2. Riva, S. 1983–2013: The long wave of biocatalysis. *Trends Biotechnol.* **2013**, *31*, 120–121.
3. Trincone, A. Potential biocatalysts originating from sea environments. *J. Mol. Catal. B-Enzym.* **2010**, *66*, 241–256.
4. Dumon, C.; Songa, L.; Bozonneta, S.; Fauréa, R.; O'Donohue, M.J. Progress and future prospects for pentose-specific biocatalysts in biorefining. *Proc. Biochem.* **2012**, *47*, 346–357.
5. Eklunda, E.A.; Bodeb, L.; Freeze, H.H. Diseases Associated with Carbohydrates/Glycoconjugates. In *Comprehensive Glycoscience Volume 4: Cell Glycobiology and Development; Health and Disease in Glycomedicine*; Kamerling, J.P., Ed.; Elsevier: NY, USA, 2007; Volume 4, pp. 339–371.
6. Kren, V. Glycoside *vs.* Aglycon: The Role of Glycosidic Residue in Biological Activity. In *Glycoscience, Chemistry and Chemical Biology*; Fraser-Reid, B.O., Tatsuta, K., Thiem, J., Eds.; Springer-Verlag: Berlin/Heidelberg, Germany, 2008; pp. 2589–2644.
7. Sears, P.; Wong, C.-H. Intervention of carbohydrate recognition by proteins and nucleic acids. *Proc. Natl. Acad. Sci. USA* **1996**, *93*, 12086–12093.
8. Wang, Q.; Dordick, J.S.; Linhardt, R.J. Synthesis and application of carbohydrate-containing polymers. *Chem. Mater.* **2002**, *14*, 3232–3244.
9. Wildman, E.C.R. Classifying Nutraceuticals. In *Handbook of Nutraceuticals and Functional Foods*; Robert, E.C., Ed.; CRC Press: Boca Raton, London, New York Washington, DC, USA, 2000; pp. 13–30.
10. Bojarova, P.; Rosencrantz, R.R.; Elling, L.; Kren, V. Enzymatic glycosylation of multivalent scaffolds. *Chem. Soc. Rev.* **2013**, *7*, 4774–4797.
11. De Roode, B.M.; Franseen, M.C.R.; van der Padt, A.; Boom, R.M. Perspectives for the industrial enzymatic production of glycosides. *Biotechnol. Prog.* **2003**, *19*, 1391–1402.
12. Trincone, A.; Giordano, A. Glycosyl hydrolases and glycosyltransferases in the synthesis of oligosaccharides. *Curr. Org. Chem.* **2006**, *10*, 1163–1193.

13. Desmet, T.; Soetaert, W.; Bojarova, P.; Kren, V.; Dijkhuizen, L.; Eastwick-Field, V.; Schiller, A. Enzymatic glycosylation of small molecules: Challenging substrates require tailored catalysts. *Chem. Eur. J.* **2012**, *18*, 10786–10801.

14. Hehre, E.J. Glycosyl transfer: A history of the concept's development and view of its major contributions to biochemistry. *Carbohydr. Res.* **2001**, *331*, 347–368.

15. Kobata, A. The history of glycobiology in Japan. *Glycobiology* **2001**, *11*, 99R–105R.

16. Koshland, D.E. Stereochemistry and the mechanism of enzymatic reactions. *Biol. Rev.* **1953**, *28*, 416–436.

17. Vivian, L.Y.; Withers, S.G. Breakdown of oligosaccharides by the process of elimination. *Curr. Opin. Chem. Biol.* **2006**, *10*, 147–155.

18. Vuong, T.V.; Wilson, D.B. Glycoside hydrolases: Catalytic base/nucleophile diversity. *Biotechnol. Bioeng.* **2010**, *107*, 195–205.

19. Thibodeaux, C.J.; Melancon, C.E.; Liu, H.-W. Unusual sugar biosynthesis and natural product glycodiversification. *Nature* **2007**, *446*, 1008–1016.

20. Hofinger, E.S.A.; Bernhardt, G.; Buschauer, A. Kinetics of Hyal-1 and PH-20 hyaluronidases: Comparison of minimal substrates and analysis of the transglycosylation reaction. *Glycobiology* **2007**, *17*, 963–971.

21. Takagaki, K.; Ishido, K.; Kakizaki, I.; Iwafune, M.; Endo, M. Carriers for enzymatic attachment of glycosaminoglycan chains to peptide. *Biochem. Biophys. Res. Comm.* **2002**, *293*, 220–224.

22. Madokoro, M.; Ueda, A.; Kiriake, A.; Shiomi, K. Properties and cDNA cloning of a hyaluronidase from the stonefish *Synanceia verrucosa* venom. *Toxicon* **2011**, *58*, 285–292.

23. Koutsioulis, D.; Landry, D.; Guthire, E.P. Novel endo-α-*N*-acetylgalactosaminidases with broader substrate specificity. *Glycobiology* **2008**, *18*, 799–805.

24. Fujita, M.; Shoda, S.; Haneda, K.; Inazu, T.; Takegawa, K.; Yamamoto, K. A novel disaccharide substrate having 1,2-oxazoline moiety for detection of transglycosylating activity of endoglycosidases. *Biochim. Biophys. Acta* **2001**, *1528*, 9–14.

25. Huang, W.; Li, J.; Wang, L.-X. Unusual transglycosylation activity of *Flavobacterium meningosepticum* endoglycosidases enables convergent chemoenzymatic synthesis of core fucosylated complex *N*-glycopeptides. *Chembiochem* **2011**, *11*, 932–941.

26. Slámová, K.; Gažák, R.; Bojarová, P.; Kulik, N.; Ettrich, R.; Pelantová, H.; Sedmera, P.; Křen, V. 4-Deoxy-substrates for β-*N*-acetylhexosaminidases: How to make use of their loose specificity. *Glycobiology* **2010**, *20*, 1002–1009.

27. Hu, Y.; Luan, H.; Liu, H.; Ge, G.; Zhou, K.; Liu, Y.; Yang, L. Acceptor specificity and transfer efficiency of a β-glycosidase from the China white jade snail. *Biosci. Biotechnol. Biochem.* **2009**, *73*, 671–676.

28. Roccatagliata, A.J.; Maier, M.S.; Seldes, A.M.; Iorizzi, M.; Minale, L. Starifhs saponins. Part II. Steroidal oligoglycosides from the starfish *Cosmasterias lurida*. *J. Nat. Prod.* **1994**, *57*, 747–754.

29. Ye, M.; Yan, L.-Q.; Li, N.; Zong, M.-H. Facile and regioselective enzymatic 5β-galactosylation of pyrimidine 2β-deoxynucleosides catalyzed by β-glycosidase from bovine liver. *J. Mol. Cat. B Enzym.* **2012**, *79*, 35–40.

30. Binder, W.H.; Kahlig, H.; Schmid, W. Galactosylation by use of β-galactosidase: Enzymatic syntheses of disaccharide nucleosides. *Tetrahedron Asymm.* **1995**, *6*, 1703–1710.

31. Andreotti, G.; Trincone, A.; Giordano, A. Convenient synthesis of β-galactosyl nucleosides using the marine β-galactosidase from *Aplysia fasciata*. *J. Mol. Catal. B-Enzym.* **2007**, *47*, 28–32.

32. Zeng, Q.M.; Li, N.; Zong, M.H. Highly regioselective galactosylation of floxuridine catalyzed by β-galactosidase from bovine liver. *Biotechnol. Lett.* **2010**, *32*, 1251–1254.

33. Andreotti, G.; Giordano, A.; Tramice, A.; Mollo, E.; Trincone, A. Hydrolyses and transglycosylations performed by purified α-D-glucosidase of the marine mollusc *Aplysia fasciata*. *J. Biotechnol.* **2006**, *122*, 274–284.

34. Manzo, E.; Tramice, A.; Pagano, D.; Trincone, A.; Fontana, A. Chemo-enzymatic preparation of α-6-sulfoquinovosyl-1,2-*O*-diacylglycerols. *Tetrahedron* **2012**, *68*, 10169–10175.

35. Remond, C.; Plantier-Royon, R.; Aubry, N.; Maes, E.; Bliard, C.; O'Donohuea, M.J. Synthesis of pentose-containing disaccharides using a thermostable α-L-arabinofuranosidase. *Carbohyd. Res.* **2004**, *339*, 2019–2025.

36. Remond, C.; Plantier-Royon, R.; Aubry, N.; O'Donohuea, M.J. An original chemoenzymatic route for the synthesis of β-D-galactofuranosides using an α-L-arabinofuranosidase. *Carbohydr. Res.* **2005**, *340*, 637–644.

37. Sandoval, M.; Civera, C.; Berenguer, J.; García-Blanco, F.; Hernaiz, M.J. Optimised *N*-acetyl-D-lactosamine synthesis using *Thermus thermophilus* β-galactosidase in bio-solvents. *Tetrahedron* **2013**, *69*, 1148–1152.

38. Mazzaferro, L.S.; Piñuel, L.; Erra-Balsells, R.; Giudicessi, S.L.; Breccia, J.D. Transglycosylation specificity of *Acremonium* sp. α-rhamnosyl- β-glucosidase and its application to the synthesis of the new fluorogenic substrate 4-methylumbelliferyl-rutinoside. *Carbohydr. Res.* **2012**, *347*, 69–75.

39. Perugino, G.; Trincone, A.; Rossi, M.; Moracci, M. Oligosaccharide synthesis by glycosynthases. *Trends Biotechnol.* **2004**, *22*, 31–37.

40. Cobucci-Ponzano, B.; Moracci, M. Glycosynthases as tools for the production of glycan analogs of natural products. *Nat. Prod. Rep.* **2012**, *29*, 697–709.

41. Schmaltz, R.M.; Hanson, S.R.; Wong, C.-H. Enzymes in the synthesis of glycoconjugates. *Chem. Rev.* **2011**, *111*, 4259–4307.

42. Mocchetti, I. Exogenous gangliosides, neuronal plasticity and repair, and the neurotrophins. *Cell. Mol. Life Sci.* **2005**, *62*, 2283–2294.

43. Vaughan, M.D.; Johnson, K.; DeFrees, S.; Tang, X.; Warren, R.A.J.; Withers, S.G. Glycosynthase-mediated synthesis of glycosphingolipids. *J. Am. Chem. Soc.* **2006**, *128*, 6300–6301.

44. Rich, J.R.; Cunningham, A-M.; Gilbert, M.; Withers, S.G. Glycosphingolipid synthesis employing a combination of recombinant glycosyltransferases and an endoglycoceramidase glycosynthase. *Chem. Commun.* **2011**, *47*, 10806–10808.

45. Okada, M.; Nakayama, T.; Noguchi, A.; Yano, M.; Hemmi, H.; Nishino, T.; Ueda, T. Site-specific mutagenesis at positions 272 and 273 of the Bacillus sp. SAM1606 α-glucosidase to screen mutants with altered specificity for oligosaccharide production by transglucosylation. *J. Mol. Catal. B-Enzym.* **2002**, *16*, 265–274.

46. Ki-Won, C.; Park, K.-M.; Jun, S.-Y.; Park, C.-S.; Park, K.-H.; Cha, J. Modulation of the regioselectivity of a *Thermotoga neapolitana* β-glucosidase by site-directed mutagenesis. *J. Microbiol. Biotechnol.* **2008**, *18*, 901–907.

47. Feng, H-Y.; Drone, J.; Hoffmann, L.; Tran, V.; Tellier, C.; Rabiller, C.; Michel Dion, M. Converting a β-glycosidase into a β-transglycosidase by directed evolution. *J. Biol. Chem.* **2005**, *280*, 37088–37097.

48. Tran, V.; Hoffmann, L.; Rabiller, C.; Tellier, C.; Dion, M. Rational design of a GH1 β-glycosidase to prevent self-condensation during the transglycosylation reaction. *Protein Eng. Des. Sel.* **2010**, *23*, 43–49.

49. Trincone, A.; Giordano, A.; Perugino, G.; Rossi, M.; Moracci, M. Highly productive autocondensation and transglycosylation reactions with *Sulfolobus solfataricus* glycosynthase. *ChemBioChem* **2005**, *6*, 1431–1437.

50. Placier, G.; Watzlawick, H.; Rabiller, C.; Mattes, R. Evolved β-galactosidases from *Geobacillus stearothermophilus* with improved transgalactosylation yield for galacto-oligosaccharide production. *App. Environ. Microbiol.* **2009**, *75*, 6312–6321.

51. Priyadharshini, R.; Hemalatha, D.; Gunasekaran, P. Role of Val289 residue in the α-amylase of *Bacillus amyloliquefaciens* MTCC 610: An analysis by site directed mutagenesis. *J. Microbiol. Biotechnol.* **2010**, *20*, 563–568.

52. Koné, F.M.T.; le Bechec, M.; Sine, J.P.; Dion, M.; Tellier, C. Digital screening methodology for the directed evolution of transglycosidases. *Prot. Engin. Des. Sel.* **2009**, *22*, 37–44.

53. Fer, M.; Préchoux, A.; Leroy, A.; Sassi, J.F.; Lahaye, M.; Boisset, C.; Nyvall-Collén, P.; Helbert, W. Medium-throughput profiling method for screening polysaccharide-degrading enzymes in complex bacterial extracts. *J. Microbiol. Meth.* **2012**, *89*, 222–229.

54. Ropartz, D.; Bodet, P.E.; Przybylski, C.; Gonnet, F.; Daniel, R.; Fer, M.; Helbert, W.; Bertrand, D.; Rogniaux, H. Performance evaluation on a wide set of matrix-assisted laser desorption ionization matrices for the detection of oligosaccharides in a high-throughput mass spectrometric screening of carbohydrate depolymerizing enzymes. *Rapid Commun. Mass Spectrom.* **2011**, *25*, 2059–2070.

Architecture of Amylose Supramolecules in Form of Inclusion Complexes by Phosphorylase-Catalyzed Enzymatic Polymerization

Jun-ichi Kadokawa

Abstract: This paper reviews the architecture of amylose supramolecules in form of inclusion complexes with synthetic polymers by phosphorylase-catalyzed enzymatic polymerization. Amylose is known to be synthesized by enzymatic polymerization using α-D-glucose 1-phosphate as a monomer, by phosphorylase catalysis. When the phosphorylase-catalyzed enzymatic polymerization was conducted in the presence of various hydrophobic polymers, such as polyethers, polyesters, poly(ester-ether), and polycarbonates as a guest polymer, such inclusion supramolecules were formed by the hydrophobic interaction in the progress of polymerization. Because the representation of propagation in the polymerization is similar to the way that a vine of a plant grows, twining around a rod, this polymerization method for the formation of amylose-polymer inclusion complexes was proposed to be named "vine-twining polymerization". To yield an inclusion complex from a strongly hydrophobic polyester, the parallel enzymatic polymerization system was extensively developed. The author found that amylose selectively included one side of the guest polymer from a mixture of two resemblant guest polymers, as well as a specific range in molecular weights of the guest polymers poly(tetrahydrofuran) (PTHF) in the vine-twining polymerization. Selective inclusion behavior of amylose toward stereoisomers of chiral polyesters, poly(lactide)s, also appeared in the vine-twining polymerization.

Reprinted from *Biomolecules*. Cite as: Kadokawa, J. Architecture of Amylose Supramolecules in Form of Inclusion Complexes by Phosphorylase-Catalyzed Enzymatic Polymerization. *Biomolecules* **2013**, *3*, 369-385.

1. Introduction

Polysaccharides are naturally occurring carbohydrate polymers, where each monosaccharide residue is linked directly through a glycosidic linkage in the main-chain [1]. The glycosidic linkage is a type of covalent bond that joins a monosaccharide residue to another group, which is typically another saccharide residue. Natural polysaccharides are found in various sources such as plant, animal, seaweed, and microbial kingdoms, which have specific and very complicated structures owing, not only to a structural diversity of monosaccharide residues, but also to the differences in stereo- and regio-configurations of glycosidic linkages. The large diversity of polysaccharide structures contributes to serve as vital materials for a range of important *in vivo* functions in host organisms, e.g., providing an energy resource, acting as a structural material, and conferring specific biological properties, and a subtle change in the chemical structure has a profound effect on the properties and functions of the polysaccharides [2–4]. Therefore, the preparation of artificial polysaccharides has attracted increasing attention because of their potential applications as materials in the fields related to medicine, pharmaceutics, cosmetics, and food industries. Polysaccharides are theoretically produced by the repeated reactions for the formation of a glycosidic linkage, so-called glycosylation of a glycosyl acceptor with a glycosyl donor [5–8]. To develop a superior method for the synthesis of polysaccharides by such repeated glycosylations, the *in vitro* approach by enzymatic catalysis *i.e.*, enzymatic polymerization, has been significantly investigated [9–15] as enzymes have remarkable catalytic advantages compared with other types of catalysts in terms of the stereo- and regioselectivities. The enzymatic polymerization, therefore, is a very powerful tool for the stereo- and regioselective construction of polysaccharides under mild conditions, where monomers can be employed in their unprotected forms, leading to the direct formation of the unprotected saccharide chains in aqueous media.

Amylose is a natural glucose polymer connected through α-(1→4)-glycosidic linkages (Figure 1) [1]. This is one component of starch and acts as an energy resource in nature with the other component of starch, that is, amylopectin, which has a branched structure composed of α-(1→4)-glucans with a small portion of α-(1→6)-glycosidic linkages [16]. Amylose has recently been recognized as a candidate as a high-performance polymeric material because it acts as a host molecule and forms polysaccharide supramolecules by inclusion complexation with various guest molecules of relatively low molecular weight (inclusion complexes) owing to the helical conformation (Figure 2a) [17]. The driving force for inclusion of guest molecules in the cavity is mainly host-guest hydrophobic interaction as the inside of the amylose helix has a hydrophobic nature due to the presence of hydrophilic hydroxy groups in the glucose residues on outer part of the helix. Therefore, hydrophobicity is generally in demand as the property of guest molecules to be included by amylose. Development of methods for the architecture of amylose supramolecules with polymeric guest molecules is a significant research topic to provide new self-assembled polymeric materials with regularly controlled nanostructures, which have potential to exhibit new high performance functions. However, only limited studies have been reported regarding the direct construction of inclusion complexes composed of amylose and polymeric molecules (Figure 2b) [18–26] as the driving force for the inclusion complexation of guest molecules into the cavity of amylose is the weak hydrophobic interaction as mentioned earlier, the amylose cavity does not have a sufficient ability to include the long chains of polymeric guests. The author has considered for the architecture of such amylose supramolecules, *i.e.*, amylose-polymer inclusion complexes in the phosphorylase-catalyzed enzymatic polymerization field [14,15,27–30] as a structurally controlled amylose is efficiently synthesized by an enzymatic polymerization through phosphorylase catalysis [31–37]. Following the recent review article on the series of these studies [30], in this article, the author would like to deal with the comprehensive results and discussion of this approach, including the further progress of the investigation to precisely architect such amylose supramolecules in form of inclusion complexes between amylose and synthetic polymers by the phosphorylase-catalyzed enzymatic polymerization [38]. Specifically, the present review article is described on the basis of the viewpoint that the precision architecture of the regularly controlled polysaccharide supramolecules has been achieved by means of the enzymatic synthesis of structurally defined polysaccharides according to Section 2.

Figure 1. Structure of amylase.

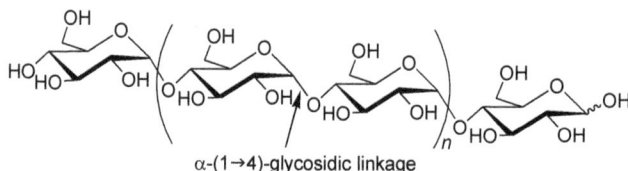

α-(1→4)-glycosidic linkage

Figure 2. Amylose forms inclusion complex with relatively low molecular weight hydrophobic molecule (**a**); but, mostly, does not form it with polymeric molecule (**b**).

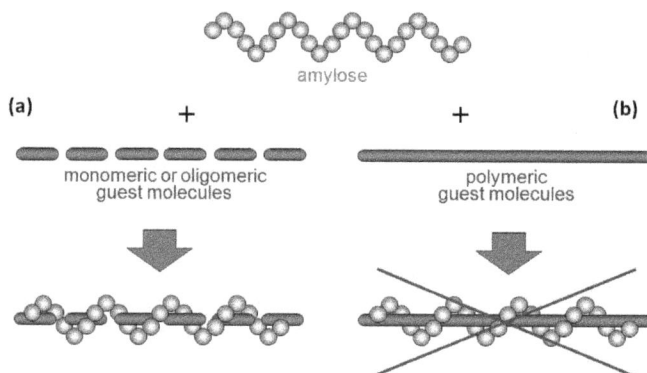

2. Characteristic Features of Phosphorylase-Catalyzed Enzymatic Polymerization to Produce Amylose

Phosphorylase catalyzes the reversible phosphorolysis of α-(1→4)-glucans at the nonreducing end, such as glycogen and starch, in the presence of inorganic phosphate to produce α-D-glucose 1-phosphate (G-1-P) [31]. By means of the reversibility of the enzymatic reaction, α-(1→4)-glycosidic linkage can be constructed by the phosphorylase-catalyzed glycosylation using G-1-P as a glycosyl donor. As a glycosyl acceptor, maltooligosaccharides with degrees of polymerization DPs higher than the smallest one recognized by phosphorylase are used. The smallest glycosyl acceptor for the phosphorylase-catalyzed glycosylation is typically known to be maltotetraose (G_4), whereas that for phosphorolysis is typically maltopentaose (G_5). In the glycosylation, a glucose unit is transferred from G-1-P to a nonreducing end of the glycosyl acceptor to form α-(1→4)-glycosidic linkage. When the excess molar ratio of G-1-P to the glycosyl acceptor is present in the reaction system, the successive glycosylations, *i.e.*, the enzymatic polymerization of G-1-P as a monomer, occurs to produce the α-(1→4)-glucan chain, that is, amylose (Figure 3) [32–37]. The polymerization is initiated from a nonreducing end of the glycosyl acceptor, and thus, it is often called a "primer." Because the phosphorylase-catalyzed enzymatic polymerization proceeds analogously to a living polymerization, the polydispersity of the amylose produced is narrow ($M_w/M_n < 1.2$) and its molecular weight can be controlled by the G-1-P/primer feed molar ratios. Phosphorylase is the only enzyme that can produce amylose with the desired average molecular weight [39].

Figure 3. Phosphorylase-catalyzed enzymatic polymerization of G-1-P to form amylase.

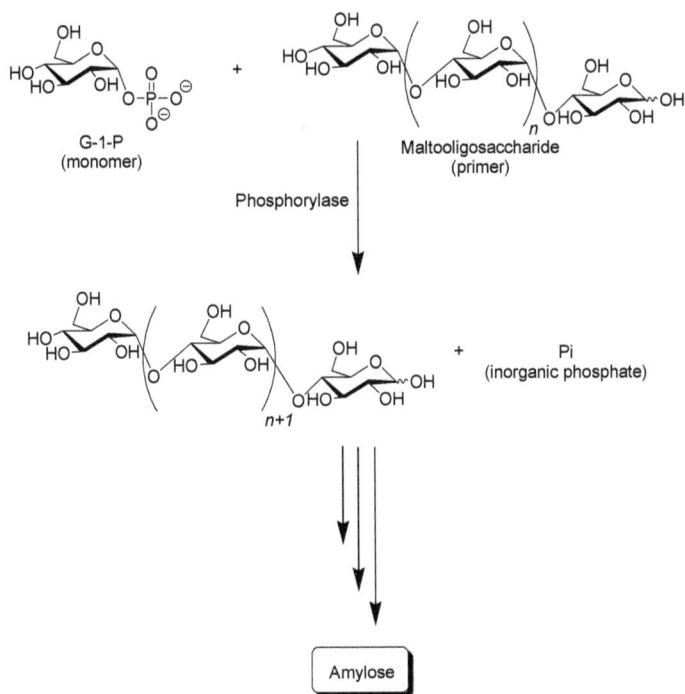

By means of the phosphorylase-catalyzed enzymatic polymerization for direct synthesis of amylose, the author has investigated developing an efficient method for the architecture of inclusion complexes of amylose with synthetic polymers. The representation of propagation in the polymerization system mirrors the way that the vine of a plant grows, twining around a rod. Accordingly, the author has proposed that this polymerization method for the architecture of amylose-polymer supramolecular inclusion complexes be named "vine-twining polymerization" (Figure 4) [14,15,27–30].

Figure 4. Image of "vine-twining polymerization".

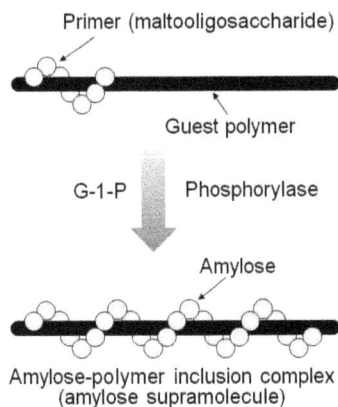

3. Architecture of Amylose-Poly(tetrahydrofuran) Inclusion Complex by Vine-Twining Polymerization

A first example of vine-twining polymerization was reported in the system using poly(tetrahydrofuran) (PTHF) as a hydrophobic guest polyether (Figure 5) [40]. When the phosphorylase-catalyzed enzymatic polymerization of G-1-P from maltoheptaose (G_7) as a primer was conducted in the presence of hydroxy-terminated telechelic PTHF, with M_n of 4000 in sodium citrate buffer, the product was gradually precipitated during the progress of the polymerization, which was isolated by filtration and characterized by ^1H NMR and powder X-ray diffraction (XRD) measurements.

Figure 5. Architecture of inclusion complexes by vine-twining polymerization using hydrophobic guest polyethers.

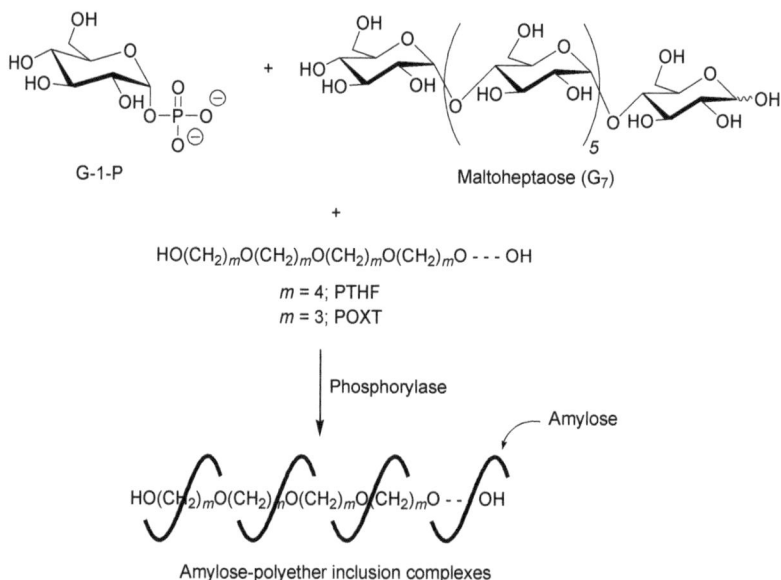

G-1-P   Maltoheptaose (G_7)

+

$HO(CH_2)_mO(CH_2)_mO(CH_2)_mO(CH_2)_mO --- OH$

$m = 4$; PTHF
$m = 3$; POXT

Phosphorylase

Amylose

$HO(CH_2)_mO(CH_2)_mO(CH_2)_mO(CH_2)_mO -- OH$

Amylose-polyether inclusion complexes

In the ^1H NMR spectrum of the product in DMSO-d_6, signals not only due to amylose but also due to PTHF were detected. Moreover, the methylene peak of PTHF was broadened and shifted to a higher magnetic field compared with that of a sole PTHF, suggesting that each methylene group in PTHF is immobile and interacts with the protons inside the amylose cavity by complexation. In addition, the NMR pattern assignable to amylose and PTHF was also observed by the measurement in NaOD/D_2O solvent. A sole PTHF was not dissolved with NaOD/D_2O, and thus, no peak due to PTHF appeared in the ^1H NMR spectrum of a mixture of PTHF with NaOD/D_2O. These NMR results indicated that PTHF in the product was solubilized in alkaline solution, probably by suppressing the formation of crystalline aggregates because of its inclusion complexation in the cavity of amylose. The XRD profile of the product showed two strong peaks at $2\theta = 12.4$ and $19.8°$ (Figure 6b), which was completely different from that of a sole amylose (Figure 6a), but similar to that of inclusion complexes of amylose with monomeric guest molecules reported in a previous study [41].

The above NMR and XRD results strongly supported that the amylose-PTHF inclusion complex was obtained by the vine-twining polymerization system.

Figure 6. XRD profiles of amylose (**a**); amylose-PTHF inclusion complex (**b**); amylose-P(GA-*co*-CL) inclusion complex (**c**); the product obtained by vine-twining polymerization using P(GA-*b*-CL) (**d**); and amylose-PLLA inclusion complex (**e**).

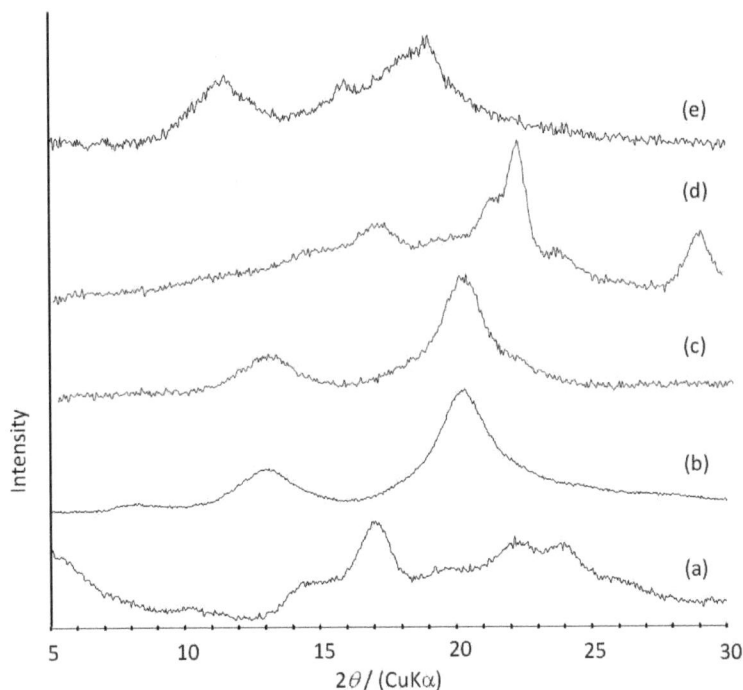

The formation of an inclusion complex was not observed by mixing amylose and PTHF in a buffer solvent, strongly suggesting its formation during the progress of the enzymatic polymerization in the above system. To additionally study the relation between the formation of an inclusion complex and the enzymatic polymerization process, the following experiment was conducted. When PTHF was added to the reaction solution immediately after the enzymatic polymerization of G-1-P had initiated, the identical inclusion complex to the aforementioned system was produced. However, the contents of PTHF in the products decreased as the time between the initiation of the enzymatic polymerization and the addition of PTHF to the solution increased. These results revealed that amylose did not sufficiently include PTHF in the cavity after the polymerization produced amylose with relatively higher molecular weight. Accordingly, it was considered that the inclusion complex had only been formed simultaneously with the progress of the enzymatic polymerization according to the "vine-twining" process.

The effect of molecular weights of PTHFs on the formation of inclusion complexes in the vine-twining polymerization was investigated by using those with various molecular weights (1000, 2000, 10,000, and 14,000) [42]. When PTHF with M_n of 1000 or 2000 was employed as the guest polymer, inclusion complexes were obtained in the vine-twining polymerization. In contrast, the use of PTHFs with higher M_ns such as 10,000 and 14,000, in the vine-twining polymerization, did not induce the formation of inclusion complexes with amylose. The PTHFs with higher M_ns were not sufficiently dispersed in buffer of the polymerization solvent, resulting in difficulty of the inclusion by amylose. To yield inclusion complexes from these PTHFs, the diethyl ether/buffer two-phase system was attempted for the vine-twining polymerization. The higher molecular weight PTHFs were first dissolved in diethyl ether, and then, buffer solvent was added to the ether solution (diethyl ether:buffer = 1:5 (v/v)). Then, the phosphorylase-catalyzed enzymatic polymerization of G-1-P was carried out with vigorously stirring the two-phase mixture. Consequently, the XRD profiles of the products from the higher molecular weight PTHFs obtained by the two-phase system indicated the formation of the inclusion complexes.

4. Architecture of Inclusion Complexes by Vine-Twining Polymerization Using Other Polyethers as Guest Polymers

To investigate the effect of alkyl chain lengths in polyethers on the formation of inclusion complexes in the vine-twining polymerization, the phosphorylase-catalyzed enzymatic polymerization of G-1-P was performed in the presence of polyethers with different alkyl chain lengths from PTHF (the number of methylenes = 4), that is, poly(oxetane) (POXT, the number of methylenes = 3) and poly(ethylene glycol) (PEG, the number of methylenes = 2) [42]. The ^{1}H NMR spectrum of the product from POXT in DMSO-d_6 showed the signals due to both amylose and POXT and its XRD pattern was same as that of the aforementioned amylose-PTHF inclusion complex. These analytical data indicated that the inclusion complex was formed by the vine-twining polymerization using POXT as the guest polyether (Figure 5). In the ^{1}H NMR spectrum of the product from PEG, on the other hand, only the signals due to amylose were detected. Moreover, the XRD profile of the product from PEG showed the pattern for amylose, but did not exhibit that for an inclusion complex. These data indicated that amylose was produced by the enzymatic polymerization in this system, but that did not induce inclusion complexation with PEG. The above results were reasonably explained by the different hydrophobicities in the polyethers. The hydrophilic nature of PEG caused much less hydrophobic interaction with the cavity of amylase, resulting in no complexation by amylose, whereas the hydrophobic polyethers such as PTHF and POXT interacted with the cavity of amylose, leading to the formation of the inclusion complexes by the vine-twining polymerization. The above results suggested that the hydrophobicity of guest polymers strongly affected whether inclusion complexation takes place in the vine-twining polymerization system.

5. Architecture of Inclusion Complexes by Vine-Twining Polymerization Using Carbonyl-Containing Hydrophobic Polymers as Guest Polymers

Based on significance in the hydrophobicity of guest polymers on the formation of inclusion complexes, well-known hydrophobic polyesters, that is, hydroxy-terminated telechelic poly(ε-caprolactone) (PCL) and poly(δ-valerolactone) (PVL) were employed as the guest polymer in the vine-twining polymerization (Figure 7) [43,44]. The phosphorylase-catalyzed enzymatic polymerization of G-1-P from G_7 was conducted in the presence of PCL or PVL in sodium citrate buffer and the precipitated products were characterized by ^1H NMR and XRD measurements. The ^1H NMR spectra of the products from PCL with M_n of 1000 and PVL with M_n of 2000 showed signals not only due to amylose but also due to the polyesters. The XRD patterns of the products were completely different from those of a sole amylose and were similar as those of the aforementioned amylose-PTHF inclusion complex. Moreover, the IR spectrum of the original PVL exhibited a strong absorption at 1728 cm^{-1} (Figure 8a), corresponding to a carbonyl group of the crystalline PVL, and which of PVL in the product shifted to the region at 1736 cm^{-1} (Figure 8b) assignable to the non-crystalline PVL. This result suggested that the crystalline PVL did not present in the product because of inclusion of a PVL chain in the cavity of amylose, suppressing the formation of crystalline aggregates among PVL chains. All the above analytical results supported the structures of the inclusion complexes of amylose with PCL and PVL.

Figure 7. Architecture of inclusion complexes by vine-twining polymerization using carbonyl-containing hydrophobic polymers.

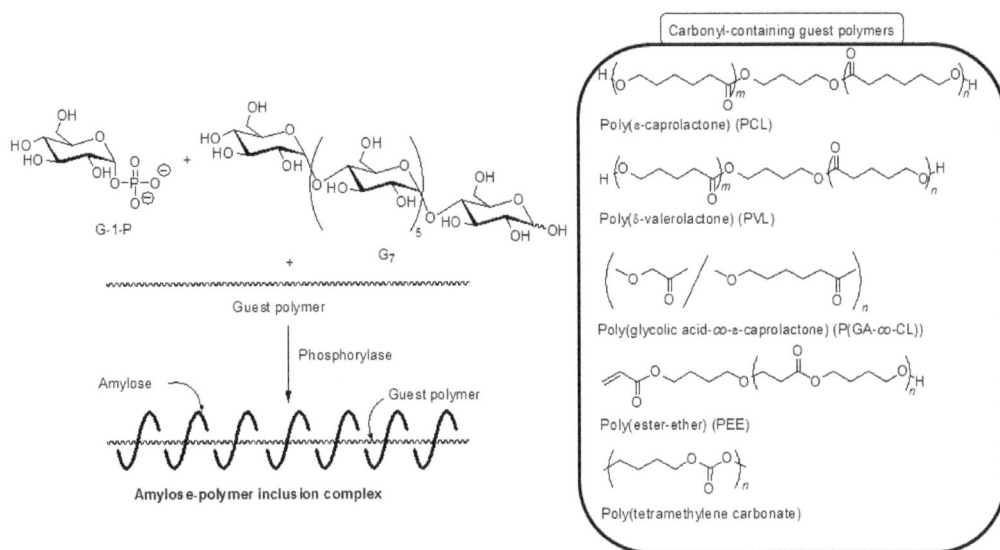

Although PCL with a higher M_n (2000) was employed as the guest polyester in the vine-twining polymerization, it was not sufficiently dispersed in sodium citrate buffer of the polymerization solvent, and accordingly, the inclusion complex was not produced. To yield the inclusion complex from such a PCL, the vine-twining polymerization was attempted in a mixed solvent of acetone and sodium citrate buffer (1:5 (v/v)) as PCL with the M_n was dispersed in the mixed solvent system. The resulting product was characterized by the ^1H NMR and XRD measurements to be the inclusion complex. As previously mentioned, the inclusion complex was formed from PVL with M_n of 2000 by the vine-twining polymerization in sodium citrate buffer, suggesting that PVL was more favorable as the guest polymer to form inclusion complex, compared with PCL by the vine-twining polymerization.

Figure 8. IR spectra of PVL (**a**); and amylose-PVL inclusion complex (**b**).

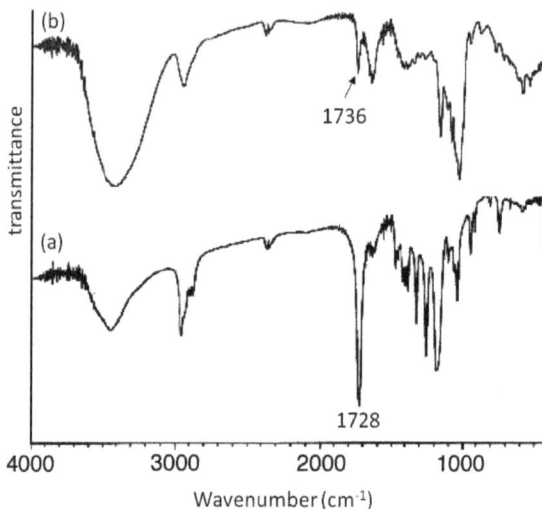

It was also found that amylose-poly(glycolic acid-*co*-ε-caprolactone) (P(GA-*co*-CL)) inclusion complexes were obtained by the vine-twining polymerization, using biodegradable P(GA-*co*-CL)s (Figure 7) [38]. As poly(glycolic acid) (PGA) shows high crystallinity and low dispersibility in aqueous buffer, resulting in the difficulty of the inclusion of PGA in the cavity of amylose, the copolyester, P(GA-*co*-CL) composed of the two biodegradable chains, was used. Thus, the vine-twining polymerization was carried out by the phosphorylase-catalyzed polymerization in the presence of P(GA-*co*-CL)s with various unit ratios in sodium acetate buffer. The ^{1}H NMR spectra of the products showed the signals due to amylose and P(GA-*co*-CL) and their XRD patterns showed the typical diffraction peaks, assignable to inclusion complexes (Figure 6c). These results indicated that the products were the inclusion complexes composed of amylose and P(GA-*co*-CL). The ratios of GA unit to CL unit in P(GA-*co*-CL)s did not affect inclusion complexation by amylose. On the other hand, an inclusion complex was not formed in the vine-twining polymerization using poly(glycolic acid-*block*-ε-caprolactone) (P(GA-*b*-CL)), as confirmed by the XRD profile of the product (Figure 6d). As P(GA-*co*-CL) and P(GA-*b*-CL) exhibit amorphous and crystalline natures, respectively, it has been considered that the crystallinity of the guest copolyesters affected inclusion complexation by amylose. In addition, lipase-catalyzed hydrolysis of P(GA-*co*-CL), in the inclusion complex, was partly inhibited, likely because amylose surrounded P(GA-*co*-CL) to prevent the approach of lipase.

As the other guest polyester, a hydrophobic poly(ester-ether) (–CH$_2$CH$_2$C(=O)OCH$_2$CH$_2$CH$_2$CH$_2$O–), which was composed of alternating ester and ether bonds, was employed for the vine-twining polymerization (Figure 7) [44]. The structure of the product was evaluated by the ^{1}H NMR and XRD measurements to be the inclusion complex. When a hydrophilic poly(ester-ether) ($-CH_2CH_2C(=O)OCH_2CH_2O-$), which had a shorter methylene length, was employed as the guest polymer, no inclusion complex was produced. This result also supported that the hydrophobicity of the guest polymers affected the formation of inclusion complexes by the vine-twining polymerization.

In addition, to no production of an inclusion complex from such a hydrophilic polymer, the formation of inclusion complexes, had not been achieved from polymers with strong hydrophobicity due to their aggregation in aqueous buffer solvent in the vine-twining polymerization, as an example using PCL with the higher M_n [44]. As the other example, the vine-twining polymerization using poly(oxepane), which was a more hydrophobic polyether owing to longer alkyl chains compared with PTHF and POXT, did not induce inclusion complexation by amylose [42].

To obtain the inclusion complex from a strongly hydrophobic polyester, the parallel enzymatic polymerization system, as an extensive approach of the vine-twining polymerization, was attempted [45]. In this system, two enzymatic polymerizations, which were the phosphorylase-catalyzed enzymatic polymerization of G-1-P from G$_7$, producing amylose and the lipase-catalyzed polycondensation of a dicarboxylic acid and a diol, giving an aliphatic polyester of the guest polymer [46,47], were simultaneously performed (Figure 9). As the monomers for the polycondensation, sebacic acid and 1,8-octanediol were used, which were converted to the strongly hydrophobic polyester by the lipase-catalyzed polycondensation under aqueous conditions. The product by the parallel enzymatic polymerization system was evaluated by the ¹H NMR and XRD measurements, which indicated the formation of the inclusion complex of amylose with the polyester. To confirm the fact that the inclusion complex was obtained only by the parallel enzymatic polymerization system, the following two experiments were conducted. When the phosphorylase-catalyzed enzymatic polymerization was carried out in the presence of such a strongly hydrophobic polyester, according to the vine-twining polymerization manner, amylose was produced, but it did not induce inclusion complexation with the polyester. As the other experiment, the lipase-catalyzed polycondensation of sebacic acid and 1,8-octanediol was carried out in the presence of amylose. Consequently, amylose included some monomers, but did not include the polyester although the enzymatic polycondensation progressed. These results concluded that the inclusion complex of amylose with such a strongly hydrophobic polyester was obtained only by the parallel enzymatic polymerization system.

Hydrophobic aliphatic polycarbonates were also used as the guest polymer in the vine-twining polymerization to prepare the corresponding inclusion complexes with amylose [48]. When the vine-twining polymerization was conducted, using poly(tetramethylene carbonate) as the guest polycarbonate in an acetone/aqueous buffer mixed solvent, the precipitated product was evaluated by ¹H NMR, XRD, and IR measurements to be the amylose-poly(tetramethylene carbonate) inclusion complex (Figure 7). The effect of the methylene chain lengths in the polycarbonates on inclusion complexation in the vine-twining polymerization was further examined by using poly(tetramethylene carbonate), poly(octamethylene carbonate), poly(decamethylene carbonate), and poly(dodecamethylene carbonate) as a guest polycarbonate. Compared with the polycarbonate with the shorter methylene chain length, such as the above mentioned poly(tetramethylene carbonate), only lesser amounts of the polycarbonates, having longer methylene chain lengths, were included in the cavity of amylose. Such strongly hydrophobic polycarbonates were not sufficiently dispersed in the acetone/aqueous buffer mixed solvent, resulting in difficulty in the inclusion complexation by amylose.

Figure 9. Architecture of inclusion complexes composed of amylose and strongly hydrophobic polyester in parallel enzymatic polymerization system.

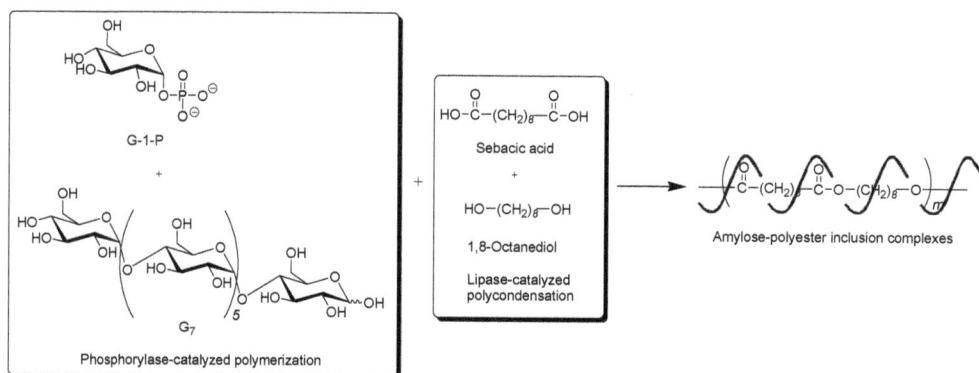

6. Selective Inclusion Complexation by Amylose in Vine-Twining Polymerization

On the basis of the aforementioned results, during the course of studies on the vine-twining polymerization, the author has considered that moderate hydrophobicity of guest polymers is in demand in deciding whether amylose includes them or not. Taking more precise information into account, amylose exhibits different inclusion behaviors depending on subtle changes in the structures of hydrophobic guest polymers. Such behavior of amylose was applied in the investigation to realize the selective inclusion complexation toward two resemblant guest polymers (Figure 10) [49,50]. For example, the selective inclusion of amylose was achieved by the vine-twining polymerization in the presence of a mixture of POXT (M_n = 1800) and PTHF (M_n = 1600) (unit molar ratio = 0.90:1.00) in sodium acetate buffer [49]. In the ^{1}H NMR spectrum of the product (DMSO-d_6), the signals due to PTHF and amylose were prominently detected, but the signals due to POXT, mostly, were not observed (POXT/PTHF = 0.02:1.00). This NMR result suggested that amylose almost selectively included PTHF from the mixture of the two resemblant polyethers in the vine-twining polymerization. The difference in the inclusion behavior of amylose toward the two polyethers was probably owing to the slight difference in their hydrophobicities. An attempt in the other selective inclusion system by amylose was made by the vine-twining polymerization in the presence of a mixture of two resemblant polyesters, that is, PVL (M_n = 830) and PCL (M_n = 930) (unit molar ratio = 1.00:0.92) [50]. In the ^{1}H NMR spectrum of the product (DMSO-d_6), the signals due to PVL and amylose were detected, whereas no signals due to PCL appeared, indicating that amylose selectively included PVL from the mixture of the two resemblant polyesters in the vine-twining polymerization.

Figure 10. Amylose selectively includes one of two resemblant polyethers or polyesters.

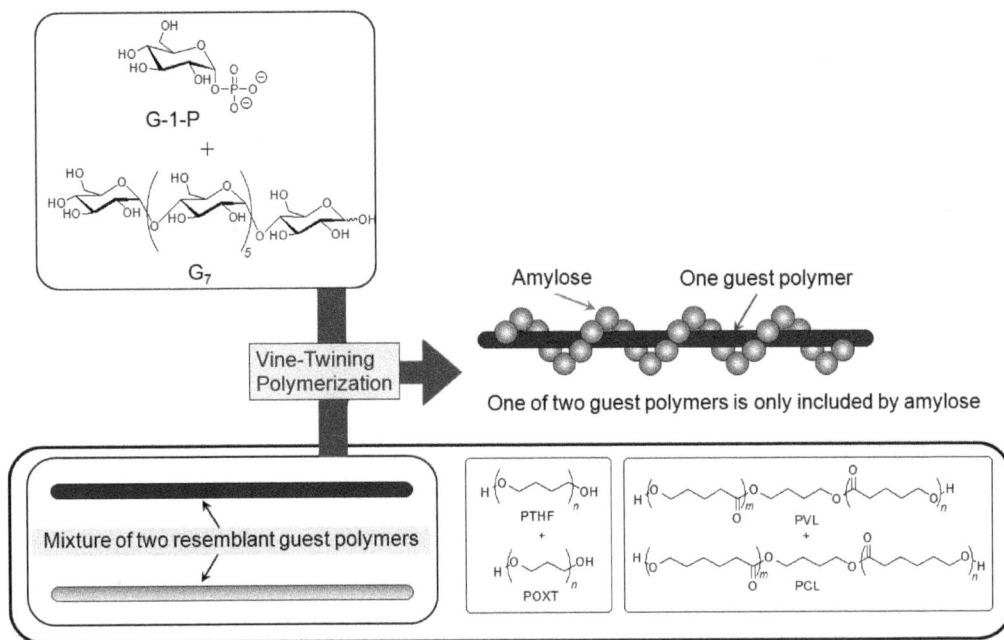

The selective inclusion complexation toward a specific range in molecular weights of synthetic guest polymers by amylose in the vine-twining polymerization was also investigated [51]. As synthetic polymers have molecular weight distribution, they are reasonably considered as mixtures of analogous molecules with different numbers of the repeating units. Moreover, the number of repeating units contributes to the exhibition of different properties of the polymers with the same repeating unit. For example, PTHF with considerably low molecular weight is soluble in water, whereas that with higher molecular weight is insoluble in water, suggesting that the molecular weight of PTHF affects its hydrophobicity. Therefore, the vine-twining polymerization in the presence of three PTHFs with different M_ns and (M_w/M_n)s (PTHF/1000; M_n and M_w/M_n = 1350 and 2.86, PTHF/3000; M_n and M_w/M_n = 3040 and 3.13, and PTHF/6000; M_n and M_w/M_n = 6330 and 2.45) was investigated. When PTHF/3000 with M_w/M_n = 3.13 was used as the guest polymer for the vine-twining polymerization, the M_w/M_n of PTHF included by amylose became narrower $(M_w/M_n$ = 1.46) although its M_n (=3590) was comparable to that of the employed one (M_n = 3040). These results indicated that amylose selectively included a specific range in molecular weights of PTHF/3000 in the vine-twining polymerization. When the vine-twining polymerization using PTHF/1000, and PTHF/6000 as the guest polymer, was conducted, the M_ns and (M_w/M_n)s of PTHFs included by amylose were similar as those using PTHF/3000 as aforementioned (the included PTHF/1000; M_n and M_w/M_n = 3120 and 1.41, the included PTHF/6000; M_n and M_w/M_n = 3700 and 1.74). Thus, it was concluded that amylose selectively included a specific range in molecular weights of PTHFs probably by the specific hydrophobic interaction.

Figure 11. Stereoselective inclusion complexation by amylose in vine-twining polymerization using poly(L-lactide) (PLLA).

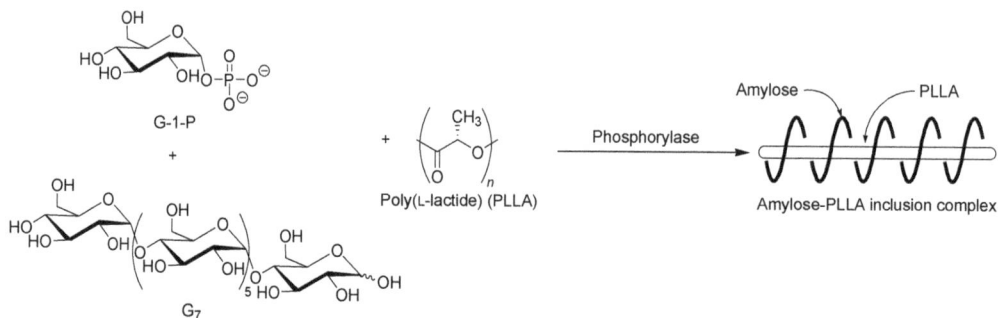

The selective inclusion complexation by amylose was also achieved in the vine-twining polymerization using chiral polyesters, *i.e.*, poly(lactide)s (PLAs) as the guest polymer (Figure 11) [52]; there are three kinds of the stereoisomers, *i.e.*, poly(L-lactide) (PLLA), poly(D-lactide) (PDLA), and racemic poly(DL-lactide) (PLDLA). When the vine-twining polymerization, using PLLA, was carried out, signals, not only due to amylose, but also due to PLLA, were observed in the ^{1}H NMR spectrum of the product in DMSO-d_6. The XRD pattern of the product showed two diffraction peaks at $2\theta = 11°–12°$ and $18°–19°$ (Figure 6e), which was completely different from that of a sole amylose (Figure 6a), supporting the inclusion complex structure of the product. Interestingly, the diffraction peaks of the product were detected at lower angles compared with those of amylase-PTHF inclusion complex (Figure 6b) [40]. This difference in the two XRD patterns reasonably suggested that the diameter of amylose helix in the product was larger by inclusion of the bulky PLLA in the cavity of amylose. These analytical results fully supported that the amylose-PLLA inclusion complex was obtained in the vine-twining polymerization using PLLA as the guest polyester. To investigate the effect of the chirality in PLAs on inclusion by amylose, the vine-twining polymerization was performed using PDLA and PDLLA. Consequently, the ^{1}H NMR spectra and the XRD patterns of the products indicated no formation of inclusion complexes. From the above results, it was concluded that amylose perfectly recognized the chirality in PLAs on inclusion complexation in the vine-twining polymerization.

7. Conclusions

In this article, the author reviewed the precision architecture of amylose supramolecules in the form of inclusion complexes by the phosphorylase-catalyzed enzymatic polymerization of G-1-P in the presence of hydrophobic synthetic polymers, such as polyethers, polyesters, a poly(ester-ether), and polycarbonates, according to the vine-twining polymerization manner. The corresponding amylose supramolecular inclusion complexes were formed in the process of the polymerization. The results in the vine-twining polymerization suggested that amylose exhibited different inclusion behaviors by the specific interactions with the guest polymers, depending on subtle changes in their structures. As of the production of the structurally defined polysaccharides by the enzymatic catalysis, the precision architecture of the regularly controlled amylose supramolecules, described herein, has been achieved. Moreover, the studies on the enzymatic architecture of the polysaccharide supramolecules have been based on the viewpoints that the greener and eco-friendly processes should be developed in the fields, not only of fundamental research, but also of practical application of the polymer and material chemistries. The polysaccharide supramolecules have increasingly been attracting a great deal of attention because of their potential for application as new functional materials in many research fields, such as medicine and pharmaceutics. Therefore, the present vine-twining polymerization method will be applied to the additional architecture of various amylose supramolecules with regularly controlled nanostructures, and accordingly contributes to providing new functional bio-based materials in the future [53,54].

Acknowledgments

The author is indebted to co-workers, whose names are found in references from his paper, for their enthusiastic collaborations. The author also gratefully thanks a Grant-in-Aid for Scientific Research from Ministry of Education, Culture, Sports, and Technology, Japan (Nos. 14550830, 17550118, 19550126, and 24350062) and Sekisui Foundation for financial supports.

Conflict of Interest

The authors declare no conflict of interest.

References

1. Schuerch, C. Polysaccharides. In *Encyclopedia of Polymer Science and Engineering*, 2nd ed.; Mark, H.F., Bilkales, N., Overberger, C.G., Eds.; John Wiley & Sons: New York, NY, USA, 1986; Volume 13, pp. 87–162.
2. *Carbohydrates in Chemistry and Biology*; Ernst, B., Hart, G.W., Sinaÿ, P., Eds.; Wiley-VCH: Weinheim, Germany, 2000.
3. *Glycoscience*, 2nd ed.; Fraser-Reid, B.O., Tatsuta, K., Thiem, J., Coté, G.L., Flitsch, S., Ito, Y., Kondo, H., Nishimura, S.-I., Yu, B., Eds.; Springer: Berlin, Germany, 2008.
4. *Essentials of Glycobiology*, 2nd ed.; Varki, A., Cummings, R.D., Esko, J.D., Freeze, H.H., Stanley, P., Bertozzi, C.R., Hart, G.W., Etzler, M.E., Eds.; Cold Spring Harbor Laboratory Press: New York, NY, USA, 2009.
5. Paulsen, H. Advances in selective chemical syntheses of complex oligosaccharides. *Angew. Chem. Int. Ed. Engl.* **1982**, *21*, 155–173.
6. Schmidt, R.R. New methods of the synthesis of glycosides and oligosaccharides—Are there alternative to the Koenigs-Knorr methods? *Angew. Chem. Int. Ed. Engl.* **1986**, *25*, 212–235.
7. Toshima, K.; Tatsuta, K. Recent progress in *O*-glycosylation methods and its application to natural products synthesis. *Chem. Rev.* **1993**, *93*, 1503–1531.
8. Mydock, L.K.; Demchenko, A.V. Mechanism of chemical *O*-glycosylation: From early studies to recent discoveries. *Org. Biomol. Chem.* **2010**, *8*, 497–510.
9. Kobayashi, S.; Uyama, H.; Kimura, S. Enzymatic polymerization. *Chem. Rev.* **2001**, *101*, 3793–3818.

32

10. Shoda, S.; Izumi, R.; Fujita, M. Green process in glycotechnology. *Bull. Chem. Soc. Jpn.* **2003**, *76*, 1–13.

11. Seibel, J.; Jördening, H.-J.; Buchholz, K. Glycosylation with activated sugars using glycosyltransferases and transglycosidases. *Biocatal. Biotranform.* **2006**, *24*, 311–342.

12. Kobayashi, S. New development of polysaccharide synthesis via enzymatic polymerization. *Proc. Jpn. Acad. Ser. B* **2007**, *83*, 215–247.

13. Kobayashi, S.; Makino, A. Enzymatic polymer synthesis: An opportunity for green polymer chemistry. *Chem. Rev.* **2009**, *109*, 5288–5353.

14. Kadokawa, J.; Kobayashi, S. Polymer synthesis by enzymatic catalysis. *Curr. Opin. Chem. Biol.* **2010**, *14*, 145–153.

15. Kadokawa, J. Precision polysaccharide synthesis catalyzed by enzymes. *Chem. Rev.* **2011**, *111*, 4308–4345.

16. Lenz, R.W. Biodegradable polymers. *Adv. Polym. Sci.* **1993**, *107*, 1–40.

17. Putseys, J.A.; Lamberts, L.; Delcour, J.A. Amylose-inclusion complexes: Formation, identity and physico-chemical properties. *J. Cereal Sci.* **2010**, *51*, 238–247.

18. Shogren, R.L.; Greene, R.V.; Wu, Y.V. Complexes of starch polysaccharides and poly(ethylene-*co*-acrylic acid)–structure and stability in solution. *J. Appl. Polym. Sci.* **1991**, *42*, 1701–1709.

19. Shogren, R.L. Complexes of starch with telechelic poly(ε-caprolactone) phosphate. *Carbohydr. Polym.* **1993**, *22*, 93–98.

20. Ikeda, M.; Furusho, Y.; Okoshi, K.; Tanahara, S.; Maeda, K.; Nishino, S.; Mori, T.; Yashima, E. A luminescent poly(phenylenevinylene)-amylose composite with supramolecular liquid crystallinity. *Angew. Chem. Int. Ed.* **2006**, *45*, 6491–6495.

21. Kida, T.; Minabe, T.; Okabe, S.; Akashi, M. Partially-methylated amyloses as effective hosts for inclusion complex formation with polymeric guests. *Chem. Commun.* **2007**, 1559–1561.

22. Kida, T.; Minabe, T.; Nakano, S.; Akashi, M. Fabrication of novel multilayered thin films based on inclusion complex formation between amylose derivatives and guest polymers. *Langmuir* **2008**, *24*, 9227–9229.

23. Frampton, M.J.; Claridge, T.D.W.; Latini, G.; Brovelli, S.; Cacialli, F.; Anderson, L. Amylose-wrapped luminescent conjugated polymers. *Chem. Commun.* **2008**, 2797–2799.

24. Kaneko, Y.; Kyutoku, T.; Shimomura, N.; Kadokawa, J. Formation of amylose-poly(tetrahydrofuran) inclusion complexes in ionic liquid media. *Chem. Lett.* **2011**, *40*, 31–33.

25. Rachmawati, R.; Woortman, A.J.J.; Loos, K. Facile preparation method for inclusion complexes between amylose and polytetrahydrofurans. *Biomacromolecules* **2013**, *14*, 575–583.

26. Rachmawati, R.; Woortman, A.J.J.; Loos, K. Tunable properties of inclusion complexes between amylose and polytetrahydrofuran. *Macromol. Biosci.* **2013**, *13*, 767–776.

27. Kaneko, Y.; Kadokawa, J. Vine-twining polymerization: A new preparation method for well-defined supramolecules composed of amylose and synthetic polymers. *Chem. Rec.* **2005**, *5*, 36–46.

28. Kaneko, Y.; Kadokawa, J. Synthesis of nanostructured bio-related materials by hybridization of synthetic polymers with polysaccharides or saccharide residues. *J. Biomater. Sci. Polym. Ed.* **2006**, *17*, 1269–1284.

29. Kaneko, Y.; Kadokawa, J. *Modern Trends in Macromolecular Chemistry*; Lee, J.N., Ed.; Nova Science Publishers, Inc.: Hauppauge, NY, USA, 2009; Chapter 8, pp. 199–217.

30. Kadokawa, J. Preparation and applications of amylose supramolecules by means of phosphorylase-catalyzed enzymatic polymerization. *Polymers* **2012**, *4*, 116–133.

31. Kitaoka, M.; Hayashi, K. Carbohydrate-processing phosphorolytic enzymes. *Trends Glycosci. Glycotechnol.* **2002**, *14*, 35–50.

32. Ziegast, G.; Pfannemüller, B. Phosphorolytic syntheses with di-, oligo- and multi-functional primers. *Carbohydr. Res.* **1987**, *160*, 185–204.

33. Gidley, M.J.; Bulpin, P.V. Aggregation of amylose in aqueous systems: The effect of chain length phase behavior and aggregation kinetics. *Macromolecules* **1989**, *22*, 341–346.

34. Niemann, C.; Sanger, W.; Pfannemüller, B.; Eigner, W.D.; Huber, A. Phospholytic synthesis of low-molecular-weight amyloses with modified terminal groups; Comparison of potato phosphorylase andmuscle phosphorylase b. In *ACS Symp. Ser. Volume 458, Biotechnology of Amylodextrin Oligosaccharides*; Friedman, R.B., Ed.; American Chemical Society: Washington, DC, USA, 1991; Chapter 13, pp. 189–204.

35. Fujii, K.; Takata, H.; Yanase, M.; Terada, Y.; Ohdan, K.; Takaha, T.; Okada, S.; Kuriki, T. Bioengineering and application of novel glucose polymers. *Biocatal. Biotransform.* **2003**, *21*, 167–172.

36. Yanase, M.; Takaha, T.; Kuriki, T. α-Glucan phosphorylase and its use in carbohydrate engineering. *J. Food Agric.* **2006**, *86*, 1631–1635.

37. Ohdan, K.; Fujii, K.; Yanase, M.; Takaha, T.; Kuriki, T. Enzymatic synthesis of amylose. *Biocatal. Biotransform.* **2006**, *24*, 77–81.

38. Nomura, S.; Kyutoku, T.; Shimomura, N.; Kaneko, Y.; Kadokawa, J. Preparation of inclusion complexes composed of amylose and biodegradable poly(glycolic acid-*co*-ε-caprolactone) by vine-twining polymerization and their lipase-catalyzed hydrolysis behavior. *Polym. J.* **2011**, *43*, 971–977.

39. Kitamura, S. Starch, Polymers, Natural and Synthetic. In *The Polymeric Materials Encyclopedia, Synthesis, Properties and Applications*; Salamone, C., Ed.; CRC Press: New York, NY, USA, 1996; Volume 10, pp. 7915–7922.

40. Kadokawa, J.; Kaneko, Y.; Tagaya, H.; Chiba, K. Synthesis of an amylose-polymer inclusion complex by enzymatic polymerization of glucose 1-phosphate catalyzed by phosphorylase enzyme in the presence of polyTHF: A new method for synthesis of polymer-polymer inclusion complexes. *Chem. Commun.* **2001**, *2001*, 449–450.

41. Seneviratne, H.D.; Biliaderis, C.G. Action of α-amylases on amylose-lipid complex superstructures. *J. Cereal Sci.* **1991**, *13*, 129–143.

42. Kadokawa, J.; Kaneko, Y.; Nagase, S.; Takahashi, T.; Tagaya, H. Vine-twining polymerization: Amylose twines around polyethers to form amylose-polyether inclusion complexes. *Chem. Eur. J.* **2002**, *8*, 3321–3326.

43. Kadokawa, J.; Kaneko, Y.; Nakaya, A.; Tagaya, H. Formation of an amylose-polyester inclusion complex by means of phosphorylase-catalyzed enzymatic polymerization of α-D-glucose 1-phosphate monomer in the presence of poly(ε-caprolactone). *Macromolecules* **2001**, *34*, 6536–6528.

44. Kadokawa, J.; Nakaya, A.; Kaneko, Y.; Tagaya, H. Preparation of inclusion complexes between amylose and ester-containing polymers by means of vine-twining polymerization. *Macromol. Chem. Phys.* **2003**, *204*, 1451–1457.

45. Kaneko, Y.; Saito, Y.; Nakaya, A.; Kadokawa, J.; Tagaya, H. Preparation of inclusion complexes composed of amylose and strongly hydrophobic polyesters in parallel enzymatic polymerization system. *Macromolecules* **2008**, *41*, 5665–5670.

46. Kobayashi, S.; Uyama, H.; Suda, S.; Namekawa, S. Dehydration polymerization in aqueous medium catalyzed by lipase. *Chem. Lett.* **1997**, 105–105.

47. Suda, S.; Uyama, H.; Kobayashi, S. Dehydration polycondensation in water for synthesis of polyesters by lipase catalyst. *Proc. Jpn. Acad. Ser. B* **1999**, *75*, 201–206.

48. Kaneko, Y.; Beppu, K.; Kadokawa, J. Preparation of amylose/polycarbonate inclusion complexes by means of vine-twining polymerization. *Macromol. Chem. Phys.* **2008**, *209*, 1037–1042.

49. Kaneko, Y.; Beppu, K.; Kadokawa, J. Amylose selectively includes one from a mixture of two resemblant polyethers in vine-twining polymerization. *Biomacromolecules* **2007**, *8*, 2983–2985.

50. Kaneko, Y.; Beppu, K.; Kyutoku, T.; Kadokawa, J. Selectivity and priority on inclusion of amylose toward guest polyethers and polyesters in vine-twining polymerization. *Polym. J.* **2009**, *41*, 279–286.

51. Kaneko, Y.; Beppu, K.; Kadokawa, J. Amylose selectively includes a specific range of molecular weights in poly(tetrahydrofuran)s in vine-twining polymerization. *Polym. J.* **2009**, *41*, 792–796.

52. Kaneko, Y.; Ueno, K.; Yui, T.; Nakahara, K.; Kadokawa, J. Amylose's recognition of chirality in polylactides on formation of inclusion complexes in vine-twining polymerization. *Macromol. Biosci.* **2011**, *11*, 1407–1415.

53. Kaneko, Y.; Fujisaki, K.; Kyutoku, T.; Furukawa, H.; Kadokawa, J. Preparation of enzymatically recyclable hydrogels through the formation of inclusion complexes of amylose in a vine-twining polymerization. *Chem. Asian J.* **2010**, *5*, 1627–1633.

54. Kadokawa, J.; Kaneko, Y. *Engineering of Polysaccharide Materials–by Phosphorylase-Catalyzed Enzymatic Chain-Elongation*; Pan Stanford Publishing Pte. Ltd.: Temasek Boulevard, Singapore, 2013.

Enzyme-Catalyzed Synthesis of Unsaturated Aliphatic Polyesters Based on Green Monomers from Renewable Resources

Yi Jiang, Albert J.J. Woortman, Gert O.R. Alberda van Ekenstein and Katja Loos

Abstract: Bio-based commercially available succinate, itaconate and 1,4-butanediol are enzymatically co-polymerized in solution via a two-stage method, using *Candida antarctica* Lipase B (CALB, in immobilized form as Novozyme® 435) as the biocatalyst. The chemical structures of the obtained products, poly(butylene succinate) (PBS) and poly(butylene succinate-*co*-itaconate) (PBSI), are confirmed by ^{1}H- and ^{13}C-NMR. The effects of the reaction conditions on the CALB-catalyzed synthesis of PBSI are fully investigated, and the optimal polymerization conditions are obtained. With the established method, PBSI with tunable compositions and satisfying reaction yields is produced. The ^{1}H-NMR results confirm that carbon-carbon double bonds are well preserved in PBSI. The differential scanning calorimetry (DSC) and thermal gravimetric analysis (TGA) results indicate that the amount of itaconate in the co-polyesters has no obvious effects on the glass-transition temperature and the thermal stability of PBS and PBSI, but has significant effects on the melting temperature.

Reprinted from *Biomolecules*. Cite as: Jiang, Y.; Woortman, A.J.J.; van Ekenstein, G.O.R.A.; Loos, K. Enzyme-Catalyzed Synthesis of Unsaturated Aliphatic Polyesters Based on Green Monomers from Renewable Resources. *Biomolecules* **2013**, *3*, 461-480.

1. Introduction

Utilizing renewable resources for the replacement of depleting fossil stocks is an appealing research topic, both in the academic and industrial areas [1–5]. It is a promising approach to solve the severe environmental problems induced by the increasing petroleum consumptions nowadays and the plausible energy shortage in the future. As abundant carbon-neutral renewable resources, biomass stocks are generated directly from solar energy in a short cycle. A great number of monomers and macromonomers can be produced from biomass stocks by natural biological activities or chemical modifications [6,7]. These bio-based monomers provide numerous opportunities for the synthesis of green and novel polymers.

Unsaturated polyesters are widely used as thermosetting resins in various industrial areas [8–10]. They are usually produced by polycondensation of diacids and diols based on petroleum stocks, using titanium or tin alkoxides as catalyst [11]. The synthesis temperature is usually above 150 °C [11,12]. Many monomers with chemically or thermally unstable moieties are not suitable for polyester synthesis, due to uncontrollable side reactions induced by such a high temperature, like gelation, decomposition and discoloration [11–13]. Besides, the residual metals from the conventional catalysts are hard to remove, which may cause undesirable pollution upon disposal [12].

Candida antarctica Lipase B (CALB) is a very versatile biocatalyst for polyester synthesis, working with various monomers and organic solvents under mild conditions [12,14–27]. CALB-catalyzed synthesis of polyesters from green monomers has recently gained increasing popularity. Succinate [28–31], fatty acids from plant oils [11,32–37], isosorbide [29,30] and 1,4-butanediol [8,28,31,38–40] are extensively studied. The bio-based polyesters produced are eco-friendly, since the monomers and the catalysts are all generated from renewable resources, and the polymers are biodegradable [9,28,39].

Itaconate is a commercially available green bio-based monomer. Its acid derivative, itaconic acid, has been industrially fermented from carbohydrates using *Aspergillus terreus* since the 1960s [41]. This monomer has interesting photoactive and biocompatible properties [9]. It is an ideal building block for constructing unsaturated polyesters with potential biomedical and engineering applications [9,42,43]. However, up until now, itaconate has not been well studied for polyester synthesis, neither by conventional catalysts nor by biocatalysts. Limited kinds of itaconate-based polyesters were synthesized using conventional chemical catalysts [8–10,43–48]. Only two papers referred to the enzymatic polymerizations of itaconate with other monomers: Barrett *et al.* reported enzymatic co-polymerizations of dimethyl itaconate and adipic acid with 1,4-cyclohexanedimethanol and poly(ethylene glycol) [9]; and Rajkhowa *et al.* reported Lipase-catalyzed polymerization of diglycidyl ether of bisphenol A and itaconic anhydride [49]. To the best of our knowledge, the enzyme-catalyzed co-polymerization of succinate, itaconate and 1,4-butanediol has not yet been studied. This is probably due to the low enzyme polymerizability of itaconate, which is caused by its short chain length [28] and the stereo-hindrance effect of the carbon-carbon double bond suspended around the carbonyl group. We believe CALB is the perfect biocatalyst for the synthesis of itaconate-based polyesters, due to its wide monomer adaptability, rendering polyesters in which the thermal unstable carbon-carbon double bonds could be preserved, since the enzymatic polymerization will be performed at mild temperatures under 100 °C [12,17].

We present an environmental friendly approach towards unsaturated aliphatic polyesters. Bio-based succinate, itaconate and 1,4-butanediol are enzymatically co-polymerized in solution via a two-stage method, using CALB as the catalyst. The general synthesis strategy is illustrated in Figure 1. Monomers are oligomerized at 80 °C under nitrogen atmosphere during the first stage. Then, the oligomers are polycondensed at the same temperature under high vacuum during the second stage. To achieve the best polymerization results, the effects of different reaction conditions on CALB-catalyzed synthesis of poly(butylene succinate-*co*-itaconate) (PBSI) are extensively investigated, and the optimal polymerization conditions are obtained. With the method we established, poly(butylene succinate) (PBS) and a series of PBSI are synthesized. The chemical structures, molecular weight and thermal properties of the co-polyesters are characterized by different methods.

Figure 1. *Candida antarctica* Lipase B (CALB)-catalyzed co-polymerization of succinate, itaconate and 1,4-butanediol.

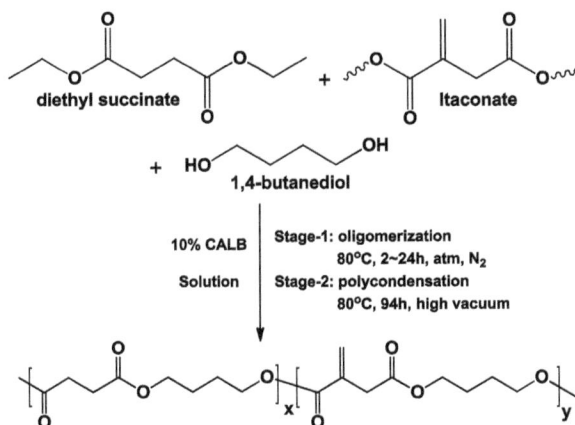

2. Results and Discussion

2.1. Effects of Polymerization Conditions on CALB-Catalyzed Co-Polymerization of Diethyl Succinate, Dimethyl Itaconate and 1,4-Butanediol

Succinic acid, itaconic acid and 1,4-butanediol are commercially available bio-based monomers. They are good building blocks for polyester synthesis. However, succinic acid has a rather low solubility in 1,4-butanediol under enzymatic polycondensation conditions, which leads to low polymerization efficiency [28]. Itaconic acid has the same problem, according to our observations reported in Section 2.2. To avoid phase separation during polymerization, diethyl succinate and dimethyl itaconate were used as the acyl donors.

For the purpose of producing PBSI with the highest amount of itaconate, molecular weight and reaction yield, the effects of several polymerization conditions on CALB-catalyzed co-polymerization of diethyl succinate, dimethyl itaconate and 1,4-butanediol were investigated, including solvent, solvent dosage, oligomerization time during the first stage and vacuum during the second stage.

2.1.1. Effect of Solvent on CALB-Catalyzed Co-Polymerization of Diethyl Succinate, Dimethyl Itaconate and 1,4-Butanediol

Dodecane, diethylene glycol dimethyl ether (diglyme) and diphenyl ether were evaluated, as they have been proven to be suitable for enzymatic synthesis of polyesters [13,28,50]. As summarized in Table 1, PBSI with the highest mole percentage of itaconate (X_I) and number average molecular weight (M_n) was synthesized using diphenyl ether as solvent. However, the highest reaction yield was obtained in diglyme; the second highest reaction yield in diphenyl ether.

As presented in Table 1, when the molar feed ratio of dimethyl itaconate was 15%, the values of product X_I obtained in diphenyl ether, dodecane and diglyme were 10.5%, 3.5% and 0.3%, respectively. The corresponding M_n calculated from ^{1}H-NMR spectra were 1304 g/mol, 963 g/mol and 854 g/mol. The reaction yields were 55.5%, 54.3% and 68.8%, respectively.

Meanwhile, when the feed ratio of dimethyl itaconate was increased to 25%, the values of product X_I achieved in diphenyl ether, dodecane and diglyme were 15.9%, 3.7% and 5.9%, respectively. The corresponding M_n were 1403 g/mol, 730 g/mol and 795 g/mol. The reaction yields were 22.6%, 18.3% and 30.2%, respectively.

Table 1. The effect of solvent on CALB-catalyzed synthesis of poly(butylene succinate-*co*-itaconate) (PBSI).

				Molar Composition					
		Feed (%)			**PBSI [a] (%)**			**Molecular Weight**	
Solvent	**log P**	**F$_S$**	**F$_I$**	**F$_B$**	**X$_S$**	**X$_I$**	**X$_B$**	**M$_n$ (g/mol) [b]**	**Yield (%)**
Diphenyl ether	4.1	35	15	50	40.5	10.5	49.0	1304	55.5
Dodecane	6.8	35	15	50	46.5	3.5	50.0	963	54.3
Diglyme	−1.3	35	15	50	49.2	0.3	50.5	854	68.8
Diphenyl ether	4.1	25	25	50	35.3	15.9	48.8	1403	22.6
Dodecane	6.8	25	25	50	46.5	3.7	49.8	730	18.3
Diglyme	−1.3	25	25	50	43.2	5.9	50.9	795	30.2

F_S, F_I, F_B: molar feed ratio of succinate, itaconate and 1,4-butanediol; X_S, X_I, X_B: mole percentage of succinate, itaconate and butylene units in PBSI; polymerization conditions: 200 wt% of solvent; Stage-1: 80 °C, 24 h, N$_2$; Stage-2: 80 °C, 94 h, vacuum 40 mmHg; [a] molar composition determined by integration of the ^{1}H-NMR spectra; [b] number average molecular weight (M_n) calculated from ^{1}H-NMR spectra; log P, logarithm of partition coefficient.

It has already been reported that diphenyl ether is the preferred solvent to achieve higher M_n for lipase-catalyzed synthesis of polyesters [13,28,50], which is in good accordance with our current results. Three factors could be attributed to our case, including the log P (logarithm of partition coefficient) value of the solvent, the accessibility of CALB and the miscibility of the intermediate and the final products in the solvent. The log P values of diphenyl ether and dodecane are higher than 1.9. They are more efficient for producing high molecular weight polyesters than diglyme. Furthermore, we found that CALB dispersed well in diphenyl ether and diglyme, but adhered tightly to the flasks in dodecane. Additionally, PBS with low molecular weight and PBSI are fully miscible in diphenyl ether at 80 °C, but precipitated fast in diglyme and dodecane. Therefore, PBSI with higher M_n is produced in diphenyl ether, since CALB is more accessible and the intermediate products are diffused better, which provide sufficient time and space for the chain growth and the transesterification of PBSI.

Moreover, we found that the enzymatic polymerizability of dimethyl itaconate was higher in diphenyl ether in comparison to the other two solvents. In addition, the molar composition of PBSI produced in diphenyl ether matched better with the feed composition of the monomers. The enzymatic polymerizability of dimethyl itaconate in dodecane and diglyme was quite low; only less than 6% of dimethyl itaconate was co-polymerized, although the reaction yield was considerably high. This is because PBS and PBSI are not soluble in dodecane and diglyme at 80 °C. In diglyme and dodecane, 1,4-butanediol prefers to react with diethyl succinate first, since the enzyme polymerizability of diethyl succinate is higher than that of dimethyl itaconate. Low molecular weight PBS and PBSI composed with a little amount of itaconate was produced and precipitated fast from the reaction.

Therefore, diphenyl ether is the most suitable solvent for CALB-catalyzed synthesis of PBSI.

2.1.2. Effect of Solvent Dosage on CALB-Catalyzed Co-Polymerization of Diethyl Succinate, Dimethyl Itaconate and 1,4-Butanediol

Figure 2 illustrates the values of product M_n, X_I and reaction yield as a function of diphenyl ether dosage. PBSI with the highest values of M_n, X_I and reaction yield was obtained from the reaction with 150 wt% of diphenyl ether (in relation to the total amount of monomers).

Figure 2. The effect of diphenyl ether dosage on CALB-catalyzed synthesis of PBSI.

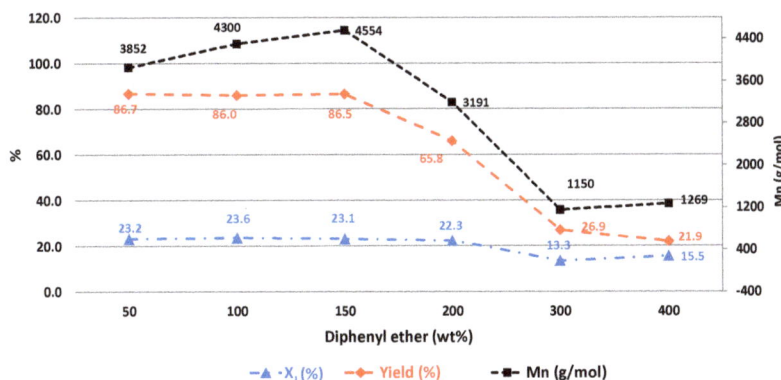

Polymerization conditions: 50%–400 wt% of diphenyl ether; $F_S/F_I/F_B$ = 25%/25%/50%; Stage-1: 80 °C, 2 h, N_2; Stage-2: 80 °C, 94 h, vacuum 2 mmHg; M_n was calculated from ^{1}H-NMR spectra.

As presented in Figure 2, the values of product X_I and reaction yield remained almost the same, when the dosage of diphenyl ether was increased from 50% to 150%. The product X_I was around 23%, and the reaction yield was close to 87%. The corresponding M_n increased from 3852 g/mol to 4554 g/mol. The X_I value calculated from ^{1}H-NMR was in good agreement with the feed ratio of itaconate. The synchronous increase of product M_n with the solvent dosage was due to the better diffusion of the reactants in dilute reaction.

By increasing the solvent dosage from 150% to 400%, the values of product M_n and reaction yield decreased significantly. The M_n reduced from 4554 g/mol to 1269 g/mol, while the reaction yield decreased from 86.5% to 21.9%. As for the X_I value, it remained similar, around 23%, when the solvent dosage was increased to 200%. On further dilution to 300%, it dropped to 13.3%, and on dilution to 400%, it remained more or less the same: 14.6%. We suspect that the increase of the residual alcohol amount and the decrease of the polymerization rate in dilute reaction could be the reasons. The alcohols were more difficult to remove by vacuum at a certain low concentration in dilute solution. The absolute amount of the residual alcohols was higher in the reactions with higher solvent dosage. At the same time, the polymerization rate was reduced, since the concentrations of

CALB and the reactants were lower. The transesterification of oligomers with itaconate was hindered, and only low molecular weight co-polyesters were produced. The low molecular weight PBSI composed with a higher amount of itaconate is soluble in methanol. In this case, only PBSI with a lower amount of itaconate was obtained after purification, which led to the lower value of the reaction yield.

As a result, the best diphenyl ether dosage for *in vitro* synthesis of PBSI is 150 wt% (in relation to the total amount of monomers).

2.1.3. Effect of Oligomerization Time during the First Stage on CALB-Catalyzed Co-Polymerization of Diethyl Succinate, Dimethyl Itaconate and 1,4-Butanediol

As shown in Table 2, the selected oligomerization time has no obvious effects on the composition and the reaction yield of PBSI. PBSI with the highest M_n was synthesized from the reaction conducting 2 h oligomerization during the first stage.

Table 2. The effect of oligomerization time on CALB-catalyzed synthesis of PBSI.

	Molar Composition							
	Feed (%)			PBSI [a](%)			Molecular Weight	
Oligomerization time	F_S	F_I	F_B	X_S	X_I	X_B	M_n (g/mol) [b]	Yield (%)
2 h	35	15	50	35.7	14.1	50.2	3936	87.7
6 h	35	15	50	35.2	14.9	49.9	3212	87.6
12 h	35	15	50	36.3	14.4	49.3	2960	84.1
2 h	25	25	50	27.0	23.1	49.9	2935	73.1
6 h	25	25	50	28.9	21.5	49.6	2459	68.5
12 h	25	25	50	27.5	22.8	49.7	2609	71.6

Polymerization conditions: 150 wt% of diphenyl ether; Stage-1: 80 °C, 2–12 h, N_2; Stage-2: 80 °C, 94 h, vacuum 2 mmHg; [a] molar composition determined by integration of the ^{1}H-NMR spectra; [b] number average molecular weight calculated from ^{1}H-NMR spectra.

When the feed ratio of dimethyl itaconate was 15%, the composition of PBSI agreed well with the feed composition of the monomers, which was independent of the time of oligomerization. The reaction yield was quite satisfying (higher than 84%). However, the product M_n decreased from 3936 g/mol to 2960 g/mol, with increasing the oligomerization time from 2 h to 12 h.

Similar trends were obtained when the feed ratio of dimethyl itaconate was 25%. In spite of increasing the oligomerization time from 2 h, 6 h and up to 12 h, the composition and reaction yield of PBSI remained almost the same. The product M_n, however, decreased a little from 2935 g/mol (2 h oligomerization) to 2609 g/mol (12 h oligomerization).

The enzymatic oligomerization process of diethyl succinate, dimethyl itaconate and 1,4-butanediol was monitored by *in situ* ^{1}H-NMR, as shown in Figure 3. The ^{1}H-NMR spectra of the intermediate products reacted for more than 30 min were almost identical, except the signals belonging to the active hydroxyl groups at 1.7–2.2 ppm. It is suspected that the monomers were fully transformed to oligomers after 30 min during the first stage.

Therefore, it can be concluded that 2 h of oligomerization during the first stage will be sufficient enough for CALB-catalyzed synthesis of PBSI.

Figure 3. *In situ* ^{1}H-NMR investigation of the oligomerization process of: (**a**) diethyl succinate (35%), dimethyl itaconate (15%) and 1,4-butanediol (50%); (**b**) diethyl succinate (25%), dimethyl itaconate (25%) and 1,4-butanediol (50%).

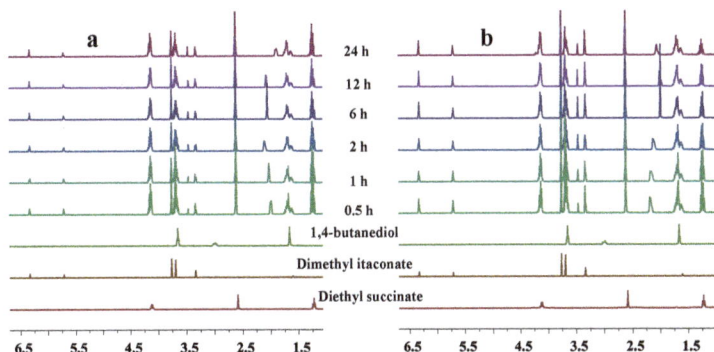

2.1.4. Effect of Vacuum during the Second Stage on CALB-Catalyzed Co-Polymerization of Diethyl Succinate, Dimethyl Itaconate and 1,4-Butanediol

As presented in Table 3, the vacuum during the second stage has a significant impact on the CALB-catalyzed co-polymerization. PBSI with the highest values of X_I, M_n and reaction yield was produced by the co-polymerizations with the highest vacuum applied (2 mmHg). Furthermore, the composition of PBSI produced under higher vacuum matched better with the feed composition of the monomers.

Table 3. The effect of vacuum on CALB-catalyzed synthesis of PBSI.

| | Molar Composition | | | | | | | |
| | Feed (%) | | | PBSI [a] (%) | | | Molecular Weight | |
Vacuum	F_S	F_I	F_B	X_S	X_I	X_B	M_n (g/mol) [b]	Yield (%)
2 mmHg	35	15	50	35.7	14.1	50.2	3936	87.7
10–20 mmHg	35	15	50	37.1	13.1	49.8	2552	56.2
40 mmHg	35	15	50	40.5	10.5	49.0	1304	55.5
2 mmHg	25	25	50	27.0	23.1	49.9	2935	73.1
10–20 mmHg	25	25	50	31.7	19.1	49.2	2328	19.5
40 mmHg	25	25	50	35.2	15.9	48.9	1203	22.6

Polymerization conditions: 150 wt% of diphenyl ether; Stage-1: 80 °C, 2 h, N_2; Stage-2: 80 °C, 94 h, vacuum at 2–40 mmHg; [a] molar composition determined by integration of the ^{1}H-NMR spectra; [b] number average molecular weight calculated from ^{1}H-NMR spectra.

When the feed ratio of dimethyl itaconate was 15%, the values of product X_I, M_n and reaction yield increased significantly with an increase of vacuum. The values of product X_I from the reactions under vacuum of 40 mmHg, 10–20 mmHg and 2 mmHg were 10.5%, 13.1% and 14.1%, respectively. The corresponding product M_n was 1304 g/mol, 2552 g/mol and 3936 g/mol. The reaction yield was 55.5%, 56.2% and 87.7%, respectively.

The same trend of product X_I, M_n and reaction yield as a function of vacuum was identified, when the feed ratio of dimethyl itaconate was 25%. By lowering the pressure from 40 mmHg to 2 mmHg, the values of product X_I increased from 15.9% to 23.1%. The product M_n increased from 1203 g/mol to 2935 g/mol. Additionally, the reaction yield increased from 22.6% to 73.1%.

The effect of vacuum is quite reasonable, since the residual alcohols and water can be further eliminated from the reaction under higher vacuum, which facilitates the chain growth of co-polyesters. It is obvious that the reduced pressure shall be regulated to 2 mmHg during the second stage for *in vitro* synthesis of PBSI in diphenyl ether.

2.2. Effect of Itaconate Structure on CALB-Catalyzed Synthesis of PBSI in Diphenyl Ether

Four itaconate derivatives were studied, namely itaconic acid, dimethyl itaconate, diethyl itaconate and dibutyl itaconate. The byproducts generated during polycondensation are water, methanol, ethanol and n-butyl alcohol, respectively.

Phase separation of itaconic acid in the presence of the other reactants was observed. This is due to the fact that itaconic acid has a rather low solubility in the mixture of diphenyl ether, diethyl succinate and 1,4-butanediol.

Dimethyl itaconate dissolved in the reaction medium when at temperatures above 60 °C. The co-polymerization with dimethyl itaconate, diethyl itaconate or dibutyl itaconate was homogeneous.

PBSI could not be obtained in a sufficient amount when using itaconic acid as the unsaturated monomer. The reaction yield was extremely low, less than 4%, as shown in Figure 4a.

Figure 4. The effect of itaconate structure on CALB-catalyzed synthesis of PBSI: (**a**) the reaction yield of PBSI as a function of the feed ratio of itaconate; (**b**) the mole percentage of itaconate in PBSI (X_I) as a function of the feed ratio of itaconate.

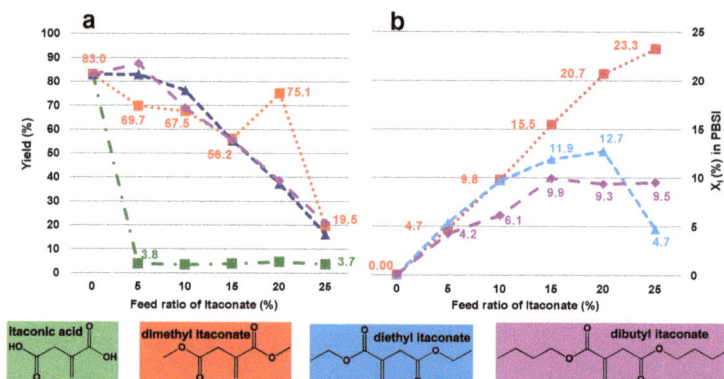

Polymerization conditions: 150 wt% of diphenyl ether; Stage-1: 80 °C, 2 h, N_2; Stage-2: 80 °C, 94 h, vacuum 10–20 mmHg.

For the co-polymerizations with dialkyl itaconate esters, the reaction yield of PBSI decreased with increasing the feed ratio of itaconate, as displayed in Figure 4a, e.g., the reaction yield decreased from 83.0% to 19.5% when the feed ratio of dimethyl itaconate increased from 0% to 25%. The same trend of the reaction yield as a function of the feed ratio of itaconate was also observed in other co-polymerizations with diethyl itaconate or dibutyl itaconate.

Moreover, for reactions with dimethyl itaconate, the value of product X_I was in good accordance with the corresponding feed ratio of itaconate, as presented in Figure 4b. While the feed ratio of itaconate was 0%, 5%, 10%, 15%, 20% and 25%, the value of product X_I was 0.0%, 4.7%, 9.8%, 15.5%, 20.7% and 23.3%, respectively. The deviation between the X_I value calculated from ^{1}H-NMR spectra and the corresponding feed ratio of itaconate was quite small.

However, for co-polymerizations with diethyl itaconate, the value of product X_I deviated obviously from the corresponding feed ratio of itaconate, especially when the feed ratio of diethyl itaconate was higher than 10%. While the feed ratio of diethyl itaconate was 0%, 5%, 10%, 15%, 20% and 25%, the corresponding product X_I was 0.0%, 5.4%, 9.7%, 11.9%, 12.7% and 4.7%, respectively. The value of product X_I only matched with the feed ratio of diethyl itaconate when less than or equal to 10% of diethyl itaconate was added. The highest X_I value was only 12.7%, which was produced from the reaction with 20% of diethyl itaconate.

For co-polymerizations with dibutyl itaconate, the highest X_I value achieved was only 9.9%. The value of product X_I increased from 0.0% to 9.9% as the corresponding feed ratio of dibutyl itaconate ascended from 0% to 15%. A plateau value was reached of around 10% when the feed ratio of dibutyl itaconate was further increased from 15% to 25%.

As a result, the enzyme polymerizability sequence of itaconate derivatives in diphenyl ether is dimethyl itaconate, diethyl itaconate, dibutyl itaconate and itaconic acid, from high to low. Itaconic acid is not favored by CALB, since it is immiscible in solution, which makes it inaccessible to the biocatalyst. Dimethyl itaconate is the most polymerizable derivative by CALB, since the reaction byproduct, methanol, can be removed easily under vacuum, because of the low boiling temperature of 64.7 °C, compared with ethanol (bp = 78.4 °C) and n-butyl alcohol (bp = 117.7 °C). Besides, the chemical reactivity of the alkyl esters is another reason. It is well known that methyl esters are chemically much more reactive than ethyl and butyl esters.

Therefore, dimethyl itaconate is the most preferred unsaturated monomer for *in vitro* synthesis of PBSI in diphenyl ether.

In conclusion, combining the results from Sections 2.1 to 2.2, we have established the optimal polymerization conditions for CALB-catalyzed co-polymerization of diethyl succinate, itaconate and 1,4-butanediol, which are as follows:

(1) using diphenyl ether as solvent;
(2) the dosage of diphenyl ether is 150 wt% (in relation to the total amount of monomers);
(3) oligomerization for 2 h during the first stage;
(4) regulating vacuum to 2 mmHg during the second stage;
(5) applying dimethyl itaconate as the unsaturated monomer.

2.3. CALB-Catalyzed Synthesis of PBSI Using Optimal Polymerization Conditions

Diethyl succinate, dimethyl itaconate and 1,4-butanediol were co-polymerized in the presence of CALB, using the optimal conditions we established. A series of co-polyesters was produced by alternating the feed ratio of dimethyl itaconate from 0% to 30%. No products were obtained if the feed ratio of dimethyl itaconate was increased to 35% and 50%. For the two control reactions without CALB, also no polymers were obtained after purification. The molar composition, reaction yield, molecular weight and the thermal properties of PBS and PBSI are summarized in Table 4.

As shown in Table 4 and plotted in Figure 5a, co-polyesters with tunable compositions and satisfying reaction yields were achieved, by adjusting the feed ratio of dimethyl itaconate from 0% to 25%. The mole percentage of itaconate in PBSI can be controlled from 0% to 23.5%. The corresponding reaction yield was quite good, higher than 75%.

Table 4. Summary of the results for the CALB-catalyzed synthesis of PBS and PBSI.

| | Molar Composition | | | | | | | | | | Molecular Weight | | | |
| | Feed (%) | | | PBSI ^{a} (%) | | | | | | | NMR | | GPC | |
Co-polyester	F_S	F_I	F_B	X_S	X_I	X_B	Yield (%)	T_g ^{b} (°C)	T_m ^{c} (°C)	T_d ^{d} (°C)	M_n ^{e}	M_n	M_w	M_w/M_n
PBS	50	0	50	50.5	0.0	49.5	85.7	−35.9	112.9	406.1	4,463	6,017	11,520	1.91
PB$_{50}$S$_{40}$I$_{10}$	40	10	50	39.7	10.4	49.9	84.6	−38.8	94.6	402.0	4,696	10,128	19,236	1.90
PB$_{50}$S$_{35}$I$_{15}$	35	15	50	35.0	15.7	49.3	90.0	−36.7	80.3	410.9	6,494	13,288	22,642	1.70
PB$_{50}$S$_{30}$I$_{20}$	30	20	50	30.9	20.1	49.0	75.1	−37.5	71.2	404.7	5,670	8,394	11,892	1.42
PB$_{50}$S$_{25}$I$_{25}$	25	25	50	27.2	23.5	49.3	86.5	−38.4	57.4	407.9	4,554	11,096	16,587	1.49
PBSI	20	30	50	36.4	15.6	48.0	20.9	−49.6	69.8	396.9	1,004	1,948	2,203	1.13
NA ^{f}	15	35	50	-	-	-	-	-	-	-	-	-	-	-
NA ^{f}	0	50	50	-	-	-	-	-	-	-	-	-	-	-
Control-1 ^{g}	50	0	50	-	-	-	-	-	-	-	-	-	-	-
Control-2 ^{g}	25	25	50	-	-	-	-	-	-	-	-	-	-	-

^{a} Molar composition determined by integration of the ^{1}H-NMR spectra; ^{b} glass-transition temperature (T_g) from differential scanning calorimetry (DSC) by a quench method; ^{c} melting temperature (T_m) from DSC measurements, first scan; ^{d} the temperature of the maximal rate of decomposition (T_d) from thermal gravimetric analysis (TGA) measurement; ^{e} number average molecular weight calculated from ^{1}H-NMR spectra; ^{f} no polymer was obtained after precipitation; ^{g} control reactions without CALB. No polymer was obtained after precipitation.

The carbon-carbon double bonds were well preserved in the unsaturated co-polyesters, as confirmed by ^{1}H-NMR spectra in Figure 6. No resonances can be assigned to the deterioration of carbon-carbon double bonds. As displayed in the ^{1}H-NMR spectra of PB$_{50}$S$_{35}$I$_{15}$ and PB$_{50}$S$_{25}$I$_{25}$, the ratio between the integration values of the two separated peaks assigned to the protons of the carbon-carbon double bonds (6.32 ppm and 5.72 ppm, respectively) and the peak assigned to the protons of the methylene group of itaconate (3.33 ppm) was close to 1:1:2, which was exactly the same as that of dimethyl itaconate. Besides, the final products were white semicrystalline powders without discoloration. It is clear that no side reaction occurred during the enzymatic co-polymerizations.

Figure 5. (a) The mole percentage of itaconate (X_I) and the reaction yield of PBSI as a function of the feed ratio of dimethyl itaconate (F_I); **(b)** Overlay of gel permeation chromatography (GPC) elution curves in chloroform; PBSI was synthesized *via* the optimal conditions.

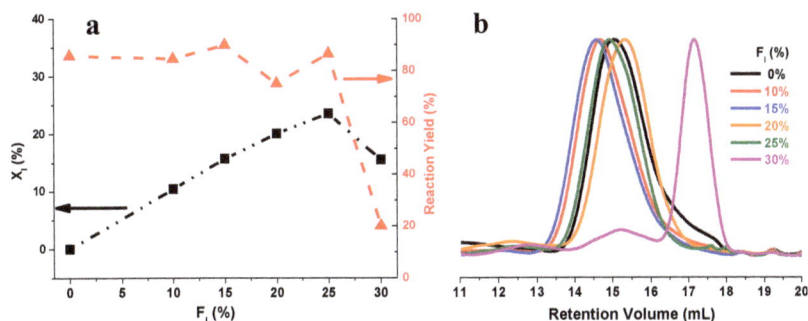

Figure 6. ^{1}H-NMR spectra of dimethyl itaconate, PB$_{50}$S$_{35}$I$_{15}$ and PB$_{50}$S$_{25}$I$_{25}$ in CDCl$_3$.

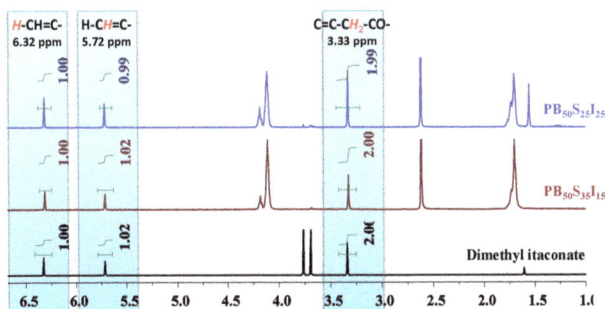

The product M_n calculated from ^{1}H-NMR was around 4000–6500 g/mol, while the feed ratio of dimethyl itaconate was less than or equal to 25%. GPC results indicate that the corresponding M_n was around 6000–14,000 g/mol. The polydispersity index (PDI, M_w/M_n) was between 1.42 and 1.91. The molecular weight of the saturated polyesters was lower than that of the unsaturated counterparts, and the PDI was higher. This is due to the higher melting temperature of PBS, which is around 112 °C. During the polycondensation step, the reaction with PBS solidified after 19 h at 80 °C. The chain growth and transesterification of PBS stopped in the solid state. In contrast to this, the reaction with PBSI proceeded continuously in the liquid state.

The highest value of X_I achieved in PBSI was 23.5%, from the reaction with 25% of dimethyl itaconate. If the feed ratio of dimethyl itaconate was increased to 30%, the product X_I reduced to 15.6%. The corresponding product M_n and the reaction yield decreased significantly to 1948 g/mol and 20.9%, as shown in Figure 5a. If the feed ratio of dimethyl itaconate was further increased to 35% and 50%, no polymer was obtained after precipitation in cold methanol.

As shown in Figure 5b, PBSI synthesized from the reaction with 30% of dimethyl itaconate had two peaks. The first peak was at a retention volume between 13.6 to 16.2 mL, similar to that of the co-polyesters with high molecular weight; however, the concentration was much lower. The major peak was at a retention volume between 16.2 to 18.2 mL, which means that the molecular weight of the most PBSI produced was quite low. It is clear that co-polyesters with two different molecular weight distributions were produced from reaction with 30% of dimethyl itaconate.

The limited incorporation of itaconate in PBSI could be attributed to the relatively low enzyme polymerizability of dimethyl itaconate compared to diethyl succinate. As shown in Figure 7, there are six possible microstructures in PBSI. It is easier for CALB to produce the microstructure of succinate-butylene-succinate (S-B-S) than that of succinate-butylene-itaconate (S-B-I) and itaconate-butylene-itaconate (I-B-I). The formation sequence from easy to difficult is S-B-S, S-B-I-1, S-B-I-2, I-B-I-1, I-B-I-2 and I-B-I-3. While the feed ratio of itaconate is 25%, the molar ratio between succinate, itaconate and 1,4-butanediol is 1:1:2. The possible dominant microstructures in PBSI could be -(S-B-I-B)$_n$-. If the feed ratio of itaconate is higher than 25%, the possible structures could be -I-B-(S-B-I-B)$_n$-I-B-, while some extra I-B-I structures are formed. However, the formation of the I-B-I microstructure is quite difficulty. Oligomers with itaconate ends will be terminated in chain growth, and the transesterification of oligomers with I-B-I structures will be hindered. Consequently, the molecular weight of PBSI will be lower. Low molecular weight PBSI is soluble in methanol and will be washed away during the purification steps. This is why we obtain only PBSI with the highest mole percentage of itaconate around 25%.

This hypothesis also explains well why PBSI obtained from the reaction with 30% of dimethyl itaconate had lower values for M_n, mole percentage of itaconate and reaction yield, as well as, had two retention volume peaks, as plotted in Figure 5.

Figure 7. Possible types of microstructures in PBSI, the formation sequence from easy to difficult: S-B-S < S-B-I-1 < S-B-I-2 < I-B-I-1 < I-B-I-2 < I-B-I-3.

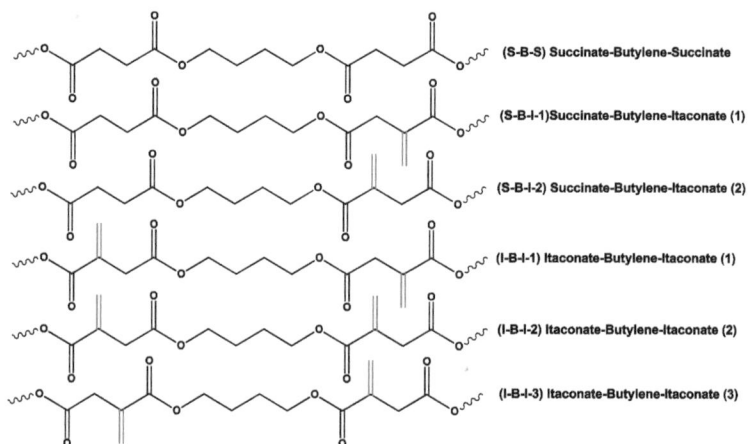

2.4. Thermal Properties of PBS and PBSI

The glass transition temperature (T_g), the melting temperature (T_m) and the temperature of the maximal rate of decomposition (T_d) of PBS and PBSI are plotted as a function of the mole percentage of itaconate in Figure 8. We found that the amount of itaconate composed in the co-polyesters has no obvious effects on the T_g and the thermal stability of PBSI. The T_g and T_d of PBS and PBSI were similar, as shown in Figure 8a. The T_g of the saturated PBS was −35.9 °C. It was slightly higher than that of the rest of the unsaturated PBSI, which was around −36—−38 °C. The T_d of all polyesters was around 400 °C.

However, the T_m of the co-polyesters is significantly affected by the amount of itaconate composed in PBSI. The T_m of the saturated PBS was 112.9 °C, which was 55.5 °C higher than that of the unsaturated counterpart with 23.5% of itaconate. The T_m of PBSI decreased almost linearly as a function of the mole percentage of itaconate, as shown in Figure 8b.

Figure 8. (a) the T_g and T_d of PBSI as a function of the mole percentage of itaconate (X_I); **(b)** the T_m of PBSI as a function of the mole percentage of itaconate (X_I); PBSI was synthesized via the optimal conditions.

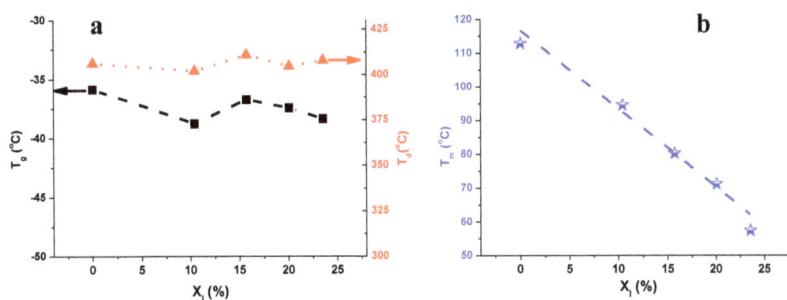

3. Experimental

3.1. Materials

Lipase acrylic resin from *Candida antarctica* Lipase B (CALB, in immobilized form as Novozyme® 435, 5000+ U/g), diethyl succinate (99%), itaconic acid (99%+), dimethyl itaconate (99%), 1,4-butanediol (99%+), dodecane (99%+, anhydrous), diethylene glycol dimethyl ether (99.5%, anhydrous) and diphenyl ether (99%) were purchased from Aldrich. Diethyl itaconate (98%+) and dibutyl itaconate (95%+) were purchased from TCI EUROPE. Diphenyl ether was vacuum distilled and stored with 4Å molecular sieves before use. The other chemicals were used as received.

3.2. General Procedure for CALB-Catalyzed Co-Polymerization of Succinate, Itaconate and 1,4-Butanediol in Solution

CALB (10 wt% in relation to the total amount of monomers, for all reactions) was first fed into a 25 mL flask and stored in a desiccator with phosphorus pentoxide at room temperature under high vacuum for 16 h. Then diethyl succinate (5.55 mmol), itaconate (5.55 mmol), 1,4-butanediol

(11.10 mmol) and the solvent (usually 150 wt% in relation to the total amount of monomers) were added. With the protection of nitrogen, the monomers were oligomerized at 80 °C for 2–24 h under atmospheric pressure during the first stage. The oligomers were further polymerized for another 94 h at the same temperature under the reduced pressure of 2–40 mmHg during the second stage.

After polymerization, chloroform (25 mL) was added into the reaction flask. CALB was filtered out and washed with chloroform (35 mL) three times. The collected solution was condensed by rotary evaporation at 40 °C under a vacuum of 300 mbar. The products were precipitated in cold methanol (−20 °C) and washed with methanol three times. Finally, the polyesters were dried in a vacuum oven at 40 °C for 2–3 days before analysis. The final polymers obtained were white semicrystalline powders.

^{1}H-NMR (400 MHz, CDCl$_3$, ppm) analysis of PBS and PBSI: 6.25–6.35 (1H, s, *H*-CH=C-CO-, from itaconate), 5.65–5.75 (1H, s, H-C*H*=C-CO-, from itaconate), 4.05–4.25 (4H, m, -CO-O-C*H*$_2$-, from 1,4-butanediol), 3.30–3.40 (2H, s, -C=C-C*H*$_2$-CO-, from itaconate), 2.58–2.68 (4H, s, -OC-C*H*$_2$-, from succinate), 1.60–1.78 (4H, m, -O-CH$_2$-CH$_2$-CH$_2$-CH$_2$-O-, from 1,4-butanediol); low intensity signals due to end group-groups were observed at 3.75–3.79 (3H, s, -O-C*H*$_3$, from itaconate), 3.63–3.73 (2H, m, -C*H*$_2$-OH, from 1,4-butanediol) and 1.15–1.32 (3H, m, -OCH$_2$C*H*$_3$, from succinate). The spectra are shown in Figure 9a.

^{13}C-NMR (100 MHz, CDCl$_3$, ppm) analysis of PBS and PBSI: 172.2 (-*C*O-, from succinate), 170.6 (-*C*O-, from itaconate), 166.0 (-C=C-*C*O-O-, from itaconate), 133.8 (-*C*=C-, from itaconate), 128.4 (-C=*C*-, from itaconate), 62.5–65.0 (-CO-*C*H$_2$-, from 1,4-butanediol), 37.6 (-*C*H$_2$-, from itaconate), 29.0 (-*C*H$_2$-, from succinate), 25.2 (-*C*H$_2$-, from 1,4-butanediol); low intensity signals assigned to end-groups were determined at 62.2 (-*C*H$_2$-, from 1,4-butanediol) and 51.8 (-*C*H$_3$, from itaconate). The spectra are shown in Figure 9b.

Figure 9. (a) ^{1}H-; (b) ^{13}C-NMR spectra of PBS and PBSI.

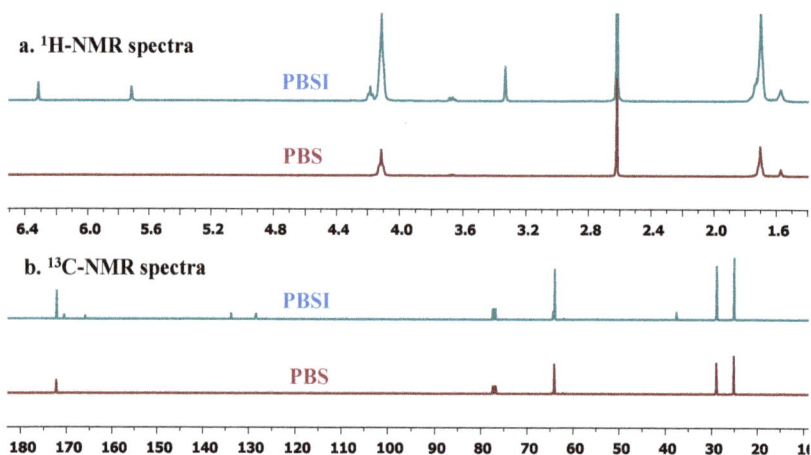

3.3. Control Reactions for Enzymatic Polymerization

Diethyl succinate, dimethyl itaconate and 1,4-butanediol were co-polymerized without CALB using the same method as we established. No polymer was obtained after precipitation.

3.4. In situ ¹H-NMR Investigation of the Oligomerization Process of Diethyl Succinate, Dimethyl Itaconate and 1,4-Butanediol in Diphenyl Ether

CALB (10 wt% in relation to the total amount of monomers) was pre-dried according to the general procedure described in Section 3.2. Diphenyl ether (150 wt% in relation to the total amount of monomers) was used in this study. Diethyl succinate, dimethyl itaconate and 1,4-butanediol were enzymatically oligomerized at 80 °C under atmospheric pressure with the protection of nitrogen for 24 h. At pre-selected time intervals, about 20 mg of the solution was withdrawn from the reaction. They were added directly into a NMR tube containing 1 g of CDCl₃ for ¹H-NMR analysis.

3.5. Instrumental Methods

¹H- and ¹³C-NMR spectra of PBS and PBSI were characterized on a Varian VXR spectrometer (400 MHz for ¹H-NMR analysis and 100 MHz for ¹³C-NMR analysis), using CDCl₃ as solvent. The chemical shifts reported were referenced to the resonances of tetramethylsilane (TMS) or the solvent.

The molecular weight (M_n and M_w) and the polydispersity index (PDI) were measured by gel permeation chromatography (GPC) using a Viscotek GPC equipped with three detectors (LS detector: Viscotek Ralls detector; VS detector: Viscotek Viscometer Model H502; RI detector: Shodex RI-71 Refractive Index detector), using a guard column (PLgel 5 μm Guard, 50 mm) and two columns (PLgel 5 μm MIXED-C, 300 mm, from Agilent Technologies) at 30 °C. Chloroform of HPLC grade was used as the eluent at a flow rate of 1.0 mL/min. The molecular weight calculations were performed based on the universal calibration. Narrow polydispersity polystyrene standards (Agilent and Polymer Laboratories), with a weight-average molecular weight from 645 to 3,001,000 g/mol, were used to generate the universal calibration curves.

The glass transition temperature and the melting temperature of the co-polyesters were measured by differential scanning calorimetry (DSC) using a TA-Instruments Q1000 DSC. A quench method was conducted for the T_g measurement. The heating rate was 20 °C/min.

Thermal gravimetric analysis (TGA) was performed on a Perkin Elmer Thermo Gravimetric Analyzer TGA7. Samples were measured at a scan rate of 10 °C/min under nitrogen environment.

3.6. Calculation of the Molar Composition of PBSI from ¹H-NMR Spectra

The molar composition of PBSI was calculated from ¹H-NMR spectra, as presented in Figure 10 and Equation (1). A_I, A_{II} and A_{III} are the integration values of Peak I, Peak II and Peak III, respectively, as displayed in Figure 10. X_S, X_I and X_B represent the mole percentage of succinate, itaconate and butylene unit in PBSI.

Figure 10. Calculation of the molar composition of PBSI from ^{1}H-NMR spectra.

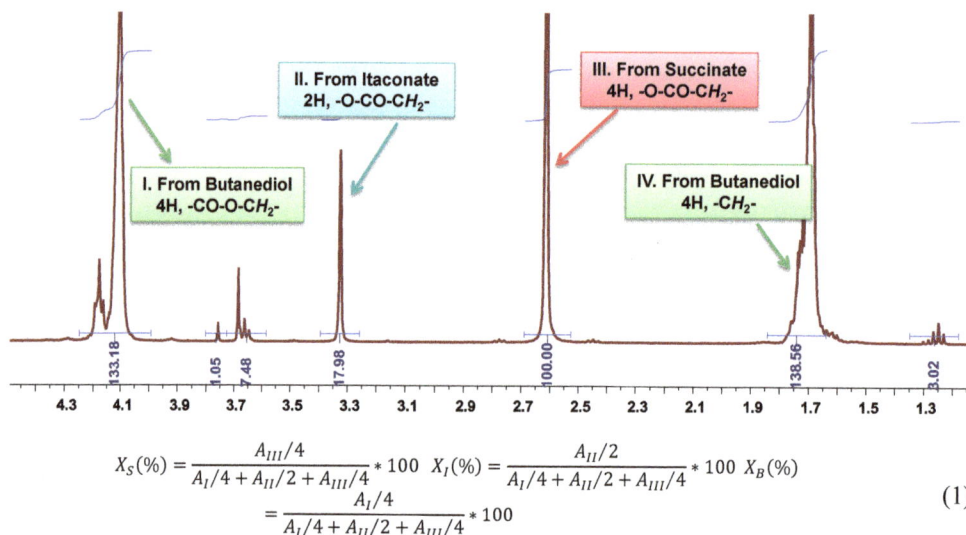

$$X_S(\%) = \frac{A_{III}/4}{A_I/4 + A_{II}/2 + A_{III}/4} * 100 \quad X_I(\%) = \frac{A_{II}/2}{A_I/4 + A_{II}/2 + A_{III}/4} * 100 \quad X_B(\%)$$
$$= \frac{A_I/4}{A_I/4 + A_{II}/2 + A_{III}/4} * 100 \tag{1}$$

3.7. Calculation of the Number Average Molecular Weight of PBSI from ^{1}H-NMR Spectra

The number average molecular weight (M_n) was characterized from ^{1}H-NMR spectra, as shown in Figure 11 and Equation (2). I_1, I_4, and I_5 are the integration values of the peaks assigned to the backbones of PBSI, which are originated from 1,4-butanediol, itaconate and succinate, respectively, as shown in Figure 11. I_2, I_3 and I_6 are the integration values of the peaks assigned to the end groups.

Figure 11. Calculation of the M_n from ^{1}H-NMR spectra.

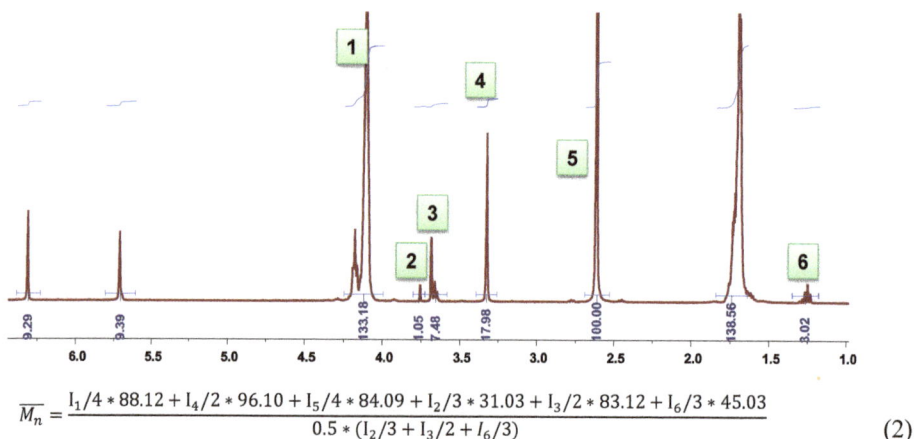

$$\overline{M_n} = \frac{I_1/4 * 88.12 + I_4/2 * 96.10 + I_5/4 * 84.09 + I_2/3 * 31.03 + I_3/2 * 83.12 + I_6/3 * 45.03}{0.5 * (I_2/3 + I_3/2 + I_6/3)} \tag{2}$$

4. Conclusions

Fully bio-based poly(butylene succinate) and poly(butylene succinate-*co*-itaconate) were synthesized by CALB-catalyzed enzymatic co-polymerizations of succinate, itaconate and 1,4-butanediol via the two-stage method. It is a totally green approach toward unsaturated aliphatic polyesters, since all the building blocks and catalysts are generated from renewable resources.

The effect of solvent on enzymatic co-polymerization was studied. We found that diphenyl ether was the most suitable solvent, resulting in the highest product M_n and mole percentage of itaconate, as well as satisfying reaction yields. We believe that such an effect could be attributed to the log *p* value of the solvent, the accessibility of CALB in the reaction medium and the solubility of the intermediate and final products in the solvent.

The study on the effect of diphenyl ether dosage indicated that the preferred solvent amount was 150 wt% (in relation to the total amount of monomers). The M_n, mole percentage of itaconate and reaction yield of PBSI increased with the increase of diphenyl ether dosage first, and then, decreased. The diffusion of the reactants, the residual byproducts amount in the reaction and the polymerization rate are the three factors contributing to such an effect.

The selected oligomerization time during the first stage had no obvious effects on CALB-catalyzed synthesis of PBSI. The *in situ* NMR investigations indicated that the oligomerization process was completed after 30 min.

We found that the vacuum during the second stage had a significant influence on enzymatic polycondensation. The best results were achieved under the highest vacuum, since the equilibrium of polycondensation was further shifted to the final products by removing the residual water and alcohols.

The enzymatic polymerizability sequence of itaconate derivatives in diphenyl ether was identified, which was dimethyl itaconate, diethyl itaconate, dibutyl itaconate and itaconic acid, from high to low. The boiling temperature of the reaction byproducts and the accessibility of itaconate to the biocatalyst are two major reasons attributed to this sequence.

With the method here, PBS and a series of PBSI were successfully synthesized with good reaction yields. The amount of itaconate in PBSI was tunable, by adjusting the feed ratio of dimethyl itaconate. The carbon-carbon double bonds of itaconate were well preserved in PBSI. The molecular weight of PBS was lower than that of the unsaturated counterparts, but the PDI was a bit higher.

The values of the product M_n, mole percentage of itaconate and reaction yield decreased significantly with the increasing of the feed ratio of dimethyl itaconate to 30%. If it was further increased to 35%, or even higher, no product was obtained.

We found that the amount of itaconate in PBSI has no obvious effects on the glass-transition temperature and the thermal stability of the co-polyesters, but has significant effects on the melting temperature. The glass transition temperature of PBS and PBSI was similar, around −35−−38 °C. The temperature of the maximal rate of decomposition remained similar, around 400 °C. However, the melting temperature of the obtained co-polyesters decreased almost linearly as the mole percentage of itaconate in PBSI increased.

52

Acknowledgments

This work forms part of the research program of the Dutch Polymer Institute (DPI), #727c Polymers Go Even Greener. The authors thank Jelena Ćirić and Joop Vorenkamp for the GPC characterizations.

Conflict of Interest

The authors declare no conflict of interest.

References

1. Gandini, A. Monomers and macromonomers from renewable resources. In *Biocatalysis in Polymer Chemistry*; Loos, K., Ed.; Wiley-VCH: Weinheim, Germany, 2010; pp. 1–34.
2. Dove, A. Polymer science tries to make it easy to be green. *Science* **2012**, *335*, 1382–1384.
3. Mathers, R.T. How well can renewable resources mimic commodity monomers and polymers? *J. Polym. Sci. Pol. Chem.* **2012**, *50*, 1–15.
4. Mülhaupt, R. Green polymer chemistry and bio-based plastics: Dreams and reality. *Macromol. Chem. Phys.* **2013**, *214*, 159–174.
5. Robert, C.; de Montigny, F.; Thomas, C.M. Tandem synthesis of alternating polyesters from renewable resources. *Nat. Commun.* **2011**, *2*, e586.
6. Werpy, T.; Petersen, G.R. *Top Value Added Chemicals from Biomass Volume I—Results of Screening for Potential Candidates from Sugars and Synthesis Gas*; US Department of Energy: Oak Ridge, TN, USA, 2004; pp. 1–67.
7. Bozell, J.J.; Petersen, G.R. Technology development for the production of biobased products from biorefinery carbohydrates—The US Department of Energy's "top 10" revisited. *Green Chem.* **2010**, *12*, 539–554.
8. Teramoto, N.; Ozeki, M.; Fujiwara, I.; Shibata, M. Crosslinking and biodegradation of poly(butylene succinate) prepolymers containing itaconic or maleic acid units in the main chain. *J. Appl. Polym. Sci.* **2005**, *95*, 1473–1480.
9. Barrett, D.G.; Merkel, T.J.; Luft, J.C.; Yousaf, M.N. One-step syntheses of photocurable polyesters based on a renewable resource. *Macromolecules* **2010**, *43*, 9660–9667.
10. Jasinska, L.; Koning, C.E. Unsaturated, biobased polyesters and their cross-linking *via* radical copolymerization. *J. Polym. Sci. Pol. Chem.* **2010**, *48*, 2885–2895.
11. Zhang, Y.-R.; Spinella, S.; Xie, W.; Cai, J.; Yang, Y.; Wang, Y.-Z.; Gross, R.A. Polymeric triglyceride analogs prepared by enzyme-catalyzed condensation polymerization. *Eur. Polym. J.* **2013**, *49*, 793–803.
12. Gross, R.A.; Ganesh, M.; Lu, W. Enzyme-catalysis breathes new life into polyester condensation polymerizations. *Trends Biotechnol.* **2010**, *28*, 435–443.
13. Mahapatro, A.; Kalra, B.; Kumar, A.; Gross, R.A. Lipase-catalyzed polycondensations: Effect of substrates and solvent on chain formation, dispersity, and end-group structure. *Biomacromolecules* **2003**, *4*, 544–551.

14. Albertsson, A.C.; Srivastava, R.K. Recent developments in enzyme-catalyzed ring-opening polymerization. *Adv. Drug Deliv. Rev.* **2008**, *60*, 1077–1093.

15. Kobayashi, S. Recent developments in lipase-catalyzed synthesis of polyesters. *Macromol. Rapid Commun.* **2009**, *30*, 237–266.

16. Uyama, H.; Kobayashi, S. Enzymatic synthesis of polyesters via polycondensation. In *Enzyme-Catalyzed Synthesis of Polymers*; Kobayashi, S., Ritter, H., Kaplan, D., Eds.; Springer-Verlag Berlin: Berlin, Germany, 2006; Volume 194, pp. 133–158.

17. Miletic, N.; Loos, K.; Gross, R.A. Enzymatic polymerization of polyester. In *Biocatalysis in Polymer Chemistry*; Loos, K., Ed.; Wiley-VCH: Weinheim, Germany, 2010; pp. 83–130.

18. Gross, R.A.; Kumar, A.; Kalra, B. Polymer synthesis by *in vitro* enzyme catalysis. *Chem. Rev.* **2001**, *101*, 2097–2124.

19. Miletic, N.; Abetz, V.; Ebert, K.; Loos, K. Immobilization of *Candida antarctica* lipase B on polystyrene nanoparticles. *Macromol. Rapid Commun.* **2010**, *31*, 71–74.

20. Matsumura, S. Enzymatic synthesis of polyesters *via* ring-opening polymerization. In *Enzyme-Catalyzed Synthesis of Polymers*; Kobayashi, S., Ritter, H., Kaplan, D., Eds.; Springer-Verlag Berlin: Berlin, Germany, 2006; Volume 194, pp. 95–132.

21. Stavila, E.; Alberda van Ekenstein, G.O.R.; Loos, K. Enzyme-catalyzed synthesis of aliphatic-aromatic oligoamides. *Biomacromolecules* **2013**, *14*, 1600–1606.

22. Miletic, N.; Fahriansyah; Nguyen, L.T.T.; Loos, K. Formation, topography and reactivity of *Candida antarctica* lipase B immobilized on silicon surface. *Biocatal. Biotransform.* **2010**, *28*, 357–369.

23. Miletic, N.; Nastasovic, A.; Loos, K. Immobilization of biocatalysts for enzymatic polymerizations: Possibilities, advantages, applications. *Bioresour. Technol.* **2012**, *115*, 126–135.

24. Stavila, E.; Arsyi, R.Z.; Petrovic, D.M.; Loos, K. Fusarium solani pisi cutinase-catalyzed synthesis of polyamides. *Eur. Polym. J.* **2013**, *49*, 834–842.

25. Stavila, E.; Loos, K. Synthesis of lactams using enzyme-catalyzed aminolysis. *Tetrahedron Lett.* **2013**, *54*, 370–372.

26. Binns, F.; Harffey, P.; Roberts, S.M.; Taylor, A. Studies of lipase-catalyzed polyesterification of an unactivated diacid/diol system. *J. Polym. Sci. Pol. Chem.* **1998**, *36*, 2069–2079.

27. Binns, F.; Harffey, P.; Roberts, S.M.; Taylor, A. Studies leading to the large scale synthesis of polyesters using enzymes. *J. Chem. Soc. Perkin Trans. 1* **1999**, 2671–2676.

28. Azim, H.; Dekhterman, A.; Jiang, Z.; Gross, R.A. *Candida antarctica* lipase B-catalyzed synthesis of poly(butylene succinate): Shorter chain building blocks also work. *Biomacromolecules* **2006**, *7*, 3093–3097.

29. Habeych, D.I.; Juhl, P.B.; Pleiss, J.; Vanegas, D.; Eggink, G.; Boeriu, C.G. Biocatalytic synthesis of polyesters from sugar-based building blocks using immobilized *Candida antarctica* lipase B. *J. Mol. Catal. B-Enzym.* **2011**, *71*, 1–9.

30. Juais, D.; Naves, A.F.; Li, C.; Gross, R.A.; Catalani, L.H. Isosorbide polyesters from enzymatic catalysis. *Macromolecules* **2010**, *43*, 10315–10319.

31. Jiang, Z. Lipase-catalyzed synthesis of aliphatic polyesters via copolymerization of lactone, dialkyl diester, and diol. *Biomacromolecules* **2008**, *9*, 3246–3251.

32. Ebata, H.; Toshima, K.; Matsumura, S. Lipase-catalyzed synthesis and properties of poly[(12-hydroxydodecanoate)-co-(12-hydroxystearate)] directed towards novel green and sustainable elastomers. *Macromol. Biosci.* **2008**, *8*, 38–45.

33. Kobayashi, T.; Matsumura, S. Enzymatic synthesis and properties of novel biodegradable and biobased thermoplastic elastomers. *Polym. Degrad. Stab.* **2011**, *96*, 2071–2079.

34. Tsujimoto, T.; Uyama, H.; Kobayashi, S. Enzymatic synthesis of cross-linkable polyesters from renewable resources. *Biomacromolecules* **2001**, *2*, 29–31.

35. Tsujimoto, T.; Uyama, H.; Kobayashi, S. Enzymatic synthesis and curing of biodegradable crosslinkable polyesters. *Macromol. Biosci.* **2002**, *2*, 329–335.

36. Uyama, H.; Kuwabara, M.; Tsujimoto, T.; Kobayashi, S. Enzymatic synthesis and curing of biodegradable epoxide-containing polyesters from renewable resources. *Biomacromolecules* **2003**, *4*, 211–215.

37. Jiang, Z.; Azim, H.; Gross, R.A.; Focarete, M.L.; Scandola, M. Lipase-catalyzed copolymerization of ω-pentadecalactone with p-dioxanone and characterization of copolymer thermal and crystalline properties. *Biomacromolecules* **2007**, *8*, 2262–2269.

38. Mazzocchetti, L.; Scandola, M.; Jiang, Z. Enzymatic synthesis and structural and thermal properties of poly(ω-pentadecalactone-co-butylene-co-succinate). *Macromolecules* **2009**, *42*, 7811–7819.

39. Liu, W.; Wang, F.; Tan, T.; Chen, B. Lipase-catalyzed synthesis and characterization of polymers by cyclodextrin as support architecture. *Carbohydr. Polym.* **2013**, *92*, 633–640.

40. Jiang, Z. Lipase-catalyzed copolymerization of dialkyl carbonate with 1,4-butanediol and omega-pentadecalactone: Synthesis of poly-(omega-pentadecalactone-co-butylene-co-carbonate). *Biomacromolecules* **2011**, *12*, 1912–1919.

41. MuralidharaRao, D.; Hussain, S.M.D.J.; Rangadu, V.P.; Subramanyam, K.; Krishna, G.S.; Swamy, A.V.N. Fermentatative production of itaconic acid by aspergillus terreus using *Jatropha* seed cake. *Afr. J. Biotechnol.* **2007**, *6*, 2140–2142.

42. Guo, B.; Chen, Y.; Lei, Y.; Zhang, L.; Zhou, W.Y.; Rabie, A.B.M.; Zhao, J. Biobased poly(propylene sebacate) as shape memory polymer with tunable switching temperature for potential biomedical applications. *Biomacromolecules* **2011**, *12*, 1312–1321.

43. Wei, T.; Lei, L.; Kang, H.; Qiao, B.; Wang, Z.; Zhang, L.; Coates, P.; Hua, K.-C.; Kulig, J. Tough bio-based elastomer nanocomposites with high performance for engineering applications. *Adv. Eng. Mater.* **2012**, *14*, 112–118.

44. Retuert, J.; Yazdanipedram, M.; Martinez, F.; Jeria, M. Soluble itaconic acid ethylene-glycol polyesters. *Bull. Chem. Soc. Jpn.* **1993**, *66*, 1707–1708.

45. Ramo, V.; Anghelescu-Hakala, A.; Nurmi, L.; Mehtio, T.; Salomaki, E.; Harkonen, M.; Harlin, A. Preparation of aqueous crosslinked dispersions of functionalized poly(d,l-lactic acid) with a thermomechanical method. *Eur. Polym. J.* **2012**, *48*, 1495–1503.

46. Sakuma, T.; Kumagai, A.; Teramoto, N.; Shibata, M. Thermal and dynamic mechanical properties of organic-inorganic hybrid composites of itaconate-containing poly(butylene succinate) and methacrylate-substituted polysilsesquioxane. *J. Appl. Polym. Sci.* **2008**, *107*, 2159–2164.

47. Brugel, W.; Demmler, K. Synthesis and properties of itaconic acid-containing polyester resins. *J. Polym. Sci. Pol. Sym.* **1969**, *22*, 1117–1137.

48. Sepulchre, M.O.; Sepulchre, M. Synthesis of unsaturated polyesters from dipotassium salts of cis-aconitic, itaconic and mesaconic acids and 1,4-dibromobutane. *Macromol. Symp.* **1997**, *122*, 291–296.

49. Rajkhowa, R.; Varma, I.K.; Albertsson, A.C.; Edlund, W. Enzyme-catalyzed copolymerization of oxiranes with dicarboxylic acid anhydrides. *J. Appl. Polym. Sci.* **2005**, *97*, 697–704.

50. Linko, Y.Y.; Wang, Z.L.; Seppala, J. Lipase-catalyzed linear aliphatic polyester synthesis in organic-solvent. *Enzyme Microb. Technol.* **1995**, *17*, 506–511.

Enantiocomplementary *Yarrowia lipolytica* Oxidoreductases: Alcohol Dehydrogenase 2 and Short Chain Dehydrogenase/Reductase

Kamila Napora-Wijata, Gernot A. Strohmeier, Manoj N. Sonavane, Manuela Avi, Karen Robins and Margit Winkler

Abstract: Enzymes of the non-conventional yeast *Yarrowia lipolytica* seem to be tailor-made for the conversion of lipophilic substrates. Herein, we cloned and overexpressed the Zn-dependent alcohol dehydrogenase ADH2 from *Yarrowia lipolytica* in *Escherichia coli*. The purified enzyme was characterized *in vitro*. The substrate scope for *Yl*ADH2 mediated oxidation and reduction was investigated spectrophotometrically and the enzyme showed a broader substrate range than its homolog from *Saccharomyces cerevisiae*. A preference for secondary compared to primary alcohols in oxidation direction was observed for *Yl*ADH2. 2-Octanone was investigated in reduction mode in detail. Remarkably, *Yl*ADH2 displays perfect (*S*)-selectivity and together with a highly (*R*)-selective short chain dehydrogenase/ reductase from *Yarrowia lipolytica* it is possible to access both enantiomers of 2-octanol in >99% ee with *Yarrowia lipolytica* oxidoreductases.

Reprinted from *Biomolecules*. Cite as: Napora-Wijata, K.; Strohmeier, G.A.; Sonavane, M.N.; Avi, M.; Robins, K.; Winkler, M. Enantiocomplementary *Yarrowia lipolytica* Oxidoreductases: Alcohol Dehydrogenase 2 and Short Chain Dehydrogenase/Reductase. *Biomolecules* **2013**, *3*, 449-460.

1. Introduction

Chiral alcohols are valuable building blocks for pharmaceuticals and agrochemicals [1] and a multitude of studies have been devoted on biocatalytic methodologies for their production. Nevertheless, there is still a high demand for new enzymes, which operate on specific substrates with high activity and selectivity. Especially, lipophilic compounds are a challenge for classical biocatalysis because substrate availability is low in the aqueous phase in which the enzymes are usually present. The non-conventional yeast *Yarrowia lipolytica* is typically found in lipid-rich media [2] and therefore its enzymes are thought to be evolved to metabolize non-polar substrates [3]. The work of Fantin *et al.* on new alcohol oxidation activities showed, for example, that *Yarrowia lipolytica* alcohol dehydrogenases (ADHs) are highly interesting candidates for biocatalysis [4]. *In vivo*, yeast ADHs are mostly responsible for ethanol formation or consumption and cofactor balance. *In vitro*, ADH1 from *Saccharomyces cerevisiae* (*Sc*ADH1; E.C: 1.1.1.1) is used for cofactor recycling with EtOH as the sacrificial substrate in order to promote NADH dependent enzyme catalyzed reduction [5]. *Sc*ADH1 is a well-studied Zn- and NAD(H) dependent enzyme [6] with known crystal structure (pdb code: 2hcy). The *Yarrowia lipolytica* genome codes for five homologous Zn-dependent ADHs. They are currently filed as putative enzymes [7]. Three of these five proteins were annotated as putative ADH1, ADH2, and ADH3, one as a protein with similarity to putative

Yarrowia lipolytica ADH3, and one as protein with similarity to mitochondrial ADH3 of *S. cerevisiae*. Of these proteins, ADH2 showed the highest similarity to *Sc*ADH1 and was therefore chosen as a target enzyme (Table 1). *Yl*ADH2 shows sequence similarity to alcohol dehydrogenases from other yeasts [8], e.g., *Pichia stipitis* ADH1 (74% identity) [9], *Candida maltosa* ADH2A [10] (73% identity), *S. cerevisiae* ADH3 (71% identity), and *Hansenula polymorpha* ADH (75% identity) [11]. Whereas *Sc*ADH3-like enzymes from different yeasts are mitochondrial enzymes [3,12], the primary sequences of *Sc*ADH1 and *Yl*ADH2have no mitochondrial targeting sequence according to the PSORTII algorithm [13]. Herein we report the heterologous expression of *Yarrowia lipolytica* ADH2, the enzyme's substrate scope and its enantioselectivity. Further, *Yl*ADH2 is compared to a *Yarrowia lipolytica* short chain dehydrogenase/ reductase (*Yl*SDR), which is enantiocomplementary and offers the possibility to synthesize the other enantiomer of 2-octanol.

Table 1. Protein similarities of *Saccharomyces cerevisiae* ADH1 and *Yarrowia lipolytica* Zn-dependent ADHs. italics: Identities (%), bold: positives (%).

	ScADH1	**YlADH1**	**YlADH2**	**YlADH3**	**YlADH**	**YlADH**
Acc. Nr.:	NP_014555	XP_503282	XP_504077	XP_500127	XP_500087	XP_503672
NP_014555	100	*68*	*68*	*69*	*66*	*54*
XP_503282	**80**	100	*94*	*98*	*81*	*57*
XP_504077	**82**	**98**	100	*94*	*79*	*56*
XP_500127	**80**	**99**	**97**	100	*82*	*58*
XP_500087	**80**	**90**	**85**	**90**	100	*53*
XP_503672	**70**	**70**	**70**	**71**	**69**	100

2. Results and Discussion

In continuation of our search for versatile oxidoreductases especially for lipophilic compounds [14], we amplified the ADH2 gene from genomic DNA of the *Yarrowia lipolytica* CLIB122 strain and cloned it into two different vector systems. In addition to the native ADH2 sequence, an *N*-terminal His-tag was introduced to facilitate enzyme purification. *Yl*ADH2 expression in the pEHisTEV vector [15]—that adds an *N*-terminal His-tag and a TEV protease cleavage site to the protein of interest—with the T7 promoter resulted in approximately identical expression level compared to untagged *Yl*ADH2 expressed from pMS470, a vector with tac promoter [16] (see Figures S1 and S2 in the supplementary information). His-tagged *Yl*ADH2 was then purified by Ni-affinity chromatography and used for *in vitro* characterization. Investigation of the cofactor specificity revealed, as expected, a strong preference of *Yl*ADH2 for NAD(H) over NADP(H) [6]. We were particularly interested in the substrate tolerance of *Yl*ADH2 and investigated the oxidation of the following substrates: EtOH, 2-propanol, 1-butanol, (2*R*,3*R*)-butanediol, cyclohexanol, 4-methyl-2-pentanol, *rac*-2-heptanol, 1-octanol, *rac*-2-octanol, (*R*)-2-octanol, (*S*)-2-octanol, 1-nonanol, *rac*-2-nonanol, 1-decanol, 1-dodecanol, 1-phenylethanol, (*R*)-2-amino-2-phenylethanol, (*S*)-2-amino-2-phenylethanol, phenylacetaldehyde, adonitol, arabitol, xylitol, sorbitol, and mannitol. Due to the lipophilicity of long chain alcohols, surfactants were used to increase their solubility under assay conditions [17].

58

Table 2. Exploration of the substrate spectrum of *Yl*ADH2.

Entry	Substrate	Relative Oxidation Activity (%)	Substrate	Relative Reduction Activity (%)
1	2-propanol	53	acetone	<5
2	1-butanol [a]	9		
3	rac-4-methyl-2-pentanol	6		
4	rac-2-heptanol [a]	64		
5	1-octanol [b]	7		
6	rac-2-octanol [a]	100 [c]	2-octanone	100 [d]
7	1-nonanol [b]	7		
8	rac-2-nonanol [a]	81	2-nonanone	106
9	1-decanol [b]	6		
10	rac-2-decanol [a]	77	2-decanone	100

[a] Tween 20 was used as solubilizer at 0.45% v/v end concentration; [b] Tween 20 was used as solubilizer at 0.75% v/v end concentration. 0.75% Tween 20 reduced the activity towards rac-2-octanol oxidation by 20% compared to 0.45%; [c] 100% corresponds to 1.1 ± 0.1 U·mg^{-1}; [d] 100% corresponds to 0.50 ± 0.06 U·mg^{-1}.

Ethanol is by far the best substrate for ADH1 from *Saccharomyces cerevisiae* [6] and *Yl*ADH2 can also oxidize EtOH, however, its specific activity is two orders of magnitude lower than that of a commercial preparation of *Sc*ADH1 (>300 U/mg as specified by the manufacturer). In this study, the above-mentioned compounds were subjected to both *Yl*ADH2 and *Sc*ADH1 oxidation. Except for EtOH (see above) and 2-propanol (197 ± 77 mU/mg), *Sc*ADH1 showed no significant activity for any substrate. *Yl*ADH2 exhibited a much broader substrate tolerance than its homolog from *Saccharomyces cerevisiae* (Table 2). Substrates which showed less than 5% of the activity towards 2-octanol oxidation are not listed in Table 2. The highest specific activity was observed for the oxidation of racemic 2-octanol (1.1 ± 0.1 U·mg^{-1}), which is a value similar to that observed for *Yarrowia lipolytica* short chain dehydrogenase/reductase *Yl*SDR (NCBI Accession Nr. XP_500963.1) [14]. Both enzymes clearly preferred secondary to primary alcohols. However, in contrast to *Yl*SDR, *Yl*ADH2 was not able to oxidize carbohydrate substrates.

The optimal reaction temperature for the oxidation of racemic-2-octanol was determined between 25 °C and 37 °C. *Yl*ADH2 showed a plateau of highest activity between 28 °C and 33 °C. The optimal pH of the reaction is strongly dependent on the reaction buffer as depicted in Figure 1. Whereas high activities were observed at pH 9.5 in carbonate and glycine buffer, the same pH was detrimental in borate buffer. A similarly negative effect of borate buffer was also observed for the *Yl*SDR enzyme.

*Yl*SDR was catalyzing the reduction of several substrates and displayed its highest activity for ribulose [14]. *Yl*ADH2, by contrast, was highly specific for medium chain lipophilic ketone substrates among those tested (see experimental section). Relative specific activities for substrate reduction are shown in Table 2 and the absolute values were approximately 0.5 U·mg^{-1}. The optimal pH of the reduction of 2-octanone appeared to be pH 6.5 (Figure 2). Interestingly, reduction reactions often proceed better at relatively low pH as compared to oxidations [18,19]. In the mechanism of a reduction reaction, a hydride is transferred from the nicotinamide donor to the substrate simultaneously to the addition of a proton. At a low pH, the amino acid residues of the protein are predominantly protonated, which facilitates the proton transfer. In oxidation direction, a proton needs to be removed from the substrate, typically from a basic amino acid residue in the active site. In this case, the deprotonated state of the protein at elevated pH seems to be beneficial.

Figure 1. pH optimum of *Yl*ADH2 catalyzed oxidation of (*S*)-2-octanol. ♦: citrate; ■: potassium phosphate; ▲: Tris-HCl; ▬: borate; X: glycine; ●: carbonate.

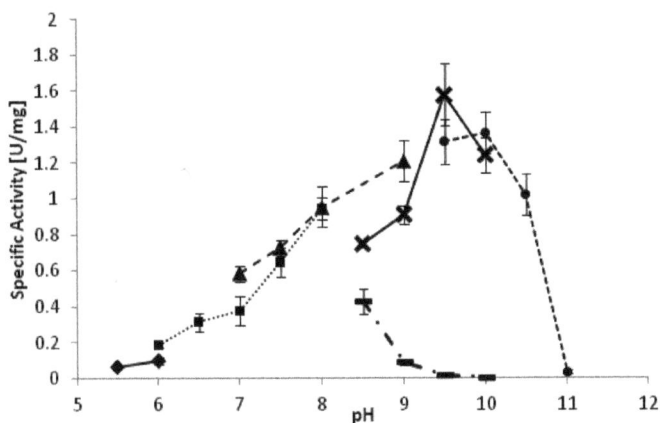

Figure 2. pH optimum of *Yl*ADH2 catalyzed reduction of 2-octanone. ♦: citrate; ■: potassium phosphate; ▲: Tris-HCl.

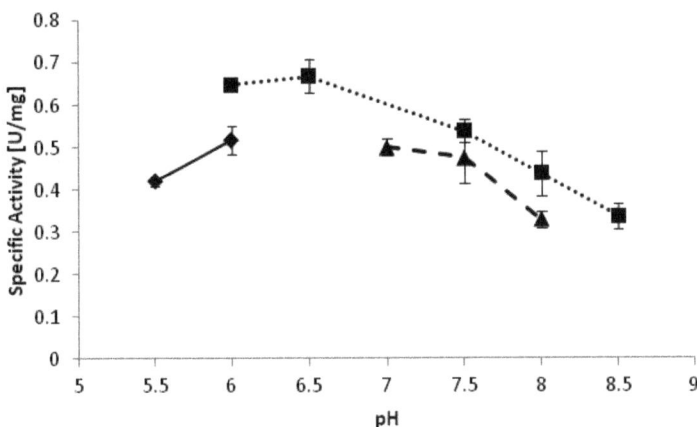

The determination of kinetic parameters for *Yl*ADH2 mediated oxidation and reduction showed that the k_{cat} value for reduction of 2-octanone is approximately half of the value of the respective oxidation (Table 3).

Table 3. Apparent kinetic parameters for *Yl*ADH2.

	Oxidation		Reduction
	(*S*)-2-octanol	NAD$^+$	2-octanone
K_m [mM]	1.42 ± 0.03	17.8 ± 1.26	5.38 ± 0.76
k_{cat} [s^{-1}]	1.05 ± 0.52	3.43 ± 0.05	0.56 ± 0.04
k_{cat}/K_m [s^{-1}·mM^{-1}]	0.74 ± 0.50	0.19 ± 0.07	0.10 ± 0.16

Alcohol dehydrogenases are often used as catalysts for enantioselective syntheses—on laboratory scale and in industrial processes [20,21]. To determine the enantiopreference of *Yl*ADH2, the single enantiomers of 2-octanol were subjected to NAD$^+$ mediated oxidation. The monitored NADH formation was significantly faster in case of (*S*)-2-octanol (1.1 U·mg^{-1}) compared to the (*R*)-enantiomer (<0.2 U·mg^{-1})—a first indication for (*S*)-selectivity of the enzyme. In order to verify this result, we investigated the reaction in reduction direction. Therefore, 2-octanone was used as the substrate and the products were analyzed by chiral gas chromatography after derivatization to the corresponding acetates. *Yl*ADH2 produced exclusively the (*S*)-enantiomer (>99% *ee*). By contrast, the (*R*)-enantiomer was obtained in >99% *ee* in case that *Yl*SDR was applied as the biocatalyst (Figure 3)

Figure 3. Time dependent formation of ♦ (*S*)-2-octanol (<99% *ee*) catalyzed by *Yl*ADH2 and ■ (*R*)-2-octanol (<99% *ee*) catalyzed by *Yl*SDR.

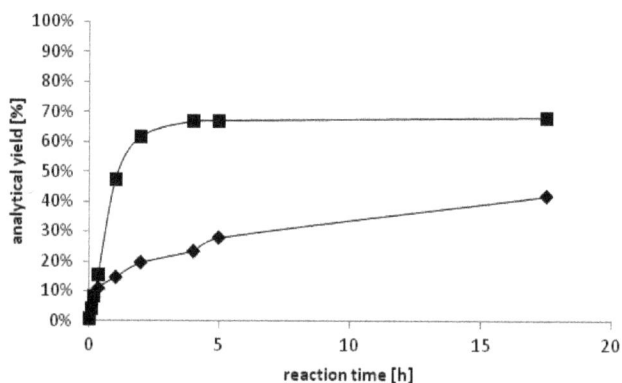

In order to improve the conversions, we applied cofactor recycling, using glucose dehydrogenase (GDH) and formate dehydrogenase (FDH) [22] in different combinations of enzyme and co-substrate concentrations. The cofactor recycling system GDH/glucose gave moderate conversions in comparison to FDH/formate. Using 0.02 U of FDH in combination with sodium formate (100 mM) at 0.5 mL scale, 70% of 2-octanone were reduced to (*S*)-2-octanol in >99% *ee* within one hour. After 2.5 h, the conversion was 83% and full conversion (>99% *ee*) was observed after a reaction time of <16 h. Enantiomerically pure lipophilic alcohols can be used as derivatizing agent for the enantioseparation of carboxylic acids [23] or e.g., for the preparation of functional materials. (*S*)-2-Octanol, for instance, was used as the chiral selector in microemulsion electrokinetic chromatography [24]. The (*R*)-enantiomer served as a precursor for chiral liquid crystals [25]. The two *Yarrowia lipolytica* oxidoreductases described herein offer the possibility to produce both enantiomers of 2-octanol in highly pure form, possibly by oxidative kinetic resolution of racemic 2-octanol, or by the reduction of prochiral 2-octanone (Scheme 1).).

Scheme 1. Routes to enantiomerically pure (S)- and (R)-2-octanol via *Yarrowia lipolytica* oxidoreductases.

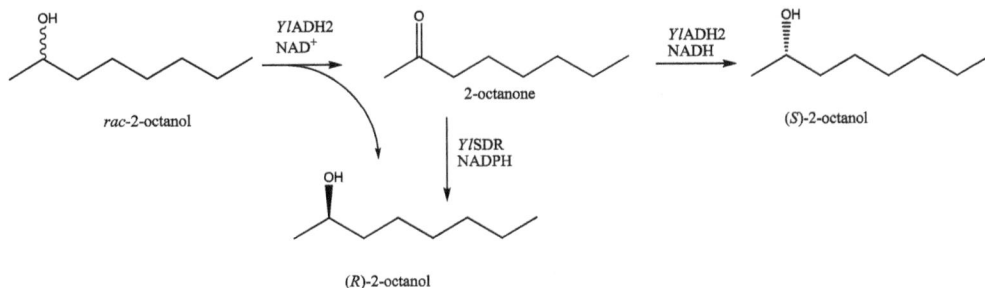

3. Experimental

3.1. General

Yarrowia lipolytica CLIB 122 (supplementary information Figure S3) was obtained from Centre International de Ressources Microbiennes (CIRM, France). *E. coli* cells were cultivated in RS 306 and Multitron shakers (Infors AG), and the cells were harvested with Avanti centrifuge J-20 (Beckman Coulter). Cell pellets were disrupted with a Branson 102C converter, power was supplied with a Branson Sonifier 250 or a French Press model and cell free extract was obtained by centrifugation in Ultracentrifuge Optima LE80K (Beckman Coulter). Enzymes were purified using a HisTrap™ FF 5 mL column on an ÄKTA Purifier 100 with Frac-950, software Unicorn 4.11, and desalted using a HiPrep™ 26/10 Desalting column on an ÄKTA Prime, software PrimeView 5.0 (GE Healthcare Life Sciences). Protein samples were analyzed with 4%–12% NuPAGE® Bis-Tris Gel (Invitrogen) and photometric measurements were carried out on Synergy Mx plate reader (BioTek) using the Gen5.11 Software. Chiral GC analyses were carried out on a Hewlett-Packard 6890 instrument. NADH and NAD$^+$ (sodium salt; 97% pure) was obtained from Roche Diagnostics. GDH was obtained from DSM Innovative Synthesis BV. 2-Nonanone and 2-decanone were purchased from Alfa Aesar and all other chemicals including alcohol dehydrogenase from *Saccharomyces cerevisiae* (lyophilized powder, ≥300 U·mg^{-1}, order number A7011) were purchased from Sigma–Aldrich/Fluka and used as received.

3.2. Isolation of Genomic DNA and Gene Cloning

Genomic DNA from *Yarrowia lipolytica* strain CLIB 122 was isolated according to the published procedure [26].

The fragment corresponding to *Yl*ADH2 was amplified from genomic DNA using Phusion® High-Fidelity DNA polymerase (Finnzymes) with the following primers: pEHisTEVmutYlADH2_f: 5'-TAC GA<u>G ATA TC</u>A TGT CTG CTC CCG TCA TCC CC-3'; pEHisTEVmutYlADH2_r:

62

5'-TAA CT<u>G CGG CCG C</u>TT ACT TGG AGG TGT-3'. The *Eco*RV and *Not*I restriction sites are underlined. The gene was cloned into the pEHisTEV vector, previously digested with *Eco*RV and *Not*I.

N-Terminally tagged and untagged *Yl*ADH2 were cloned into vector pMS470 as follows: the fragments were amplified from pEHisTEV:ADH2 using Phusion® High-Fidelity DNA polymerase (Finnzymes) and following primers: pMS470d8ADH2_f 5'-TAT CA<u>C ATA TG</u>T CTG CTC CCG TCA TC-3'; pMS470d8ADH2_r 5'-TTT CT<u>G CAT GC</u>T TAC TTG GAG GTG TC-3'; pMS470d8_HIS-TEVADH2_f 5'-ATA <u>CAT ATG</u> TCG TAC TAC CAT CAC CAT CAC C-3' and pMS470d8_HIS-TEVADH2_r 5'-ATA <u>GCA TGC</u> TTA CTT GGA GGT GTC CAG-3'; The restriction sites *Nde*I and *Sph*I are underlined. Amplification conditions were: 98 °C for 5 min, followed by 30 cycles of 98 °C for 30 s, 55 °C for 30 s, and 72 °C for 30 s, then a final incubation of 72 °C for 7 min. The PCR products were gel separated and the excised DNA was purified with the QIAquick Gel Extraction Kit. The DNA was digested with *Nde*I and *Sph*I restriction enzymes (Fermentas) in the presence of Tango buffer (Fermentas) and column purified according to QIAquick PCR purification protocol. The genes were cloned into the pMS470 vector, previously digested with *Nde*I and *Sph*I and dephosphorylated with Calf Intestine Alkaline Phosphatase (Fermentas) in the presence of FastDigest buffer (Fermentas), using T4 polymerase (Fermentas) in T4 DNA ligase buffer (Fermentas), at room temperature for 1 h.

The fragment corresponding to *Yl*SDR was amplified using Phusion® High-Fidelity DNA polymerase (Finnzymes) with the following primers: YaliSDR2470_f: 5'-AAT CA<u>C ATA TGC</u> CTG CAC CAG CAA CCT AC-3' and YaliSDR2470_r: 5'-AAT CA<u>G CAT GC</u>T CAA GGA CAA CAG TAG CC-3'. The *Nde*I and *Sph*I restriction sites are underlined. Amplification conditions were: 98 °C for 30 s, followed by 30 cycles of 98 °C for 10 s, 58 °C for 20 s, and 72 °C for 30 s, then a final incubation of 72 °C for 7 min. The PCR products were gel separated and the excised DNA was purified with the QIAquick Gel Extraction Kit (QIAGEN). The DNA was digested with *Nde*I and *Sph*I restriction enzymes (Fermentas) in the presence of Tango buffer (Fermentas) and column purified according to the QIAquick PCR purification protocol. The gene was cloned into the pK470 vector, which contained an *N*-terminal His-Tag (for the vector map, see Figure S4 supplementary information). The pK470 vector was digested with *Nde*I and *Sph*I and gel purified according the procedure described above, prior to the ligation. Ligation was carried out with T4 polymerase (Fermentas) in T4 DNA ligase buffer (Fermentas), at room temperature for 1 h.

The constructs were transformed into electrocompetent *E. coli* TOP10 F' cells (Invitrogen) and cells were plated out on LB with 50 µg/mL kanamycin (for pEHisTEV and pK470) or 100 µg/mL ampicillin (for pMS470). The plasmids were isolated with the GeneJET™ Plasmid Miniprep Kit (Fermentas) and the sequences confirmed by LGC genomics. The plasmids were then transformed into electrocompetent *E. coli* BL21 (DE3) Gold cells (Stratagen).

3.3. Expression and Purification

Expression and purification of *Yl*SDR was carried out as described previously (supplementary information Figure S5) [14]. *E. coli* BL21 (DE3) Gold harboring ADH2 plasmids were cultivated as follows: overnight cultures [50 mL LB with 50 µg/mL kanamycin (for pEHisTEV) or 100 µg/mL ampicillin (for pMS470)] were inoculated with a single colony and grown overnight at

37 °C in an orbital shaker at 110 rpm. 500 mL LB medium with the appropriate antibiotic in 2-L baffled Erlenmeyer flasks were inoculated to an OD of 0.1. These main cultures were grown at 37 °C and 110 rpm to an OD of 0.4–0.6, cooled on ice for 30 min, induced with 0.5 mM of IPTG and supplemented with 0.25 mM $ZnSO_4$ [27]. The cultures were incubated for 20 h at 16 °C and $23 \times g$. The cells were harvested by centrifugation ($2{,}831 \times g$, 4 °C, 10 min), washed with buffer, and disrupted by sonication or French press treatment in Tris/HCl buffer (40 mM; 0.3 M NaCl, pH 8.5). After centrifugation at $72{,}647 \times g$, 4 °C for 1 h, the cell free extract was either stored at −20 °C or subjected to Ni-affinity chromatography, re-buffered into potassium phosphate buffer (50 mM, 500 mM NaCl, 40 mM KCl pH 8.5), concentrated with Vivaspin 20 (Sartorius Stedim Biotech S.A), shock frozen in liquid nitrogen, and stored at −80 °C. Protein concentrations were determined using the Bradford method.

3.4. Substrate Scope

Alcohol dehydrogenase activity of recombinant *Yl*ADH2 and commercial *Sc*ADH1 were determined by following the reduction of $NAD(P)^+$ at 340 nm in UV-Star Polystyrene plates (Greiner Bio-One). Specifically, 20 µL substrate solution (various alcohols and sugars, 100 mM in 50 mM potassium phosphate, 40 mM KCl, pH 8.5) was added to 140 µL potassium phosphate (50 mM, 40 mM KCl, pH 8.5), followed by 20 µL enzyme solution (0.05–0.1 mg/mL; *Sc*ADH1 dissolved freshly in 10 mM sodium phosphate, pH 7.5; purified *Yl*ADH2 was thawed on ice and diluted appropriately). The reaction was started by addition of 20 µL NAD^+ (or $NADP^+$; 10 mM in water) and monitored at 28 °C for *Yl*ADH2 and 30 °C for *Sc*ADH1 for 10 min. The following substrates were investigated: EtOH, 2-propanol, 1-butanol, (2R,3R)-butanediol, cyclohexanol, 4-methyl-2-pentanol, *rac*-2-heptanol, 1-octanol, *rac*-2-octanol, (R)-2-octanol, (S)-2-octanol, 1-nonanol, *rac*-2-nonanol, 1-decanol, 1-dodecanol, 1-phenylethanol, (R)-2-amino-2-phenylethanol, (S)-2-amino-2-phenylethanol, phenylacetaldehyde, adonitol, arabitol, xylitol, sorbitol, and mannitol. To substrates with limited water solubility, 4.5% or 7.5% v/v of Tween 20 was added to the 100 mM substrate stock. In case of phenylacetaldehyde, the addition of 50% DMSO was necessary to ensure a homogenous reaction mixture. Each reaction was performed at least in two sets of quadruple measurements. Blanks without substrate were subtracted. Activity units are defined as the amount of enzyme producing 1 µmol of NADH per min. Specific activity was expressed as units per mg of protein.

The reduction of acetone, cyclohexanone, octanal, 2-octanone, 2-nonanone, 2-decanone, 2-dodecanone, acetophenone, phenylacetaldehyde, ribose, arabinose, xylose, glucose, mannose, lactose, and fructose was monitored at 340 nm *via* the oxidation of NADH in UV-Star Polystyrene plates (Greiner Bio-One). The conditions above were used with the following modifications: 4.5% v/v of Tween 20 was added to the 100 mM substrate stock solution of 2-ketones and 10% Triton to octanal. The reaction was carried out at pH 7.0 and 28 °C and it was started by addition of 20 µL NADH (7.5 mM in water). Activity units are defined as the amount of enzyme consuming 1 µmol of NADH per min.

3.5. Determination of pH Optima

Optimal oxidation pH was determined by following the reduction of NAD^+ as described in section "substrate scope". (S)-2-Octanol was used as the substrate. For the different pH points, the following buffers were used, each in 50 mM concentration containing 40 mM KCl: citrate (pH 5.5–6.0), potassium phosphate buffer (pH 6.0–8.0), TrisHCl (pH 7.0–9.0), borate (pH 8.5–10.0), glycine (pH 8.5–10.0), and carbonate buffer (pH 9.5–11.0). Similarly, the optimal pH for reduction was determined using 2-octanone as the substrate with above mentioned buffers.

3.6. Determination of Kinetic Parameters

The kinetic parameters for (S)-2-octanol oxidation and 2-octanone reduction as well as NAD^+ reduction were determined. (S)-2-octanol was used in concentrations from 0.5 mM to 15 mM and assayed in potassium phosphate buffer (50 mM, 40 mM KCl, pH 8.5). 2-Octanone was used in concentrations from 1 mM to 40 mM and assayed in potassium phosphate buffer (50 mM, 40 mM KCl, pH 7.0). The stock solutions contained 4.5% Tween 20 or less. Kinetic parameters for NAD^+ were determined by oxidation of (S)-2-octanol (10 mM) in potassium phosphate buffer (50 mM, 40 mM KCl, pH 8.5) with concentrations of NAD^+ from 200 µM to 50 mM. All assays were performed as described in section "substrate scope" at 28 °C. The results were evaluated based on Michaelis - Menten kinetics, using SigmaPlot™ version 11.0 for non-linear fitting.

3.7. Determination of Enantioselectivity

(**S**)-**2-octanol** was prepared under the following conditions: purified YlADH2 in potassium phosphate buffer (50 mM, containing 40 mM KCl, pH 6.5) was mixed with 2-octanone (100 mM in the same buffer with 7.5% v/v Tween 20) and NADH (100 mM in water) to give 0.16 mg/mL, 10 mM and 11 mM end concentration, respectively, in total volumes of 500 µL. The reaction proceeded at 28 °C in an Eppendorf Thermomixer at 600 rpm. For each time-point, an extra sample was sacrificed. Substrate and products were extracted into 500 µL of ethyl acetate. A triethylamine-4-(dimethylamino)-pyridine stock solution [TEA-DMAP stock solution: DMAP (8.9 mg, 73.2 µmol) dissolved in TEA (2.00 mL, 14.3 mmL)] was added to the sodium sulfate-dried ethyl acetate extract of the reaction (500 µL, contains ≤10.0 mM of 2-octanol) (TEA: 68.3 µL, 490 µmol, 98 equivalents.; DMAP: 0.31 mg, 2.5 µmol, 0.5 equivalents) and acetic anhydride (23.6 µL, 250 µmol, 50 equivalents). After keeping the mixture at 40 °C for 3 h, the reaction was quenched by adding saturated sodium chloride solution (300 µL) and subsequent vigorous shaking. Finally, the ethyl acetate layer was directly subjected to GC analysis on a Chirasil-Dex CB column (25 m × 0.32 mm; 0.25 µm film; Varian). The GC settings were as follows: injector 220 °C; 1.0 bar constant pressure H_2 flow; temperature program: initial temperature 60 °C, 85 °C/rate 1.5 °C per min, hold 3 min; The absolute configuration of 2-octanol was assigned by comparison of the elution order on chiral GC with literature known data [28] and by derivatization of commercial (R)- and (S)-2-octanol. Retention times were 8.0 min for 2-octanone, 13.9 min for (S)-octan-2-yl acetate and 17.2 min for (R)-octan-2-yl acetate.

For cofactor recycling, the same conditions as describe above were used, with the exception that also 0.03 U of FDH and 100 mM of sodium formate were added to the reaction and the content of NADH cofactor was reduced to 1 mM.

(**R**)-**2-octanol** was prepared under the following conditions: purified *Yl*SDR in citrate buffer (50 mM, pH 5.0) was mixed with 2-octanone (100 mM in the same buffer with 3% v/v Tween 20) and NADPH (100 mM in water) to give 0.11 mg/mL, 10 mM and 11 mM end concentration, respectively, in total volumes of 500 μL. The reaction proceeded at 28 °C in an Eppendorf Thermomixer at 600 rpm. Workup and analysis were carried out as described for (*S*)-2-octanol.

4. Conclusions

In conclusion, we have shown that *Yarrowia lipolytica* harbors versatile oxidoreductases that catalyze selective oxidation and reduction reactions. From the two enzymes described herein, secondary alcohols are the preferred substrates in the oxidation direction compared to primary alcohols and aldehydes. Medium chain length ketones with the carbonyl function at position C-2 are reduced to the corresponding secondary alcohols in enantio-complementary form: whereas *Yl*ADH2 produced the (*S*)-enantiomer in >99% *ee*, the (*R*)-enantiomer was obtained with *Yl*SDR.

Acknowledgments

We are grateful to Regina Kratzer for providing the FDH expressing strain as published in [22]. Sarah S. Schindlbacher, Natalia Pankiewicz, Dorota K. Pomorska, Gerlinde Offenmüller and Thorsten Bachler are kindly acknowledged for technical support. This work has been supported by the Austrian BMWFJ, BMVIT, SFG, Standortagentur Tirol, and ZIT through the Austrian FFG-COMET-Funding Program.

Conflict of Interest

The authors declare no conflict of interest.

References

1. DeWildeman, S.M.A.; Sonke, T.; Schoemaker, H.E.; May, O. Biocatalytic reductions: From lab curiosity to first choice. *Acc. Chem. Res.* **2007**, *40*, 1260–1266.
2. Barth, G.; Gaillardin, C. Yarrowia lipolytica. In *Nonconventional Yeasts in Biotechnology*; Wolf, K., Ed.; Springer-Verlag: Berlin/Heidelberg, Germany; New York, NY, USA, 1996; pp. 313–388.
3. Fickers, P.; Benetti, P.-H.; Waché, Y.; Marty, A.; Mauersberger, S.; Smit, M.S.; Nicaud, J.-M. Hydrophobic substrate utilisation by the yeast *Yarrowia lipolytica*, and its potential applications. *FEMS Yeast Res.* **2005**, *5*, 527–543.
4. Fantin, G.; Fogagnolo, M.; Medici, A.; Pedrini, P.; Fontana, S. Kinetic resolution of racemic secondary alcohols via oxidation with *Yarrowia lipolytica* strains. *Tetrahedron-Asymmetry* **2000**, *11*, 2367–2373.

5. Kroutil, W.; Mang, H.; Edegger, K.; Faber, K. Biocatalytic oxidation of primary and secondary alcohols. *Adv. Synth. Catal.* **2004**, *346*, 125–142.

6. Leskovac, V.; Trivic, S.; Pericin, D. The three zinc-containing alcohol dehydrogenases from baker's yeast. *FEMS Yeast Res.* **2002**, *2*, 481–494.

7. Dujon, B.; Sherman, D.; Fischer, G.; Durrens, P.; Casaregola, S.; Lafontaine, I.; de Montigny, J.; Marck, C.; Neuveglise, C.; Talla, E.; *et al.* Genome evolution in yeasts. *Nature* **2004**, *430*, 35–44.

8. Reid, M.F.; Fewson, C.A. Molecular characterization of microbial alcohol dehydrogenases. *Crit. Rev. Microbiol.* **1994**, *20*, 13–56.

9. Passoth, V.; Schäfer, B.; Liebel, B.; Weierstall, T.; Klinner, U. Yeast sequencing reports–molecular cloning of alcohol dehydrogenase genes of the yeast *Pichia stipitis* and identification of the fermentative ADH. *Yeast* **1998**, *14*, 1311–1325.

10. Lin, Y.; He, P.; Wang, Q.; Lu, D.; Li, Z.; Wu, C.; Jiang, N. The alcohol dehydrogenase system in the xylose-fermenting yeast *Candida maltosa*. *PLoS One* **2010**, *5*, e11752.

11. Suwannarangsee, S.; Oh, D.-B.; Seo, J.-W.; Kim, C.H.; Rhee, S.K.; Kang, H.A.; Chulalaksananukul, W.; Kwon, O. Characterization of alcohol dehydrogenase 1 of the thermotolerant methylotrophic yeast *Hansenula polymorpha*. *Appl. Microbiol. Biotechnol.* **2010**, *88*, 497–507.

12. Yurimoto, H.; Lee, B.; Yasuda, F.; Sakai, Y.; Kato, N. Alcohol dehydrogenases that catalyse methyl formate synthesis participate in formaldehyde detoxification in the methylotrophic yeast *Candida boidinii*. *Yeast* **2004**, *21*, 341–350.

13. PSORT II Prediction. Available online: http://psort.hgc.jp/form2.html (accessed on 12 September 2012).

14. Napora, K.; Wrodnigg, T.M.; Kosmus, P.; Thonhofer, M.; Robins, K.; Winkler, M. *Yarrowia lipolytica* dehydrogenase/reductase: An enzyme tolerant for lipophilic compounds and carbohydrate substrates. *Bioorg. Med. Chem. Lett.* **2013**, *23*, 3393–3395.

15. Huanting, L.; Naismith, J.H. A simple and efficient expression and purification system using two newly constructed vectors. *Protein Expr. Purif.* **2009**, *63*, 102–111.

16. Balzer, D.; Ziegelin, G.; Pansegrau, W.; Kruft, V.; Lanka, E. Kor B protein of promiscuous plasmid RP4 recognizes inverted sequence repetitions in regions essential for conjugative plasmid transfer. *Nucleic Acid Res.* **1992**, *20*, 1851–1858.

17. Saerens, K.; van Bogaert, I.; Soetaert, W.; Vandamme, E. Production of glucolipids and specialty fatty acids from sophorolipids by *Penicillium decumbens* naringinase: Optimization and kinetics. *Biotechnol. J.* **2009**, *4*, 517–524.

18. Kosjek, B.; Stampfer, W.; Pogorevc, M.; Goessler, W.; Faber, K.; Kroutil, W. Purification and characterization of a chemotolerant alcohol dehydrogenase applicable to coupled redox reactions. *Biotechnol. Bioeng.* **2004**, *86*, 55–62.

19. Pennacchio, A.; Sannino, V.; Sorrentino, G.; Rossi, M.; Raia, C.A.; Esposito, L. Biochemical and structural characterization of recombinant short-chain NAD(H)-dependent dehydrogenase/reductase from *Sulfolobus acidocaldarius* highly enantioselective on diaryl diketone benzyl. *Appl. Microbiol. Biotechnol.* **2013**, *97*, 3949–3964.

20. DeWildeman, S.; Sereinig, N. Enzymatic Reduction of Carbonyl Groups. In *Science of Synthesis, Stereoselective Synthesis*; de Vries, J.G., Molander, G.A., Evans, P.A., Eds.; Georg Thieme-Verlag: Stuttgart, Germany, 2011; pp. 113–208.

21. Hollmann, F.; Arends, I.W.C.E.; Buehler, K.; Schallmey, A.; Buehler, B. Enzyme-mediated oxidations for the chemist. *Green Chem.* **2011**, *13*, 226–265.

22. Mädje, K.; Schmölzer, K.; Nidetzky, B.; Kratzer, R. Host cell and expression engineering for development of an *E. coli* ketoreductase catalyst: Enhancement of formate dehydrogenase activity for regeneration of NADH. *Microb. Cell Fact.* **2012**, *11*, 1–7.

23. Anelli, P.L.; Tomba, C.; Uggeri, F. Optical resolution of 2-chloro-3-phenylmethoxypropanoic acid after derivatization with (*S*)-2-octanol by high-performance liquid chromatography. *J. Chromatogr.* **1992**, *589*, 346–348.

24. Threeprom, J. (*S*)-(+)-2-Octanol as a chiral oil core for the microemulsion electrokinetic chromatographic separation of chiral basic drugs. *Anal. Sci.* **2007**, *23*, 1071–1075.

25. Parra, M.; Vergara, J.; Hildalgo, P.; Barbera, J.; Sierra, T. (*S*)-Isoleucine and (*R*)-2-octanol as chiral precursors of new chiral liquid crystalline thiadiazoles: Synthesis, mesomorphic and ferroelectric properties. *Liquid Cryst.* **2006**, *33*, 739–745.

26. Hoffman, C.S.; Winston, F. A ten-minute DNA preparation from yeast efficiently releases autonomous plasmids for transformation of *Escherichia coli*. *Gene* **1987**, *57*, 267–272.

27. Brouns, S.J.; Turnbull, A.P.; Willemen, H.L.; Akerboom, J.; van der Oost, J. Crystal structure and biochemical properties of the D-arabinose dehydrogenase from *Sulfolobus solfataricus*. *J. Mol. Biol.* **2007**, *371*, 1249–1260.

28. Silva, C.R.; Souza, J.C.; Araújo, L.S.; Kagohara, E.; Garcia, T.P.; Pelizzari, V.H.; Andrade, L.H. Exploiting the enzymatic machinery of *Arthrobacter atrocyaneus* for oxidative kinetic resolution of secondary alcohols. *J. Mol. Catal. B: Enzym.* **2012**, *83*, 23–28.

Lipases Immobilization for Effective Synthesis of Biodiesel Starting from Coffee Waste Oils

Valerio Ferrario, Harumi Veny, Elisabetta De Angelis, Luciano Navarini, Cynthia Ebert and Lucia Gardossi

Abstract: Immobilized lipases were applied to the enzymatic conversion of oils from spent coffee ground into biodiesel. Two lipases were selected for the study because of their conformational behavior analysed by Molecular Dynamics (MD) simulations taking into account that immobilization conditions affect conformational behavior of the lipases and ultimately, their efficiency upon immobilization. The enzymatic synthesis of biodiesel was initially carried out on a model substrate (triolein) in order to select the most promising immobilized biocatalysts. The results indicate that oils can be converted quantitatively within hours. The role of the nature of the immobilization support emerged as a key factor affecting reaction rate, most probably because of partition and mass transfer barriers occurring with hydrophilic solid supports. Finally, oil from spent coffee ground was transformed into biodiesel with yields ranging from 55% to 72%. The synthesis is of particular interest in the perspective of developing sustainable processes for the production of bio-fuels from food wastes and renewable materials. The enzymatic synthesis of biodiesel is carried out under mild conditions, with stoichiometric amounts of substrates (oil and methanol) and the removal of free fatty acids is not required.

Reprinted from *Biomolecules*. Cite as: Ferrario, V.; Veny, H.; De Angelis, E.; Navarini, L.; Ebert, C.; Gardossi, L. Lipases Immobilization for Effective Synthesis of Biodiesel Starting from Coffee Waste Oils. *Biomolecules* **2013**, *3*, 514-534.

1. Introduction

Next generation biofuels is about utilization of non-food based feedstock and more sustainable process technology. The biodiesel industrial production worldwide is predominantly by chemical transesterification from food based feedstock. This is because with chemical transesterification the highest yield can be achieved in a relatively short reaction time. However, the current major cost of biodiesel production is from the feedstock [1]. Therefore, various non food feedstocks, such as waste oil and non edible oil, have been considered and studied in view of their potential use as raw materials [2–6].

In most cases the chemical process is performed by an alkaline catalyst, so that acid impurities and especially free fatty acids (FFA) contained in feedstock must be removed before transesterification to avoid the formation of saponification products. For instance, a basic solution is mixed with the extracted oil so that additional pre-treatments steps are introduced in the productive cycle [7]. In this regard, lipase-catalyzed transesterification of non food feedstock is becoming more attractive for the biodiesel industry, not only because it is sustainable and environmental friendly, but also because the free fatty acids can be esterified by lipases. Recently, attention has been given to oil extracted from coffee waste and examples of chemical conversion of oil from spent coffee ground into biodiesel have been reported [8,9]. The coffee grounds are mainly composed of proteins, carbohydrates, and lipids. It must be underlined that coffee is one of the largest agricultural products and, according to the U.S. Department of Agriculture, the world's coffee production is 16.34 billion pounds per year [8].

The spent coffee grounds contain, on an average, 15% (w/w) oil, which can be extracted by solvents such as trichloroethylene [10], *n*-hexane, ether and dichloromethane [10,11] with yields ranging from 6%–28% (w/w) [9,10]. This is quite significant as compared to other major biodiesel feedstock such as rapeseed oil (37%–50%), palm oil (20%), and soybean oil (20%) [12]. Furthermore, the biodiesel from coffee possesses better stability than biodiesel from other sources due to its high antioxidant content, which hinders the rancimat process [13,14].

The work of Kondamundi reports the extraction of 15% (w/w) of oil from spent ground, which was dried prior to extraction in order to reduce the moisture content. A small amount of FFA, monoglycerides (MG), and diglycerides (DG) was also observed in the oil but a conversion in biodiesel of 100% was obtained by chemical transesterification. The oil and biodiesel formed in that process were found to be stable over one month without any observable physical changes and analysis demonstrated that biodiesel obtained from spent coffee grounds is a strong candidate as an alternative to diesel [8].

One additional issue in the development of an economically sustainable production of biodiesel by enzymatic transesterification is represented by the cost of the biocatalyst. The economic impact of biocatalysts can be reduced by immobilizing the lipases on solid supports and then recycling them. Therefore, it is important to select immobilized lipases that not only express high activity but also allow for repeated use thanks to improved stability.

Lipases are one of the classes of enzymes most largely employed in industry also because of their potential to work in non-aqueous environments [15] and they are applied at industrial scale for the transesterification of fats and oils in the food sector [16]. However, to the best of our knowledge, there is still a lack of immobilized lipases commercially available and suitable for application in biodiesel synthesis [17].

Indeed, in most cases, the lipase catalyzed synthesis of biodiesel has been studied by employing biocatalysts originally developed for interesterification of food oils [7]. However, the latter process implies the application of lipases in highly hydrophobic environments whereas biodiesel synthesis involves the use of relatively high percentages of hydrophilic short chain alcohols that have inactivating effects on enzymes [18,19]. Moreover, as the reaction proceeds, glycerol is produced. Consequently, the biocatalyst will behave quite differently in the two processes. Phenomena, such as partition of hydrophilic components, will deserve explicit attention and investigation when planning a methanolysis process.

By analyzing the immobilized lipases available on the market, Lipozyme TL IM (lipase from *Thermomyces lanuginosa*) results probably the most widely applied at industrial scale in triglyceride transformations in the food sector. It is immobilized by spraying the liquid lipase concentrate onto silica particles together with food grade granulation additives. After subsequent drying in fluid beds, the granules are ready for use in interesterification of triglycerides. However, Lipozyme TL IM will disintegrate when dispersed into water or hydrophilic media [20].

In the present work, the enzymatic synthesis of biodiesel was approached by studying immobilized biocatalysts specifically developed for this application. A particular attention was devoted to the nature of the immobilization carrier and the prevention of aggregation and methanol aspecific adsorption, phenomena that might cause enzyme inactivation. Finally, the selected biocatalysts were applied in the transesterification of oil extracted from spent coffee ground. Factors affecting the efficiency of lipase immobilization were also analyzed.

2. Results and Discussion

2.1. Selection of Lipases and Immobilization Supports

The present work follows our previous detailed investigation of structural and conformational properties of a series of lipases [21]. Lipases have been evolved for transforming insoluble hydrophobic substrates so that their surface present unusual features that make these proteins adapt for approaching lipophilic surfaces. Accommodation and transformation of bulky triglycerides is strictly related to the accessibility of the active site. The latter, as also the surrounding superficial area, is hydrophobic. A flexible protein domain, called lid, shields the opening of the active site when the protein is exposed to a hydrophilic environment, thus occluding the substrate access. Therefore, in principle, the immobilized lipase should maintain an open active conformation throughout the alcoholysis process despite the presence of polar hydrophilic components, such as the alcohol and the glycerol, in the reaction mixture.

The present study focuses attention on two lipases that demonstrated different conformational behavior when exposed to a hydrophilic environment, namely lipase B from *Candida antarctica* (CaLB) and *Burkholderia* (*Pseudomonas*) *cepacia* (PcL) (Figure 1). P revious MD simulations indicated that, upon exposure to water, the accessibility of the active site of these lipases is affected only at a minor extent when exposed to polar (e.g., aqueous) media [21].

CaLB is characterized by a small lid [22] and we have previously demonstrated that after 10 ns of MD simulations in explicit water the small lid domain undergoes only some modest conformational changes. Moreover, because of the small size of the lid, there is no closing of the active site. Indeed, the final conformation presents no significant difference in the hydrophobic surface exposed to the bulky aqueous medium [21].

Regarding PcL, MD simulations demonstrated that a β-hairpin domain contributes to the stabilization of a "putative" second lid of PcL in its open conformation by forming two hydrogen bonds between Asn257-Thr224 and between Gln262-Gln215. Only the first one is lost during 20 ns MD in water, so that the upper part of the hairpin moves away from the α-helix but this second putative lid does not change its position considerably and does not occlude the active site [21].

Here, we show (Figure 2) the starting open conformation and the result after 20 ns MD simulations. No significant variation of the superficial domains occurs when the protein is embedded in water and, most importantly, the conformation achieved leads to a partial coverage of the active site. This can be deduced from the mapping of the hydrophobic/hydrophilic areas performed by GRID analysis [23], which reveals how a considerable part of the hydrophobic active site remains exposed to the solvent (Figure 2b).

Figure 1. Tridimensional models of CaLB (**a**) (PDB code 1TCA) and PcL (**b**) (PDB code 1YS1). The structures are colored according to their secondary structures; lids are highlighted in red. PcL (**b**) has the second "putative" lid highlighted in green and the Ca^{2+} ion represented as orange sphere.

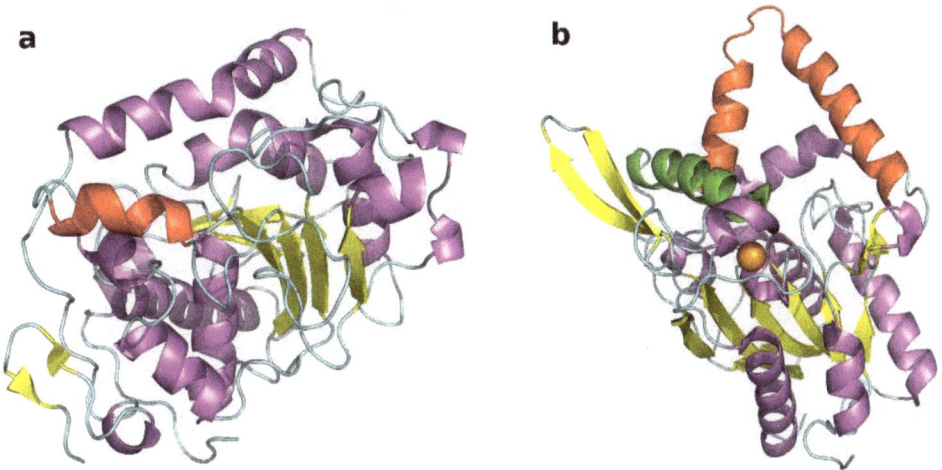

Figure 2. GRID analysis of hydrophobic (yellow) and hydrophilic (blue) surface of PcL. On the left: open conformation corresponding to the crystal structure obtained in the presence of an inhibitor (PDB code 1YS1). On the right: partially closed conformation computed after 20 ns MD simulation in explicit water.

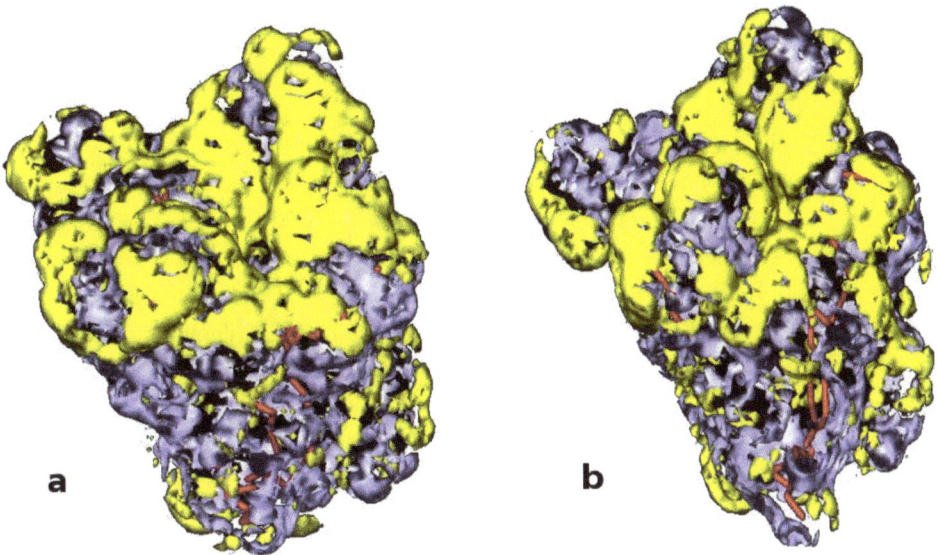

From the point of view of substrate specificity, lipase B from *Candida antarctica* (CaLB) shows a preference towards short and medium size fatty acids, although it has been investigated extensively also in biodiesel applications [24,25]. It is recognized that the active site of CaLB is situated in the core of the protein, the binding site has a funnel-like shape and highly hydrophobic amino acid residues envelop the cavity inner walls. Consequently, CaLB has, compared to other lipases, a very limited available space in the active site pocket that explains its substrate specificity [26].

Lipase from *Burkholderia cepacia* (PcL), instead, displays a marked specificity for long chain fatty acids and therefore, it appears to be a promising lipase for applications in biodiesel synthesis, as also reported in the literature [27].

In the present investigation, the selection and study of immobilized lipases suitable for biodiesel synthesis was guided by several considerations. Firstly, it must be taken into account that the enzymatic synthesis of biodiesel, unlike oil interesterification, involves the use of relatively high percentages of hydrophilic short chain alcohols that have inactivating effects on enzymes [19]. Moreover, as the reaction proceeds, glycerol is produced. Therefore, the immobilization of lipases for biodiesel synthesis should aim at preventing any detrimental interaction between the biocatalysts and these hydrophilic components, such as aspecific adsorption that might accentuate enzyme inactivation. Moreover, hydrophilic particles generally aggregate in hydrophobic media. On that basis, hydrophobic supports should be preferred.

However, it must be underlined that lipases recognize and accept very hydrophobic substrates that interact with the lipophilic area corresponding to the opening of the active site. As a continuation of our previous work, we have simulated the behavior of PcL at a water-octane interface (Figure 3) by carrying out a molecular dynamic (MD) simulation using a *coarse grained force field* (MARTINI) [28]. At the beginning of the MD simulation the opening of the active site (yellow dots) is oriented towards the aqueous phase; at the end, the lipase orients the opening of the active site towards the hydrophobic phase. This simulation suggests that the hydrophobic region of the enzyme will be also responsible for the establishment of hydrophobic interactions with hydrophobic supports. Indeed, this feature enables the exploitation of polymeric resins for achieving lipase purification and immobilization in one single step starting from crude enzymatic solutions, where lipases represent the only hydrophobic component [29]. Therefore, such interactions would promote an unfavorable orientation of the enzyme and scarce substrate accessibility.

On that basis, it seems difficult to define an ideal support for lipase immobilization *a priori*.

In order to elucidate the effect of the hydrophilic/hydrophobic nature of the carriers, the present study evaluated three different biocatalysts immobilized on highly and medium hydrophobic organic resins specifically developed by Sprin S.p.A. (Trieste, Italy) for biodiesel synthesis (Table 1). Then, the biocatalysts were compared with two preparations immobilized on hydrophilic siliceous carriers, namely diatomaceous earth (Celite). Table 1 reports the characterization of all the biocatalysts using standard assays.

A commercial formulation of PcL, Lipase PS-IM, was initially considered. It is commercialized by Amano and it consists in lipase PcL adsorbed on diatomaceous earth powder. However, despite the high hydrolytic activity expressed by the enzyme, the preparation was unsuitable for the methanolysis because the hydrophilic powder formed aggregates upon addition of the methanol to the oil.

Figure 3. Molecular dynamic (MD) simulation of PcL embedded in an explicit bi-phasic system octane-water. The hydrophobic side of the enzyme, corresponding to the opening of the active site, is highlighted in yellow beads. The octane phase is in grey points in the figure. At the starting point of the simulation (**a**) the water-octane interface is not completely defined; during the simulation the interface was formed (**b**) and the enzyme is oriented with its active site towards the octane part.

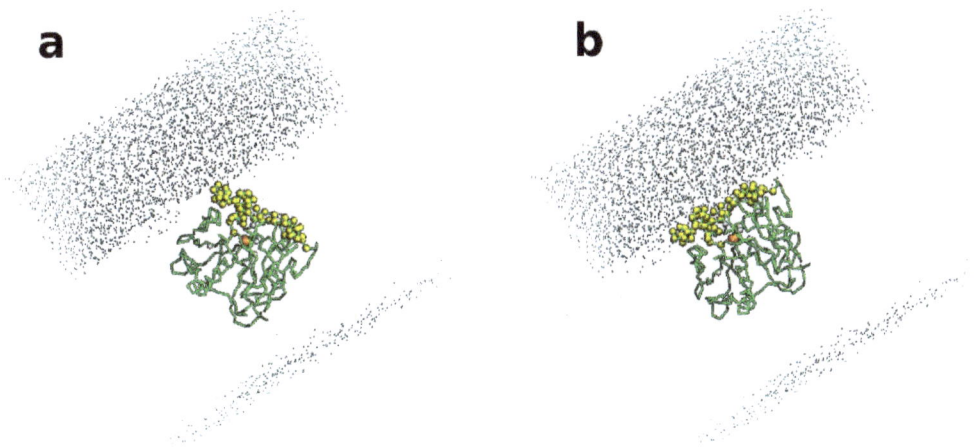

Table 1. Activity of immobilized lipases tested in the study. CaL = lipase B from *Candida antarctica*. PcL = lipase from *Pseudomonas cepacia*.

Immobilized Formulation	Carrier	Hydrophylicity	Particle Size	Residual Water [a] (%)	Synthetic Activity (U/g dry)	Hydrolitic Activity [d] (U/g dry)
PcL-S	Styrenic Porous	---	Beads, 300–500 μm	<5	159 [b]	463
PcL PS-IM	Siliceous Non porous	++	Powder <20 μm	<5	820 [b]	15,400
CaL-S	Styrenic Porous	--	Beads, 300–500 μm	<5	3450 [c]	978
CaL-M	Methacrylic Porous	-	Beads, 300–500 μm	<5	3020 [c]	490
CaLB on Celite® R-640	Siliceous Porous	+++	Rods 5 × 3 mm	15	2050 [c]	274

[a] The residual water content in the final immobilized preparation was determined on aluminum plates. A known amount of biocatalyst is dried at 110 °C for 6 h. Solvent content is defined as the % of weight loss after drying. [b] Synthetic activity: transesterification of vinyl acetate with 1-phenyl-1-ethanol. [c] Synthetic activity: esterification of lauric acid with 1-propanol. [d] Hydrolysis of tributyrin.

In light of the aggregation observed using the fine Celite particles, the immobilization of CaLB on hydrophilic carrier was carried out by selecting a commercial porous product, Celite® R-640 (Fluka), which consists in calcined Celite extruded in the form of big porous rods (5 mm high with a diameter of 3 mm). Porosity confers to the immobilization matrix a remarkable ability of adsorbing more than 100% of water (w/w) as well as a cumulative pore volume of 0.8 cm^3/g [30]. Immobilization was carried out by following a protocol previously developed in our lab for application of biocatalysts in low water media [31].

CaL-S and PcL-S are lipases adsorbed on highly hydrophobic styrenic resin whereas CaL-M corresponds to CaLB covalently immobilized on a methacrylic polymer [32]. It appears clear that there is no linear correlation between hydrolytic and synthetic activity. It must be also underlined that no direct comparison is possible between the hydrolytic activity of CaL-S and CaL-M since all enzymes immobilized through physical adsorption undergo partial leaching when suspended in aqueous media and this interfere with kinetic evaluation.

Moreover, the different substrate specificity of CaLB and PcL makes impracticable any direct comparison between the two enzymes.

2.2. Methanolysis of Triolein and Effect of Methanol Concentration

Methanolysis was conducted at 30 °C by using PcL-S (10% w/w of triolein) and by adding three equivalents of methanol obtaining 13% of conversion after 6 h and only 35% after 26 h. The data confirm the severe inactivating effect of methanol. Therefore, in the following experiments, multistep additions of methanol were used, by adding one equivalent molar of methanol at 0, 100 and 200 min. Proton NMR of the crude mixture (see Electronic Supplementary Information, Figure S1) showed the disappearance of the triglyceride peak already after 6 h of reaction. However, upon recycling, the biocatalyst displayed less than 40% of the initial activity. The recycles were carried out by introducing fresh triolein in each cycle and by determining the residual methyl oleate content prior to addition of methanol. Therefore, the PcL-S preparation, although very active, appeared unsuitable for multiple applications in biodiesel synthesis.

This unexpected behavior might be ascribable to different factors deserving specific investigations, which, however, are out of the scope of the present work. Since PcL displayed such poor efficiency when immobilised on the same support used for CaLB, the cause might reside either in the inherent properties of the protein or in the composition of the crude enzymatic formulation used for the immobilization. PcL is commercialized as a powder containing roughly 1% of protein diluted with cyclodextrins. The effect of this large amount of additives on the final immobilized formulation deserves further attention, although, it must be underlined that purification steps would cause an unacceptable increase of the cost of the biocatalyst.

One further point of attention is represented by the presence of a calcium ion in the structure of PcL (Figure 1b), which strongly affects the protein stability and this might be lost upon recycling [33].

Finally, a specific effect of some micro-components of triglyceride mixture on PcL stability cannot be excluded. Actually, several compounds generated by atmospheric oxidation of triglycerides, such as hydroperoxides and secondary products, may cause significant lipase inactivation in low water medium. Activity decay is usually time-dependent and shows a non-linear dependence on inactivating compound concentration [34].

When methanolysis was catalyzed by CaLB immobilized on Celite® R-640 (10% w/w of triolein) conversions lower than 5% were observed after 48 h. By adding 2.5% w/w of enzyme at the end of the reaction, there was no improvement in the conversion. It must be underlined that the biocatalyst was able to catalyze tributirin hydrolysis and propil laurate synthesis as shown in Table 1. The data indicate that the stop of reaction is not due to inactivation of enzyme but rather to some other factor connected to the reaction system. Most probably, the hydrophilic and hydrated pores (15% water by weight) of Celite® R-640 do not favor the partition of the oil towards the lipase.

Finally, the two preparations CaL-S and CaL-M immobilized on polymeric organic resins were monitored at different methanol to triolein molar ratios. Figure 4 reports the percentage of activity of the two CaLB formulations, defined as percentage of methyl ester yield evaluated after 25 h of reaction (theoretical maximum conversion in methyl ester is 33%, 66% and 100% for methanol to triolein molar ratio of 1:1, 2:1 and 3:1, respectively). Results indicate that the lipase activity of both CaL-S and CaL-M decreased with the increase of methanol concentration. By using a molar ratio of 3:1 the enzyme inactivation is so fast and severe that the reaction stops after 29% and 5% of conversion, respectively. CaL-S appears more resistant to the inactivating effect of methanol, since a conversion of 54% is achieved at a molar ratio of 2:1.

Figure 4. Effect of methanol concentration on CaL-S (star) and CaL-M (square) expressed as the conversion in methyl ester achieved after 25 h. The transesterification of triolein was carried out at 30 °C with molar ratios of 1:1, 2:1 and 3:1. Therefore, theoretical maximum conversions achievable were 33%, 66% and 100%, respectively.

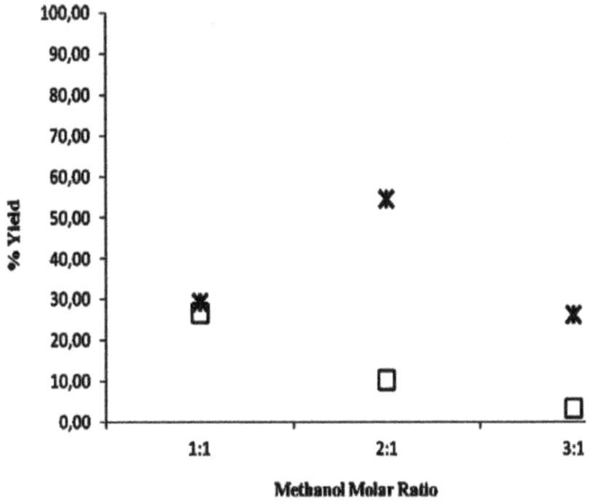

The different behavior of the two preparations is visible also from the kinetic profile of the reactions carried out at 1:1 molar ratio of triolein and methanol and 10% of biocatalyst (w/w % of triolein) (Figure 5). Apparently, the CaL-M preparation is less efficient even at such low concentration of methanol. In fact, as expected, initial rates are similar since comparable enzymatic units were employed. However the reaction profile of CaL-M indicates that the reaction slows down and, surprisingly, a lower final conversion is achieved, although the thermodynamic equilibrium of the reaction does not depend on the biocatalyst by definition. No further increase of the yield could be achieved upon addition of fresh enzyme and this would suggest that the poorer performance of CaL-M is not due to enzyme inactivation.

76

Figure 5. Reaction profiles (24 h) of transesterification of triolein using a 1:1 molar ratio of oil and methanol (30 °C). CaL-S (star) and CaL-M (square). The maximum theoretical yield is 33%.

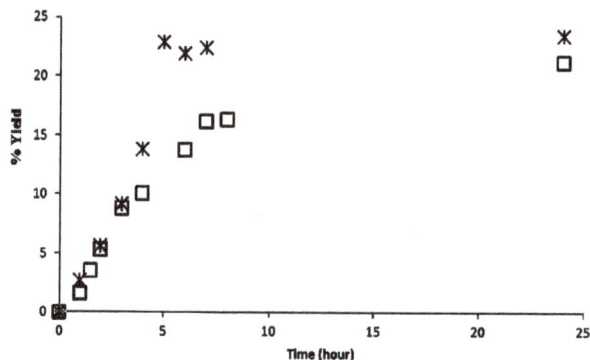

CaL-S and CaL-M show a good dispersion of the polymeric supports throughout the reaction with no formation of aggregates. Figure 6 illustrates the appearance of the reaction system at the end of transesterification with stepwise additions of methanol (molar ratio 1:1).

Figure 6. The appearance of the reaction system at the end of the methanolysis using the three preparations of CaLB considered in the study.

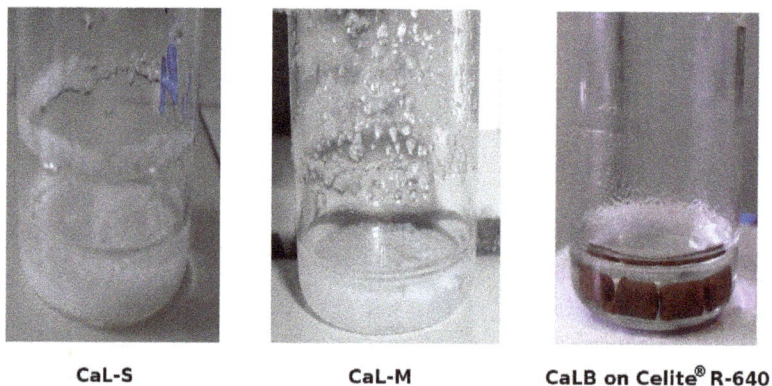

CaL-S   CaL-M   CaLB on Celite® R-640

Methanolysis reaction (molar ratio 1:1) using CaL-S gives 24% of conversion after 6 h. It must be underlined that we also carried out methanolysis under the same conditions by using *Novozyme 435* obtaining about 10% of formation of methyl oleate.

As reported before, the transesterification catalyzed by CaL-S and CaL-M did not achieve a quantitative conversion of the triglyceride. In order to verify whether some methanol was lost during the reaction and the sampling procedure, the transesterification was conducted for 48 h under similar operating conditions but without sampling. The final yield of methyl oleate was 29% for CaL-S but the NMR analysis proved no presence of residual methanol in the reaction medium (see Electronic Supplementary Information, Figure S2). The data suggest that during the transesterification process, some methanol is adsorbed on the immobilization support and this phenomenon is more pronounced in the case of CaL-M, as indicated by the lower conversion achieved. Therefore, the nature of the support appears to play a major role, since an increased local concentration of methanol is expected to be detrimental for the stability of the lipase. This is also in accordance with the lower efficiency of CaL-M observed at higher methanol concentration, as illustrated in Figure 5 above.

The effect of the nature of the immobilization carrier on the partition of hydrophilic components was studied by measuring the water activity of the multiphase reaction systems. Water activity was measured before and after the addition of the immobilized enzymes by means of a hygrometer and after 24 h equilibration as described previously [30,35]. The initial reaction system was a mixture of triolein and methanol with molar ratio 1:1. The values of water activity of the different reaction systems are shown in Table 2.

Table 2. Water activity of reaction systems in the presence of different preparations of immobilized CaLB.

Reaction System	Water Activity (a_w)
Reactants mixture	0.64
CaL-S	0.48
CaL-M	0.27
CaLB on Celite® R-640	0.27

All the supports here considered are porous and have the ability to bind a significant amount of water (from 50%–100% of their weight) although the residual water (evaluated by weight variation upon drying) resulted to be <5% (w/w) in CaL-S and CaL-M (Table 1). Results show that no immobilized enzyme brings free water to the reaction system that could cause competing hydrolytic reactions [36].

On the contrary, the hydrophilic carriers adsorb some water from the reactants, as indicated by the decrease of a_w values, even in the case of Celite R-640, which contains a residual 15% of water in its pores. Significantly, CaL-S, which is the most hydrophobic support, can bind a lower amount of water and, most probably, less methanol as well.

In order to investigate in more detail the effect of methanol on CaL-S, the kinetic profile of the methanolysis at different concentrations of methanol was studied. Figure 7 shows how, by working with three equivalents of methanol, the inactivating effect is visible already after the first hour of reaction. The residual activity of CaL-S after 1 h of reaction at a methanol/triglyceride molar ratio of 3:1 was assayed also by using the method of propil laurate synthesis (see materials and methods). Data indicates that the activity of CaL-S decreases from the initial 3450–1600 (U/g dry), thus confirming the partial inactivation of the enzyme. In the other two cases, the reaction proceeded until the equilibrium was reached and no appreciable variation of conversion was observed by adding fresh enzyme at the end of the reaction (2.5% w/w). This also confirms that the stopping of the reaction was not due to lipase inactivation.

Figure 7. Effect of methanol concentration on CaL-S evaluated at 30 °C by monitoring the transesterification of triolein at different methanol/oil molar ratio.

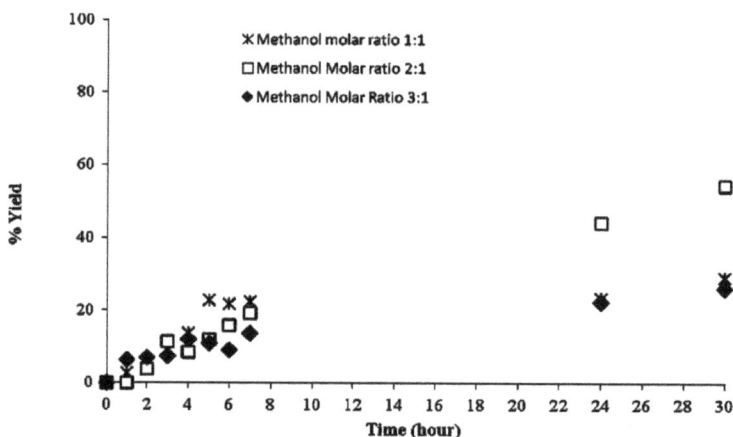

2.3. Recyclability of Cal-S

The stability study was performed using a methanol to oil molar ratio of 1:1 and by stopping the reaction after 4 h in each cycle and measuring the conversion in terms of formation of methyl oleate. Then, the biocatalyst was recovered and reused without further treatment/rinsing by simply introducing fresh triolein and methanol. It must be noted that for each cycle, after introducing fresh triolein, the residual methyl oleate content deriving from the previous cycle was determined prior to the addition of methanol and the starting of the methanolysis. The results indicate that CaLB on styrene is stable after 10 cycles, without any rinsing treatment (Figure 8). Moreover, the biocatalyst has shown its stability even after 22 days of exposure to the reaction conditions. Therefore, no appreciable inhibition due to oil, glycerol or product was detected. Importantly, no aggregation of the particle was observed. The behavior of the preparation indicates that the styrenic resin prevents the undesirable hydrophilic interactions (glycerol and methanol adsorption, protein aggregation, particle aggregation) which are likely to occur in the hydrophobic oils.

Notably, Liù and co-workers reported how CaLB Novozymes 435 undergoes a severe inactivation under comparable conditions, with a loss of roughly 10% of activity after each synthetic cycle [24].

2.4. Enzymatic Methanolysis of Oil Extracted from Espresso Spent Coffee Ground

As a final step in the investigation of lipase catalyzed methanolysis, the immobilized CaLB was applied to the transformation of a non-edible oil from food waste. The oil was extracted from espresso spent coffee ground properly dried [8] according to the procedure already reported [37]. The oil from spent coffee ground appears as a transparent homogeneous amber colored liquid (see Electronic Supplementary Information, Figure S3). Table 3 illustrates the composition in terms of fatty acids determined by GC-MS and compared to the oil used in the work of Kondamundi. Of course, fatty acids can vary not only as a function of the type of coffee used but also as consequence of the method used for coffee brewing.

Figure 8. Recyclability of CalB immobilized on styrenic support expressed as the percentage of methyl oleate formed after 4 h at 30 °C in the transesterification of triolein with methanol (1:1 molar ratio).

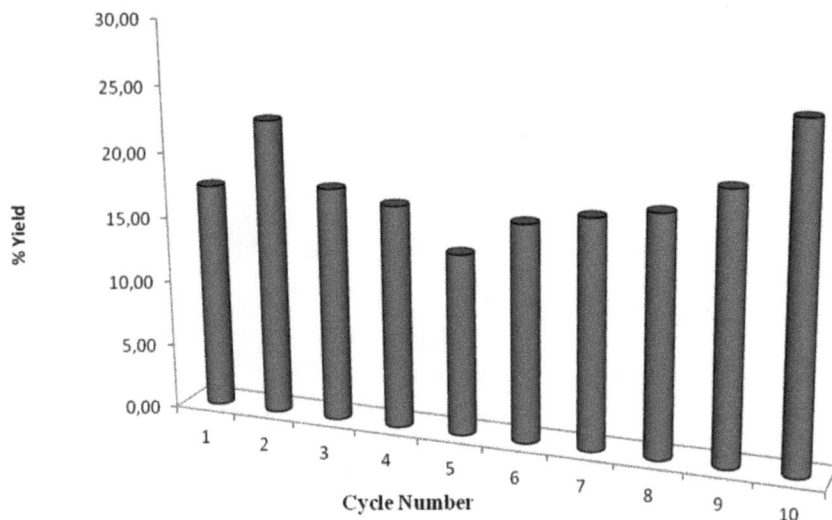

Table 3. Composition of the oil from espresso spent coffee ground in terms of fatty acids and compared to the oil used in the work of Kondamundi *et al.* [8].

Fatty acids	Oil from spent coffee ground as in [8]	Oil from espresso spent coffee ground
C14	n.d.	n.d.
C16	51.4	58.29
C18	8.3	8.79
C18:1	n.d.	3.41
C18:2	40.3	27.80
C18:3	n.d.	0.09
C20	n.d.	1.61
C22	n.d.	n.d.

The transesterification was carried out using CaL-S on oil from espresso spent coffee ground without pretreatment of free fatty acid and at 30 °C.

The reaction was monitored via HPLC by evaluating the formation of the methyl esters of the main fatty acids (palmitic, oleic, linoleic, linolenic, stearic, arachidonic). Because of the complexity of the reaction mixture, a semi-quantitative evaluation of the conversion was obtained by summing the areas of these products of the conversion. About 55% of biodiesel yield was achieved by performing one single addition of three equivalents of methanol at the beginning of the reaction whereas multistep additions of one equivalent of methanol (time = 0, 100 min, 200 min) led to 72% conversion after 30 h of reaction. No optimization of the process (e.g., range of time for addition of methanol) was carried out.

The decrement of the H^1-NMR signals relative to the triglycerides was used as a further indicator of the proceeding of the reaction. The area of the protons at 2.5 ppm (signal related to two protons in α-position to carbonyl group of fatty acid) and the area of the protons at 3.6 ppm (signal related to the three protons of methyl esters) indicate that the conversion is nearly quantitative within 24 h (Figure 9).

Figure 9. H^1-NMR spectra of the oil from espresso spent coffee ground (**a**) and of the reaction mixture after 5 h (**b**) and 24 h (**c**).

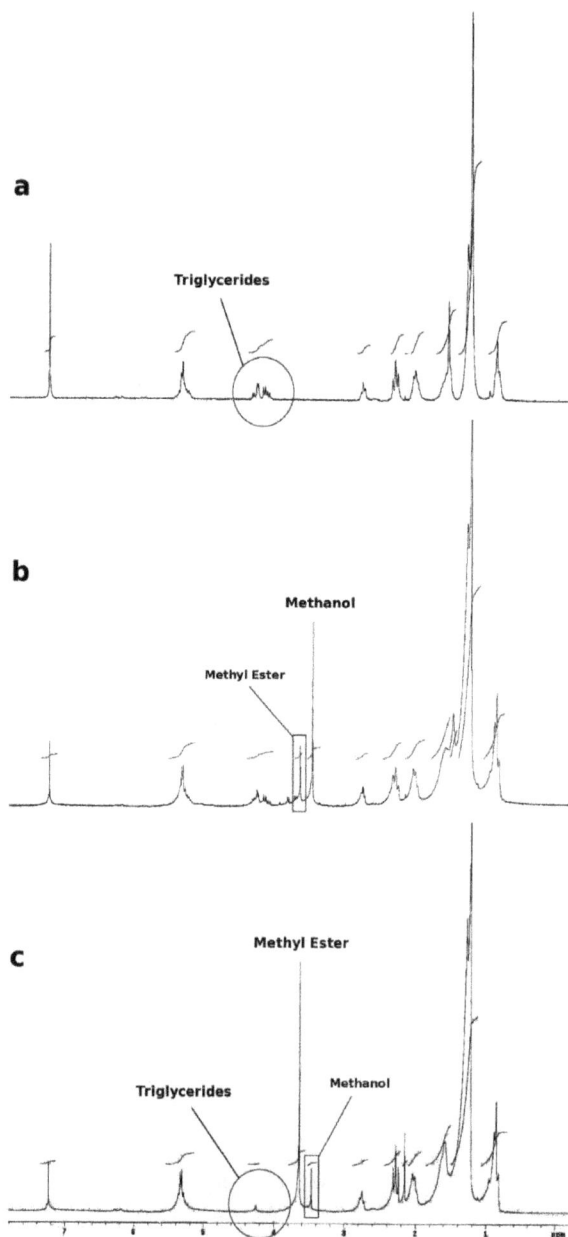

The GC-MS analysis of the products obtained from the methanolysis (see Electronic Supplementary Information, Figure S4) confirms the formation of the methyl esters of all the fatty acids present in the oil from spent coffee ground, as reported in Table 3. Therefore, CaLB demonstrates to be a versatile biocatalyst, accepting all the different fatty acids present in the oil from spent coffee ground.

It must be underlined that the chemical (KOH) methanolysis of oil from spent coffee ground reported by Kondamudi required the use of an excess of 40 volumes of methanol and was carried out under reflux at 70 °C. The process described in the present manuscript is carried out at 30 °C and requires no excess of methanol, so that the only co-product of the reaction is the glycerol. Moreover, at the end of the reaction the biocatalyst can be simply filtrated and no acid must be used to neutralize the reaction mixture.

3. Experimental Sections

3.1. Enzymes

Native CaLB employed during this study was Lipozyme CalB L from Novozyme (DK). The commercial preparation is constituted by CaLB (11 mg/mL) diluted in a solution of glycerol, sorbitol and salts to stabilize the protein. The pH value of the enzymatic solution is about 4.2.

Native PcL was Lipase PS "AMANO" SD from AMANO (Japan). The commercial preparation is a yellowish lyophilized powder constituted by PcL (about 1%) diluted with dextrins.

Immobilized CaL-M (methacrylic) [32] and CaL-S (styrenic) were kindly donated by Sprin S.p.A. (Trieste, Italy). Organic polymeric resins are in the form of beads with particle size of 300–500 µm. Characterization is reported in Table 1.

The residual water content in the final immobilized preparation was determined on aluminum plates. A known amount of biocatalyst was dried at 110 °C for 6 h. Water content is defined as the % of weight loss after drying.

3.2. Immobilization of CalB on Celite®R-640

The immobilization was done according to the procedure already reported [31]. The Lipozyme solution was adjusted to pH 8 prior to immobilization. 2.5 mL of enzymatic solution, 1 g of dry Celite® R640 and 12 mL of dry toluene were mixed and kept at 25 °C for one day. The organic solvent was removed and the enzymatic preparation was washed with acetone on a büchner filter under reduced pressure for three times (support/solvent ratio 1/2 w/v). The residual water content was then evaluated as reported above.

3.3. Chemicals

Triolein (99%), methyl esters standards and all other chemical reagents are from Sigma Aldrich.

3.4. Monitoring the Formation of Fatty acid Methyl Ester (Biodiesel)

Methyl oleate formed from transesterification of triolein was measured by Gilson HPLC equipped with an auto injector. The column was ODS Hypersil SUPERCHROM set at isothermal oven temperature of 54 °C. The detector was UV/VIS-155 with dual wavelength of 200 nm and 210 nm. The mobile phase was 100% Acetonitrile and 0.05% of TFA with flow of 1 mL/min. Biodiesel (methyl esters of fatty acids-FAME) was analyzed by following methods from ref. [10]. Biodiesel yield was calculated by summing the areas of methyl esters present in the reaction mixture and on the basis of calibration curves built up with standards FAME.

3.5. Synthetic Activity of PcL

Activity was determined by transesterification reaction of vinyl acetate with 1-phenyl-1-ethanol, which is a standard synthetic method reported by AMANO Enzymes company. Transesterification reaction was carried out at 25 °C and mixing at 200 rpm. 1-phenylethyl acetate formed during the reaction was measured by Gilson HPLC equipped with an auto injector. The column was ODS Hypersil SUPERCHROM set at isothermal oven temperature of 30 °C. The detector was a Gilson UV/VIS-155 with dual wavelength of 210 nm and 260 nm. The mobile phase was 40% acetonitrile and 0.05% of TFA and 60% H_2O with a flow of 1 mL/min.

3.6. Synthetic Activity of CaLB

The assay allows the determination of enzymatic activity through the synthesis of propyl laurate formed by enzymatic esterification of lauric acid and 1-propanol. One unit corresponds to the amount of enzyme that produces 1 μmol of propyl laurate in one minute at 55 °C without solvent. In a vial of 20 mL, 1.2 g of lauric acid and 0.36 g of 1-propanol were added. The reaction mixture was thermostated at 55 °C and mixed at 250 rpm in order to allow the melting of lauric acid. A withdrawal of 0.1 mL was diluted in 1.3 mL of hexane. 0.2 mL of this solution was added to 1.6 mL of hexane and analyzed by HPLC ($t = 0$). The reaction was started by adding 40–50 mg of biocatalyst to the main solution and maintained under continuous stirring at 250 rpm. Withdrawals were performed at different times and analysed by HPLC.

3.7. Hydrolytics Activity of Lipases

The activity of enzymatic preparations was assayed by following the tributyrin hydrolysis and by titrating, with 0.1 M sodium hydroxide, the butyric acid that is released during the hydrolysis. An emulsion composed by 1.5 mL tributyrin, 5.1 mL gum arabic emulsifier (0.6% w/v) and 23.4 mL water was prepared in order to obtain a final molarity of tributyrin of 0.17 M. Successively, 2 mL of K-phosphate buffer (0.1 M, pH 7.0) were added to 30 mL of tributyrin emulsion and the mixture was incubated in a thermostated vessel at 30 °C, equipped with a mechanical stirrer. After pH stabilization, about 50 mg of immobilized protein were added. The consumption of 0.1 M sodium hydroxide was monitored for 15–20 min. One unit of activity was defined as the amount of immobilized enzyme required to produce 1 μmol of butyric acid per min at 30 °C.

3.8. Water Activity

Water activity of the reaction system was determined at 30 °C by using a hygrometer (DARAI-Trieste, Italy) as previously described [30]. Measurements were carried out by sealing the sensor into the open end of 5 mL glasses vials, thermostated at 30 °C, until constant reading. All samples were previously equilibrated for 24 h. The hygrometer was firstly calibrated for 24 h with saturated salt solution of $MgCl_2$ ($a_w = 0.3273$), NaCl ($a_w = 0.7532$) and NH_4NH_2 $(a_w = 0.927)$ using ultrapure water [30,35]. The values of standard salt solution from calibrated hygrometer were 0.39, 0.74 and 0.87.

3.9. Monitoring the Methanolysis by HPLC

Methyl esters formed from the transesterification were evaluated by means of a Gilson HPLC equipped with auto injector. The column was ODS Hypersil SUPERCHROM set at isothermal oven temperature of 54 °C. The detector was UV/VIS-155 with dual wavelength of 200 nm and 210 nm. The mobile phase was 100% acetonitrile and 0.05% of TFA with flow of 1 mL/min. Biodiesel (FAME) content and its standards were analyzed by following methods from [38]. Biodiesel yield was calculated based on total area of the methyl ester mixture in the final product.

3.10. Lipase Catalyzed Methanolysis

Transesterification was carried out in 10 mL screw capped vials in orbital shaker with temperature control. The temperature was set at 30 °C with shaking rate of 250 rpm. Prior to addition of methanol, the immobilized lipase (10% w/w of oil) was mixed with the feedstock (2 g) for a few minutes. 10 μL samples were withdrawn and analyzed by HPLC.

3.11. Recycling of CaL-S

The stability study was performed using a methanol to oil molar ratio of 1:1, stopping the reaction after 4 hours in each cycle and by measuring the conversion in terms of formation of methyl oleate. Then, the biocatalyst was recovered and reused without further treatment/rinsing by simply introducing fresh triolein and methanol. For each cycle, in order to avoid overestimation of the product concentration, after introducing fresh triolein, the residual methyl oleate content deriving from the previous cycle was determined prior to the addition of methanol and the starting of the new methanolysis cycle. The reactions were performed at 30 °C.

3.12. ^{1}H-NMR

Spectra were recorded on a NMR Varian 200 Gemini, operating at 200 MHz. Samples were prepared by diluting 10 μL of the reaction mixture in 700 μL of $CDCl_3$.

3.13. Extraction of Oil and GC-MS Analysis of Fatty Acids

The spent coffee ground was dried [8] and extracted according to the procedure already reported [37], obtaining yields around 20% (w/w). Characterization was performed according to a method previously described [39] by mean of GC MS Agilent technologies 6890 N and Agilent 5973 MSD as detector. The column was a Zebron ZB-FFAP Capillary Column 60 m × 0.25 mm × 0.25 μm. For the analysis, the temperature raised from 170–235 °C by increasing 2 °C/min. Gas phase was helium at constant flow of 1.3 mL/min.

3.14. Computational Study: Molecular Dynamic Simulations

The molecular dynamic (MD) simulations to analyse the behaviour of lipases upon water exposure were performed using the software GROMACS 4 with the GROMOS-96 53a6 force field. The crystal structure of *Pseudomonas cepacia* lipase (PDB 1YS1) and the crystal structure of *Candida antarctica* lipase B (PDB 1TCA) were implemented in the force field in *gro* file format by using the tool pdb2gmx of the GROMACS software package, which also adds the necessary hydrogen atoms. The proteins were solvated separately with explicit SPC water in a virtual box of 343 nm^3 each. The molecular dynamic simulations were performed in an NPT environment simulating the temperature of 300 K and keeping the pressure constant (Berendsen thermostat and pressure); the cut-off for electrostatic interactions was set to 1.4 nm and the limit for the Van der Waals interactions set to 1.4 nm. For the minimization procedures, the PME (Particle Mesh Ewald) algorithm was used for the calculation of the electrostatic interactions, setting the limit at 1.0 nm. Before the MD simulation, the systems were minimized at least for 10,000 steps.

The MD simulation of *Pseudomonas cepacia* lipase at water-octane interface was performed using the software GROMACS 4 with the MARTINI force field. Crystal structure of *Pseudomonas cepacia* lipase (PDB 1YS1) was implemented in the MARTINI force field in *gro* file format by using the necessary scripts available on the MARTINI web site [40] and the DSSP program [41] for the necessary secondary structure definition. The protein was solvated with explicit water-octane 1:1 mixture in virtual cubic boxes of 512 nm^3. The MD simulation was performed in a NPT environment and in conditions specified above. The time step for integration was set to 4 fs (usually this value is set to 2 fs). Minimization procedures were performed before the MD simulation using a cut-off for electrostatic interactions and by setting the threshold at 1.4 nm. The steepest descendent algorithm was used. Minimization was performed for at least 10,000 steps.

3.15. Computational Study: GRID Mapping of Surface of Proteins

The GRID analysis [32] was performed on the output of the dinamised crystal structure of *Pseudomonas cepacia* lipase (PDB code 1YS1) by choosing a cage big enough to include the whole protein. The grid nodes were set every 0.5 Å. The probes used for the calculation of the molecular interaction fields were DRY (hydrophobic probe) and WATER (H2O probe). Isopotential surfaces were visualized by setting energy values of −0.3 kcalmol^{-1} for the DRY probe and −2.5 kcalmol^{-1} for the WATER probe.

4. Conclusions

The present study shows that immobilization plays a major role in determining the efficiency of lipases in the methanolysis of oils. Information on the structure and conformation of lipases provides a rational basis for the selection of biocatalysts and their immobilization. *Ad hoc* immobilization methodologies are necessary for fully exploiting the catalytic potential of lipases while favoring effective mass transfer and partition of substrates/products.

Lipase B from *Candida antartica* (CaLB) displayed the highest efficiency when immobilized on the most hydrophobic supports (CaL-S). The biocatalyst showed good stability after 10 cycles of reaction in presence of equimolar concentration of methanol. Hydrophilic immobilization supports demonstrated to be less suitable for reactions involving the bulky and hydrophobic triglycerides, most probably because of unfavorable partition phenomena. Moreover, data suggest that these porous carriers are more prone to absorb water or other hydrophilic components such as methanol, which affect negatively the stability of lipases.

The study of methanolysis of oil from spent coffee ground indicates that new types of non-edible oils can be considered for developing competitive and sustainable enzymatic biodiesel synthesis. Immobilized CaLB was able to catalyze the conversion of all different fatty acids present in the raw material. Optimization studies will be required for implementing appropriate feed-batch processes to decrease the reaction time and for the evaluation of various types of oils from different coffee wastes.

Acknowledgments

Harumy Veny is grateful to ICS-UNIDO (Trieste, Italy) for a fellowship. Thanks are due to Sara Cantone and Diana Fattor (SPRIN S.p.A., Technology for Sustainable Chemistry, Trieste, Italy) for enzyme samples and useful discussions.

References

1. Medina, A.R.; González-Moreno, P.A.; Esteban-Cerdán, L.; Molina-Grima, E. Biocatalysis: Towards ever greener biodiesel production, *Biotechnol. Adv.* **2009**, *27*, 398–408.
2. Mittelbach, M.; Remschmidt, C. *Biodiesel—The Comprehensive Handbook*, 1st ed.; Börsedruk Ges. m.b.H., Vienna, 2004.
3. Uma, B.H.; Kim, Y.S. Review: A chance for Korea to advance algal-biodiesel technology. *J. Ind. Eng. Chem.* **2009**, *15*, 1–7.
4. Chisti, Y. Biodiesel from Microalgae. *Biotechnol. Adv.* **2007**, *25*, 294–306.
5. Shah, S.; Sharma, S.; Gupta, M.N. Biodiesel preparation by lipase-catalyzed transesterification of jatropha oil. *Energy Fuels* **2004**, *18*, 154–159.
6. Oliveira, L.S.; Franca, A.S.; Camargos, R.R.S.; Ferraz, V.P. Coffee oil as a potential feedstock for biodiesel production. *Bioresour. Technol.* **2008**, *99*, 3244–3250.
7. Calabrò, V.; Ricca, E.; de Paola, M.G.; Curcio, S.; Iorio, G. Kinetics of enzymatic trans-esterification of glycerides for biodiesel production. *Bioprocess Biosyst. Eng.* **2010**, *33*, 701–710.

8. Kondamundi, N.; Mohapatra, S.K.; Misra, M. Spent coffee grounds as a versatile source of green energy. *J. Agric. Food Chem.* **2008**, *56*, 11757–11760.

9. Caetano, N.S.; Silva, V.F.M.; Mata, T.M. Valorization of coffee grounds for biodiesel production. *Chem. Eng. Trans.* **2012**, *26*, 267–272.

10. Khan, N.A.; Brown, J.B. The composition of coffee oil and its component fatty acids. *J. Am. Oil Chem. Soc.* **1953**, *30*, 606–609.

11. Nunes, A.A.; Franca, A.S.; Oliveira, L.S. Activated carbons from waste biomass: An alternative use for biodiesel production solid residues. *Bioresour. Technol.* **2009**, *100*, 1786–1792.

12. Gui, M.M.; Lee, K.T.; Bhata, S. Feasibility of edible oil *vs.* non-edible oil *vs.* waste edible oil as biodiesel feedstock. *Energy* **2008**, *33*, 1646–1653.

13. Yanagimoto, K.; Ochi, H.; Lee, K.G.; Takayuki, S. Antioxidative activities of fractions obtained from brewed coffee. *J. Agric. Food Chem.* **2004**, *52*, 592–596.

14. Campo, P.; Zhao, Y.; Suidan, M.T.; Venosa, A.D.; Sorial, G.A. Biodegradation kitetics and toxicity of vegetable oils triacylglycelols under aerobic conditions. *Chemosphere* **2007**, *68*, 2054–2062.

15. Schmid, R.D.; Verger, R. Lipases: Interfacial enzyme with attractive application. *Angew. Chem. Int. Ed.* **1998**, *37*, 1608–1633.

16. Mittelbach, M. Lipase-catalyzed alcoholysis of sunflower oil. *J. Am. Chem. Soc.* **1990**, *67*, 168–170.

17. Nielsen, P.M.; Brask, J.; Fjerbaek, L. Enzymatic biodiesel production: Technical and economical considerations. *Eur. J. Lipid Sci. Technol.* **2008**, *110*, 692–700.

18. Du, W.; Xu, Y.Y.; Liu, H.; Li, Z.B. Study on acyl migration in immobilized lipozyme TL-catalyzed transesterification of soybean oil for biodiesel production. *J. Mol. Catal. B Enzym.* **2005**, *37*, 68–71.

19. Du, W.; Xu, Y.; Liu, D.; Zeng, J. Comparative study on lipase-catalyzed transformation of soybean oil for biodiesel production with different acyl acceptors. *J. Mol. Catal. B Enzym.* **2004**, *30*, 125–129.

20. Christensen, M.W.; Andersen, L.; Husum, T.L.; Kirk, O. Industrial lipase immobilization. *Eur. J. Lipid Sci. Technol.* **2003**, *105*, 318–321.

21. Ferrario, V.; Ebert, C.; Knapic, L.; Fattor, D.; Basso, A.; Spizzo, P.; Gardossi, L. Conformational changes of lipases in aqueous media: A comparative computational study and experimental implications. *Adv. Synth. Catal.* **2011**, *353*, 2466–2480.

22. Skjot, M.; de Maria, L.; Chatterjee, R.; Svendsen, A.; Patkar, S.A.; Ostergraad, P.R.; Brask, J. Understanding the plasticity of the alpha/beta hydrolase fold: Lid swapping on the Candida antarctica lipase B results in chimeras with interesting biocatalytic properties. *ChemBioChem* **2009**, *10*, 520–527.

23. Goodford, P.J. A computational procedure for determining energetically favorable binding sites on biologically important macromolecules. *J. Med. Chem.* **1985**, *28*, 849–857.

24. Xu, Y.; Du, W.; Liu, D. Study on the kinetics of enzymatic interesterification of triglycerides for biodiesel production with methyl acetate as the acyl acceptor. *J. Mol. Catal. B Enzym.* **2005**, *32*, 241–245.

25. Watanabe, Y.; Shimada, Y.; Sugihara, A.; Tominaga, Y. Conversion of degummed soybean oil to biodiesel fuel with immobilized *Candida antartica* lipase. *J. Mol. Catal. B Enzym.* **2002**, *17*, 151–155.

26. Anderson, E.; Larsson, K.; Kirk, O. One biocatalyst—Many applications: The use of Candida antarctica. *Biocatal. Biotransform.* **1998**, *16*, 181–204.

27. Salis, A.; Pinna, M.; Monduzzi, M.; Solinas, V. Biodiesel production from triolein and short chain alcohols through biocatalysis. *J. Biotechnol.* **2005**, *119*, 291–299.

28. Marrink, S.J.; Tieleman, D.P. Perspective on the Martini model. *Chem. Soc. Rev.* **2013**, doi:10.1039/C3CS60093A.

29. Friedrich, T.; Stuermer, R. Production of immobilized lipase from Pseudomonas and application for enantioselective reactions. U.S. Patent 6 596 520, 2003.

30. Gardossi, L. Immobilization of Enzymes and Control of Water Activity in Low-Water Media: Properties and Applications of Celite R-640 (Celite Rods). In *Methods in Biotechnology: Enzyme in Non-Aqueous Solvents: Methods and Protocols*; Vulfson, E.N., Halling, P.J., Holland, H., Eds.; Humana Press, Inc.: Totowa, NJ, USA, 2001; pp. 151–172.

31. Basso, A.; de Martin, L.; Ebert, C.; Gardossi, L.; Linda, P. High isolated yields in thermodynamically controlled peptide synthesis in toluene catalysed by thermolysin adsorbed on Celite R-640. *Chem. Commun.* **2000**, *6*, 467–468.

32. Basso, A.; Braiuca, P.; Cantone, S.; Ebert, C.; Linda, P.; Spizzo, P.; Caimi, P.; Hanefeld, U.; Degrassi, G.; Gardossi, L. *In silico* analysis of enzyme surface and glycosylation effect as a tool for efficient covalent immobilization of CalB and PGA on Sepabeads®. *Adv. Synth. Catal.* **2007**, *349*, 877–886.

33. Tanaka, A.; Sugimoto, H.; Muta, Y.; Mizuno, T.; Senoo, K.; Obata, H.; Inouye, K. Differential scanning calorimetry of the effects of Ca2+ on the thermal unfolding of Pseudomonas cepacia lipase. *Biosci. Biotechnol. Biochem.* **2003**, *67*, 207–210.

34. Pirozzi, D. Improvement of lipase stability in the presence of commercial triglycerides. *Eur. J. Lipid Sci. Technol.* **2003**, *105*, 608–613.

35. Ulijn, R.V.; de Martin, L.; Halling, P.J.; Janssen, A.E.M.; Gardossi, L.; Moore, B.D. Solvent selection for solid-to-solid synthesis. *Biotechnol. Bioeng.* **2002**, *80*, 509–515.

36. Kaeida, M.; Samukawa, T.; Kondo, A.; Fukuda, H. Effect of methanol and water contents on production of biodiesel fuel from plant oil catalyzed by various lipases in a solvent-free system. *J. Biosci. Bioeng.* **2001**, *91*, 12–15.

37. Ferrari, M.; Ravera, F.; De Angelis, E.; Suggi Liverani, F.; Navarini, L. Interfacial properties of coffee oils. *Colloids Surf. A Physicochem. Eng. Aspects* **2010**, *365*, 79–82.

38. Holcapek, M.; Jandera, P.; Fischer, J.; Prokes, B. Analytical monitoring of the production of biodiesel by high-performance liquid chromatography with various detection methods. *J. Chromatogr. A* **1999**, *858*, 13–31.

39. D'Amelio, N.; de Angelis, E.; Navarini, L.; Schievano, E.; Mammi, S. Green coffee oil analysis by high-resolution nuclear magnetic resonance spectroscopy. *Talanta* **2013**, *110*, 118–127.
40. Available online: http://md.chem.rug.nl/cgmartini/index.php/home (accessed on 12 May 2010).
41. Wolfgang, K.; Sander, C. Dictionary of protein secondary structure: Pattern recognition of hydrogen-bonded and geometrical features. *Biopolymers* **1983**, *22*, 2577–2637.

Pyranose Dehydrogenase from *Agaricus campestris* and *Agaricus xanthoderma*: Characterization and Applications in Carbohydrate Conversions

Petra Staudigl, Iris Krondorfer, Dietmar Haltrich and Clemens K. Peterbauer

Abstract: Pyranose dehydrogenase (PDH) is a flavin-dependent sugar oxidoreductase that is limited to a rather small group of litter-degrading basidiomycetes. The enzyme is unable to utilize oxygen as an electron acceptor, using substituted benzoquinones and (organo) metal ions instead. PDH displays a broad substrate specificity and intriguing variations in regioselectivity, depending on substrate, enzyme source and reaction conditions. In contrast to the related enzyme pyranose 2-oxidase (POx), PDHs from several sources are capable of oxidizing α- or β-1→4-linked di- and oligosaccharides, including lactose. PDH from *A. xanthoderma* is able to perform C-1 and C-2 oxidation, producing, in addition to lactobionic acid, 2-dehydrolactose, an intermediate for the production of lactulose, whereas PDH from *A. campestris* oxidizes lactose nearly exclusively at the C-1 position. In this work, we present the isolation of PDH-encoding genes from *A. campestris* (Ac) and *A. xanthoderma* (Ax) and a comparison of other so far isolated PDH-sequences. Secretory overexpression of both enzymes in *Pichia pastoris* was successful when using their native signal sequences with yields of 371 $U \cdot L^{-1}$ for AxPDH and 35 $U \cdot L^{-1}$ for AcPDH. The pure enzymes were characterized biochemically and tested for applications in carbohydrate conversion reactions of industrial relevance.

Reprinted from *Biomolecules*. Cite as: Staudigl, P.; Krondorfer, I.; Haltrich, D.; Peterbauer, C.K. Pyranose Dehydrogenase from *Agaricus campestris* and *Agaricus xanthoderma*: Characterization and Applications in Carbohydrate Conversions. *Biomolecules* **2013**, *3*, 535-552.

1. Introduction

Pyranose dehydrogenase (PDH, EC 1.1.99.29) is a monomeric extracellular glycoprotein of around 75 kDa, carrying a covalently bound FAD cofactor (8α-N3-histidyl-FAD) [1]. It is a member of the glucose-methanol-choline (GMC) family together with other sugar oxidoreductases like the catalytically related enzymes glucose oxidase, cellobiose dehydrogenase and pyranose-2 oxidase. PDH was first described in 1997 when it was isolated from the edible basidiomycete fungus *Agaricus bisporus* [2]. Later, the enzyme from other members of the family of *Agaricaceae* like *Macrelepiota rhacodes* [3], *A. xanthoderma* [4] and *A. meleagris* [5,6] was investigated. Recently, the crystal structure of *A. meleagris* PDH (AmPDH) was resolved and revealed a two-domain structure consisting of the ADP-binding Rossman domain and a sugar-binding domain [1].

The biological function of PDH is still not fully clear. As the enzyme is limited to litter-decomposing fungi of the family *Agaricaceae* and is not able to utilize molecular oxygen as electron acceptor, the reduction of quinones and radicals formed during lignin degradation were proposed as its natural role [3]. Other possible functions like a participation in Fenton's reaction or the defense against antimicrobial (quinone) substances produced by plants were reported [7].

As the production of the enzyme in basidiomycete fungi is quite laborious and time-consuming [2,4,5], approaches for heterologous expression in *Aspergillus nidulans* and *A. niger* [8], *E. coli* and *P. pastoris* [9] were tested. Attempts to solubly express PDH in *E. coli* did not succeed due to the formation of inactive inclusion bodies whereas an expression in *P. pastoris* yielded high levels of recombinant protein with properties equal to the wild-type [9]. Therefore, the methylotrophic yeast was the expression host of choice for the heterologous production of *A. campestris* and *A. xanthoderma* PDH in this study.

The oxidation products of PDH depend on the source of the enzyme, the substrate and the reaction conditions. The enzyme is able to oxidize free, non-phosphorylated sugars in pyranose form, heteroglycosides, disaccharides and glucooligosaccharides at the C-1, C-2, C-3 and also at C-1,2, C-2,3 and C-3,4 atom [2,3,10–14]. The oxidation products of D-glucose and D-galactose, 2-keto-D-glucose and 2-keto-D-galactose, represent industrially relevant intermediates for the production of the high-value sugars D-fructose and D-tagatose [15,16]. An easily available disaccharide lactose, can be oxidized by PDH to the corresponding C-1, C-2 or C-2,3 product. Depending on the source of the enzyme, 2-keto-lactose and lactobionic acid, the hydrolysis product of lactobionolactone, are formed in different ratios. Volc and coworkers screened various *Agaricus sp.* for their PDH oxidation products and observed that *A. campestris* PDH almost exclusively oxidizes lactose at the C-1 position, yielding lactobionic acid, whereas 2-keto-lactose was the main product of *A. xanthoderma* PDH [12]. Lactobionic acid has numerous applications in the pharmaceutical-, cosmetic- and food-industry, such as in organ preservation solutions and macrolide antibiotics, skin care cosmetics or as an acidulant or flavor enhancer in food [17]. The C-2 oxidation product 2-keto-lactose can be used for the production of lactulose, a prebiotic carbohydrate administered against obstipation and hepatic encephalopathy which has beneficial effects on the gastrointestinal microbiota [18]. Here, we describe for the first time the heterologous expression of PDH genes from *Agaricus campestris* and *Agaricus xanthoderma* in the methylotrophic yeast *Pichia pastoris* and present a detailed characterization of both enzymes. Furthermore, we performed comprehensive studies on the conversion of lactose and present a novel alternative for the production of lactobionic acid and 2-dehydrolactose, a key intermediate for the isomerization to lactulose.

2. Results and Discussion

2.1. Expression of Acpdh and Axpdh in P. pastoris

To obtain the PDH-encoding gene from *A. campestris*, different oligonucleotide primers were designed based on conserved regions from already known sequences (accession numbers are given in paragraph 3.8.). PCRs were performed using different forward primers, the anchor primer and first-strand-cDNA as template. Resulting fragments were sequenced and used to design sequence specific primers for identification of the 5′-flanking region by primer walking using the DNA Walking SpeedUp Premix Kit. The nucleotide sequence of the AcPDH cDNA contains an ORF of 1788 bp encoding a polypeptide of 595 amino acids. Two primers based on the cDNA sequence and containing restriction sites for ligation into the pPICZb vector were designed, and used to re-amplify the cDNA and construct the expression vector under control of the methanol-inducible AOX promoter.

The previously unknown signal sequence and the 5'-flanking region of AxPDH were analogously identified using the DNA Walking SpeedUp Premix Kit and three specific reverse primers (AxTSP1-3). The purified fragments were sequenced, and based on these results, the full-length cDNA could be amplified. The AxPDH encoding cDNA contains an ORF of 1803 bp encoding a polypeptide of 600 amino acids. The cDNA fragment was re-amplified with two primers containing restrictions sites for ligation into the pPICZb vector. The plasmids were transformed into *E. coli* NEB5α for proliferation. Isolated plasmids were linearized with *SacI* and transformed into the expression host *P. pastoris* and cultivated in 96-well deep well plates and screened for PDH activity. To confirm the results from the first round of screening, a rescreening experiment with multiple parallel determinations was performed. The clones with the highest activity were selected for further studies.

2.2. Multiple Sequence Alignment

To compare the amino acid sequences of the PDHs isolated and characterized so far in our group (*A. meleagris* PDH1 [5,6,9], *A. bisporus* (our unpublished information) *A. campestris* (this work) and *A. xanthoderma* PDH [4]), a multiple sequence alignment was constructed using the MUSCLE algorithm (Figure S1). The PDHs from different sources show a sequence identity between 74% and 78%. From the crystal structure of AmPDH1 [1], His 512 and His 556 were identified as the catalytic pair of major importance for sugar substrate oxidation. These two amino acids and His 103, where the FAD cofactor is covalently bound, are highly conserved among PDHs (Figure S1, highlighted in red). Docking experiments with several electron donors in different oxidation poses revealed that the principal sugar interaction partners are the two catalytic histidines but also Gln 392 and Tyr 510 (Figure S1, highlighted in green). The fact that these amino acids are conserved in all four PDHs supports these findings.

All PDHs are glycoproteins with different degrees of glycosylation. Putative *N*- and *O*-glycosylation sites predicted by NetNGlyc 1.0 server and NetOGlyc 3.1 server [19] are highlighted in red and green, respectively.

2.3. Heterologous Protein Production

The cultivation of *P. pastoris* cells expressing the *acpdh*- and *axpdh*-encoding gene was carried out in a 7-L stirred and aerated bioreactor and lasted 187 and 161 h, respectively (Figure 1). The initial glycerol batch phase produced 113 $g \cdot L^{-1}$ and 75 $g \cdot L^{-1}$ wet biomass in 27 h and 25 h (its end was indicated by an increase in dissolved oxygen concentration). The following feed with 50% glycerol was maintained for 17 h and 19 h and resulted in a final biomass of 156 $g \cdot L^{-1}$ and 155 $g \cdot L^{-1}$, respectively. A methanol feed was initiated for induction, and at the end of this phase, the biomass reached a level of 260 $g \cdot L^{-1}$ and 293 $g \cdot L^{-1}$. The activity of the extracellular enzyme fraction finally reached 35 $U \cdot L^{-1}$ for AcPDH and 371 $U \cdot L^{-1}$ for AxPDH, while the level of extracellular protein increased to 345 $mg \cdot L^{-1}$ and 350 $mg \cdot L^{-1}$.

Figure 1. Large scale production of pyranose dehydrogenases (PDHs) in *P. pastoris*. Black circles, wet biomass; grey triangles, extracellular protein concentration; black squares, volumetric activity.

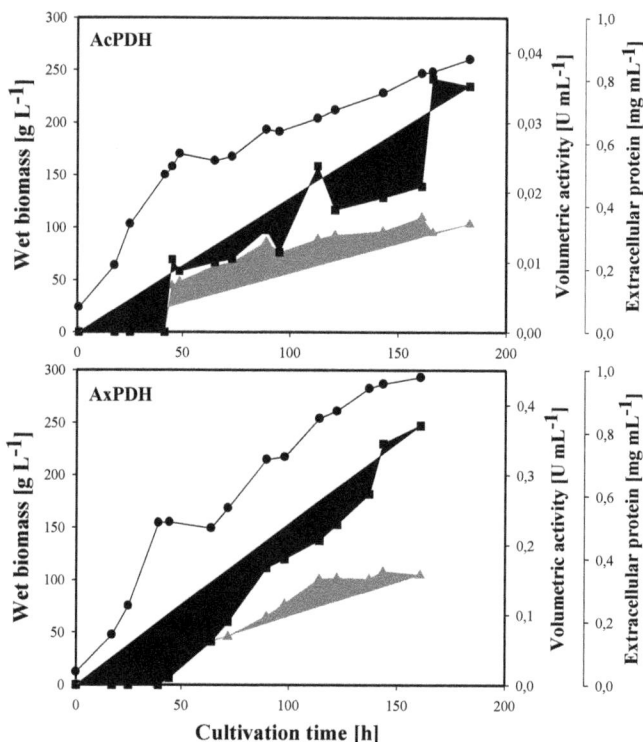

2.4. Purification of Recombinant PDHs

Recombinant AcPDH was purified from the cultivation broth in a four-step protocol (Table 1) including an additional hydrophobic interaction chromatography step (phenyl-source) compared to the three-step purification of AxPDH, which consisted of hydrophobic interaction chromatography, anion exchange chromatography and gel filtration as a polishing step. Before the AcPDH pool was loaded on the phenyl-source column, solid ammonium sulfate was added to a saturation of 40%, similar to the first purification step. Unexpectedly, the protein did not bind to the column in this case, and the whole PDH activity was found in the flow-through. This purification step indeed increased the specific activity from 0.4 U mg^{-1} to 2.8 U mg^{-1} but the flow-through still contained impurities due to the lack of restrictive pooling. Therefore, a subsequent gel filtration step was conducted, resulting in apparent homogeneity for both AcPDH and AxPDH (Figure 2), with final specific activities of 4.9 U mg^{-1} and 16.6 U mg^{-1}, respectively. For AcPDH, two pools with different specific activities were formed due to rather low overall yields. Pool 1 represented the center of the elution peak and all further analyses were performed with this enzyme preparation. The low purification yield for AcPDH corresponds to the fact that PDH accounted only for 0.1% of the total protein in the extracellular fraction, whereas AxPDH accounted for more than 2%. The purification step that decreased the yield most dramatically is the first for both enzymes. As the starting volume for purification after centrifugation was around 4 L in both cases, the calculation of the total activity based on the activity per mL could lead to imprecise results. This is especially true in the case of AcPDH, where the volumetric activity per mL was below the detection limit of the standard ferrocenium/glucose activity assay and only represents an estimate. A reduction of the volume and therefore concentration of the cultivation broth would have been useful for more precise measurements of the initial volumetric activity. The higher degree of glycosylation of AcPDH could also play a disadvantageous role for the purification (Figure 2, Table 2). All concentrated protein pools showed the typical light yellow color of flavoproteins and were stable over several months at 4 °C in 65 mM sodium phosphate buffer pH 7.5.

Table 1. Purification schemes of recombinant PDHs.

Purification Step	Total Protein [mg]	Total Activity [U]	Specific Activity [U mg^{-1}]	Purification [-fold]	Yield [%]
AcPDH					
Crude extract	1730	154.4	0.1	1	100
Phenyl sepharose	124.4	27.4	0.2	2.5	18
DEAE sepharose	28.2	21.5	0.4	4.1	14
Phenyl source	5.5	15.2	2.8	31.0	10
Gel filtration pool 1	1.2	5.6	4.9	54.5	4
Gel filtration pool 2	0.4	1.5	3.7	41.9	1
AxPDH					
Crude extract	1226.4	1298.9	1.1	1	100
Phenyl sepharose	109.9	538.6	4.9	4.6	41
DEAE sepharose	40.2	524.9	13.1	12.3	40
Gel filtration	25.8	428.8	16.6	15.7	33

Figure 2. SDS-PAGE of purified PDHs. M, molecular marker; 1, AcPDH; 2, AcPDH deglycosylated; 3, Ax PDH; 4, AxPDH deglycosylated.

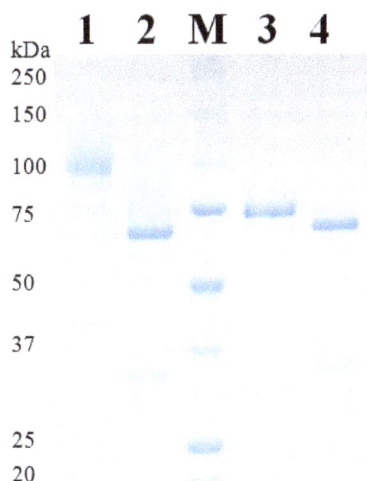

Table 2. Molecular properties of recombinant PDHs.

PDH	Mass SDS-PAGE [kDa]	Mass SDS-PAGE Deglyc. [kDa]	Theor. Mass [kDa]	Glycan Mass [%]	N-Glyc sites Predicted	O-Glyc Sites Predicted
Ac	98	68	61.8	31	6	3
Ax	73	68	62.3	7	5	0

2.5. Molecular Properties

The molecular masses of AcPDH and AxPDH were determined by SDS-PAGE (Figure 2) and native PAGE (Figure 3). AcPDH formed a diffuse band around 98 kDa (Figure 2, lane 1), after deglycosylation with PNGase F under denaturing conditions, a sharp band at 68 kDa could be observed (lane 2). AxPDH showed a band at 73 kDa (lane 4); after deglycosylation, the band shifted to around 68 kDa (lane 5). The high degree of glycosylation of AcPDH compared to AxPDH (Table 2) is also observed in native PAGE (Figure 3). From the migration difference of the glycosylated and deglycosylated protein band in the gel, a glycan mass of 31% for AcPDH and 7% for AxPDH could be calculated (Table 2). The native AxPDH [4] showed a slightly smaller mass on the SDS-PAGE compared to the recombinant protein (around 65 kDa). This is most likely due to a difference in glycosylation in basidiomycete fungi compared to the yeast *P. pastoris*. Whereas proteins in (homo) basidiomycete fungi carry *N*-glycans of the oligomannosidic type (4–9 mannoses), *P. pastoris* tends to produce hyper-mannosylated glycans [20–22]. The NetNGlyc 1.0 server found nine glycosylation motifs in the sequence of AxPDH, five of them putatively glycosylated, and nine for AcPDH with six of them likely to carry a glycan structure. Concerning *O*-glycosylation, NetOGlyc 3.1 server predicted three sites for AcPDH with potential above the threshold and none for AxPDH. The potentially higher degree of *O*-glycosylation of AcPDH compared to AxPDH cannot account for the large difference in glycan mass between the two proteins. The deglycosylation was carried out using PNGase F, which exclusively removes *N*-glycans, and the deglycosylated proteins have a quite similar molecular mass. Furthermore, *O*-glycans in *P. pastoris* mostly consist of up to three, rarely four, mannose units in contrast to hyper-mannosylated *N*-glycans [23]. A substantial over-glycosylation with a comparable glycan content of approximately 30% of protein expressed in *P. pastoris* was also observed for AmPDH [9]. PDH is one of the rare flavoproteins carrying a covalently bound cofactor [24]. Covalent incorporation was proven by the method of Scrutton [25], the flavin associated with the protein gives a fluorescent signal when exposed to UV-light. The positive control (AmPDH), AcPDH and AxPDH showed a bright band under UV-light whereas the negative control glucose oxidase (GOx) from *A. niger* [26] did not give any signal (Figure S2).

UV-Vis spectra of AcPDH and AxPDH in the oxidized state were recorded; typical flavoprotein absorbance maxima around 450 nm and 340 nm could be observed (Figure S3; AxPDH: data not shown).

Figure 3. Native PAGE of purified PDHs. M, molecular marker; 1, AcPDH; 2, AxPDH.

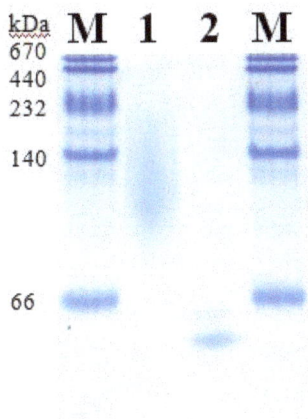

2.6. Kinetic Properties

Catalytic constants for selected sugar substrates and electron acceptors were determined and are summarized in Tables 3 and 4. For both enzymes, D-glucose represents the preferred electron donor. This is mainly due to the K_m value, which displays a more than 10 times higher affinity for this substrate compared to e.g., D-galactose. The pentose sugar D-xylose is the second best substrate for Ac and AxPDH. This finding stands in contrast to the catalytic efficiencies of other so-far characterized PDHs like from *Agaricus meleagris* [5] and the native *A. xanthoderma* PDH [4], where L-arabinose and D-galactose are preferred over D-xylose. The catalytic efficiency of AxPDH with D-xylose is more than 75% of the catalytic efficiency for the main substrate D-glucose, whereas for AcPDH it is only 13%. The k_{cat}/K_m-values of AcPDH are in general lower for all sugar substrates. Remarkable here is that the catalytic efficiencies of Ac and AxPDH are similar for lactose but the K_m of AcPDH is 5.5-times lower than the K_m of AxPDH, whereas the k_{cat} behaves the opposite way.

Table 3. Apparent kinetic constants for selected electron donors determined at 30 °C with 0.2 mM ferrocenium hexafluorophosphate as the electron acceptor.

	AcPDH			AxPDH		
	K_m [mM]	k_{cat} [s^{-1}]	k_{cat}/K_m [mM^{-1} s^{-1}]	K_m [mM]	k_{cat} [s^{-1}]	k_{cat}/K_m [mM^{-1} s^{-1}]
D-glucose	0.35 ± 0.06	4.10 ± 0.19	11.7	0.49 ± 0.03	13.02 ± 0.38	26.6
D-galactose	7.13 ± 0.19	5.23 ± 0.53	0.7	4.99 ± 0.16	24.77 ± 2.23	5.0
D-xylose	4.19 ± 0.26	6.37 ± 0.05	1.5	1.44 ± 0.07	29.16 ± 0.25	20.3
L-arabinose	4.23 ± 0.02	3.05 ± 0.04	0.7	4.16 ± 0.58	22.90 ± 2.23	5.5
Lactose	53.16 ± 0.10	3.12 ± 0.17	0.1	293.84 ± 8.00	24.65 ± 0.37	0.1

Table 4. Apparent kinetic constants for selected electron acceptors determined at 30 °C with 25 mM D-glucose as the electron donor.

	AcPDH			AxPDH		
	K_m [mM]	k_{cat} [s^{-1}]	k_{cat}/K_m [mM^{-1} s^{-1}]	K_m [mM]	k_{cat} [s^{-1}]	k_{cat}/K_m [mM^{-1} s^{-1}]
Fc$^+$PF$_6$ (pH 8.5)	1.19 ± 0.17	19.92 ± 2.87	16.7	0.03 ± 0.00	22.07 ± 0.05	735.7
1,4-BQ (pH 4)	0.12 ± 0.01	34.82 ± 1.02	302.8	3.25 ± 0.51	12.89 ± 1.56	4.0
DCIP (pH 4)	0.11 ± 0.00	10.56 ± 0.57	96.0	0.09 ± 0.01	7.65 ± 0.66	85.0

Concerning the kinetic constants for the electron acceptors, the two enzymes have quite different preferences (Table 4). For AcPDH 1,4-benzoquinone is the favored substrate whereas AxPDH shows a clear preference for ferrocenium hexafluorophosphate. All PDHs that have been characterized to date show a higher catalytic activity with ferrocenium compared to 1,4-benzoquinone; AcPDH is the first PDH where a clear preference for 1,4-benzoquinone was observed [4,5]. The catalytic efficiencies for DCIP are nearly equal for both PDHs. In general, PDH shows activity only with a limited group of electron acceptors whereas it oxidizes a very broad range of sugar substrates. Many major mono- and oligosaccharide components of lignocellulose can be utilized as substrates, giving evidence for the putative biological function of PDH in lignin degradation [7]. Recently, the molecular mechanism of glucose oxidation by *A. meleagris* PDH was explored using MD simulation; the findings support the experimentally observed promiscuity of PDH concerning sugars [27].

The pH dependence of PDH activity was tested for the electron acceptors ferrocenium hexafluorophosphate and 1,4-benzoquinone with D-glucose as the electron donor (Figure 4). Using 1,4-benzoquinone as the electron acceptor, AcPDH displayed maximum activity at pH 7 (phosphate buffer) and already reached 95% activity at pH 5.5 (citrate buffer). AxPDH showed the highest activity at pH 5.5 (citrate buffer). With ferrocenium hexafluorophosphate, the optimum pH for AcPDH was 8.5 and 9 for AxPDH (borate buffer). Compared to the native AxPDH [4], the pH optimum for ferrocenium hexafluorophosphate is comparable but with 1,4-benzoquinone the native AxPDH exhibited highest activity at pH 2.5 and around 70% activity at pH 8. The recombinant AxPDH showed less than 2.5% activity at pH 2.5. In general, it can be observed that the pH optimum is highly dependent on the electron acceptor used. PDHs from *Agaricus* sp. showed pH optima in the basic region when using ferrocenium hexafluorophosphate whereas with 1,4-benzoquinone the enzymes were more active under acidic conditions and in some cases showed a second maximum in the alkaline region, which could be due to high blank readings caused by the formation of quinhydrone [2,4,5].

2.7. Batch Carbohydrate Conversion Experiments

Both enzymes were used for the conversion of 25 mM lactose together with equimolar amounts of the electron acceptor 1,4-benzoquinone in 1 mL batch experiments and the reaction products were analyzed by HPLC (Figure 5). Conversions were carried out in water due to interference of buffer salts with the HPLC analysis. 10 U of AxPDH converted lactose to nearly 100% (97%), producing 69% (67%) lactobionic acid and 31% (30%) 2-dehydrolactose (Figure 5a). Due to the fact that the cultivation yield of AcPDH was quite low, only one unit of the purified protein was used for the conversion experiment. Therefore, only 48% of the lactose was converted and yielded 88% (42%) lactobionic acid and only 12% (6%) 2-dehydrolactose (Figure 5b). These results confirm the preference for C-1 oxidation in AcPDH-catalyzed conversions of lactose (the ratio of C-1 to C-2 oxidation is 7:1), compared to the AxPDH-catalyzed reaction where the ratio of C-1 to C-2 oxidation is only 2:1. C-2,3 oxidation, which can occur when oxidation at C-2 is complete under excess of 1,4-benzoquinone, could not be observed [12]. For industrial use, there is still need for improvement of the conversion yield. Acidification due to spontaneous hydrolysis of lactobionolactone to lactobionic acid slowed down the enzyme activity at the end of the conversion but could be avoided by buffering.

Figure 4. pH optima of AcPDH (black squares) and AxPDH (grey triangles) with the electron acceptors ferrocenium hexafluorophosphate and 1,4-benzoquinone; D-glucose as electron donor.

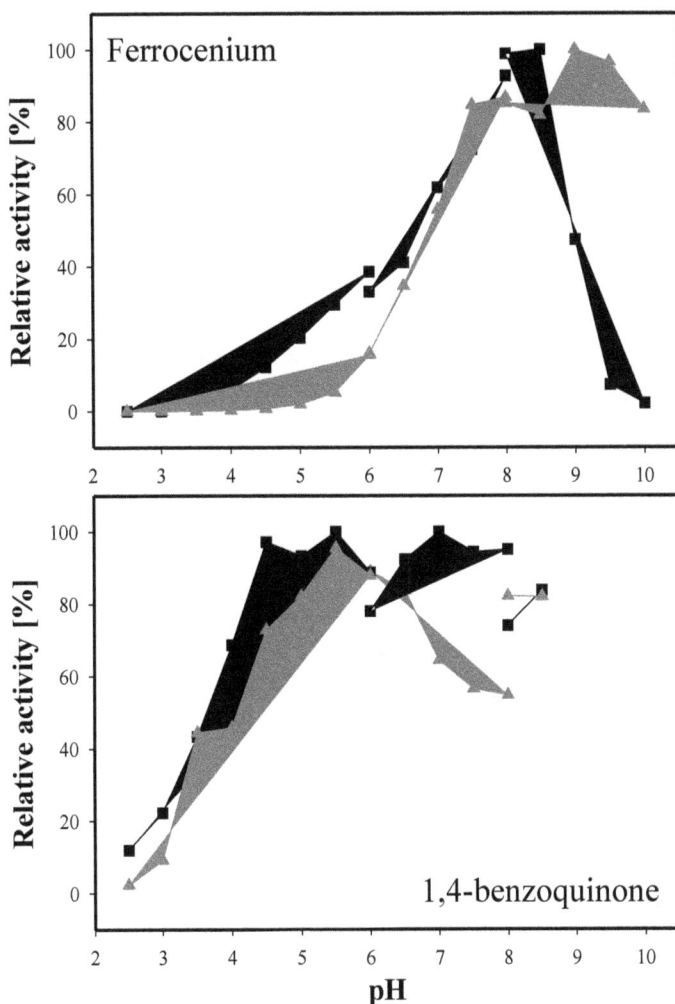

Figure 5. (a) HPLC analysis of lactose conversion by AcPDH; **(b)** and AxPDH at 0 h **(A)**, 1 h **(B)**, 3 h **(C)** and 7 h **(D)** incubation. Peaks: I, residual salt from enzyme preparation; II, lactobionic acid; III, lactose; IV, 2-dehydrolactose.

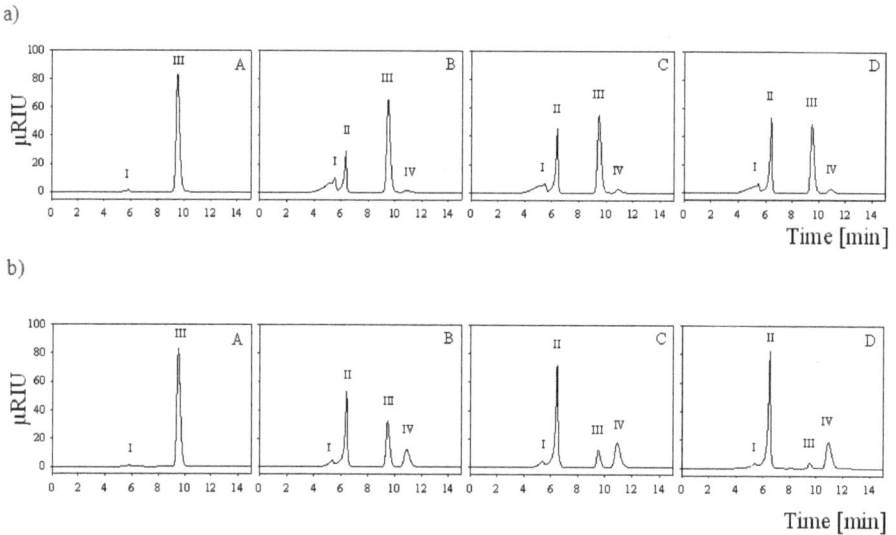

3. Experimental Section

3.1. Chemicals and Microorganisms

All chemicals, sugar standards for HPLC and media components were purchased from Sigma (Steinheim, Germany) unless otherwise stated and were of the highest purity available. Restriction endonucleases, T4 DNA ligase and Phusion High-Fidelity DNA Polymerase were obtained from Fermentas (St. Leon-Rot, Germany) unless otherwise stated and were used according to the manufacturer's instructions. *Agaricus campestris* (strain CCBAS 20649) and *Agaricus xanthoderma* (strain CCBAS 225) were obtained from the Culture Collection of Basidiomycetes of the Academy of Sciences (Prague, Czech Republic). *Escherichia coli* strain NEB5α (New England Biolabs, Ipswich, MA, USA) was used for subcloning, *Pichia pastoris* strain X-33 (Invitrogen, Carlsbad, CA, USA) was used for expression. Ferrocenium hexafluorophosphate and the various substituted quinones were obtained from Aldrich (Steinheim, Germany). Phenyl-Sepharose Fast Flow resin was purchased from Amersham Pharmacia Biotech (Uppsala, Sweden), DEAE Sepharose Fast Flow resin and Sephacryl S300-HR resin were from GE Healthcare (Chalfont St. Giles, UK). GOx from *Aspergillus niger* was from Sigma.

3.2. Isolation of Genomic DNA and RNA

For DNA- and RNA-isolation, approximately 10 mL liquid Sabouraud medium was inoculated with mycelial fragments from freshly grown malt extract agar plates. The cultivations were performed in petri dishes at 25 °C without shaking over 3 weeks. Mycelia were harvested, squeezed dry between filter paper and shock-frozen in liquid nitrogen. Portions of approximately 100 mg of mycelium were used for DNA- and RNA-isolation. Genomic DNA extraction was performed according to Liu *et al.* [28]. Total RNA was extracted using Trizol reagent (Invitrogen) according to the manufacturer's instructions. To remove genomic DNA, the samples were incubated with *DNAseI* as recommended by the manufacturer. The isolated mRNA was reverse-transcribed using RevertAid First Strand cDNA Synthesis kit (Thermo Fisher Scientific, Waltham, MA, USA) and the anchor primer (Table S1).

3.3. Cloning and Sequencing of AcPDH Encoding Gene

Nucleic acid amplifications were done using Phusion High-Fidelity Polymerase, GC-Buffer, dNTP mix, oligonucleotide primers (VBC Biotech, Vienna, Austria) and a BioRad C-1000 thermocycler (BioRad, Vienna, Austria). Nucleotide sequences of all primers used in this work are shown in Table S1. To obtain the PDH-encoding gene from *A. campestris* degenerate primers (AcPDHfwd1-3) were designed according to a sequence analysis of conserved regions in *pdh* genes from *A. meleagris* and *A. bisporus* and used for the amplification of cDNA fragments of various lengths. 35 PCR cycles at temperatures of 98 °C (10 s), 57 °C (20 s) and 72 °C (1 min) and an initial denaturation at 98 °C (2 min) and a final extension at 72 °C (7 min), were employed with cDNA as template and "universal" as reverse primer. The amplicons were purified and sequenced by a commercial sequencing service (LGC Genomics, Berlin, Germany). For identification of the 5' flanking region, including the native signal sequence, the DNA Walking SpeedUp Premix Kit (Seegene, Seoul, South Korea) was used. Target-specific reverse primers (AcTSP1-3) were designed, genomic DNA was used as template and the PCRs were done according to the manufacturer's guidelines. The resulting PCR products were purified by using the illustra GFX PCR DNA and Gel Band Purification Kit (GE Healthcare) and sequenced. To obtain full-length cDNA clones a PCR was performed with the primer pair AcPDHfwd and AcPDHrev and cDNA as template. The resulting fragment was cloned into the pJET1.2 vector (Fermentas) according to the instructions in the manual and sequenced.

3.4. Cloning and Sequencing of AxPDH Encoding Gene

To obtain the 5'- flanking region, including the native signal sequence, the DNA Walking SpeedUp Premix Kit (Seegene) was used. Target-specific reverse primers (AxTSP1-3) were designed according to *A. xanthoderma* PDH gene sequence, genomic DNA was used as template and the PCRs were done according to the manufacturer's guidelines. The resulting PCR products were purified and sequenced. To obtain full-length cDNA clones a PCR was performed with the primer pair AxPDHfwd and AxPDHrev and cDNA as template. The amplified sequence was temporarily cloned into the pJET1.2 vector (Fermentas) according to the instructions in the manual and sequenced.

3.5. Construction of Expression Vectors for P. pastoris

The *acpdh* gene (in the pJET1.2 vector) was re-amplified with the primers AcPDHKpnIfwd and AcPDHNotIrev. The re-amplification of the *axpdh* gene was performed using the primer pair AxKpnIfwd and AxNotIrev. The resulting PCR products were digested with *KpnI* and *NotI* and ligated into the equally treated vector pPICZb (Invitrogen). After transformation into chemically competent *E. coli* NEB5α, according to the manufacturer's instructions, the plasmids were proliferated, linearized with *SacI* and transformed into electrocompetent *P. pastoris*, which were prepared according to Lin-Cereghino *et al.* [29]. For selection the Luria Bertani (LB) medium contained 25 µg mL^{-1} Zeocin in case of *E. coli*, while the YPD-medium contained 100 µg mL^{-1}. The resulting colonies were picked and grown in 96-well deep well plates.

3.6. Microscale Screening for High-Producing PDH Transformants

Microscale cultivation and expression in 96-well deep well plates was done according to Weis *et al.* [30] with some modifications. Cells were grown in 250 µL BMD1 (13.4 g·L^{-1} yeast nitrogen base, 0.4 mg·L^{-1} biotin, 10 g·L^{-1} D-glucose, 200 mM potassium phosphate [pH 6.0]) at 25 °C, 385 rpm and 60% humidity for approximately 60 h to reach the stationary growth phase. Induction was started by the addition of 250 µL of BMM2 medium (13.4 g·L^{-1} yeast nitrogen base, 0.4 mg·L^{-1} biotin, 1% methanol, 200 mM potassium phosphate [pH 6.0]) to reach a final concentration of 0.5% methanol. After 70, 82, and 108 h of incubation, 50 µL BMM10 (BMM2 with 5% methanol) were added to maintain inducing conditions. The cultivation was stopped after 130 h by centrifugation of the deep-well plates at 3000 rpm at room temperature for 20 min. PDH activity was measured using 2,6-dichloroindophenol (DCIP, $\varepsilon520 = 6.8$ mM^{-1} cm^{-1}) as electron acceptor and D-glucose as donor. Fifty µL of the supernatant were transferred to the 96-well screening plates and the time-dependent reduction of 300 µM DCIP in 100 mM sodium acetate buffer pH 4 containing 50 mM D-glucose was followed at 520 nm with a PerkinElmer EnSpire plate reader. The reaction was started by addition of 150 µL of the DCIP assay mixture to the screening plate and end-point measurements were carried out after incubation at 30 °C for 2 and 4 h.

3.7. Sequence Analysis

The translated amino acid sequences of the obtained cDNAs were analyzed using the programs Translate, Compute pI/MW and SignalP at http://www.expasy.org/ [31]. A multiple sequence alignment of AmPDH1, AbPDH, AcPDH and AxPDH was created using the MUSCLE algorithm (EMBL-EBI, Cambridgeshire, UK). Sequence identities were determined by BLAST search [32]. Predictions for *N*- and *O*-glycosylation sites were performed on the NetNGlyc 1.0 Server and the NetOGlyc 3.1 Server [19] of the Center for Biological Sequence Analysis (CBS) at the Technical University of Denmark (http://www.cbs.dtu.dk/services/). All predicted *N*- and *O*-glycosylation sites with a threshold above 0.5 except for Asn-Pro-sites were displayed.

3.8. Nucleotide and Protein Sequence Accession Numbers

The NCBI accession numbers for the sequences in this work are: AY53306, AY753308, DQ117577, AAW82996, AAW82997, AAW82998, AAW82999, AAZ94874, AAZ94875 (*A. meleagris* PDHs); AY764148, AAW92124, EKV41672 (*A. bisporus* PDH); AY764147, AAW92123, KF534751 (*A. xanthoderma* PDH); KF534750 (*A. campestris* PDH).

3.9. Recombinant Protein Production in P. pastoris

AxPDH and AcPDH were produced in a 7-L bioreactor (MBR, Wetzikon, Switzerland) with an initial volume of 4 L basal salts cultivation medium, according to the "*Pichia* Fermentation Process Guidelines" (Invitrogen) with slight modifications. After autoclaving the bioreactor, the temperature was set to 30 °C, the pH was adjusted to 5 and maintained by addition of 28% ammonium hydroxide solution during the cultivation. Dissolved oxygen was regulated to 4% by supplying filtered air and adjusting the stirrer velocity (around 800 rpm). Two shaking flasks with 20 mL YPD-Zeocin medium each were inoculated with the colony-PCR-verified *P. pastoris* clones and grown overnight at 30 °C and 120 rpm. The cultures were transferred to two shaking flasks with 200 mL YPD medium each and again grown overnight at 30 °C and 120 rpm. This culture (400 mL) was used to inoculate the bioreactor. After consumption of the glycerol in the batch medium (indicated by an O_2 spike), a feed of 50% glycerol containing 12 mL L^{-1} PTM1 trace salts was initiated with around 20 mL h^{-1} over night. Protein production was induced by changing to a feed of 100% methanol containing 12 mL PTM1 trace elements per liter. The feed rate was adjusted to maintain a dissolved oxygen concentration of around 4%. Samples were taken at least twice a day and biomass wet weight, PDH activity and total protein concentration was determined. The formation of foam was avoided by daily manual addition of approximately 10 mL a 10% antifoam 204 solution (Sigma). When no further increase in the specific activity could be observed, the bioreactor was harvested and the cultivation broth was centrifuged at 4 °C and 6000 rpm in a Sorvall Evolution RC centrifuge (Thermo Fisher Scientific).

3.10. Protein Purification

Solid ammonium sulfate was added to the cultivation supernatants to a saturation of 40%. The crude extracts (approximately 4 L) were applied to a 750 mL phenyl-sepharose FF column (GE Healthcare), and washed with binding buffer (50 mM potassium phosphate, pH 6.5 containing 1.5 M ammonium sulfate). The protein was eluted using a linear gradient from 0%–100% elution buffer (50 mM potassium phosphate, pH 6.5) in 1 column volume (CV). Prior to the next purification step, the pooled fractions were desalted using cross-flow filtration (SpectrumLabs, Houston, TX, USA) to a conductivity equal to or less than 2 mS/cm. The pools of desalted fractions were loaded to a 60 mL DEAE sepharose column (GE Healthcare), washed with binding buffer (50 mM BisTris, pH 6) and eluted with a linear gradient from 0%–100% elution buffer (50 mM BisTris, 1 M NaCl, pH 6) in 4 column volumes. For AcPDH, the concentrated pool from the anion exchange chromatography was subjected to a second hydrophobic interaction chromatography step using a 70 mL phenyl-source column (GE Healthcare). The purification was conducted similar to the first hydrophobic interaction chromatography step except for the elution of the protein, which was carried out in 5 CV.

The fractions with the highest Ax- and AcPDH activities were pooled and concentrated to a volume of around 2 mL using an Amicon Ultra Centrifugal Filter Unit (EMD Millipore, Billerica, MA, USA). The concentrated pools were applied to a 190 mL Sephacryl S300 gel filtration column (GE healthcare) equilibrated with 50 mM potassium phosphate buffer (pH 7.5) containing 150 mM NaCl. Fractions with the highest purity were pooled, concentrated for buffer exchange (65 mM sodium phosphate buffer, pH 7.5) and stored at 4 °C.

3.11. Enzyme Assay, Molecular Properties

Standard PDH activity was measured by following spectrophotometrically the D-glucose dependent reduction of the ferrocenium ion (Fc+) to ferrocene at 300 nm and 30 °C as described before [4] with modifications: The standard reaction mixture (1 mL) contained 50 μmol sodium phosphate buffer pH 7.5, 0.2 μmol of ferrocenium hexafluorophosphate and 25 μmol D-glucose. Protein concentration was determined using the method of Bradford using a BSA standard curve and a prefabricated assay solution (BioRad). Enzymatic deglycosylation and SDS-PAGE were carried out as described in Sygmund *et al.*, using the Precision Plus Protein Unstained Standard (BioRad) [9]. 1.5–2 μg of the protein samples were loaded in each lane. Native PAGE was performed using 10% and 5% polyacrylamide as the separation and stacking gels, respectively, and Tris-glycine buffer (pH 8.3) as the electrode buffer [33]. 5–10 μg of the protein samples were loaded in each lane. Staining procedure was carried out using Bio-Safe Coomassie (BioRad) according to the manufacturer's instructions. For determination of molecular weight, HMW Native Marker Kit (GE Healthcare) was used. To proof the covalent linkage of the FAD cofactor an additional SDS-PAGE was performed according to Scrutton [25]. 10 μg of the protein samples were loaded in each lane, the covalently linked FAD was visualized by exposure of the gel to UV-light (λ 302 nm, GelDoc2000, BioRad). As a positive control, recombinant *A. meleagris* PDH was loaded [1]; glucose oxidase from *A. niger* was used as a negative control.

Molecular masses of the proteins were calculated from their migration distances on the SDS-PAGE; the theoretical mass was derived from ExPASy ProtParam tool (http://web.expasy.org/protparam/) [31]. The glycan mass in% was calculated from the difference of the masses of the glycosylated and deglycosylated proteins on the SDS-PAGE.

UV-Vis absorbance spectra of 13 μM AcPDH and AxPDH were recorded in 65 mM sodium phosphate buffer pH 7.5 at room temperature using a U-3000 spectrophotometer (Hitachi, Tokyo, Japan) from 300–700 nm.

3.12. Kinetic Properties

Apparent kinetic constants for electron donors were measured using the standard activity assay with ferrocenium hexafluorophosphate as described above. Kinetic constants for ferrocenium hexafluorophosphate, 1,4-benzoquinone and 2,6-dichloroindophenol were determined using 25 mM D-glucose as electron donor. The observed data were fitted to the Michaelis-Menten equation and kinetic constants were calculated by nonlinear least-squares regression. Using the molecular mass, turnover numbers (k_{cat}) and catalytic efficiencies (k_{cat}/K_m) were calculated. The pH optima with the electron acceptors ferrocenium hexafluorophosphate (0.2 mM) and 1,4-benzoquinone (2 mM) were determined with the following buffers: 100 mM citrate (pH 2.5–6), 100 mM potassium phosphate (pH 6–8) and 100 mM borate (pH 8–10) and 25 mM D-glucose as the electron donor. Activities with 1,4-benzoquinone were not determined above pH 8.5 due to the formation of quinhydrone under basic conditions.

3.13. Batch Conversion Experiments

Small-scale lactose conversions were carried out in 1.5 mL Eppendorf vials containing 25 mM 1,4-benzoquinone, 25 mM lactose monohydrate and 1 U of purified AcPDH or 10 U of purified AxPDH in 1 mL deionized water. The vials were incubated at 30 °C and 400 rpm in a thermomixer, samples were taken in regular time intervals (50 μL). Immediately after sampling, PDH activity was stopped by heating the sample to 99 °C for 3 min. The samples were centrifuged, diluted 1:2 and subjected to HPLC analysis.

3.14. HPLC Analysis of Batch Conversion Products

HPLC analysis of the batch conversion products was performed on a Dionex Summit HPLC system (Thermo Fisher Scientific) fitted with a Shodex RI-101 refractive index detector (Shoko Scientific, Yokohama, Japan) using an Aminex HPX 87-K column (BioRad) with a guard column. Samples and standards were eluted at 80 °C with deionized water (0.5 mL min^{-1}). For the calculation of lactose and lactobionic acid concentrations, standards were included in the run. As there was no standard available for 2-dehydrolactose, the ratio of 2-dehydrolactose to lactobionic acid was estimated by comparing the peak areas.

4. Conclusions

This study demonstrates the successful expression of the PDH-encoding genes from the litter-degrading basidiomycetes *A. campestris* and *A. xanthoderma*, in the eukaryotic host organism *P. pastoris*. Small-scale conversion experiments with lactose as substrate revealed that AcPDH has a strong preference for C-1 oxidation, resulting in the production of lactobionic acid. Compared to AxPDH, which produces mixtures of C-2/C-1 oxidation products in a 1:2 ratio, AcPDH is a very attractive biocatalyst for the production of lactobionic acid. Further research towards a better expression yield is required for industrial applications/purposes.

Acknowledgments

The authors thank Cindy Lorenz for technical assistance and performing the HPLC analysis. This work was supported by the Austrian Science Fund FWF (grant P22094 to CKP), IK is a member of the doctoral program BioToP (Biomolecular Technology of Proteins) of the Austrian Science Fund (W1224).

Conflict of Interest

The authors declare no conflict of interest.

104

References

1. Tan, T.C.; Spadiut, O.; Wongnate, T.; Sucharitakul, J.; Krondorfer, I.; Sygmund, C.; Haltrich, D.; Chaiyen, P.; Peterbauer, C.K.; Divne, C. The 1.6 Å crystal structure of pyranose dehydrogenase from *Agaricus meleagris* rationalizes substrate specificity and reveals a flavin intermediate. *PLoS One* **2013**, *8*, e53567.

2. Volc, J.; Kubátová, E.; Wood, D.A.; Daniel, G. Pyranose 2-dehydrogenase, a novel sugar oxidoreductase from the basidiomycete fungus *Agaricus bisporus*. *Arch. Microbiol.* **1997**, *167*, 119–125.

3. Volc, J.; Kubátová, E.; Daniel, G.; Sedmera, P.; Haltrich, D. Screening of basidiomycete fungi for the quinone-dependent sugar C-2/C-3 oxidoreductase, pyranose dehydrogenase, and properties of the enzyme from *Macrolepiota rhacodes*. *Arch. Microbiol.* **2001**, *176*, 178–186.

4. Kujawa, M.; Volc, J.; Halada, P.; Sedmera, P.; Divne, C.; Sygmund, C.; Leitner, C.; Peterbauer, C.; Haltrich, D. Properties of pyranose dehydrogenase purified from the litter-degrading fungus *Agaricus xanthoderma*. *FEBS J.* **2007**, *274*, 879–894.

5. Sygmund, C.; Kittl, R.; Volc, J.; Halada, P.; Kubátová, E.; Haltrich, D.; Peterbauer, C.K. Characterization of pyranose dehydrogenase from *Agaricus meleagris* and its application in the C-2 specific conversion of D-galactose. *J. Biotechnol.* **2008**, *133*, 334–342.

6. Kittl, R.; Sygmund, C.; Halada, P.; Volc, J.; Divne, C.; Haltrich, D.; Peterbauer, C.K. Molecular cloning of three pyranose dehydrogenase-encoding genes from *Agaricus meleagris* and analysis of their expression by real-time RT-PCR. *Curr. Genet.* **2008**, *53*, 117–127.

7. Peterbauer, C.K.; Volc, J. Pyranose dehydrogenases: Biochemical features and perspectives of technological applications. *Appl. Microbiol. Biotechnol.* **2010**, *85*, 837–848.

8. Pisanelli, I.; Kujawa, M.; Gschnitzer, D.; Spadiut, O.; Seiboth, B.; Peterbauer, C. Heterologous expression of an *Agaricus meleagris* pyranose dehydrogenase-encoding gene in *Aspergillus* spp. and characterization of the recombinant enzyme. *Appl. Microbiol. Biotechnol.* **2010**, *86*, 599–606.

9. Sygmund, C.; Gutmann, A.; Krondorfer, I.; Kujawa, M.; Glieder, A.; Pscheidt, B.; Haltrich, D.; Peterbauer, C.; Kittl, R. Simple and efficient expression of *Agaricus meleagris* pyranose dehydrogenase in *Pichia pastoris*. *Appl. Microbiol. Biotechnol.* **2012**, *94*, 695–704.

10. Volc, J.; Sedmera, P.; Halada, P.; Přikrylová, V.; Daniel, G. C-2 and C-3 oxidation of D-glc, and C-2 oxidation of D-gal by pyranose dehydrogenase from *Agaricus bisporus*. *Carbohydr. Res.* **1998**, *310*, 151–156.

11. Volc, J.; Sedmera, P.; Halada, P.; Prikrylová, V.; Haltrich, D. Double oxidation of D-xylose to D-glycero-pentos-2,3-diulose (2,3-diketo-D-xylose) by pyranose dehydrogenase from the mushroom *Agaricus bisporus*. *Carbohydr. Res.* **2000**, *329*, 219–225.

12. Volc, J.; Sedmera, P.; Kujawa, M.; Halada, P.; Kubátová, E.; Haltrich, D. Conversion of lactose to β-D-galactopyranosyl-(1→4)-D-arabino-hexos-2-ulose-(2-dehydrolactose) and lactobiono-1,5-lactone by fungal pyranose dehydrogenase. *J. Mol. Catal. B Enzym.* **2004**, *30*, 177–184.

13. Sedmera, P.; Halada, P.; Peterbauer, C.; Volc, J. A new enzyme catalysis: 3,4-dioxidation of some aryl β-D-glycopyranosides by fungal pyranose dehydrogenase. *Tetrahedron. Lett.* **2004**, *45*, 8677–8680.

14. Sedmera, P.; Halada, P.; Kubátová, E.; Haltrich, D.; Přikrylová, V.; Volc, J. New biotransformations of some reducing sugars to the corresponding (di)dehydro(glycosyl) aldoses or aldonic acids using fungal pyranose dehydrogenase. *J. Mol. Catal. B Enzym.* **2006**, *41*, 32–42.

15. Haltrich, D.; Leitner, C.; Neuhauser, W.; Nidetzky, B.; Kulbe, K.D.; Volc, J. A convenient enzymatic procedure for the production of aldose-free D-tagatose. *Ann. N. Y. Acad. Sci.* **1998**, *864*, 295–299.

16. Leitner, C.; Neuhauser, W.; Volc, J.; Kulbe, K.D.; Nidetzky, B.; Haltrich, D. The cetus process revisited: A novel enzymatic alternative for the production of aldose-free D-fructose. *Biocatal. Biotransform.* **1998**, *16*, 365–382.

17. Gutiérrez, L.F.; Hamoudi, S.; Belkacemi, K. Lactobionic acid: A high value-added lactose derivative for food and pharmaceutical applications. *Int. Dairy J.* **2012**, *26*, 103–111.

18. Schuster-Wolff-Bühring, R.; Fischer, L.; Hinrichs, J. Production and physiological action of the disaccharide lactulose. *Int. Dairy J.* **2010**, *20*, 731–741.

19. Julenius, K.; Mølgaard, A.; Gupta, R.; Brunak, S. Prediction, conservation analysis, and structural characterization of mammalian mucin-type o-glycosylation sites. *Glycobiology* **2005**, *15*, 153–164.

20. Berends, E.; Ohm, R.A.; de Jong, J.F.; Rouwendal, G.; Wösten, H.A.B.; Lugones, L.G.; Bosch, D. Genomic and biochemical analysis of *N* glycosylation in the mushroom-forming basidiomycete *Schizophyllum commune*. *Appl. Environ. Microbiol.* **2009**, *75*, 4648–4652.

21. Gemmill, T.R.; Trimble, R.B. Overview of *N*- and *O*-linked oligosaccharide structures found in various yeast species. *Biochim. Biophys. Acta* **1999**, *1426*, 227–237.

22. Wilson, I.B.; Zeleny, R.; Kolarich, D.; Staudacher, E.; Stroop, C.J.; Kamerling, J.P.; Altmann, F. Analysis of asn-linked glycans from vegetable foodstuffs: Widespread occurrence of lewis a, core alpha1,3-linked fucose and xylose substitutions. *Glycobiology* **2001**, *11*, 261–274.

23. Duman, J.G.; Miele, R.G.; Liang, H.; Grella, D.K.; Sim, K.L.; Castellino, F.J.; Bretthauer, R.K. *O*-mannosylation of *Pichia pastoris* cellular and recombinant proteins. *Biotechnol. Appl. Biochem.* **1998**, *28*, 39–45.

24. Heuts, D.P.H.M.; Scrutton, N.S.; McIntire, W.S.; Fraaije, M.W. What's in a covalent bond? On the role and formation of covalently bound flavin cofactors. *FEBS J.* **2009**, *276*, 3405–3427.

25. Scrutton, S. Identification of Covalent Flavoproteins and Analysis of the Covalent Link. In *Methods in Molecular Biology: Flavoprotein Protocols*; Chapman, K., Reid, A., Eds.; Humana Press Inc.: Totowa, NJ, USA, 1999; Volume 131, pp. 181–193.

26. Hecht, H.J.; Kalisz, H.M.; Hendle, J.; Schmid, R.D.; Schomburg, D. Crystal structure of glucose oxidase from *Aspergillus niger* refined at 2.3 å resolution. *J. Mol. Biol.* **1993**, *229*, 153–172.

27. Graf, M.M.; Bren, U.; Haltrich, D.; Oostenbrink, C. Molecular dynamics simulations give insight into D-glucose dioxidation at C2 and C3 by *Agaricus meleagris* pyranose dehydrogenase. *J. Comput. Aided Mol. Des.* **2013**, *27*, 295–304.

28. Liu, D.; Coloe, S.; Baird, R.; Pedersen, J. Rapid mini-preparation of fungal DNA for PCR. *J. Clin. Microbiol.* **2000**, *38*, 471.

29. Lin-Cereghino, J.; Wong, W.W.; Xiong, S.; Giang, W.; Luong, L.T.; Vu, J.; Johnson, S.D.; Lin-Cereghino, G.P. Condensed protocol for competent cell preparation and transformation of the methylotrophic yeast *Pichia pastoris*. *BioTechniques* **2005**, *38*, 44–48.

30. Weis, R.; Luiten, R.; Skranc, W.; Schwab, H.; Wubbolts, M.; Glieder, A. Reliable high-throughput screening with *Pichia pastoris* by limiting yeast cell death phenomena. *FEMS Yeast Res.* **2004**, *5*, 179–189.

31. Artimo, P.; Jonnalagedda, M.; Arnold, K.; Baratin, D.; Csardi, G.; de Castro, E.; Duvaud, S.; Flegel, V.; Fortier, A.; Gasteiger, E.; *et al.* Expasy: Sib bioinformatics resource portal. *Nucleic Acids Res.* **2012**, *40*, W597–W603.

32. Altschul, S.F.; Madden, T.L.; Schäffer, A.A.; Zhang, J.; Zhang, Z.; Miller, W.; Lipman, D.J. Gapped blast and psi-blast: A new generation of protein database search programs. *Nucleic Acids Res.* **1997**, *25*, 3389–3402.

33. Laemmli, U.K. Cleavage of structural proteins during the assembly of the head of bacteriophage t4. *Nature* **1970**, *227*, 680–685.

Carbonic Anhydrases and Their Biotechnological Applications

Christopher D. Boone, Andrew Habibzadegan, Sonika Gill and Robert McKenna

Abstract: The carbonic anhydrases (CAs) are mostly zinc-containing metalloenzymes which catalyze the reversible hydration/dehydration of carbon dioxide/bicarbonate. The CAs have been extensively studied because of their broad physiological importance in all kingdoms of life and clinical relevance as drug targets. In particular, human CA isoform II (HCA II) has a catalytic efficiency of 10^8 M^{-1} s^{-1}, approaching the diffusion limit. The high catalytic rate, relatively simple procedure of expression and purification, relative stability and extensive biophysical studies of HCA II has made it an exciting candidate to be incorporated into various biomedical applications such as artificial lungs, biosensors and CO_2 sequestration systems, among others. This review highlights the current state of these applications, lists their advantages and limitations, and discusses their future development.

Reprinted from *Biomolecules*. Cite as: Boone, C.D.; Habibzadegan, A.; Gill, S.; McKenna, R. Carbonic Anhydrases and Their Biotechnological Applications. *Biomolecules* **2013**, *3*, 553-562.

1. Introduction

Three analogous families of carbonic anhydrases (CA) exist within nature: α-CAs (predominant within animals), β-CAs (predominant within plants), and the γ-CAs (predominant within Archaea) [1–5]. In total, there are 15 human α-CA isoforms, all of which differ in their catalytic rates, inhibitor sensitivity and selectivity, cellular localization and tissue distribution [1,6,7]. The 12 catalytically active human isoforms (HCAI–VA, VB–VII, IX, XII–XIV) exhibit a wide range of catalytic efficiencies ($k_{cat}/K_M = 10^3-10^8$ M^{-1} s^{-1}). The acatalytic human CA-related proteins (HCA-RPs VIII, X and XI) are inactive due to the evolutionarily loss of one or more of the zinc-coordinating histidine residues, leading to loss of the zinc metal from the active site [1,8].

CAs are involved in various physiological roles fluid secretion, acid/base balance and thus pH regulation, gluconeogenesis, ureagenesis, gastric acid production, and transport of CO_2 from tissues to the lungs (in the form of bicarbonate) through blood [4,9,10]. CO_2 released as a part of respiration by tissues is not very soluble in blood and thus, in order to be transported, is converted to HCO_3^- by HCA II. Furthermore, the role of CA in diseases such as glaucoma has long been known. Over secretion of aqueous humor in the eye causes increased intra-ocular pressures consequently leading to a condition called glaucoma. Reduction in CA activity decreases the secretion of HCO_3^- and aqueous humor, thereby reducing the pressure [1,7,11,12].

The best characterized of these enzymes is HCA II, found within the cytosol of many cells and organs [9,13–15]. Known to possess a remarkably high catalytic efficiency, with a k_{cat} of 1.4×10^6 s^{-1} and a k_{cat}/K_M of 1.5×10^8 $M^{-1}s^{-1}$ [6,16,17], HCA II aids in the conversion of water and carbon dioxide into bicarbonate and a proton through a two-step ping pong mechanism:

$$H_2O$$

$$\text{E:Zn-OH}^- + \text{CO}_2 \rightleftarrows \text{E:Zn-H}_2\text{O} + \text{HCO}_3^- \qquad\qquad \text{(reaction 1)}$$

$$\text{E:Zn-H}_2\text{O} + \text{B} \rightleftarrows \text{E:ZnOH}^- + \text{BH}^+ \qquad\qquad \text{(reaction 2)}$$

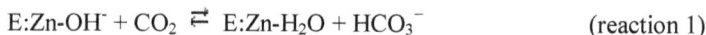

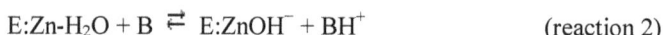

In the hydration direction shown, in the first step the zinc-bound hydroxide acts as a nucleophile, attacking the carbon dioxide and ultimately forming bicarbonate. This leads to a water molecule bound to the zinc (reaction 1). The second step (reaction 2) regenerates the zinc-bound hydroxide through a proton transfer mechanism via His64 in HCA II [18] to solvent, B [19–22].

This review will discuss the current state of utilizing HCA II in the biomedical field to aid in the development of an artificial lung system, as a biosensor for trace elements in complex media and in CO_2 sequestration among confined spaces, followed by a short discussion on other systems. HCA II is a particularly attractive candidate for these applications because of its relatively high stability [23], ability to be expressed in large quantities from *E. coli* [24], and the relatively easy purification from either affinity or conventional chromatography [25,26]. Additionally, the available high-resolution X-ray and medium neutron crystallographic structures of HCA II [27–30] allow for the rational engineering via site-directed mutagenesis for enhanced catalytic activity [31,32] and stability [33–35] for various industrial [36,37] and medical [1,38–40] applications.

2. Artificial Lungs

One of the current prevailing health problems within the United States is respiratory failure [41]. A common treatment for this condition is the utilization of mechanical ventilators [42]. Unfortunately, these ventilators can create many problems for patients who are treated with them, including decreased lung efficacy because of over-pressurized or over-distended lung tissue [43]. An artificial lung is a device capable of assisting with respiration without input from the lungs. This technology could supersede ventilators in treating respiratory failure. There are still many challenges facing this new technology, however, that must be dealt with before artificial lungs replace mechanical ventilators [44].

As of now, the main issue preventing effective artificial lungs concerns inadequate transfer of CO_2 per square inch across the polymetric hollow fiber membranes (HFM) present within this technology. Currently, a 1–2 m^2 surface area is required to sufficiently transfer CO_2 through the membrane [45–48]. A surface area of this size lacks the practicalities of functioning effectively within the human body [49,50]. One way that has been effective at increasing the transfer of CO_2 lies in immobilizing CA onto the HFM. The enzyme, dissolved in a phosphate buffer, is added to the surface of the HFM. Cyanogen bromide within acetonitrile activates the HFM, allowing covalent bonds to form between CA and the HFM. Transfer rates of CO_2 measured with CA treated compared to untreated HFM show a 75% higher rate of CO_2 removal rate present in with the treated HFM. This finding indicates the possibilities for smaller artificial lungs to be engineered with CA incorporation, which could function effectively within the human body [51].

Another method that has been shown to also increase CO_2 transfer across the HFM of artificial lungs relies on impeller devices that increase the rate of blood mixing. Unfortunately, this method cannot be combined with the CA method at this time. When these two methods were combined, the shear forces of the impeller device denatured CA, leading to a loss of enzyme function. This creates the need for a more stable form of CA that will not be denatured by the shear forces. If such a stable CA variant can be engineered, these methods might be combined, which could lead to smaller more efficient artificial lungs [52].

3. Biosensors

Quantification of trace analytes in complex media containing chemically similar molecules is lacking in many traditional chemical systems. As such, the development of sensors based on biological molecules, termed biosensors, can achieve such specificity and sensitivity [53]. The high affinity of HCA II for zinc (4 pM) [54] has been used to quantify trace amounts of zinc in sea and waste water [55] for concerns over toxicity to certain plants, invertebrates and fish [56,57]. Optimally, this biosensor would operate along the sea bed and relay a fluorescence signal up to the ocean surface that is released upon binding of a strong inhibitor, dansylamide, upon binding of zinc in the active site of apo-CA [58]. However, the slow dissociation rate of zinc from the CA active site ($t_{1/2} \approx 90$ days [54]) limits the reusability and efficiency of the system. The relative abundance of natural zinc in the environment compared to that of the binding affinity also limits the production of apo-HCA II [23]. As such, an HCA II variant (E117Q) that contained both a lowered binding affinity (nM) and a much faster dissociation time ($t_{1/2} \approx 3$ sec) for zinc was developed to circumvent these limitations [59]. Other studies have aimed to improve the fluorescence signaling upon zinc binding in the active site of HCA II via incorpororation of the H36C variant, which then selectively labeled with a thiol-reactive fluorophore [60] that would interact upon ligation of an inhibitor, azosulfonamide, acting as a fluorescence acceptor [61].

Other metals that bind to HCA II consist primarily of transition metals in the +2 oxidation state, which include: Cd^{2+}, Co^{2+}, Cu^{2+}, Hg^{2+}, Fe^{2+}, Mn^{2+}, Ni^{2+}, Pb^{2+} and In^{3+} [53,54,60,62]. However, only the binding affinity of HCA II for Cu^{2+} and Hg^{2+} is greater than that of Zn^{2+} [54], so variants with a lowered binding affinity for these metals would have to be developed before detection of other metals is feasible. Sulfonamide inhibitors, however, do not bind tightly to CA with metals other than Zn^{2+} or Co^{2+} bound in the active site [63], promoting the need for a novel development of metal ligation. This limitation can been superseded because several of these divalent ions (Cu^{2+}, Co^{2+} and Ni^{2+}) exhibit weak d-d absorbance bands in the visible regions that can be directly measured via fluorescence energy transfer lifetimes [60]. This can be extended to the other metals that do not exhibit d-d absorbance bands, (Hg^{2+} and Cd^{2+}) since the binding of these metals to apo-CA causes a quenching of the fluorescence of an active site fluorophore [64]. Since biologically prevalent divalent metals such as Mg^{2+} and Ca^{2+} do not bind to CA and interfere with the assay, biosensors employed in biomedical applications are especially useful [65–70].

4. CO$_2$ Sequestration

Elevated CO_2 levels in the human body have detrimental effects ranging from impaired judgment to death. CO_2 control is important in confined spaces where there is little buffering ability to absorb this gas, such as spacecraft or submarines. These life support systems employ a small amount of CA dissolved in thin aqueous buffered films and compressed between porous polypropylene

110

membranes [71]. The concentrations of CO_2 commonly experienced in these systems (~0.1% v/v) are ideal for selective capture by CA. Analysis of the produced (scrubbed) gas shows that the CA-containing setup selectively lets N_2 and O_2 through, with ratios of 1400:1 and 900:1, respectively [71,72]. The relatively low concentration of CO_2 readily dissolves in the thin layer of enzyme containing buffer and across the membrane, where it is removed via vacuum or carrier gas. Engineered CA-based bioreactors outperformed chemical methods using diethylamine solutions, with much higher selectivity, 400:1 and 300:1 for N_2 and O_2, respectively [72]. In addition, the presence of CA increased CO_2 transport across the polypropylene membrane by ~70% [71]. Another benefit of these CA-bioreactor systems is that they are very efficient at ambient pressures and temperatures [72], improving overall cost-efficiency. However, the longevity of the systems has raised concerns as the need to keep the membranes wet, or at least humid, will add cost and operational difficulties to their practical use.

5. Pharmalogical Considerations

CAs have been employed in CO_2-responsive cationic hydrogels in antidote delivery to treat analgesic overdose without losing therapeutic levels of drug [73]. Alternate medicines, such as opioids, have very potent analgesic effects but overdoses can cause respiratory hypoventilation, which leads to increased CO_2 and decreased O_2 levels in the body ultimately leading to an acidosis-induced death. The CA treatment involves a feedback-regulated antidote delivery system that responds to high CO_2 levels or decrease in pH [73]. The cationic hydrogel is based on N,N-dimethylaminoethyl methacrylate (DMAEMA) polymers that have modified to have a pK_a ~ 7.5, which makes it an adequate blood pH monitor. Incorporation of CA as a CO_2 sensor improved the efficiency of these antidote-delivery systems [73]. Other hydrogels have been designed with a switchable co-block polymer can undergo a transition change from gel to sol upon exposure to CO_2 [74]. This study demonstrates that stimuli-triggered drug delivery could be incorporated with CAs utilizing CO_2, bicarbonate or pH changes as signaling molecules.

High-resolution X-ray [75,76] and neutron structures [29] of HCA II in complex with acetazolamide (Diamox), a tight binding inhibitor used in the treatment of glaucoma [12,77], has accelerated research into structural-based rational design of an isozyme specific inhibitor. Current research interest includes specific inhibition of HCA IX, which has been shown to be overexpressed in a wide array of cancer cell lines [11,39,78–80]. In short, tumor cells proliferate in acidic environments which could be presumably due to the catalytic activity of HCA IX on the cell surface. Selective inhibition of HCA IX could provide a means for targeted tumor eradication. A suitable drug candidate has not been discovered as of yet, but an impressive library of inhibitors designed from different functional groups with varying binding affinities and specificities for various CA isoforms has been steadily growing with entries and has been summarized elsewhere [2,10,38,40,81,82].

6. Blood Substitutes

A continual source of blood is required for use in trauma injuries or major surgeries, and, as natural blood is often in limited supply, there has been progress in the development of blood substitutes which primarily consist of 4–5 cross-linked stroma-free hemoglobin (polySFHb) molecules [83]. The major drawback of these substitutes, however, was the inadequate CO_2 removal rates. Increased CO_2 levels in the body leads to acidosis, and if left untreated will end up in coma and death [9]. Incorporation of catalase (CAT), superoxide dismutase (SOD) and CA to the PolySFHb substitute (PolySFHb-SOD-CAT-CA) was introduced to overcome this limitation with encouraging activity [84]. Blood substitutes have also been shown to be advantageous over transfused whole blood in that they can be sterilized, stored for long periods and contains no blood antigens [83].

7. Conclusions

The various aforementioned biotechnological aspects of the different CA-associated systems emphasize the usefulness of this enzyme. The advancement of fast and cost-effective genome sequencing, molecular biology techniques that boost overexpression of protein and direct evolution techniques that can select for highly active and stable CAs provide an optimistic view as to the advancement in the efficiency and selectivity in current systems. It is also likely that further developments in these fields will lead to novel biomedical applications of CAs.

Conflict of Interest

The authors declare no conflict of interest.

References

1. Aggarwal, M.; Boone, C.D.; Kondeti, B.; McKenna, R. Structural annotation of human carbonic anhydrases. *J. Enzyme Inhib. Med. Chem.* **2013**, *28*, 267–277.
2. Krishnamurthy, V.M.; Kaufman, G.K.; Urbach, A.R.; Gitlin, I.; Gudiksen, K.L.; Weibel, D.B.; Whitesides, G.M. Carbonic anhydrase as a model for biophysical and physical-organic studies of proteins and protein-ligand binding. *Chem. Rev.* **2008**, *108*, 946–1051.
3. Rowlett, R.S. Structure and catalytic mechanism of the beta-carbonic anhydrases. *Biochim. Biophy. Acta* **2010**, *1804*, 362–373.
4. Supuran, C.T. Carbonic anhydrases—An overview. *Curr. Pharm. Des.* **2008**, *14*, 603–614.
5. Hewett-Emmett, D.; Tashian, R.E. Functional diversity, conservation, and convergence in the evolution of the alpha-, beta-, and gamma-carbonic anhydrase gene families. *Mol. Phylogenetics Evolut.* **1996**, *5*, 50–77.
6. Lindskog, S. Structure and mechanism of carbonic anhydrase. *Pharmacol. Ther.* **1997**, *74*, 1–20.
7. Alterio, V.; Di Fiore, A.; D'Ambrosio, K.; Supuran, C.T.; de Simone, G. Multiple binding modes of inhibitors to carbonic anhydrases: How to design specific drugs targeting 15 different isoforms? *Chem. Rev.* **2012**, *112*, 4421–4468.
8. Bergenhem, N.C.; Hallberg, M.; Wisén, S. Molecular characterization of the human carbonic anhydrase-related protein (hca-rp viii). *Biochim. Biophy. Acta* **1998**, *1384*, 294–298.

9. Sly, W.S.; Hu, P.Y. Human carbonic anhydrases and carbonic anhydrase deficiencies. *Annu. Rev. Biochem.* **1995**, *64*, 375–401.

10. Supuran, C.T.; Scozzafava, A. Carbonic anhydrases as targets for medicinal chemistry. *Bioorganic Med. Chem.* **2007**, *15*, 4336–4350.

11. Pastorekova, S.; Parkkila, S.; Pastorek, J.; Supuran, C.T. Carbonic anhydrases: Current state of the art, therapeutic applications and future prospects. *J. Enzyme Inhib. Med. Chem.* **2004**, *19*, 199–229.

12. Aggarwal, M.; McKenna, R. Update on carbonic anhydrase inhibitors: A patent review (2008–2011). *Expert Opin. Ther. Pat.* **2012**, *22*, 903–915.

13. Chegwidden, W.R.; Carter, N.D. Introduction to the Carbonic Anhydrases. In *The Carbonic Anhdyrases: New horizons*; Chegwidden, W.R., Carter, N.D., Edwards, Y.H., Eds.; Birkhäuser Verlag: Boston, MA, USA, 2000; pp. 13–29.

14. Christianson, D.W.; Fierke, C.A. Carbonic anhydrase: Evolution of the zinc binding site by nature and design. *Acc. Chem. Res.* **1996**, *29*, 331–339.

15. Duda, D.; McKenna, R. Carbonic Anhydrase, α-class. In *Handbook of Metalloproteins*; Messerschmidt, A., Ed.; John Wiley & Sons: New York, NY, USA, 2004; pp. 249–263.

16. Lindskog, S.; Coleman, J.E. Catalytic mechanism of carbonic-anhydrase. *Proc. Natl. Acad. Sci. USA* **1973**, *70*, 2505–2508.

17. Lindskog, S.; Silverman, D.N. The Catalytic Mechanism of Mammalian Carbonic Anhydrases. In *The Carbonic Anhdyrases: New Horizons*; Chegwidden, W.R., Carter, N.D., Edwards, Y.H., Eds.; Birkhäuser Verlag: Boston, MA, USA, 2000; pp. 175–195.

18. Tu, C.K.; Silverman, D.N.; Forsman, C.; Jonsson, B.H.; Lindskog, S. Role of histidine 64 in the catalytic mechanism of human carbonic anhydrase ii studied with a site-specific mutant. *Biochemistry* **1989**, *28*, 7913–7918.

19. Mikulski, R.L.; Silverman, D.N. Proton transfer in catalysis and the role of proton shuttles in carbonic anhydrase. *Biochim. Biophy. Acta* **2010**, *1804*, 422–426.

20. Silverman, D.N. Carbonic anhydrase: Oxygen-18 exchange catalyzed by an enzyme with rate-contributing proton-transfer steps. *Methods Enzymol.* **1982**, *87*, 732–752.

21. Silverman, D.N.; Lindskog, S. The catalytic mechanism of carbonic anhydrase: Implications of a rate-limiting protolysis of water. *Acc. Chem. Res.* **1988**, *21*, 30–36.

22. Silverman, D.N.; McKenna, R. Solvent-mediated proton transfer in catalysis by carbonic anhydrase. *Acc. Chem. Res.* **2007**, *40*, 669–675.

23. Avvaru, B.S.; Busby, S.A.; Chalmers, M.J.; Griffin, P.R.; Venkatakrishnan, B.; Agbandje-McKenna, M.; Silverman, D.N.; McKenna, R. Apo-human carbonic anhdrase II revisited: Implications of the loss of a metal in protein structure, stability, and solvent network. *Biochemistry* **2009**, *48*, 7365–7372.

24. Murakami, H.; Marelich, G.P.; Grubb, J.H.; Kyle, J.W.; Sly, W.S. Cloning, expression, and sequence homologies of cdna for human carbonic anhydrase II. *Genomics* **1987**, *1*, 159–166.

25. Krebs, J.F.; Fierke, C.A. Determinants of catalytic activity and stability of carbonic anhydrase II as revealed by random mutagenesis. *J. Biol. Chem.* **1993**, *268*, 27458–27466.

26. Osborne, W.R.; Tashian, R.E. An improved method for the purification of carbonic anhydrase isozymes by affinity chromatography. *Anal. Biochem.* **1975**, *64*, 297–303.

27. Avvaru, B.S.; Kim, C.U.; Sippel, K.H.; Gruner, S.M.; Agbandje-McKenna, M.; Silverman, D.N.; McKenna, R. A short, strong hydrogen bond in the active site of human carbonic anhydrase II. *Biochemistry* **2010**, *49*, 249–251.

28. Eriksson, A.E.; Jones, T.A.; Liljas, A. Refined structure of human carbonic anhydrase II at 2.0 a resolution. *Proteins* **1988**, *4*, 274–282.

29. Fisher, S.Z.; Aggarwal, M.; Kovalesky, A.; Silverman, D.N.; McKenna, R. Neutron-diffraction of acetazolamide-bound human carbonic anhydrase II reveals atomic details of drug binding. *J. Am. Chem. Soc.* **2012**, *134*, 14726–14729.

30. Fisher, S.Z.; Kovalevsky, A.Y.; Domsic, J.F.; Mustyakimov, M.; McKenna, R.; Silverman, D.N.; Langan, P.A. Neutron structure of human carbonic anhydrase II: Implications for proton transfer. *Biochemistry* **2010**, *49*, 415–421.

31. Fisher, S.Z.; Tu, C.; Bhatt, D.; Govindasamy, L.; Agbandje-McKenna, M.; McKenna, R.; Silverman, D.N. Speeding up proton transfer in a fast enzyme: Kinetic and crystallographic studies on the effect of hydrophobic amino acid substitutions in the active site of human carbonic anhydrase ii. *Biochemistry* **2007**, *46*, 3803–3813.

32. Mikulski, R.; West, D.; Sippel, K.H.; Avvaru, B.S.; Aggarwal, M.; Tu, C.; McKenna, R.; Silverman, D.N. Water networks in fast proton transfer during catalysis by human carbonic anhydrase ii. *Biochemistry* **2013**, *52*, 125–131.

33. Fisher, Z.; Boone, C.D.; Biswas, S.M.; Venkatakrishnan, B.; Aggarwal, M.; Tu, C.; Agbandje-McKenna, M.; Silverman, D.; McKenna, R. Kinetic and structural characterization of thermostabilized mutants of human carbonic anhydrase ii. *Protein Eng. Des. Sel. PEDS* **2012**, *25*, 347–355.

34. Mårtensson, L.-G.; Karlsson, M.; Carlsson, U. Dramatic stabilization of the native state of human carbonic anhydrase ii by an engineered disulfide bond. *Biochemistry* **2002**, *41*, 15867–15875.

35. Boone, C.D.; Habibzadegan, A.; Tu, C.; Silverman, D.N.; McKenna, R. Structural and catalytic characterization of a thermally stable and acid-stable variant of human carbonic anhydrase II containing an engineered disulfide bond. *Acta Crystallogr. Sect. D Biol. Crystallogr.* **2013**, *69*, 1414–1422.

36. Boone, C.D.; Gill, S.; Habibzadegan, A.; McKenna, R. Carbonic anhydrases and their industrial applications. *Curr. Top. Biochem. Res.* **2013**, *14*, 1–10.

37. Christianson, D.W.; Fierke, C.A. Carbonic anhydrase: Evolution of the zinc binding site by nature and by design. *Acc. Chem. Res.* **1996**, *29*, 331–339.

38. Supuran, C.T. Carbonic anhydrase inhibitors. *Bioorganic Med. Chem. Lett.* **2010**, *20*, 3467–3474.

39. Supuran, C.T. Inhibition of carbonic anhydrase ix as a novel anticancer mechanism. *World J. Clin. Oncol.* **2012**, *3*, 98–103.

40. Supuran, C.T. Carbonic anhydrases: Novel therapeutic applications for inhibitors and activators. *Nat. Rev. Drug Discov.* **2008**, *7*, 168–181.

41. Ware, L.B.; Matthay, M.A. The acute respiratory distress syndrome. *N. Engl. J. Med.* **2000**, *342*, 1334–1349.

42. Esteban, A.; Anzueto, A.; Frutos, F.; Alia, I.; Brochard, L.; Stewart, T.E.; Benito, S.; Epstein, S.K.; Apezteguia, C.; Nightingale, P.; *et al.* Characteristics and outcomes in adult patients receiving mechanical ventilation: A 28-day international study. *JAMA* **2002**, *287*, 345–355.

43. Maggiore, S.M.; Richard, J.C.; Brochard, L. What has been learnt from p/v curves in patients with acute lung injury/acute respiratory distress syndrome. *Eur. Respir. J.* **2003**, *22*, 22s–26s.

44. Haft, J.W.; Griffith, B.P.; Hirschl, R.B.; Bartlett, R.H. Results of an artificial-lung survey to lung transplant program directors. *J. Heart Lung Transplant.* **2002**, *21*, 467–473.

45. Hattler, B.G.; Federspiel, W.J. Gas Exchange in the Venous System: Support for the Failing Lung. In *The Artificial Lung*; Vaslef, S.N., Anderson, R.W., Eds.; Landes Bioscience: Georgetown, DC, USA, 2002; pp. 133–174.

46. Wegner, J.A. Oxygenator anatomy and function. *J. Cardiothorac. Vasc. Anesth.* **1997**, *11*, 275–281.

47. Federspiel, W.J.; Henchir, K.A. Artificial Lungs: Basic Principles and Current Applications. In *Encyclopedia of Biomaterials and Biomedical Engineering*; Wnek, G.E., Bowlin, G.L., Eds.; Marcel Dekker, Inc: New York, NY, USA, 2004; pp. 922–931.

48. Beckley, P.D.; Holt, D.W.; Tallman, R.D. Oxygenators for Extracorporeal Circulation. In *Cardiopulmonary Bypass: Principles and Techniques of Extracorporeal Circulation*; Mora, C.T., Ed.; Springer-Verlag: New York, NY, USA, 1995; pp. 199–219.

49. Okamoto, T.; Tashiro, M.; Sakanashi, Y.; Tanimoto, H.; Imaizumi, T.; Sugita, M.; Terasaki, H. A new heparin-bonded dense membrane lung combined with minimal systemic heparinization prolonged extracorporeal lung assist in goats. *Artif. Organs* **1998**, *22*, 864–872.

50. Watnabe, H.; Hayashi, J.; Ohzeki, H.; Moro, H.; Sugawara, M.; Eguchi, S. Biocompatibility of a silicone-coated polypropylene hollow fiber oxygenator in an in vitro model. *Ann. Thorac. Surg.* **1999**, *67*, 1315–1319.

51. Kaar, J.L.; Oh, H.-I.; Russell, A.J.; Federspiel, W.J. Towards improved artificial lungs through biocatalysis. *Biomaterials* **2007**, *28*, 3131–3139.

52. Arazawa, D.T.; Oh, H.-I.; Ye, S.-H.; Johnson, C.A., Jr.; Woolley, J.R.; Wagner, W.R.; Federspiel, W.J., Immobilized carbonic anhydrase on hollow fiber membranes accelerates CO_2 removal from blood. *J. Membr. Sci.* **2012**, *404*, 25–31.

53. Hunt, J.A.; Lesburg, C.A.; Christianson, D.W.; Thompson, R.B.; Fierke, C.A. Active-site Engineering of Carbonic Anhydrase and Its Applications to Biosensors. In *The Carbonic Anhydrases: New horizons*; Chegwidden, W.R., Carter, N.D., Edwards, Y.H., Eds.; Birkhäuser Verlag: Boston, MA, USA, 2000; pp. 221–240.

54. Lindskog, S.; Nyman, P.O. Metal-binding properties of human erythrocyte carbonic anhydrase. *Biochem. Biophys. Acta* **1964**, *85*, 462–474.

55. Thompson, R.B.; Jones, E.R. Enzyme-based fiber optic zinc biosensor. *Anal. Chem.* **1993**, *65*, 730–734.

56. Rout, G.R.; Das, P. Effect of metal toxicity on plant growth and metabolism: I. Zinc. *Agronomie* **2003**, *23*, 3–11.

57. Muyssen, B.T.; de Schamphelaere, K.A.; Janssen, C.R. Mechanisms of chronic waterborne zn toxicity in daphnia magna. *Aquat. Toxicol.* **2006**, *77*, 393–401.

58. Chen, R.F.; Kernohan, J.C. Combination of bovine carbonic anhydrase with a fluorescence sulfonamide. *J. Biol. Chem.* **1967**, *242*, 5813–5823.

59. Huang, C.-C.; Lesburg, C.A.; Kiefer, L.L.; Fierke, C.A.; Christianson, D.W. Reversal of the hydrogen bond to zinc ligand histidine-119 dramatically diminishes catalysis and enhances metal equilibriation kinetics in carbonic anhydrase. *Biochemistry* **1996**, *35*, 3439–3446.

60. Thompson, R.B.; Ge, Z.; Patchan, M.W.; Kiefer, L.L.; Fierke, C.A. Performance enhancement of fluorescence energy transfer-based biosensors by site-directed mutagenesis of the transducer. *SPIE* **1996**, *2508*, 136–144.

61. Thompson, R.B.; Patchan, M.W. Lifetime-based fluorescence energy transfer biosensing of zinc. *Anal. Biochem.* **1995**, *227*, 123–128.

62. Demille, G.R.; Larlee, K.; Livesey, D.L.; Mailer, K. Conformational change in carbonic anhydrase studied by perturbed directional correlations of gamma rays. *Chem. Phys. Lett.* **1979**, *64*, 534–539.

63. Harrington, P.C.; Wilkins, R.G. Interaction of acetazolamide and 4-nitrothiophenolate ion with bivalent metal ion derivatives of bovine carbonic anhydrase. *Biochemistry* **1977**, *16*, 448–454.

64. Thompson, R.B.; Ge, Z.; Patchan, M.W.; Huang, C.-C.; Fierke, C.A. Fiber optic biosensor for co(II) and cu(II) based on fluorescence energy transfer with an enzyme transducer. *Biosens. Bioelectron.* **1996**, *11*, 557–564.

65. Frederickson, C.J.; Giblin, L.J.; Krezel, A.; McAdoo, D.J.; Mueller, R.N.; Zeng, Y.; Balaji, R.V.; Masalha, R.; Thompson, R.B.; Fierke, C.A.; *et al.* Concentrations of extracellular free zinc (pzn)e in the central nervous system during simple anesthetization, ischemia and reperfusion. *Exp. Neurol.* **2006**, *198*, 285–293.

66. Thompson, R.B.; Peterson, D.; Mahoney, W.; Cramer, M.; Maliwal, B.P.; Suh, S.W.; Frederickson, C.; Fierke, C.; Herman, P. Fluorescent zinc indicators for neurobiology. *J. Neurosci. Methods* **2002**, *118*, 63–75.

67. Thompson, R.B.; Whetsell, W.O., Jr.; Maliwal, B.P.; Fierke, C.A.; Frederickson, C.J. Fluorescence microscopy of stimulated zn(II) release from organotypic cultures of mammalian hippocampus using a carbonic anhydrase-based biosensor system. *J. Neurosci. Methods* **2000**, *96*, 35–45.

68. Bozym, R.; Hurst, T.K.; Westerberg, N.; Stoddard, A.; Fierke, C.A.; Frederickson, C.J.; Thompson, R.B. Chapter 14 determination of zinc using carbonic anhydrase-based fluorescence biosensors. *Methods Enzymol.* **2008**, *450*, 287–309.

69. Wang, D.; Hurst, T.K.; Thompson, R.B.; Fierke, C.A. Genetically encoded ratiometric biosensors to measure intracellular exchangeable zinc in escherichia coli. *J. Biomed. Opt.* **2011**, *16*, doi:10.1117/1.3613926.

70. McCranor, B.J.; Bozym, R.A.; Vitolo, M.I.; Fierke, C.A.; Bambrick, L.; Polster, B.M.; Fiskum, G.; Thompson, R.B. Quantitative imaging of mitochondrial and cytosolic free zinc levels in an in vitro model of ischemia/reperfusion. *J. Bioenerg. Biomembr.* **2012**, *44*, 253–263.

71. Simsek-Ege, F.A.; Bond, G.M.; Stringer, J. Matrix molecular weight cut-off for encapsulation of carbonic anhydrase in polyelectrolyte beads. *J. Biomater. Sci. Polym. Ed.* **2002**, *13*, 1175–1187.

72. Cowan, R.M.; Ge, J.; Qin, Y.J.; McGregor, M.L.; Trachtenberg, M.C. CO_2 capture by means of an enzyme-based reactor. *Ann. N. Y. Acad. Sci.* **2003**, *984*, 453–469.

73. Satav, S.S.; Bhat, S.; Thayumanavan, S. Feedback regulated drug delivery vehicles: Carbon dioxide responsive cationic hydrogels for antidote release. *Biomacromol* **2010**, *11*, 1735–1740.

74. Han, D.; Boissiere, O.; Kumar, S.; Tong, X.; Tremblay, L.N.; Zhao, Y. Two-way co2-switchable triblock copolymer hydrogels. *Macromol* **2012**, *45*, 7440–7445.

75. Aggarwal, M.; Boone, C.D.; Kondeti, B.; Tu, C.; Silverman, D.N.; McKenna, R. Effects of cryoprotectants on the structure and thermostability of the human carbonic anhydrase ii-acetazolamide complex. *Acta Crystallogr. Sect. D Biol. Crystallogr.* **2013**, *69*, 860–865.

76. Sippel, K.H.; Robbins, A.H.; Domsic, J.; Genis, C.; Agbandje-McKenna, M.; McKenna, R. High-resolution structure of human carbonic anhydrase ii complexed with acetazolamide reveals insights into inhibitor drug design. *Acta Crystallogr. Sect. F Struct. Biol. Cryst. Commun.* **2009**, *65*, 992–995.

77. Aggarwal, M.; Kondeti, B.; McKenna, R. Insights towards sulfonamide drug specificity in alpha-carbonic anhydrases. *Bioorganic Med. Chem.* **2013**, *21*, 1526–1533.

78. Svastová, E.; Huliková, A.; Rafajová, M.; Zat'ovicová, M.; Gibadulinová, A.; Casini, A.; Cecchi, A.; Scozzafava, A.; Supuran, C.T.; Pastorek, J.; *et al.* Hypoxia activates the capacity of tumor-associated carbonic anhydrase ix to acidify extracellular ph. *FEBS lett.* **2004**, *577*, 439–445.

79. Vullo, D.; Franchi, M.; Gallori, E.; Pastorek, J.; Scozzafava, A.; Pastorekova, S.; Supuran, C.T. Carbonic anhydrase inhibitors: Inhibition of the tumor-associated isozyme ix with aromatic and heterocyclic sulfonamides. *Bioorganic Med. Chem. Lett.* **2003**, *13*, 1005–1009.

80. Winum, J.Y.; Rami, M.; Scozzafava, A.; Montero, J.L.; Supuran, C. Carbonic anhydrase ix: A new druggable target for the design of antitumor agents. *Med. Res. Rev.* **2008**, *28*, 445–463.

81. Supuran, C.T. Carbonic anhydrase inhibitors: An editorial. *Expert Opin. Ther. Pat.* **2013**, *23*, 677–679.

82. Supuran, C.T.; Scozzafava, A.; Casini, A. Carbonic anhydrase inhibitors. *Med. Res. Rev.* **2003**, *23*, 146–189.

83. Gould, S.A.; Moore, E.E.; Hoyt, D.B.; Ness, P.M.; Norris, E.J.; Carson, J.L.; Hides, G.A.; Freeman, I.H.; deWoskin, R.; Moss, G.S. The life-sustaining capacity of human polymerized hemoglobin when red cells might be unavailable. *J. Am. Coll. Surg.* **2002**, *195*, 445–452.

84. Bian, Y.; Rong, Z.; Chang, T.M. Polyhemoglobin-superoxide dismutase-catalase-carbonic anhydrase: A novel biotechnology-based blood substitute that transports both oxygen and carbon dioxide and also acts as an antioxidant. *Artif. Cells Blood Substit. Immobil. Biotechnol.* **2012**, *40*, 28–37.

A Sensitive DNA Enzyme-Based Fluorescent Assay for Bacterial Detection

Sergio D. Aguirre, M. Monsur Ali, Bruno J. Salena and Yingfu Li

Abstract: Bacterial detection plays an important role in protecting public health and safety, and thus, substantial research efforts have been directed at developing bacterial sensing methods that are sensitive, specific, inexpensive, and easy to use. We have recently reported a novel "mix-and-read" assay where a fluorogenic DNAzyme probe was used to detect model bacterium *E. coli*. In this work, we carried out a series of optimization experiments in order to improve the performance of this assay. The optimized assay can achieve a detection limit of 1000 colony-forming units (CFU) without a culturing step and is able to detect 1 CFU following as short as 4 h of bacterial culturing in a growth medium. Overall, our effort has led to the development of a highly sensitive and easy-to-use fluorescent bacterial detection assay that employs a catalytic DNA.

Reprinted from *Biomolecules*. Cite as: Aguirre, S.D.; Ali, M.M.; Salena, B.J.; Li, Y. A Sensitive DNA Enzyme-Based Fluorescent Assay for Bacterial Detection. *Biomolecules* **2013**, *3*, 563-577.

1. Introduction

Infectious agents, such as foodborne pathogens, have caused numerous large-scale and costly outbreaks in the human history and will continue to be a major public health threat and financial burden for our society [1–4]. Early detection of pathogens, as the first step to prevent such outbreaks, has become increasingly more important today because the globalization of commerce and speedy travel have significantly increased the rate and breadth of the spread of infectious agents. Thus, the demand for faster, simpler, less expensive and more reliable pathogen testing methods has become ever greater.

Although the traditional culture method continues to be the "gold standard" for bacterial detection, it is time-consuming and requires days or even weeks to complete (depending on the specific pathogen in question) [5]. Modern methods take advantage of well-established biomolecular techniques, such as polymerase chain reaction (PCR) and immunoassay (where an antibody is used as molecular recognition element), to achieve faster and more sensitive pathogen detection [5–11]. Despite the popularity of these techniques, they also come with certain drawbacks, such as the need for costly instrumentation and highly trained personnel to isolate or purify relevant targets (DNA for PCR and proteins for immunoassays). Thus, the entire test using such methods often still needs one or more days to complete. Detection sensitivity (for immunoassay) and tendency to generate false-positive results (for PCR) are also issues of concerns. For these considerations, we recently began to examine the utility of RNA-cleaving fluorogenic DNAzyme (RFD) probes for bacterial detection [12–14]. RFDs can be isolated from random-sequence DNA pools to perform three linked functions: ligand binding, catalysis and fluorescence generation. Each RFD cleaves a synthetic nucleic acid substrate containing a single ribonucleotide as the cleavage site embedded in a DNA sequence, and the cleavage site is located between two nucleotides modified with a matching pair of fluorophore and quencher [12–21]. Because of these two features, these reporter molecules emit an increasing level of fluorescence when they carry out the catalytic cleavage of the RNA linkage. In other words, the cleavage event results in separation of the fluorophore from the quencher, accompanied by the increase of fluorescence intensity in real time.

More recently, we developed a method of isolating novel DNAzyme probes against the crude extracellular mixture (CEM) left behind by a specific type of bacteria in their environment or in the media they are cultured [12]. The CEM is rich in diverse targets, including small molecules and proteins. Thus the use of the crude mixture as the complex target to conduct *in vitro* selection [22–24] experiment circumvents the tedious process of purifying and identifying a suitable target from the microbe of interest for biosensor development, and provides a subsequent assaying procedure that is simple because it does not require steps to purify a target of interest. Using this approach, we have isolated an RFD that cleaves its substrate only in the presence of the CEM produced by *E. coli* (CEM-EC) [12]. This *E. coli*-sensing RFD, named RFD-EC1, was found to be highly selective to CEM-EC but nonresponsive to CEMs from many other Gram-negative and Gram-positive bacteria. We have also shown that the DNAzyme-based assay is capable of reporting the presence of a single *E. coli* cell after 12 h of culturing. These experiments have illustrated the utility of RFDs as fluorogenic bacterial indicators. In this work we carried out a thorough investigation to characterize this bacterial detection system with a goal to further improve the detection sensitivity.

2. Results and Discussion

2.1. Establishing a Trans-Acting DNAzyme

Our previously reported RFD-EC1 is a *cis*-acting DNAzyme that cleaves a covalently attached substrate. However, a *trans*-acting DNAzyme where the DNAzyme cleaves a detached substrate has an additional advantage such as ease-of-synthesis, thus lowering the cost and labor. Synthesis of long DNA chain modified with fluorophore, quencher and ribonucleotide is associated with lower yields and higher costs. Therefore, in this study, we first examined the possibility of converting it into a *trans*-acting catalyst by detaching the substrate portion of the sequence, FS1, from the DNAzyme portion, EC1 (Figure 1A). We found that EC1 was indeed able to cleave FS1 in *trans*, even at 1:1 ratio (50 nM each of EC1 and FS1), in a CEM-EC dependent manner (Figure 1B). Note that the reaction mixtures were analyzed by denaturing polyacrylamide gel electrophoresis (dPAGE).

We next tested a second *trans* construct, named EC1T (Figure 1A), by truncating 28 nucleotides from the two ends of EC1 (italic letters, Figure 1A) that were used as the primer-binding sites for polymerase chain reaction during the original *in vitro* selection experiment. Interestingly, EC1T was found to be considerably more active than EC1 (comparing Lanes 3 and 5, Figure 1B; *i.e.*, 45% *vs.* 72%). As a control, we also tested a mutant sequence, EC1TM, with 10 nucleotides (lower-case letters, Figure 1A) mutated from EC1T. These mutations rendered EC1TM completely inactive in the presence of CEM-EC (Figure 1B).

Figure 1. Design of *trans*-acting DNAzymes. (**A**) The sequences of EC1, EC1T, EC1TM and FS1. EC1 is the full length DNAzyme including two primer binding sites (nucleotides in italic) for polymerase chain reaction used in the original *in vitro* selection experiment. EC1T is the shortened version of EC1 with deleted primer binding sites. EC1TM is a mutant of EC1T wherein the nucleotides shown as lower-case letters are altered. The substrate FS1 contains an adenosine ribonucleotide (R) flanked by a fluorescein-dT (F) and a DABCYL-dT (Q); (**B**) dPAGE analysis of the cleavage reaction mixtures of FS1 with EC1, EC1T, or EC1TM in the absence (−) and presence (+) of CEM-EC. P1 represents the 5′-cleavage product, which can be observed by fluorescence scan as it contains the F unit. MK (marker) is a sample of FS1 fully cleaved by NaOH. Clv% for each sample was calculated following our previously reported method [20].

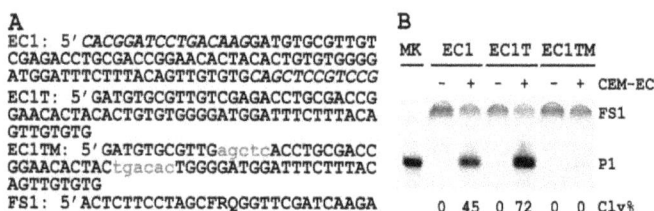

A
```
EC1: 5' CACGGATCCTGACAAGGATGTGCGTTGT
CGAGACCTGCGACCGGAACACTACACTGTGTGGGG
ATGGATTTCTTTACAGTTGTGTGCAGCTCCGTCCG
EC1T: 5' GATGTGCGTTGTCGAGACCTGCGACCG
GAACACTACACTGTGTGGGGATGGATTTCTTTACA
GTTGTGTG
EC1TM: 5' GATGTGCGTTGagctcACCTGCGACC
GGAACACTACtgacacTGGGGATGGATTTCTTTAC
AGTTGTGTG
FS1: 5' ACTCTTCCTAGCFRQGGTTCGATCAAGA
```

B
MK EC1 EC1T EC1TM

− + − + − + CEM-EC

FS1

P1

0 45 0 72 0 0 Clv%

2.2. Comparing DNAzyme Activity Using Crude Extracellular Mixture (CEM) and Crude Intracellular Mixture (CIM) of E. coli

The original DNAzyme RFD-EC1 was isolated to cleave in the presence of CEM of *E. coli*. We hypothesized that the target that activates the DNAzyme might be more abundant inside the cellular environment. To test this idea, we made an *E. coli* culture and used it to prepare the CEM-EC and CIM-EC as follows: the cells were precipitated by centrifugation and the supernatant was taken as the CEM-EC. The cell pellet was re-suspended in the reaction buffer, heat-treated, and then centrifuged; the remaining supernatant was taken as the CIM-EC (see experimental section for details). The CEM-EC and CIM-EC were then used to induce the cleavage activity of EC1T towards FS1, and the results are illustrated in Figure 2A. It is clear that the CIM-EC indeed contained a much higher amount of the target than the CEM-EC as it induced much stronger cleavage of FS1 by EC1T (45% *vs.* 1%). Note that much lower cleavage in this experiment with CEM-EC is due to the shorter culture time (7 h) with low number of *E. coli* cells (50,000 colony forming units). For the remaining experiments, the CIM-EC was used as the target of interest.

2.3. Searching for an Optimal Culture Broth

We next investigated the effect of bacterial growth media on the quality of CIM (as measured by the cleavage activity of EC1T/FS1) in order to establish an optimal culture broth. Seven common growth media were chosen for this analysis and they were: Luria Bertani (LB), Terrific Broth (TB), Todd-Hewitt (TH), Lysogeny Broth Miller (LBM), Tryptic Soy Broth (TSB), Super Optimal Broth (SOB) and Super Optimal Broth with Catabolic repressor (SOC). 250 *E. coli* cells were allowed to grow in 1 mL of each broth for 7 h at 37 °C, from which CIM was prepared and used to induce the cleavage of EC1T/FS1; the results are illustrated as Figure 2B. The CIMs from SOB and SOC produced the highest activity (~26% cleavage), followed by those from LB, LBM, and THB (10%–16%). The CEMs from TSB and TB were least effective (≤5%). Based on these results, SOB was chosen as the broth for the remaining experiments.

Figure 2. Cleavage reactions of EC1T/FS1 with (**A**) crude extracellular mixture (CEM)-EC and CIM-EC and (**B**) crude intracellular mixture (CIM)-EC collected from *E. coli* cells grown in various culture broths. NC is a negative control where the reaction was conducted in the absence of CEM-EC and CIM-EC. Each reaction mixture was analyzed by 10% dPAGE, followed by fluorimaging. NC: negative control where the reaction was conducted in RB without CEM-EC or CIM-EC.

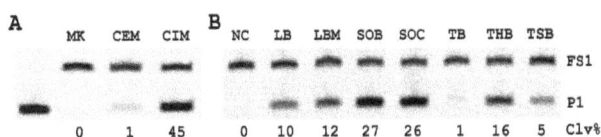

2.4. Effects of Divalent Metal Ions

Divalent metal ions play crucial roles in catalytic functions of DNAzymes and it has been shown that different metal ions can significantly affect the catalytic activity of a DNAzyme [25–28]. For example, 8–17, a well-studied RNA-cleaving DNAzyme, exhibits the highest activity in presence of lead ions even though it was originally isolated using Mg^{2+} [29] or Zn^{2+} [30]. A recent study has revealed that Pb^{2+} promotes the most favorable folding of 8–17 [31]. Therefore, we sought to compare the effects of various divalent metal ions on the activity of our *E. coli*-sensing DNAzyme although the original DNAzyme RFD-EC1 was obtained by *in vitro* selection in the presence of 15 mM $MgCl_2$ [12]. Nine different divalent metal ions were tested and they were: Ba^{2+}, Cd^{2+}, Co^{2+}, Mg^{2+}, Mn^{2+}, Ni^{2+}, Cu^{2+}, Zn^{2+}, and Ca^{2+}; the results are given in Figure 3A. We found that Ba^{2+}, Ca^{2+}, Mg^{2+} and Mn^{2+} all induced a robust cleavage activity of the DNAzyme (causing 56%–68% of cleavage). In contrast, Cd^{2+}, Co^{2+}, Ni^{2+}, Cu^{2+}, and Zn^{2+} resulted in weak cleavage (1%–2%). It is possible that Ba^{2+} Mg^{2+}, Mn^{2+} and Ca^{2+} fit into the catalytic core better than the other divalent metal ions. However, this should be experimentally verified.

It is noteworthy that we have previously shown that Mn^{2+} exhibits potent fluorescence quenching effect, resulting in significantly reduced signal magnitude when the fluorescence intensity is measured in a fluorimeter [32]. We also found a similar effect of Mn^{2+} in our assay (data not shown). In contrast, Ba^{2+} produced no quenching effect. This observation indicates that Ba^{2+} is a more suitable divalent metal ion for our assay. Thus, Ba^{2+} was chosen for further experiments. In order to establish the optimal Ba^{2+} concentration we investigated the effect of Ba^{2+} concentration on EC1T's activity. The data presented in Figure 3B indicates that the catalytic activity of EC1T reaches a plateau at 15 mM Ba^{2+}.

122

Figure 3. (A) Cleavage activity of EC1T/FS1 in the presence of CEM-EC and various divalent metal ions; (B) Effect of the Ba^{2+} concentration.

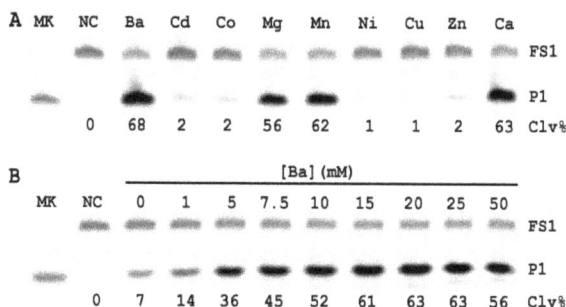

2.5. Varying Reaction Temperature

We examined the cleavage activity of EC1T/FS1 at different temperatures and the results are provided in Figure 4A. A robust cleavage activity was observed at both 15 and 23 °C. In contrast, reduced activity was observed when the reaction temperature was decreased to 4 °C or increased to 37 °C and 50 °C. Interestingly, although CIM was absolutely required to induce the cleavage at 4, 15 and 23 °C, EC1T can cleave FS1 in the absence of CIM at both 37 °C and 50 °C (grey bars in Figure 4A). Since room temperature is the most ideal condition to conduct assays avoiding the requirements of heating and cooling system, we chose 23 °C as the reaction temperature for the remaining experiments.

Figure 4. Cleavage activity of EC1T/FS1 with varying temperature (A); pH (B); and EC1T/FS1 ratio (C). The data are the average of two independent experiments.

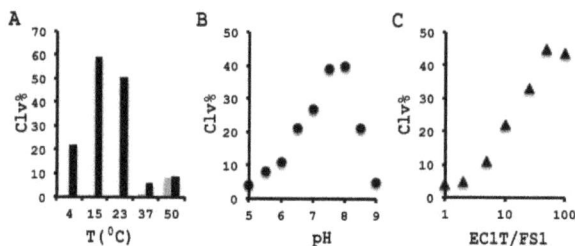

2.6. pH Effect

We next examined the activity of EC1T/FS1 when the reaction pH was varied between 5.0 and 9.0; the results are shown in Figure 4B. Although EC1T was able to cleave FS1 in the entire pH range tested, the highest activity was observed at pH 7.5–8.0. Since the original DNAzyme was isolated at pH 7.5, it is not surprising that EC1T exhibits such a narrow pH preference.

2.7. DNAzyme/Substrate Ratio

We also examined the cleavage activity at different ratios of EC1T/FS1. For this experiment, the concentration of FS1 was kept at 50 nM while the DNAzyme concentration was changed from 0 to 5 μM; the results are shown in Figure 4C. The cleavage activity reached the plateau at a ratio of 50:1. Thus, this ratio was used for the remaining experiments.

2.8. Specificity

With the significant changes of the reaction conditions, we wondered if EC1T was still able to maintain its specificity for *E. coli*. Four other gram-negative bacteria and four gram-positive bacteria were arbitrarily chosen for comparison. Each bacterium was cultured in SOB for a different period of time until the OD_{600} (optical density at 600 nm) of each culture reached ~1. The CIM was then prepared and tested with EC1T/FS1 under the optimal reaction buffer (50 mM HEPES, pH 7.5, 150 mM NaCl and 15 mM $BaCl_2$, room temperature, EC1T/FS1 = 50/1). None of the CIMs from other bacteria was able to induce cleavage (Figure 5), indicating that EC1T/FS1 retained the specificity for *E. coli*.

Figure 5. Specificity of EC1T/FS1 for various gram-negative and gram-positive bacteria. PP: *Pseudomonas peli*, YR: *Yersinia rukeri*, HA: *Hafnea alvei*, AX: *Achromobacter xylosoxidans*, EC: *Escherichia coli*, BS: *Bacillus subtilis*, LM: *Leuconostoc mesenteroides*, LP: *Lactobacillus planturum*, PA: *Pediococcus acidilactici*.

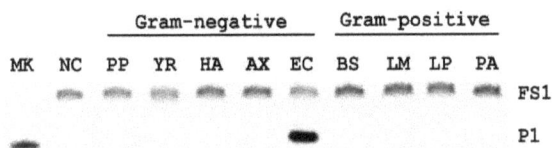

2.9. Detection Sensitivity

To test the detection sensitivity of EC1T/FS1, we prepared a series of *E. coli* stock solutions from which CIM samples were prepared as described in experimental section. These samples were then assessed for inducing the cleavage of EC1T/FS1 under the optimal reaction condition established above. These reactions were monitored in a fluorimeter in real time for 60 min (Figure 6A). The reaction mixtures were also analyzed by dPAGE (Figure 6B). We found that the fluorimeter method was able to detect 10^5 cells while the dPAGE method can detect 10^4 cells.

We also tested the detection sensitivity of the original *cis*-acting DNAzyme RFD-EC1 using the optimal reaction condition. Interestingly, RFD-EC1 showed better sensitivities: the fluorimeter method can detect 10^4 cells (Figure 6C) while the dPAGE method was able to detect 10^3 cells (Figure 6D).

Figure 6. Sensitivity test. (**A**) Real-time fluorescence monitoring and (**B**) dPAGE analysis of EC1T/FS1 in the presence of CIMs prepared from 10^3–10^7 *E. coli* cells. (**C**) and (**D**) Similar experiments using RNA-cleaving fluorogenic DNAzyme (RFD-EC1) with CIMs prepared from 10^2–10^7 *E. coli* cells. The data in (A) and (C) are the average of two independent experiments.

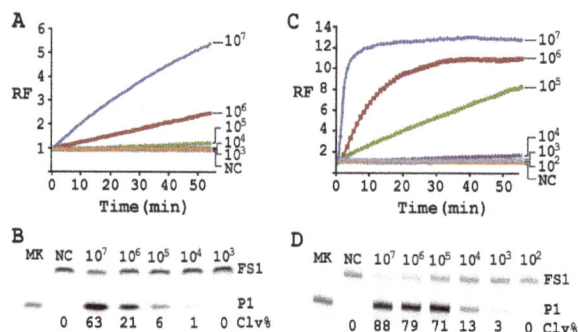

2.10. Detection of a Single Cell via Culturing

Finally we determined the time required to enrich a single live bacterium (*i.e.*, one colony forming unit or 1 CFU) via culturing in SOB. Following a previous protocol [12], we inoculated a single *E. coli* cell in SOB and cultured for 2, 4, 6, 8 and 10 h at 37 °C. CIMs were prepared for the samples collected at each time point and tested with both *trans* and *cis* constructs. These samples were then assessed for inducing the cleavage of EC1T/FS1 under the optimal reaction condition. Each reaction was examined both in a fluorimeter (Figure 7A) and by dPAGE (Figure 7B). Using EC1T/FS1, 8 h of culturing was sufficient for detection by the fluorimeter method (Figure 7A) and 6 h by dPAGE method (Figure 7B). Using RFD-EC1, however, only 6 h and 4 h of culturing were required to achieve the detection by the fluorimeter (Figure 7C) and dPAGE (Figure 7D) method, respectively. The lower activity of EC1T/FS1 in comparison to the *cis*-acting RFD-EC1 might be due to the weakened interaction between enzyme and substrate strands when they were separated from each other.

3. Experimental Section

3.1. Synthesis and Purification of Oligonucleotides

The standard DNA oligonucleotides (EC1, EC1T, EC1TM and EC1LT) were purchased from Integrated DNA Technologies (IDT, Coralville, IA, USA) and purified by 10% denaturing polyacrylamide gel electrophoresis (dPAGE). The modified oligonucleotide FS1 was acquired from W. M. Keck Oligonucleotide Synthesis Facilities (Yale University, New Haven, CT, USA), deprotected and purified by 10% dPAGE following a previously reported protocol [15].

Figure 7. Culturing time required to detect a single *E. coli* cell (1 CFU). (**A**) Monitoring fluorescence of EC1T/FS1 with CIMs prepared from samples taken after a culturing time of 2, 4, 6, 8 and 10 h; (**B**) dPAGE analysis of the reaction mixtures in (A). (**C**) and (**D**) are equivalent experiments in which RFD-EC1 was used to replace EC1T/FS1. The data in (A) and (C) are the average of two independent experiments.

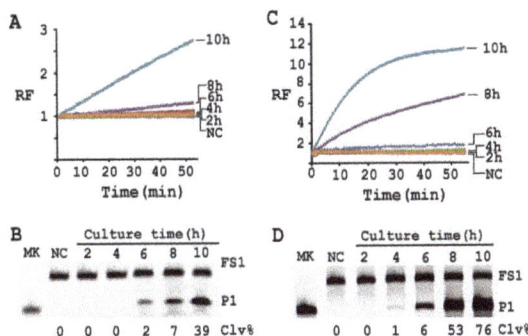

3.2. Enzymes and Chemical Reagents

T4 DNA ligase and T4 polynucleotide kinase (PNK) were purchased from MBI Fermentas (Burlington, ON, Canada). Tryptone and yeast extract was acquired from BD Biosciences (Mississauga, ON, Canada). All other chemical reagents were purchased from Sigma-Aldrich (Oakville, ON, Canada) and were used without further purification.

3.3. Growth Media

Luria Bertani (LB), Terrific Broth (TB), and Todd-Hewitt (TH) were purchased from Sigma-Aldrich. Lysogeny Broth Miller (LBM) was obtained from EMD Canada (Mississauga, ON, Canada). Tryptic Soy Broth (TSB) was acquired from BD Biosciences. Super Optimal Broth (SOB) and Super Optimal Broth with Catabolic repressor (SOC) were made in house. SOB contains 2% (w/v) tryptone, 0.5% (w/v) yeast extract, 10 mM NaCl and 2.5 mM KCl. SOC has the same ingredients as SOB but also contains 20 mM glucose and 10 mM $MgCl_2$.

3.4. Preparation of Cis-Acting RFD-EC1

RFD-EC1 was generated by template-mediated ligation of FS1 to EC1. In brief, 200 pmol of FS1 were treated with 1× PNK buffer A (MBI Fermentas), 1 mM ATP and 20 U (units) of PNK for 30 min at 37 °C (reaction volume = 50 µL). The reaction was quenched by heating at 90 °C for 5 min. Equimolar EC1 and EC1LT (5'-CTAGG AAGAG TCGGA CGGAG CTG; the ligation template) were then added to this solution and was heated at 90 °C for 30 s and cooled to room temperature for 10 min. Afterwards, 10 µL of 10× T4 DNA ligase buffer (MBI Fermentas), 39 µL of deionized distilled water (ddH$_2$O) and 1 µL of T4 DNA ligase (10 U/µL) were added. After incubation at room temperature (RT) for 2 h, the ligated EC1-FS1 was purified by 10% dPAGE.

3.5. Bacterial Cells

Gram-negative bacteria *Pseudomonas peli*, *Yersinia rukeri*, *Hafnea alvei*, and *Achromobacter xylosoxidans* were donated by Dr. Gerard Wright (Micheal G. DeGroote Institute for Infectious Disease Research, McMaster University). Gram-positive bacteria *Leuconostoc mesenteroides*, *Lactobacillus planturum* and *Pediococcus acidilactici* (PA) were gifts from Dr. Brian Coombes and Dr. Russel Bishop (Department of Biochemistry and Biomedical Sciences, McMaster University). *E. coli* K12 (MG1655) and *Bacillus subtilis* 168 are regularly maintained in our laboratory.

3.6. Comparison of the Cleavage Activity of EC1, EC1T and EC1TM in the Presence of CEM-EC

E. coli was plated onto a TSB agar (1.5%) plate and grown for 14 h at 37 °C. A single colony was taken and inoculated into 2 mL of TSB and grown for 14 h at 37 °C with shaking at 250 rpm. A 1% fresh culture was made by re-inoculating 20 μL of the above culture into 2 mL of TSB. The re-inoculation was allowed to grow at 37 °C with shaking at 250 rpm until the culture reached an OD_{600} of ~1. 1 mL of this culture was centrifuged at 11,000 g for 5 min at room temperature; the supernatant was taken as the crude extracellular mixture (CEM-EC) and stored at −20 °C.

For each candidate DNAzyme construct, two reactions were set up, a control and a test. For the test, 25 μL of 2× reaction buffer (2× RB; 100 mM HEPES, 300 mM NaCl, 30 mM $MgCl_2$, pH 7.5) was mixed with 23 μL of the CEM-EC prepared above, 1 μL of 2.5 μM FS1 and 1 μL of 2.5 μM EC1, EC1T or EC1TM. For the control, TSB was used to substitute the CEM-EC. Each reaction mixture was incubated at RT for 60 min, followed by quenching with 5 μL of 3 M NaOAc (pH 5.5) and 135 μL of cold ethanol. DNA was recovered by centrifugation and analyzed by 10% dPAGE. DNA bands in the gel were visualized by Typhoon 9200 (GE Healthcare) and quantified by ImageQuant software (Molecular Dynamics).

3.7. Comparison of the Cleavage Activity of EC1T in the Presence of CEM-EC and CIM-EC

100 μL of 50,000 CFU/mL glycerol stock of *E. coli* was inoculated into 2 mL of TSB and grown at 37 °C for 7 h with shaking at 250 rpm. 1 mL of this culture was centrifuged at 11,000 g for 5 min at room temperature; the supernatant was taken as the CEM-EC for this experiment. The cell pellet was suspended in 200 μL of 1× RB and heated at 50 °C for 15 min. The heat-treated cell suspension was then centrifuged at 11,000 g for 5 min at RT. The clear supernatant was taken as the CIM-EC for the experiment.

The cleavage reaction with the CEM-EC was carried out by mixing 25 μL of 2× RB, 23 μL of the CEM-EC prepared above, 1 μL of 2.5 μM FS1 and 1 μL of 2.5 μM EC1T. The reaction concerning the CIM-EC was conducted by mixing 41 μL of 1× RB, 5 μL of CIM-EC, 1 μL of 2.5 μM FS1, 1 μL of 2.5 μM EC1T and 2 μL of 2× RB (note that the CIM-EC was made by suspending the cell pellet from originally 1 mL of *E. coli* culture in 200 μL of 1× RB, which translates into a concentrating factor of 5). A control experiment without the CEM-EC and CIM-EC was also conducted. Each reaction mixture was incubated at RT for 60 min, followed by 10% dPAGE analysis as described above.

3.8. Comparison of the Cleavage Activity of EC1T in the Presence of CIM-EC Obtained from E. coli Grown in Various Growth Media

100 μL of 2500 CFU/mL glycerol stock of *E. coli* was inoculated into 2 mL of LB, LBM, SOB, SOC, TB, TH, or TSB. Following 7 h incubation at 37 °C, 1 mL of each culture was taken and centrifuged at 11,000 g for 5 min at RT. The cell pellet was re-suspended in 200 μL of 1× RB. Cleavage reactions were then conducted by mixing 41 μL of 1× RB, 5 μL of each CIM-EC, 1 μL of 2.5 μM FS1, 1 μL of 2.5 μM EC1T and 2 μL of 2× RB. Each reaction mixture was incubated at RT for 60 min, followed by 10% dPAGE analysis as described above.

3.9. Comparison of the Cleavage Activity of EC1T in the Presence of Different Divalent Metals

First, stocks of 2× RB′ (100 mM HEPES, 300 mM NaCl, pH 7.5) and 150 mM MCl_2 (M = Cd, Co, Mg, Mn, Ni, Cu, Zn and Ca) were prepared. The CIM-EC was also prepared from *E. coli* grown in SOB in the same way as described immediately above except for the use of 1× RB′ instead of 1× RB. The cleavage reactions as shown in Figure 3A were set up by mixing 15.5 μL of water, 22.5 μL of 2× RB′, 5 μL of a relevant MCl_2 stock, 1 μL of 2.5 μM FS1, 1 μL of 2.5 μM EC1T, and 5 μL of the CIM-EC. The cleavage reactions as shown in Figure 3B were set up similarly except that the volume of water and 150 mM $BaCl_2$ were co-varied to achieve a final $[BaCl_2]$ of 0, 1, 5, 7.5, 10, 15, 20, 25 and 50 mM. Each reaction mixture was incubated at RT for 60 min, followed by 10% dPAGE analysis as described above.

3.10. Comparison of the Cleavage Activity of EC1T at Different Reaction Temperature

A 2× RB_{Ba} stock (100 mM HEPES, 300 mM NaCl, 30 mM $BaCl_2$, pH 7.5) was first prepared. Five cleavage reaction mixtures were then set up by mixing 19.5 μL of water, 22.5 μL of 2× RB_{Ba}, 1 μL of 2.5 μM FS1, 1 μL of 2.5 μM EC1T, and 5 μL of the CIM-EC prepared with 1× RB_{Ba}. These mixtures were incubated, respectively, at 4, 15, 23, 37 and 50 °C for 60 min, followed by 10% dPAGE analysis as described above.

3.11. Comparison of the Cleavage Activity of EC1T at Different pH

A series of 2× RB_{Ba}′ stock (300 mM NaCl, 30 mM $BaCl_2$, along with a chosen buffering agent at 100 mM) were first prepared with pH being varied from 5.0 to 9.0 at an increasing interval of 0.5 units. MES was used for pH 5.0, 5.5 and 6.0; HEPES was used for pH 6.5, 7.0, 7.5 and 8.0; Tris was used for pH 8.5 and 9.0. The cleavage reactions were then conducted in a similar fashion as described in the section immediately above. Note that the CIM-EC for a given pH was prepared with a relevant 1× RB_{Ba}′.

3.12. Comparison of the Cleavage Activity of EC1T at Varying FS1/EC1T Ratios

Stocks of EC1T at 2.5, 5, 12.5, 25, 62.5, 125, and 250 μM were first prepared. Cleavage reactions were then conducted by mixing 19.5 μL of water, 22.5 μL of 2× RB_{Ba}, 1 μL of 2.5 μM FS1, 1 μL of a given EC1T stock, and 5 μL of the CIM-EC prepared with $1\times$ RB$_{Ba}$. Each reaction mixture was incubated at RT for 60 min, followed by 10% dPAGE analysis as described above.

3.13. Specificity Test

Five Gram-negative bacteria (*P. peli, Y. rukeri, H. alvei, A. xylosoxidans* and *E. coli*) and four Gram-positive bacteria (*L. mesenteroides, L. planturum, P. acidilactici* and *B. subtilis*) were tested in this experiment. Each bacterium was cultured in SOB for a different period of time until the OD600 reached ~1. The CIM was then prepared with $1\times$ RB$_{Ba}$ and tested with EC1T/FS1 under the optimal reaction condition (50 mM HEPES, pH 7.5, 150 mM NaCl and 15 mM BaCl$_2$, room temperature, EC1T/FS1 = 50/1). Each reaction mixture was incubated at RT for 60 min, followed by 10% dPAGE analysis as described above.

3.14. Detection Sensitivity

First, a single colony of *E. coli* from an agar plate was taken, inoculated into 2 mL of SOB and grown for 14 h at 37 °C with shaking at 250 rpm. 10-fold serial dilution was then carried out as follows: 100 μL of the 14-h culture was mixed with 900 μL of fresh SOB. 100 μL of the diluted culture was again taken and mixed with 900 μL of fresh SOB. This process was repeated 7 times. 100 μL of the final dilution were plated onto a TSB agar plate (done in triplicate), which was incubated at 37 °C for 15 h. Colonies in each plate were counted; the average number of colonies from the three plates was taken as the number of cells for this final dilution. This number was then used to calculate the number of cells for the other dilutions. 500 μL of each dilution was taken and centrifuged at 11,000 g for 5 min at RT. The cell pellet was re-suspended in 100 μL of $1\times$ RB$_{Ba}$ and used as the CEM-EC for this experiment (done in triplicate).

Cleavage reactions concerning EC1T/FS1 were set up and monitored as follows: 19.5 μL of water, 22.5 μL of $2\times$ RB$_{Ba}$, 1 μL of 2.5 μM FS1, 1 μL of 125 μM EC1T were mixed in a quartz crystal cuvette, which was placed in a fluorimeter (Cary Eclipse Fluorescence Spectrophotometer; excitation wavelength = 488 nm and emission wavelength = 520 nm) set at RT. Fluorescence intensity was recorded every minute for 5 min; 5 μL of a relevant CIM-EC was then added into the cuvette and the solution was quickly mixed by pipetting the mixture up and down a few times. Following this step, the fluorescence intensity of the solution was recorded for 55 more minutes. All the reactions were conducted in 3 replicates and the average data are shown in Figure 6A. The final reaction mixture was also taken and analyzed by 10% dPAGE and data are shown in Figure 6B.

Cleavage reactions concerning RFD-EC1 were set up and monitored similarly: 20.5 μL of water, 22.5 μL of $2\times$ RB$_{Ba}$, 1 μL of 2.5 μM RFD-EC1 was mixed in a cuvette. After reading fluorescence intensity for 5 min, 5 μL of a relevant CIM-EC was then added, followed by fluorescence intensity reading for 55 more minutes (Figure 6C). The final reaction mixture was also analyzed by 10% dPAGE (Figure 6D).

3.15. Single Cell Detection via Culturing

For isolating a single cell we followed our previously reported protocol [12]. Briefly, a glycerol stock containing 2 CFU/mL of *E. coli* was prepared. 100 μL of this stock was distributed to 10 culture tubes each with 2 mL of SOB. Since the concentration of the stock was 2 CFU/mL, only 2 out of the 10 tubes contained a single seeding cell (2 CFU/mL × 0.1 mL = 2). All the tubes were incubated at 37 °C with shaking at 250 rpm. At 2, 4, 6, 8 and 10 h, 200 μL of culture was harvested from each culture tube and CIMs were prepared (40 μL of 1× RB_{Ba} was used to dissolve the cell pellet). All the tubes were further incubated for 20 h to identify the two tubes containing *E. coli* cell (the culture in these tubes turned turbid while that in other 8 tubes stayed clear). Each CIM from *E. coli*-containing tubes was used to initiate the cleavage reaction by mixing 19.5 μL of water, 22.5 μL of 2× RB_{Ba}, 1 μL of 2.5 μM FS1, 1 μL of 125 μM EC1T, and 5 μL of a relevant CIM. The reaction and dPAGE analysis procedures were same as described above.

4. Conclusions

We recently described an RNA-cleaving fluorogenic DNAzyme, named RFD-EC1, which is active in the presence of the crude extracellular mixture (CEM) of the model Gram-negative bacterium *E. coli* [12–14]. RFD-EC1 was found to be highly active with CEM of *E. coli* but inactive with CEMs from a host of other Gram-negative and Gram-positive bacteria, and thus, RFD-EC1 can be used to develop a simple, "mix-and-read" fluorescence assay to achieve selective detection of *E. coli*. However, several parameters that are particularly relevant to the performance of this assay remained to be investigated. In this study we sought to establish a *trans*-acting DNA catalyst that cleaves an external substrate, optimize the reaction conditions that best support the catalytic activity of the DNAzyme, and determine the culturing conditions that enable the quickest detection of a single live bacterial cell.

The *trans*-acting DNAzyme was successfully established by segregating the substrate sequence domain from the sequence of the original DNA library. Also the two fixed sequence domains flanking the random-sequence domain could be removed without affecting the catalytic performance of the DNAzyme. The shortened, *trans*-acting DNAzyme, named EC1T, now contains 70 nucleotides.

Originally, the DNAzyme was isolated to cleave in the presence of the crude extracellular mixture (CEM) of *E. coli* and it has been determined that the target that activates the DNAzyme is a protein molecule based on the observation that the treatment of the CEM with proteases abolishes the DNAzyme activity [12]. Although the identity of this target is yet to be determined, we found that the target protein is much more abundant intracellularly and could be retrieved with a simple heating step (50 °C; 15 min). This led us to the use of the crude intracellular mixture (CIM) as the target of detection, translating into a better assay sensitivity.

Our results revealed that the nutritional factors in culture media played a vital role in growing the cells in faster rate (varying by as much as ~25-fold) with super Optimal Broth (SOB) which can substantially reduce the time required for single cell detection.

In order to establish an optimal reaction condition for EC1T, we examined the following reaction parameters: choice of divalent metal ions, reaction temperature and pH as well as the ratio between the substrate and the DNAzyme. Although EC1T was found to be active in the absence of any divalent ion, it exhibited much stronger activity in the presence of Ba^{2+}, Ca^{2+}, Mn^{2+} or Mg^{2+}. We chose Ba^{2+} as the divalent metal ion cofactor because this metal ion does not impose any fluorescence quenching effect. The DNAzyme was originally derived at room temperature (~23 °C) and a solution pH of 7.5 and therefore it was not surprising that EC1T exhibited the strongest activity at 23 °C and pH 7.5. We further found that when the concentration of FS1 was kept at 50 nM, 2.5 μM EC1T was required to reach the optimal cleavage activity. All the above optimization experiments led to the establishment of the optimal reaction condition for EC1T: 50 mM HEPES, 150 mM NaCl, 15 mM $BaCl_2$, pH 7.5, DNAzyme: substrate ratio = 50:1.

Under the above optimal reaction condition, the *trans*-acting system was able to detect 10^5 cells when the reaction was monitored in a fluorimeter. If the reaction mixture was analyzed by dPAGE (which separates the reaction product from the substrate), the system can detect 10^4 cells. When the original RFD-EC1 was used for the assay, the detection sensitivity was further improved: the fluorimeter method was able to detect 10^4 cells while the dPAGE method was able to detect as low as 10^3 cells. Importantly, the optimized assay did not compromise the specificity.

With a culturing step, the optimized assay is able to achieve the detection of *E. coli* from a single colony forming unit in 4–6 h (dependent on the method of choice), which represents a significant deduction in time (12 h) required by the same probe under unoptimized conditions. Overall, we have significantly improved the performance of our DNAzyme probe and demonstrate the utility of such probes as simple biosensors to achieve sensitive and speedy detection of bacterial pathogens.

Acknowledgments

This work was supported by research grants from the Natural Sciences and Research Council of Canada (NSERC) and Sentinel Bioactive Paper Network. We would like to thank Gerard Wright, Brian Coombes and Russell Bishop for providing various bacterial cells.

Conflict of Interest

The authors declare no conflict of interest.

References

1. World Health Organization (WHO). Fact sheet N^{0}237. Available online: https://apps.who.int/inf-fs/en/fact237.html (accessed on 16 August 2013).
2. Osterholm, M.T. Foodborne disease in 2011—The rest of the story. *N. Engl. J. Med.* **2011**, *364*, 889–891.
3. Scallan, E.; Hoekstra, R.M.; Angulo, F.J.; Tauxe, R.V.; Widdowson, M.A.; Roy, S.L.; Griffin, P.M. Foodborne illness acquired in the United States-major pathogens. *Emerg. Infect. Dis.* **2011**, *17*, 7–15.

4. Newell, D.G.; Koopmans, M.; Verhoef, L.; Duizer, E.; Aidara-Kane, A.; Sprong, H.; Opsteegh, M.; Langelaar, M.; Threfall, J.; Scheutz, F.; *et al.* Food-borne diseases—The challenges of 20 years ago still persist while new ones continue to emerge. *Int. J. Food Microbiol.* **2010**, *139*, S3–S15.

5. Zourob, M.; Elwary, S.; Turner, A. *Principles of Bacterial Detection: Biosensors, Recognition Receptors and Microsystems*; Springer: New York, NY, USA, 2008.

6. Velusamy, V.; Arshak, K.; Korostynska, O.; Oliwa, K.; Adley, C. An overview of foodborne pathogen detection: In the perspective of biosensors. *Biotechnol. Adv.* **2010**, *28*, 232–254.

7. Lazcka, O.; Campo, F.J.D.; Muñoz, F.X. Pathogen detection: A perspective of traditional methods and biosensors. *Biosens. Bioelectron.* **2007**, *22*, 1205–1217.

8. Wright, A.C.; Danyluk, M.D.; Otwell, W.S. Pathogens in raw foods: What the salad bar can learn from the raw bar. *Curr. Opin. Biotechnol.* **2009**, *20*, 172–177.

9. Call, D.R. Challenges and opportunities for pathogen detections using DNA microarrays. *Crit. Rev. Microbiol.* **2005**, *31*, 91–99.

10. Yagi, K. Applications of whole-cell bacterial sensors in biotechnology and environmental science. *Appl. Microbiol. Biotechnol.* **2007**, *73*, 1251–1258.

11. Laberge, I.; Griffiths, M.W. Prevalence, detection and control of *Cryptosporidium parvum* in food. *Int. J. Food Microbiol.* **1996**, *32*, 1–26.

12. Ali, M.M.; Aguirre, S.D.; Lazim, H.; Li, Y. Fluorogenic DNAzyme probes as bacterial indicators. *Angew. Chem. Int. Ed.* **2011**, *50*, 3751–3754.

13. Aguirre, S.D.; Ali, M.M.; Li, Y. Detection of bacteria using fluorogenic DNAzymes. *J. Vis. Exp.* **2012**, e3961, doi:10.3791/3961.

14. Li, Y. Advancements in using reporter DNAzymes for identifying pathogenic bacteria at speed and with convenience. *Future Microbiol.* **2011**, *6*, 973–976.

15. Mei, S.H.; Liu, Z.; Brennan, J.D.; Li, Y. An efficient RNA-cleaving DNA enzyme that synchronizes catalysis with fluorescence signaling. *J. Am. Chem. Soc.* **2003**, *125*, 412–420.

16. Liu, Z.; Mei, S.H.; Brennan, J.D.; Li, Y. Assemblage of signalling DNA enzymes with intriguing metal specificity and pH dependences. *J. Am. Chem. Soc.* **2003**, *125*, 7539–7545.

17. Shen, Y.; Brennan, J.D.; Li, Y. Characterizing the secondary structure and identifying functionally essential nucleotides of pH6DZ1, a fluorescence-signaling and RNA-cleaving deoxyribozyme. *Biochemistry* **2005**, *44*, 12066–12076.

18. Kandadai, S.A.; Li, Y. Characterization of a catalytically efficient acidic RNA-cleaving deoxyribozyme. *Nucleic Acids Res.* **2006**, *33*, 7164–7175.

19. Shen, Y.; Chiuman, W.; Brennan, J.D.; Li, Y. Catalysis and rational engineering of trans-acting pH6DZ1, an RNA-cleaving and fluorescence-signaling deoxyribozyme with a four-way junction structure. *ChemBioChem* **2006**, *7*, 1343–1348.

20. Ali, M.M.; Kandadai, S.A.; Li, Y. Characterization of pH3DZ1—An RNA-Cleaving deoxyribozyme with optimal activity at pH 3. *Can. J. Chem.* **2007**, *85*, 261–273.

21. Kandadai, S.A.; Mok, W.W.K.; Ali, M.M.; Li, Y. Characterization and optimization of an RNA-cleaving deoxyribozyme active at pH 5. *Biochemistry* **2009**, *48*, 7383–7391.

22. Tuerk, C.; Gold, L. Systematic evolution of ligands by exponential enrichment: RNA ligands to bacteriophage T4 DNA polymerase. *Science* **1990**, *249*, 505–510.

23. Ellington, A.D.; Szostak, J.W. *In vitro* selection of RNA molecules that bind specific ligands. *Nature* **1990**, *346*, 818–822.

24. Joyce, G.F. Forty years of *in vitro* evolution. *Angew. Chem. Int. Ed.* **2007**, *46*, 6420–6436.

25. Okumoto, Y.; Sugimoto, N. Effects of metal ions and catalytic loop sequences on the complex formation of a deoxyribozyme and its RNA substrate. *J. Inorg. Biochem.* **2000**, *82*, 189–195.

26. He, Q.C.; Zhou, J.M.; Zhou, D.M.; Nakamatsu, Y.; Baba, T.; Taira, K. Comparison of metal-ion-dependent cleavages of RNA by a DNA enzyme and a hammerheadribozyme. *Biomacromolecules* **2002**, *3*, 69–83.

27. Brown, A.K.; Li, J.; Pavot, C.M.; Lu, Y. A lead-dependent DNAzyme with a two-step mechanism. *Biochemistry* **2003**, *42*, 7152–7161.

28. Lan, T.; Lu, Y. Metal ion-dependent DNAzymes and their applications as biosensors. *Met. Ions Life Sci.* **2012**, *10*, 217–248.

29. Santoro, S.W.; Joyce, G.F. A general purpose RNA-cleaving DNA enzyme. *Proc. Natl. Acad. Sci. USA* **1997**, *94*, 4262–4266.

30. Li, J.; Zheng, W.; Kwon, A.H.; Lu, Y. *In vitro* selection and characterization of a highly efficient Zn(II)-dependent RNA-cleaving deoxyribozyme. *Nucleic Acids Res.* **2000**, *28*, 481–488.

31. Kim, H.K.; Liu, J.; Li, J.; Nagraj, N.; Li, M.; Pavot, C.M.; Lu, Y. Metal-dependent global folding and activity of the 8–17 DNAzyme studied byfluorescence resonance energy transfer. *J. Am. Chem. Soc.* **2007**, *129*, 6896–6902.

32. Rupcich, N.; Chiuman, W.; Nutiu, R.; Mei, S.; Flora, K.K.; Li, Y.; Brennan, J.D. Quenching of fluorophore-labeled DNA oligonucleotides by divalent metal ions: Implications for selection, design and applications of signaling aptamers and signaling deoxyribozymes. *J. Am. Chem. Soc.* **2006**, *128*, 780–790.

Decarboxylation of Pyruvate to Acetaldehyde for Ethanol Production by Hyperthermophiles

Mohammad S. Eram and Kesen Ma

Abstract: Pyruvate decarboxylase (PDC encoded by *pdc*) is a thiamine pyrophosphate (TPP)-containing enzyme responsible for the conversion of pyruvate to acetaldehyde in many mesophilic organisms. However, no *pdc*/PDC homolog has yet been found in fully sequenced genomes and proteomes of hyper/thermophiles. The only PDC activity reported in hyperthermophiles was a bifunctional, TPP- and CoA-dependent pyruvate ferredoxin oxidoreductase (POR)/PDC enzyme from the hyperthermophilic archaeon *Pyrococcus furiosus*. Another enzyme known to be involved in catalysis of acetaldehyde production from pyruvate is CoA-acetylating acetaldehyde dehydrogenase (AcDH encoded by *mhpF* and *adhE*). Pyruvate is oxidized into acetyl-CoA by either POR or pyruvate formate lyase (PFL), and AcDH catalyzes the reduction of acetyl-CoA to acetaldehyde in mesophilic organisms. AcDH is present in some mesophilic (such as clostridia) and thermophilic bacteria (e.g., *Geobacillus* and *Thermoanaerobacter*). However, no AcDH gene or protein homologs could be found in the released genomes and proteomes of hyperthermophiles. Moreover, no such activity was detectable from the cell-free extracts of different hyperthermophiles under different assay conditions. In conclusion, no commonly-known PDCs was found in hyperthermophiles. Instead of the commonly-known PDC, it appears that at least one multifunctional enzyme is responsible for catalyzing the non-oxidative decarboxylation of pyruvate to acetaldehyde in hyperthermophiles.

Reprinted from *Biomolecules*. Cite as: Eram, M.S.; Ma, K. Decarboxylation of Pyruvate to Acetaldehyde for Ethanol Production by Hyperthermophiles. *Biomolecules* **2013**, *3*, 578–596.

1. Introduction

Thermophilic microorganisms can be categorized into several groups: moderate thermophiles, or simply thermophiles, are those that grow optimally between 50–64 °C, extreme thermophiles are those with optimal growth temperatures between 65–79 °C. Finally, the organisms that can grow optimally above 80 °C are called hyperthermophiles. Hyperthermophiles can survive at room temperature for long periods of time, but cannot propagate at temperatures lower than 50 °C [1–5].

Hyperthermophilic microorganisms are widely studied for their remarkable scientific values and industrial potential. It is generally accepted that hyperthermophilic enzymes have very similar functions and catalytic mechanisms to their mesophilic ones. However, most of the hyperthermophilic enzymes characterized so far have optimum temperatures close to the host organism's growth requirements; thus, due to their intrinsic properties, the enzymes are stable and active under conditions that are detrimental to their mesophilic counterparts. Interestingly, enzymes from such extremophiles usually show increased stability not to one, but to several environmental factors. There are a number of advantages for using the hyper/thermophilic enzymes (especially for industrial applications) over their mesophilic partners, including the reduced risk of contamination during industrial processes, the possibility of self-distillation of the products at high temperatures, decreased viscosity and increased solubility/bioavailability of both the enzyme' and the substrate(s) leading to minimization of the diffusion limitations, and elimination of the costly transportation under cold temperature-controlled environment [6–10].

The aforementioned properties along with high demand from the biotech industries for the development of "tailor-made" bio-catalysts have created significant attention on the biochemistry and physiology of these organisms. Enzymes such as proteases, polymerases, hydrolases, isomerases, lipases, and oxidases are studied for their potential biotechnological exploitation, with the ultimate goal of using them or their products (mainly enzymatic) for biotechnological applications.

It is also appealing to determine the molecular, biochemical, physiological, and evolutionary mechanisms that enable these organisms to adapt to such hostile environments. Furthermore, hyperthermophilic proteins serve as models to study enzyme evolution, structure-function relationships and catalytic mechanisms. The findings of these studies can benefit the design of highly stable and active enzymes to be used for many applications [6,11,12].

2. Microbial Production of Ethanol

Demand for biofuel as substitutes for oil-based fuels is increasing due to concerns related to national security, economic stability, environmental impacts, and global warming. The national research council of the United States has predicted that, by 2020, half of all organic chemicals and materials will be produced by bioconversion. Bio-ethanol can also be used as a precursor for many other commodity chemicals, such as acetaldehyde, acetic acid and their derivatives [13–15].

The most commonly used ethanologenic organisms being intensively studied or already in use for industrial-scale production are *Zymomonas mobilis*, *Saccharomyces cervisiae*, *Escherichia coli*, and *Klebsiella oxytoca*. Substantial attention and effort have been dedicated to redirecting the metabolic pathways of these and others towards higher yield of ethanol production, by means of metabolic engineering [16–18].

However, lack of suitable microorganisms that can efficiently convert the raw biomaterials to bio-ethanol has been one of the main obstacles to widespread use of bio-fuels. In addition to the ability to ferment a wide variety of sugars, some other features must be considered when choosing organisms for industrial-scale bio-ethanol production. These important features include but are not limited to the ability to have high ethanol yield, tolerance to fermentation products/by-products, simple growth requirements, and the ability to grow under conditions that prevent contaminating organisms from growing [14,16].

Production of bio-ethanol using thermophilic and hyperthermophilic organisms is the focus of many research groups. Extremophiles in general and hyperthermophiles in particular are outstanding organisms that produce highly stable enzymes due to their natural habitats, and many of them are able to tolerate changes in environment; making them good candidates for bio-ethanol production [19].

Several distinct advantages are associated with using thermophiles over mesophiles, including high temperatures and the mostly anaerobic nature of thermophilic organisms, which result in elimination of oxygenation and cooling of the fermenter. Another aspect is improved solubility of many reaction components at elevated temperatures [20]. In addition, the high temperature of the process leads to lowering the viscosity of reaction mixtures, causing improved production yields. Various thermophiles can ferment hexose and/or pentose sugars, as well as more complex substrates such as cellulose and xylan in some cases. Many of these organisms and their enzymes are relatively resistant to sudden pH or temperature changes and high concentrations of solvents [21–23]. High temperatures can result in lower gas solubility and significantly decrease the risk of process failure and product loss due to contamination that is the common problem in the yeast-based fermentation system. At the same time, high temperatures lower the cost of ethanol recovery due to the high volatility of ethanol at high fermentation temperatures [14,19,24,25]. However, there are some disadvantages associated with using hyperthermophiles, the most important one being their intrinsic low substrate tolerance and product/by-product inhibition [26,27]. Moreover, some of these organisms are mixed-fermenters that result in production of sometimes too many types of products during growth [14,16].

Application of metabolic engineering approaches has had a great impact on elimination of the problems associated with using thermophiles, and led to development of strains with bio-ethanol yields that are almost equal to those of the yeast-based systems. Members of the genus *Clostridium*, especially thermophilic members such as *Clostridium thermocellum*, have been studied intensively due to their competence in production substantial amounts of ethanol, butanol and hydrogen [24,28,29]. Members of the genus *Thermoanaerobacter*, including *T. ethanolicus*, *T. tengcongensis*, and *T. pentosaceus* are extremely thermophilic bacteria that are well studied for their high ethanol production potential especially from pentoses [30–34]. The genus *Geobacillus* has been studied widely for bio-ethanol production potential [19,29,35,36]. Production of ethanol, although at lower concentrations, has also been reported for the extremely thermophilic *Caldicellulosiruptor* species that includes *C. owensensis* [37], *C. kristjanssonii* [38], and *C. saccharolyticus* [39].

Compared to the thermophilic ethanol producers, very little is known about the ethanol production levels and pathways in the extremely thermophilic and hyperthermophilic microorganisms. It was shown that the peptide- and carbohydrate-fermenting hyperthermophilic archaeon *Pyrococcus furiosus* can produce H_2, CO_2, acetate, alanine, and small amounts of ethanol [40]. The strictly anaerobic archaeon *Thermococcus* sp. strain ES1 produced some ethanol and butanol when cultures were grown at low concentrations of elemental sulfur [41]. The production of ethanol as an end product of fermentation was also shown in the hyperthermophilic anaerobic archaeon *Thermococcus guaymasensis* [42] and more recently in the autotrophic hyperthermophile, *Thermococcus onnurineus* [43]. Within the bacterial hyperthermophiles, traces of ethanol have been reported in cultures of different Thermotogales including *T. hypogea* [44], *T. lettingae* [45], *T. neapolitana* [46], *Kosmotoga olearia* [47], and *Thermosipho affectus* [48].

3. Key Enzymes Involved in Ethanol Production

One of the key enzymes in both ethanol production pathways is alcohol dehydrogenase. Alcohol dehydrogenases are members of the oxidoreductase family and are present in all three domains of life [49,50]. They belong to the dehydrogenase/reductase superfamily of enzymes and catalyze the reversible inter-conversion of alcohols to corresponding aldehydes or ketons. ADHs can be classified based on their cofactor requirements: (I) the flavin adenine di-nucleotide (FAD)-dependent

ADHs; (II) the pyrollo-quinoline quinone (PQQ), heme or cofactor F_{420} dependent ADHs; (III) NAD(P)-dependent ADHs [49,51]. Alternatively, they can be divided into three major groups based on their molecular size and metal contents: the first group is known as zinc-dependent long chain alcohol dehydrogenase; which have sizes of 300–900 amino acids, the second group is the short chain alcohol dehydrogenase: which contain no metal ions and have approximate lengths of 250 amino acids; and the third group is the long-chain iron dependent ADHs; with a length of 385–900 residues [49–52].

Many different ADHs have been characterized from various thermophilic and hyperthermophilic bacteria and archaea, with a majority of them being NAD(P)-dependent. Some of the more recently characterized hyper/thermophilic ADHs are those from *P. furiosus* [53,54], *Thermococcus hydrothermalis* [55], *Thermococcus kodakarensis* [56–58], *Thermococcus sibiricus* [59,60], *Thermococcus guaymasensis* [42], *Sulfolobus acidocaldarius* [61], *Thermococcus* strain ES1 [62], *Aeropyrum pernix* [63], *Thermotoga hypogea* [64], and *Pyrobaculum aerophilum* [65].

Although there is a relatively long list of ADHs isolated and characterized from thermophilic and hyperthermophilic archaea and bacteria, with the physiological roles of several proposed to be in the reduction of aldehydes to alcohols, other enzymes involved in the ethanol production pathways are not well characterized, especially the enzyme(s) that catalyze the production of acetaldehyde from pyruvate.

4. Pathways for the Production of Acetaldehyde from Pyruvate

Pyruvate is an intermediate in the central metabolism of carbohydrates [66,67], and it can be converted to acetaldehyde that will eventually be reduced to ethanol using one of the following two pathways:

(1) A two-step pathway that is used by yeast and a few bacteria like *Zymomonas mobilis* [68] and *Sarcina ventriculi* [69]. In this pathway pyruvate is non-oxidatively decarboxylated to acetaldehyde and carbon dioxide, which is catalyzed by pyruvate decarboxylase (PDC). Acetaldehyde is then converted to ethanol that is catalyzed by ADH (Figure 1);

(2) A three-step pathway that is more widespread in bacteria. Pyruvate is oxidatively decarboxylated to acetyl-coenzyme A (acetyl-CoA) by the metalloenzyme pyruvate ferredoxin oxidoreductase (POR) and/or pyruvate formate lyase (PFL). Acetyl-CoA is then converted to acetaldehyde by a CoA-dependent-acetylating acetaldehyde dehydrogenase (AcDH). Finally, acetaldehyde is reduced to ethanol by ADH.

The key metabolite for the two known pathways is acetaldehyde. The thiamine pyrophosphate (TPP)-dependent enzyme pyruvate decarboxylase is the only enzyme proficient at direct conversion of pyruvate to acetaldehyde. Interestingly, a majority (but not all) of the enzymes which are involved in the acetaldehyde production pathways are members of the superfamily of TPP-dependent enzymes, which includes PDC, POR, and PFL [70,71].

Figure 1. Two pathways of ethanol production from pyruvate. POR; Pyruvate ferredoxin oxidoreductase; PFL; Pyruvate formate lyase, AcDH; Acetaldehyde dehydrogenase, ADH; Alcohol dehydrogenase, PDC; pyruvate decarboxylase; CoASH; coenzyme A, Fd_{ox}; oxidized ferredoxin, Fd_{red}; reduced ferredoxin.

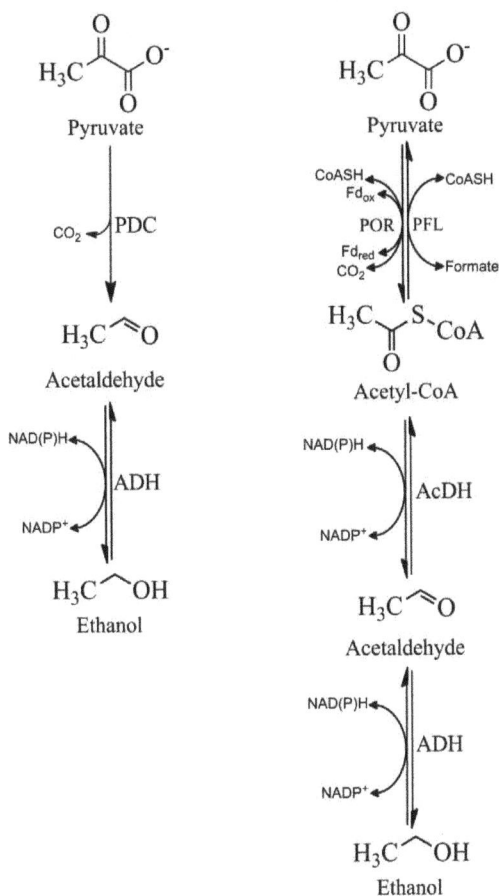

TPP, also known as thiamine diphosphate (ThDP), is composed of an aromatic methylaminopyrimidine ring, linked to a methyl thiazolium ring via. a methylene group with a pyrophosphate group attached to a hydroxylethyl side chain. TPP is derived from the water-soluble vitamin B1 and is the most common cofactor for enzymes that catalyze the cleavage and formation of carbon-carbon bonds next to a carbonyl group; hence TPP-dependent enzymes are involved in a wide range of metabolic pathways. Unlike many other cofactors (e.g., nicotinamide adenine dinucleotide, NADH) which are basically co-reactants, TPP remains at the enzymes' catalytic center and is directly involved in the catalysis of the reaction [72]. The reactions catalyzed by TPP-dependent enzymes can be divided into at least three groups: the oxidative reactions, non-oxidative reactions, and carboligation reactions [73].

5. Pyruvate Decarboxylase (PDC)

In 1911, Neuberg and Karczag for the first time described the decarboxylation of pyruvate to acetaldehyde in *S. cerevisiae*. In 1922, the same research group detected the potential of yeast in the formation of C-C bonds. Neuberg named the new enzyme "carboligase", and assumed it to exist apart from "α-carboxylase" (PDC) in yeast [74]. However, the preliminary characterization of the enzymes' cofactor was delayed until 1937, when Lohmann and Schuster analyzed structure of the enzymes' cofactor to be "cocarboxylase" or "aneurinpyrophosphate" or thiamin diphosphate [73].

The enzyme catalyzes non-oxidative decarboxylation of α-keto acids to produce a corresponding aldehyde and carbon dioxide. The most extensively examined enzymes of this group are the ones from *Saccharomyces cerevisiae* and its bacterial counterpart *Z. mobilis*. In addition to decarboxylation of pyruvate, PDC also catalyzes the enantio-selective formation of 2-hydroxy ketons via. carboligase side reactions.

PDC, or its gene (*pdc*), is found to be widely distributed in fungi and higher plants but it is relatively rare in prokaryotes and unknown in animals. In fungi, PDC is found in *Saccharomyces cerevisiae*, *Saccharomyces carlsbergensis* (also known as *S. pastorianus*) and *Saccharomyces uvarum*, *Neurospora crassa*, members of the *Kluyveromyces* species, members of the *Aspergillus* species, *Hanseniaspora uvarum*, *Schizosaccharomyces pombe*, and in *Candida* (*Torulopsis*) *glabrata*. PDC is present in a variety of plants, including maize (*Zea maize*), parsnip, orange, pea (*Pisum sativum*), jack bean, sweet potato, wheat, cotton wood, soybean and rice (*Oryza sativa*). In prokaryotes, PDC is found and studied in *Z. mobilis*, *Sarcina ventriculi*, *Clostridium botulinum*, *Acetobacter* species, *Zymobacter palmae*, and in *Erwinia amylovora* [75–79]. So far there has been no report on finding PDC/*pdc* homolog in thermophilic or hyperthermophilic bacteria or in any of the members of the third major evolutionary lineage of life, archaea as a whole [76–78,80].

PDCs from different organisms show at least a 30% identity at the amino acid level and most of them are composed of subunits of 562–610 amino acid residues. The holoenzyme is usually composed of four identical or non-identical subunits of approximately 60 kDa (ensuing in a total mass of about 240 kDa) in which every two subunits binds tightly (but not covalently) to a set of cofactors including TPP and Mg^{2+} ion. PDCs with four subunits are often arranged as a dimer of dimers, with multiple close contacts within the dimers and several contacts between the dimers. The contact area between two related dimers forms the "V" conformation that is a common property of all TPP-dependent enzymes studied so far, and it also has an essential role in cofactor binding for this group of enzymes [81,82].

The catalytic mechanism of PDC for the most part follows the principles of catalytic mechanisms of other TPP-dependent enzymes: in brief, carbonyl addition of pyruvate to the reactive C2 atom of the cofactor thiazolium ring [73] yields the intermediate 2-(2-lactyl)-TDP (LTDP). The subsequent release of carbon dioxide produces resonating carbanion/enamine forms of 2-(1-hydroxyethyl)-TDP (HETDP, also known as hydroxyethylidene-TPP). The resonating form is considered to be a central and highly reactive intermediate state in TPP-dependent enzymes acting on pyruvate. However, unlike most other TPP-dependent enzymes in which the intermediate is oxidized, the carbanion/enamine in PDC is protonated at the C2α position, yielding C2α-hydroxylethylthiamine diphosphate (HETDP) before the final release of acetaldehyde completes the reaction [72,83,84].

Crystal structures of several pyruvate decarboxylases are solved particularly from yeasts and *Z. mobilis* [81,85–87]. The active sites of these enzymes are also studied comprehensively using site-directed mutagenesis [88–90].

6. Pyruvate Ferredoxin Oxidoreductase (POR)

The enzyme pyruvate ferredoxin oxidoreductase (also known as pyruvate synthase as the reaction is reversible) is one of the best studied members of the 2-oxoacid oxidoreductase family [91–93]. The enzyme catalyzes coenzyme A and TPP-dependent oxidative decarboxylation of pyruvate to acetyl-CoA, releasing a molecule of CO_2 and transferring the reducing equivalents to the electron acceptor ferredoxin or flavodoxin. Alternatively, in other pyruvate oxidizing enzymes, the reducing equivalents are transferred to NAD^+ (in the case of pyruvate dehydrogenase using lipoate as oxidizing agent for the production of acetyl-CoA), to molecular-oxygen-producing hydrogen peroxide (in the case of pyruvate oxidase), or to the carbonyl groups producing formate (in case of pyruvate formate lyase) [94–96]. In acetaldehyde- and ethanol-producing organisms, acetyl-CoA is usually converted to acetaldehyde via. the CoA-dependent (acetylating) acetaldehyde dehydrogenase.

POR uses iron-sulfur cluster chemistry to catalyze the pyruvate decarboxylation and release of acetyl-CoA. POR is an ancient molecule, and it seems to have existed even before the divergence of the domains of the bacteria and archaea [97]. The enzyme is present in all three domains of life. All archaea catalyze the conversion of pyruvate to acetyl-CoA using POR, and all of the archaeal genomes sequenced so far contain hetero-tetrameric PORs, which have been proposed to be the closest to the POR common ancestor [97,98].

POR is prevalent mainly in anaerobic bacteria and infrequently found in anaerobic protozoa, for example, in *Giardia duodenalis* [99] and *Enthamoeba histolytica* [100,101]. The enzyme has been isolated and studied from many different anaerobic or microaerophilic microorganisms including anaerobic bacteria like the genera *Clostridium* [102], *Moorella thermoacetica* [103] and anaerobic sulphate-reducing bacteria *Desulfovibrio africanus* [104–107]. In hyperthermophiles, PORs are characterized from the hyperthermophilic bacterium *Thermotoga maritima* [108] and hyperthermophilic archaea *Pyrococcus furiosus* [109] and *Archaeoglobus fulgidus* [110], as well as the methanogenic archaea *Methanosarcina barkeri* [111,112] and *Methanobacterium thermoautotrophicum* [113].

The quaternary oligomeric structure of the POR is variable depending on the source microorganism and can be homo-dimeric (e.g., most bacterial PORs), hetero-dimeric (e.g., POR of *Halobacterium salinarium*), hetero-tetrameric (archaeal PORs), and heteropentameric (anabolic PORs), although all of the PORs studied so far, regardless of their source and structure, seem to be phylogenetically related and derived from a common archaeal-type heterotetrameric ancestor [97,98].

The crystal structures of several POR have been determined. PORs from *Desulfovibrio africanus* (with and without bound substrate) and *Desulfovibrio vulgaris* [114–116] are among the most extensively studied PORs. POR is a metalloenzyme and all PORs studied so far contained between one and three [4Fe-4S] clusters arranged in a spatial order from the TPP located at the active center of the enzyme toward its surface, suggesting that they are part of an electron transfer pathway [117,118].

POR can also catalyze the reaction to form pyruvate from acetyl-CoA and carbon dioxide, which is the basis of the carbon dioxide fixation in many autotrophic microorganisms [119]. This type represents the so-called "anabolic" PORs that are studied from the thermophilic facultative aerobic bacterium *Hydrogenobacter thermophilus* [120–122], as well as the hydrogenotrophic methanoarchaeon *Methanococcus maripaludis* [123,124]. Interestingly, in the case of the heteropentameric POR of *M. maripaludis*, four subunits are very closely related to the archaeal heterotetrameric (ancestral) PORs, the fifth subunit has no known homologue within PORs.

The general steps of the POR catalytic reactions follow the same principles as those of other TPP-dependent enzymes. However, the enzyme is unique in one aspect: unlike most other TPP-dependent enzymes, POR takes advantage of free radical chemistry to catalyze the decarboxylation reaction [94,125].

Pyruvate dehydrogenase complexes (PDH), which also catalyze the oxidative decarboxylation of pyruvate to acetyl-CoA using NAD^+ as an electron acceptor, are normally present in aerobic organisms [126,127], which have been found in some thermopiles [128–130]. But no PDH has been identified in hyperthermophiles [131]. Since PDH does not play any significant role in the production of acetaldehyde and ethanol, no further description of this enzyme complex will be given in this review.

7. POR/PDC Bi-Functional Enzyme

In 1997, it was reported that the POR was also capable of converting pyruvate to acetaldehyde in the hyperthermophilic anaerobic archaeon *Pyrococcus furiosus* [80]. Unlike the commonly-known PDCs, which employ chemical rather than radical intermediates and therefore are oxygen insensitive, the reported PDC activity was highly oxygen sensitive. Both the POR and PDC activities of the hyperthermophilic enzyme were TPP- and coenzyme A-dependent. By using the coenzyme A analogue (desulfocoenzyme A), it was shown that coenzyme A has only a structural, and not a catalytic role in the catalyzed PDC reaction. Consequently, a "switch" mechanism was proposed for the enzyme's bi-functionality, suggesting the conversion of active aldehyde to either acetyl-CoA or acetaldehyde, depending on the binding of CoA. According to the proposed model, binding of coenzyme A causes conformational changes in the intermediate structure, causing its protonation and generation of hydroxyethyl-TPP (HETDP). This reaction leads to release of acetaldehyde, allowing for the regeneration of TPP and possible release of CoA [80]. Ferredoxin is not required for its full PDC activity nor has any inhibitory effect when tested under *in vitro* conditions. However, it is likely that the *in vivo* PDC activity might be dependent on the availability of oxidized ferredoxin, which means that a lower ratio of oxidized to reduced ferredoxin may favor the PDC activity and *vice versa*. Therefore, it can be predicted that more acetaldehyde would be produced for being reduced to ethanol if the ratio of the oxidized to reduced ferredoxin would be kept very low under the anaerobic growth condition. Such a low ratio may also require a relatively low activity of the ferredoxin-oxidizing hydrogenases present in *P. furiosus* [132,133].

To date there has been no further study on the bi-functionality of the POR enzyme or the physiological relevance of such bifunctionality in any other organisms. It is not clear whether this bi-functionality is only a trait of *Pyrococcales*' POR or a common property of all hyper/thermophilic PORs.

8. Acetaldehyde Dehydrogenase (CoA-Acetylating)

Acetaldehyde dehydrogenase (CoA-acetylating, EC 1.2.1.10) is a member of a very divergent superfamily of enzymes known as the "aldehyde dehydrogenases". The prototype enzyme (*adhE*) was first discovered in *Escherichia coli* and is required for its anaerobic growth [134]. It was then discovered in the strictly anaerobic bacterium *Clostridium kluyveri* [135]. The enzyme is responsible for the conversion of acetyl-coenzyme A (acetyl-CoA) to acetaldehyde that is eventually converted to ethanol. Two forms of the enzyme are available: one is the monofunctional enzyme with only AcDH activity (*mhpF*) and the other is the bifunctional enzyme with both AcDH and ADH activities (*adhE*). The latter group is composed of an ADH active *C*-terminal and an AcDH active *N*-terminal, a structure believed to be the result of gene fusion between the genes encoding for each single enzyme [136,137].

Reports are available on isolation and characterization of the bifunctional NADP-dependent alcohol/acetaldehyde dehydrogenase (CoA-acetylating) from mesophilic microorganisms including *Giardia lamblia* [138] and *Enthamoeba histolytica* [101,139]. They are also present in some thermophiles, including *T. ethanolicus* [140,141], *T. mathranii* [32] and members of the genus *Geobacillus* [19]. However, no mono- or bi-functional AcDH activity was characterized from hyperthermophiles. Survey of the fully sequenced genomes of hyperthermophilic archaea and bacteria has shown no *adhE* or *mhpF* homologue either (Eram and Ma, unpublished data).

9. Conclusions

Many hyperthermophilic microorganisms produce ethanol as an end metabolic product. Although alcohol dehydrogenase and pyruvate ferredoxin oxidoreductase are found to be present, enzymes catalyzing the production of acetaldehyde from pyruvate are not well characterized. The commonly-known pyruvate decarboxylase and coenzyme A-dependent aldehyde dehydrogenase have not been identified. The only report of a bi-functional pyruvate decarboxylase is the POR/PDC from *P. furiosus*, which is thermostable but oxygen-sensitive. Therefore, it is likely that they use a two-step pathway to convert pyruvate to ethanol. The regulation of each of the POR/PDC activities is not clear but it may be related to the redox states inside the cells. To date, it appears that at least one multifunctional enzyme is responsible for catalyzing the non-oxidative decarboxylation of pyruvate to acetaldehyde in hyperthermophiles, and further study is needed to understand the catalysis of acetaldehyde production from pyruvate at high temperatures.

Acknowledgments

This work was supported by research grants from the Natural Sciences and Engineering Research Council (Canada), Genome Canada/Genome Prairie and Canada Foundation for Innovation to KM.

Conflicts of Interest

The authors declare no conflict of interest.

References

1. Wiegel, J. Temperature spans for growth: Hypothesis and discussion. *FEMS Microbiol. Lett.* **1990**, *75*, 155–169.
2. Charlier, D.; Droogmans, L. Microbial Life at high temperature, the challenges, the strategies. *Cell. Mol. Life Sci.* **2005**, *62*, 2974–2984.
3. Stetter, K. History of discovery of the first hyperthermophiles. *Extremophiles* **2006**, *10*, 357–362.
4. Lebedinsky, A.; Chernyh, N.; Bonch-Osmolovskaya, E. Phylogenetic systematics of microorganisms inhabiting thermal environments. *Biochemistry (Mosc.)* **2007**, *72*, 1299–1312.
5. Wagner, I.D.; Wiegel, J. Diversity of Thermophilic Anaerobes. *Ann. NY Acad. Sci.* **2008**, *1125*, 1–43.
6. Morozkina, E.; Slutskaya, E.; Fedorova, T.; Tugay, T.; Golubeva, L.; Koroleva, O. Extremophilic microorganisms: Biochemical adaptation and biotechnological application. *Appl. Biochem. Microbiol.* **2010**, *46*, 1–14.
7. Sommer, P.; Georgieva, T.; Ahring, B.K. Potential for using thermophilic anaerobic bacteria for bioethanol production from hemicellulose. *Biochem. Soc. Trans.* **2004**, *32*, 283–289.
8. Vieille, C.; Zeikus, G.J. Hyperthermophilic enzymes: Sources, uses, and molecular mechanisms for thermostability. *Microbiol. Mol. Biol. Rev.* **2001**, *65*, 1–43.
9. Haki, G.D.; Rakshit, S.K. Developments in industrially important thermostable enzymes: A review. *Bioresour. Technol.* **2003**, *89*, 17–34.
10. Egorova, K.; Antranikian, G. Industrial relevance of thermophilic Archaea. *Curr. Opin. Microbiol.* **2005**, *8*, 649–655.
11. Van den Burg, B. Extremophiles as a source for novel enzymes. *Curr. Opin. Microbiol.* **2003**, *6*, 213–218.
12. Atomi, H.; Sato, T.; Kanai, T. Application of hyperthermophiles and their enzymes. *Curr. Opin. Biotechnol.* **2011**, *22*, 618–626.
13. Lynd, L.R.; Wyman, C.E.; Gerngross, T.U. Biocommodity engineering. *Biotechnol. Prog.* **1999**, *15*, 777–793.
14. Zaldivar, J.; Nielsen, J.; Olsson, L. Fuel ethanol production from lignocellulose: A challenge for metabolic engineering and process integration. *Appl. Microbiol. Biotechnol.* **2001**, *56*, 17–34.
15. Mabee, W.E.; Saddler, J.N. Bioethanol from lignocellulosics: Status and perspectives in Canada. *Bioresour. Technol.* **2010**, *101*, 4806–4813.
16. Dien, B.S.; Cotta, M.A.; Jeffries, T.W. Bacteria engineered for fuel ethanol production: Current status. *Appl. Microbiol. Biotechnol.* **2003**, *63*, 258–266.
17. Buschke, N.; Schäfer, R.; Becker, J.; Wittmann, C. Metabolic engineering of industrial platform microorganisms for biorefinery applications-optimization of substrate spectrum and process robustness by rational and evolutive strategies. *Bioresour. Technol.* **2012**, *135*, 544–554.

18. Jang, Y.-S.; Park, J.M.; Choi, S.; Choi, Y.J.; Seung, D.Y.; Cho, J.H.; Lee, S.Y. Engineering of microorganisms for the production of biofuels and perspectives based on systems metabolic engineering approaches. *Biotechnol. Adv.* **2012**, *30*, 989–1000.

19. Taylor, M.P.; Eley, K.L.; Martin, S.; Tuffin, M.I.; Burton, S.G.; Cowan, D.A. Thermophilic ethanologenesis: Future prospects for second-generation bioethanol production. *Trends Biotechnol.* **2009**, *27*, 398–405.

20. Bustard, M.T.; Burgess, J.G.; Meeyoo, V.; Wright, P.C. Novel opportunities for marine hyperthermophiles in emerging biotechnology and engineering industries. *J. Chem. Technol. Biotechnol.* **2000**, *75*, 1095–1109.

21. Huber, H.; Stetter, K.O. Hyperthermophiles and their possible potential in biotechnology. *J. Biotechnol.* **1998**, *64*, 39–52.

22. Schiraldi, C.; de Rosa, M. The production of biocatalysts and biomolecules from extremophiles. *Trends Biotechnol.* **2002**, *20*, 515–521.

23. Hough, D.W.; Danson, M.J. Extremozymes. *Curr. Opin. Chem. Biol.* **1999**, *3*, 39–46.

24. Lamed, R.; Zeikus, J.G. Ethanol production by thermophilic bacteria: Relationship between fermentation product yields of and catabolic enzyme activities in *Clostridium thermocellum* and *Thermoanaerobium brockii*. *J. Bacteriol.* **1980**, *144*, 569–578.

25. Klapatch, T.R.; Hogsett, D.A.L.; Baskaran, S.; Pal, S.; Lynd, L.R. Organism development and characterization for ethanol production using thermophilic bacteria. *Appl. Biochem. Biotechnol.* **1994**, *45–46*, 209–223.

26. Chang, T.; Yao, S. Thermophilic, lignocellulolytic bacteria for ethanol production: Current state and perspectives. *Appl. Microbiol. Biotechnol.* **2011**, *92*, 13–27.

27. Zeikus, J.G.; Ben-Bassat, A.; Ng, T.K.; Lamed, R.J. Thermophilic ethanol fermentations. In *Trends in the Biology of Fermentations for Fuels and Chemicals*; Hollaender, A., Rabson, R., Rogers, P., Pietro, A.S., Valentine, R., Wolfe, R., Eds.; Springer: New York, NY, USA, 1981; pp. 441–461.

28. Demain, A.L.; Newcomb, M.; Wu, J.H.D. Cellulase, clostridia, and ethanol. *Microbiol. Mol. Biol. Rev.* **2005**, *69*, 124–154.

29. Barnard, D.; Casanueva, A.; Tuffin, M.; Cowan, D. Extremophiles in biofuel synthesis. *Environ. Technol.* **2010**, *31*, 871–888.

30. Tomás, A.F.; Karagöz, P.; Karakashev, D.; Angelidaki, I. Extreme thermophilic ethanol production from rapeseed straw: Using the newly isolated *Thermoanaerobacter pentosaceus* and combining it with *Saccharomyces cerevisiae* in a two-step process. *Biotechnol. Bioeng.* **2013**, *110*, 1574–1582.

31. Shaw, A.J.; Podkaminer, K.K.; Desai, S.G.; Bardsley, J.S.; Rogers, S.R.; Thorne, P.G.; Hogsett, D.A.; Lynd, L.R. Metabolic engineering of a thermophilic bacterium to produce ethanol at high yield. *Proc. Natl. Acad. Sci. USA* **2008**, *105*, 13769–13774.

32. Yao, S.; Mikkelsen, M.J. Identification and overexpression of a bifunctional aldehyde/alcohol dehydrogenase responsible for ethanol production in *Thermoanaerobacter mathranii*. *J. Mol. Microbiol. Biotechnol.* **2010**, *19*, 123–133.

144

33. Svetlitchnyi, V.; Kensch, O.; Falkenhan, D.; Korseska, S.; Lippert, N.; Prinz, M.; Sassi, J.; Schickor, A.; Curvers, S. Single-step ethanol production from lignocellulose using novel extremely thermophilic bacteria. *Biotechnol. Biofuels* **2013**, *6*, 1–15.

34. Yao, S.; Mikkelsen, M. Metabolic engineering to improve ethanol production in *Thermoanaerobacter mathranii*. *Appl. Microbiol. Biotechnol.* **2010**, *88*, 199–208.

35. Thompson, A.; Studholme, D.; Green, E.; Leak, D. Heterologous expression of pyruvate decarboxylase in *Geobacillus thermoglucosidasius*. *Biotechnol. Lett.* **2008**, *30*, 1359–1365.

36. Cripps, R.E.; Eley, K.; Leak, D.J.; Rudd, B.; Taylor, M.; Todd, M.; Boakes, S.; Martin, S.; Atkinson, T. Metabolic engineering of *Geobacillus thermoglucosidasius* for high yield ethanol production. *Metab. Eng.* **2009**, *11*, 398–408.

37. Huang, C.-Y.; Patel, B.K.; Mah, R.A.; Baresi, L. *Caldicellulosiruptor owensensis* sp. nov., an anaerobic, extremely thermophilic, xylanolytic bacterium. *Int. J. Syst. Bacteriol.* **1998**, *48*, 91–97.

38. Bredholt, S.; Sonne-Hansen, J.; Nielsen, P.; Mathrani, I.M.; Ahring, B.K. *Caldicellulosiruptor kristjanssonii* sp. nov., a cellulolytic, extremely thermophilic, anaerobic bacterium. *Int. J. Syst. Bacteriol.* **1999**, *49*, 991–996.

39. Van Niel, E.W.J.; Claassen, P.A.M.; Stams, A.J.M. Substrate and product inhibition of hydrogen production by the extreme thermophile, *Caldicellulosiruptor saccharolyticus*. *Biotechnol. Bioeng.* **2003**, *81*, 255–262.

40. Kengen, S.; de Bok, F.; van Loo, N.; Dijkema, C.; Stams, A.; de Vos, W. Evidence for the operation of a novel Embden-Meyerhof pathway that involves ADP-dependent kinases during sugar fermentation by *Pyrococcus furiosus*. *J. Biol. Chem.* **1994**, *269*, 17537–17541.

41. Ma, K.; Loessner, H.; Heider, J.; Johnson, M.; Adams, M. Effects of elemental sulfur on the metabolism of the deep-sea hyperthermophilic archaeon *Thermococcus* strain ES-1: Characterization of a sulfur-regulated, non-heme iron alcohol dehydrogenase. *J. Bacteriol.* **1995**, *177*, 4748–4756.

42. Ying, X.; Ma, K. Characterization of a zinc-containing alcohol dehydrogenase with stereoselectivity from the hyperthermophilic archaeon *Thermococcus guaymasensis*. *J. Bacteriol.* **2011**, *193*, 3009–3019.

43. Moon, Y.-J.; Kwon, J.; Yun, S.-H.; Lim, H.L.; Kim, M.-S.; Kang, S.G.; Lee, J.-H.; Choi, J.-S.; Kim, S.L.; Chung, Y.-H. Proteome analyses of hydrogen-producing hyperthermophilic archaeon *Thermococcus onnurineus* NA1 in different one-carbon substrate culture conditions. *Mol. Cell. Proteomics* **2012**, doi:10.1074/mcp.M111.015420.

44. Fardeau, M.L.; Ollivier, B.; Patel, B.K.C.; Magot, M.; Thomas, P.; Rimbault, A.; Rocchiccioli, F.; Garcia, J.L. *Thermotoga hypogea* sp. nov., a xylanolytic, thermophilic bacterium from an oil-producing well. *Int. J. Syst. Bacteriol.* **1997**, *47*, 1013–1019.

45. Balk, M.; Weijma, J.; Stams, A.J.M. *Thermotoga lettingae* sp. nov., a novel thermophilic, methanol-degrading bacterium isolated from a thermophilic anaerobic reactor. *Int. J. Syst. Evol. Microbiol.* **2002**, *52*, 1361–1368.

46. De Vrije, T.; Bakker, R.; Budde, M.; Lai, M.; Mars, A.; Claassen, P. Efficient hydrogen production from the lignocellulosic energy crop *Miscanthus* by the extreme thermophilic bacteria *Caldicellulosiruptor saccharolyticus* and *Thermotoga neapolitana*. *Biotechnol. Biofuels* **2009**, *2*, e12.

47. DiPippo, J.L.; Nesbo, C.L.; Dahle, H.; Doolittle, W.F.; Birkland, N.-K.; Noll, K.M. *Kosmotoga olearia* gen. nov., sp. nov., a thermophilic, anaerobic heterotroph isolated from an oil production fluid. *Int. J. Syst. Evol. Microbiol.* **2009**, *59*, 2991–3000.

48. Podosokorskaya, O.A.; Kublanov, I.V.; Reysenbach, A.L.; Kolganova, T.V.; Bonch-Osmolovskaya, E.A. *Thermosipho affectus* sp. nov., a thermophilic, anaerobic, cellulolytic bacterium isolated from a Mid-Atlantic Ridge hydrothermal vent. *Int. J. Syst. Evol. Microbiol.* **2011**, *61*, 1160–1164.

49. Reid, M.F.; Fewson, C.A. Molecular characterization of microbial alcohol dehydrogenases. *Crit. Rev. Microbiol.* **1994**, *20*, 13–56.

50. Littlechild, J.A.; Guy, J.E.; Isupov, M.N. Hyperthermophilic dehydrogenase enzymes. *Biochem. Soc. Trans.* **2004**, *32*, 255–258.

51. Radianingtyas, H.; Wright, P.C. Alcohol dehydrogenases from thermophilic and hyperthermophilic archaea and bacteria. *FEMS Microbiol. Rev.* **2003**, *27*, 593–616.

52. Korkhin, Y.; Kalb, A.J.; Peretz, M.; Bogin, O.; Burstein, Y.; Frolow, F. NADP-dependent bacterial alcohol dehydrogenases: Crystal structure, cofactor-binding and cofactor specificity of the ADHs of *Clostridium beijerinckii* and *Thermoanaerobacter brockii*. *J. Mol. Biol.* **1998**, *278*, 967–981.

53. Machielsen, R.; Uria, A.R.; Kengen, S.W.M.; van der Oost, J. Production and characterization of a thermostable alcohol dehydrogenase that belongs to the aldo-keto reductase superfamily. *Appl. Environ. Microbiol.* **2006**, *72*, 233–238.

54. Van der Oost, J.; Voorhorst, W.G.B.; Kengen, S.W.M.; Geerling, A.C.M.; Wittenhorst, V.; Gueguen, Y.; de Vos, W.M. Genetic and biochemical characterization of a short-chain alcohol dehydrogenase from the hyperthermophilic archaeon *Pyrococcus furiosus*. *Eur. J. Biochem.* **2001**, *268*, 3062–3068.

55. Antoine, E.; Rolland, J.-L.; Raffin, J.-P.; Dietrich, J. Cloning and over-expression in *Escherichia coli* of the gene encoding NADPH group III alcohol dehydrogenase from *Thermococcus hydrothermalis*. *Eur. J. Biochem.* **1999**, *264*, 880–889.

56. Bashir, Q.; Rashid, N.; Jamil, F.; Imanaka, T.; Akhtar, M. Highly thermostable L-threonine dehydrogenase from the hyperthermophilic archaeon *Thermococcus kodakaraensis*. *J. Biochem. (Tokyo)* **2009**, *146*, 95–102.

57. Bowyer, A.; Mikolajek, H.; Stuart, J.W.; Wood, S.P.; Jamil, F.; Rashid, N.; Akhtar, M.; Cooper, J.B. Structure and function of the l-threonine dehydrogenase (TkTDH) from the hyperthermophilic archaeon *Thermococcus kodakaraensis*. *J. Struct. Biol.* **2009**, *168*, 294–304.

58. Wu, X.; Zhang, C.; Orita, I.; Imanaka, T.; Fukui, T.; Xing, X.-H. Thermostable alcohol dehydrogenase from *Thermococcus kodakarensis* KOD1 for enantioselective bioconversion of aromatic secondary alcohols. *Appl. Environ. Microbiol.* **2013**, *79*, 2209–2217.

59. Stekhanova, T.N.; Mardanov, A.V.; Bezsudnova, E.Y.; Gumerov, V.M.; Ravin, N.V.; Skryabin, K.G.; Popov, V.O. Characterization of a thermostable short-chain alcohol dehydrogenase from the hyperthermophilic archaeon *Thermococcus sibiricus*. *Appl. Environ. Microbiol.* **2010**, *76*, 4096–4098.

60. Lyashenko, A.V.; Bezsudnova, E.Y.; Gumerov, V.M.; Lashkov, A.A.; Mardanov, A.V.; Mikhailov, A.M.; Polyakov, K.M.; Popov, V.O.; Ravin, N.V.; Skryabin, K.G.; *et al.* Expression, purification and crystallization of a thermostable short-chain alcohol dehydrogenase from the archaeon *Thermococcus sibiricus*. *Acta Crystallogr. F Struct. Biol. Cryst. Commun.* **2010**, *66*, 655–657.

61. Pennacchio, A.; Giordano, A.; Pucci, B.; Rossi, M.; Raia, C. Biochemical characterization of a recombinant short-chain NAD(H)-dependent dehydrogenase/reductase from *Sulfolobus acidocaldarius*. *Extremophiles* **2010**, *14*, 193–204.

62. Ying, X.; Grunden, A.; Nie, L.; Adams, M.; Ma, K. Molecular characterization of the recombinant iron-containing alcohol dehydrogenase from the hyperthermophilic Archaeon, *Thermococcus* strain ES1. *Extremophiles* **2009**, *13*, 299–311.

63. Guy, J.E.; Isupov, M.N.; Littlechild, J.A. The structure of an alcohol dehydrogenase from the hyperthermophilic archaeon *Aeropyrum pernix*. *J. Mol. Biol.* **2003**, *331*, 1041–1051.

64. Ying, X.; Wang, Y.; Badiei, H.; Karanassios, V.; Ma, K. Purification and characterization of an iron-containing alcohol dehydrogenase in extremely thermophilic bacterium *Thermotoga hypogea*. *Arch. Microbiol.* **2007**, *187*, 499–510.

65. Vitale, A.; Thorne, N.; Lovell, S.; Battaile, K.P.; Hu, X.; Shen, M.; D'Auria, S.; Auld, D.S. Physicochemical characterization of a thermostable alcohol dehydrogenase from *Pyrobaculum aerophilum*. *PLoS One* **2013**, *8*, e63828.

66. Verhees, C.H.; Kengen, S.W.M.; Tuininga, J.E.; Schut, G.J.; Adams, M.W.W.; de Vos, W.M.; van der Oost, J. The unique features of glycolytic pathways in Archaea. *Biochem. J.* **2003**, *375*, 231–246.

67. Siebers, B.; Schönheit, P. Unusual pathways and enzymes of central carbohydrate metabolism in Archaea. *Curr. Opin. Microbiol.* **2005**, *8*, 695–705.

68. Buchholz, S.E.; Dooley, M.M.; Eveleigh, D.E. *Zymomonas*—An alcoholic enigma. *Trends Biotechnol.* **1987**, *5*, 199–204.

69. Canale-Parola, E. Biology of the sugar-fermenting *Sarcinae*. *Microbiol. Mol. Biol. Rev.* **1970**, *34*, 82–97.

70. Duggleby, R.G. Domain relationships in thiamine diphosphate-dependent enzymes. *Acc. Chem. Res.* **2006**, *39*, 550–557.

71. Costelloe, S.; Ward, J.; Dalby, P. Evolutionary analysis of the TPP-dependent enzyme family. *J. Mol. Evol.* **2008**, *66*, 36–49.

72. Kluger, R.; Tittmann, K. Thiamin diphosphate catalysis: Enzymic and nonenzymic covalent intermediates. *Chem. Rev.* **2008**, *108*, 1797–1833.

73. Schellenberger, A. Sixty years of thiamin diphosphate biochemistry. *Biochim. Biophys. Acta* **1998**, *1385*, 177–186.

74. Iding, H.; Siegert, P.; Mesch, K.; Pohl, M. Application of alpha-keto acid decarboxylases in biotransformations. *Biochim. Biophys. Acta* **1998**, *1385*, 307–322.

75. Bringer-Meyer, S.; Schimz, K.L.; Sahm, H. Pyruvate decarboxylase from *Zymomonas mobilis*. Isolation and partial characterization. *Arch. Microbiol.* **1986**, *146*, 105–110.

76. Raj, K.C.; Ingram, L.O.; Maupin-Furlow, J.A. Pyruvate decarboxylase: A key enzyme for the oxidative metabolism of lactic acid by *Acetobacter pasteurianus*. *Arch. Microbiol.* **2001**, *176*, 443–451.

77. Raj, K.C.; Talarico, L.A.; Ingram, L.O.; Maupin-Furlow, J.A. Cloning and characterization of the *Zymobacter palmae* pyruvate decarboxylase gene (*pdc*) and comparison to bacterial homologues. *Appl. Environ. Microbiol.* **2002**, *68*, 2869–2876.

78. Talarico, L.A.; Ingram, L.O.; Maupin-Furlow, J.A. Production of the Gram-positive *Sarcina ventriculi* pyruvate decarboxylase in *Escherichia coli*. *Microbiology* **2001**, *147*, 2425–2435.

79. Wang, Q.; He, P.; Lu, D.; Shen, A.; Jiang, N. Purification, characterization, cloning and expression of pyruvate decarboxylase from *Torulopsis glabrata* IFO005. *J. Biochem. (Tokyo)* **2004**, *136*, 447–455.

80. Ma, K.; Hutchins, A.; Sung, S.-J.S.; Adams, M.W.W. Pyruvate ferredoxin oxidoreductase from the hyperthermophilic archaeon, *Pyrococcus furiosus*, functions as a CoA-dependent pyruvate decarboxylase. *Proc. Natl. Acad. Sci. USA* **1997**, *94*, 9608–9613.

81. Dobritzsch, D.; Konig, S.; Schneider, G.; Lu, G. High resolution crystal structure of pyruvate decarboxylase from *Zymomonas mobilis*. Implications for substrate activation in pyruvate decarboxylases. *J. Biol. Chem.* **1998**, *273*, 20196–20204.

82. Jordan, F. Current mechanistic understanding of thiamin diphosphate-dependent enzymatic reactions. *Nat. Prod. Rep.* **2003**, *20*, 184–201.

83. Kluger, R. Thiamin diphosphate: A mechanistic update on enzymic and nonenzymic catalysis of decarboxylation. *Chem. Rev.* **1987**, *87*, 863–876.

84. Candy, J.M.; Duggleby, R.G. Structure and properties of pyruvate decarboxylase and site-directed mutagenesis of the *Zymomonas mobilis* enzyme. *Biochim. Biophys. Acta* **1998**, *1385*, 323–338.

85. Kutter, S.; Weiss, M.S.; Wille, G.; Golbik, R.; Spinka, M.; König, S. Covalently bound substrate at the regulatory site of yeast pyruvate decarboxylases triggers allosteric enzyme activation. *J. Biol. Chem.* **2009**, *284*, 12136–12144.

86. Siegert, P.; McLeish, M.J.; Baumann, M.; Iding, H.; Kneen, M.M.; Kenyon, G.L.; Pohl, M. Exchanging the substrate specificities of pyruvate decarboxylase from *Zymomonas mobilis* and benzoylformate decarboxylase from *Pseudomonas putida*. *Protein Eng. Des. Sel.* **2005**, *18*, 345–357.

87. Arjunan, P.; Umland, T.; Dyda, F.; Swaminathan, S.; Furey, W.; Sax, M.; Farrenkopf, B.; Gao, Y.; Zhang, D.; Jordan, F. Crystal structure of the thiamin diphosphate-dependent enzyme pyruvate decarboxylase from the yeast *Saccharomyces cerevisiae* at 2.3 Å resolution. *J. Mol. Biol.* **1996**, *256*, 590–600.

88. Pohl, M. Protein design on pyruvate decarboxylase (PDC) by site-directed mutagenesis. *Adv. Biochem. Eng. Biotechnol.* **1997**, *58*, 15–43.

89. Liu, M.; Sergienko, E.A.; Guo, F.; Wang, J.; Tittmann, K.; Hubner, G.; Furey, W.; Jordan, F. Catalytic acid-base groups in yeast pyruvate decarboxylase. 1. Site-directed mutagenesis and steady-state kinetic studies on the enzyme with the D28A, H114F, H115F, and E477Q substitutions. *Biochemistry (Mosc.)* **2001**, *40*, 7355–7368.

90. Schenk, G.; Layfield, R.; Candy, J.M.; Duggleby, R.G.; Nixon, P.F. Molecular evolutionary analysis of the thiamine-diphosphate-dependent enzyme, transketolase. *J. Mol. Evol.* **1997**, *44*, 552–572.

91. Raeburn, S.; Rabinowitz, J.C. Pyruvate: Ferredoxin oxidoreductase: II. Characteristics of the forward and reverse reactions and properties of the enzyme. *Arch. Biochem. Biophys.* **1971**, *146*, 21–33.

92. Uyeda, K.; Rabinowitz, J.C. Pyruvate-ferredoxin oxidoreductase. IV. Studies on the reaction mechanism. *J. Biol. Chem.* **1971**, *246*, 3120–3125.

93. Uyeda, K.; Rabinowitz, J.C. Pyruvate-ferredoxin oxidoreductase. III. Purification and properties of the enzyme. *J. Biol. Chem.* **1971**, *246*, 3111–3119.

94. Ragsdale, S.W. Pyruvate ferredoxin oxidoreductase and its radical intermediate. *Chem. Rev.* **2003**, *103*, 2333–2346.

95. Ragsdale, S.W.; Pierce, E. Acetogenesis and the Wood-Ljungdahl pathway of CO_2 fixation. *Biochim. Biophys. Acta* **2008**, *1784*, 1873–1898.

96. Tittmann, K. Reaction mechanisms of thiamin diphosphate enzymes: Redox reactions. *FEBS J.* **2009**, *276*, 2454–2468.

97. Kletzin, A.; Adams, M. Molecular and phylogenetic characterization of pyruvate and 2- ketoisovalerate ferredoxin oxidoreductases from *Pyrococcus furiosus* and pyruvate ferredoxin oxidoreductase from *Thermotoga maritima*. *J. Bacteriol.* **1996**, *178*, 248–257.

98. Zhang, Q.; Iwasaki, T.; Wakagi, T.; Oshima, T. 2-Oxoacid: Ferredoxin oxidoreductase from the thermoacidophilic archaeon, *Sulfolobus* sp. strain 7. *J. Biochem. (Tokyo)* **1996**, *120*, 587–599.

99. Townson, S.M.; Upcroft, J.A.; Upcroft, P. Characterisation and purification of pyruvate: Ferredoxin oxidoreductase from *Giardia duodenalis*. *Mol. Biochem. Parasitol.* **1996**, *79*, 183–193.

100. Horner, D.S.; Hirt, R.P.; Embley, T.M. A single eubacterial origin of eukaryotic pyruvate: Ferredoxin oxidoreductase genes: Implications for the evolution of anaerobic eukaryotes. *Mol. Biol. Evol.* **1999**, *16*, 1280–1291.

101. Pineda, E.; Encalada, R.; Rodríguez-Zavala, J.S.; Olivos-García, A.; Moreno-Sánchez, R.; Saavedra, E. Pyruvate: Ferredoxin oxidoreductase and bifunctional aldehyde-alcohol dehydrogenase are essential for energy metabolism under oxidative stress in *Entamoeba histolytica*. *FEBS J.* **2010**, *277*, 3382–3395.

102. Wahl, R.C.; Orme-Johnson, W.H. Clostridial pyruvate oxidoreductase and the pyruvate-oxidizing enzyme specific to nitrogen fixation in *Klebsiella pneumoniae* are similar enzymes. *J. Biol. Chem.* **1987**, *262*, 10489–10496.

103. Meinecke, B.; Bertram, J.; Gottschalk, G. Purification and characterization of the pyruvate-ferredoxin oxidoreductase from *Clostridium acetobutylicum. Arch. Microbiol.* **1989**, *152*, 244–250.

104. Pieulle, L.; Magro, V.; Hatchikian, E. Isolation and analysis of the gene encoding the pyruvate-ferredoxin oxidoreductase of *Desulfovibrio africanus*, production of the recombinant enzyme in *Escherichia coli*, and effect of carboxy-terminal deletions on its stability. *J. Bacteriol.* **1997**, *179*, 5684–5692.

105. Pieulle, L.; Guigliarelli, B.; Asso, M.; Dole, F.; Bernadac, A.; Hatchikian, E.C. Isolation and characterization of the pyruvate-ferredoxin oxidoreductase from the sulfate-reducing bacterium *Desulfovibrio africanus. Biochim. Biophys. Acta* **1995**, *1250*, 49–59.

106. Pieulle, L.; Charon, M.-H.; Bianco, P.; Bonicel, J.; Petillot, Y.; Hatchikian, E.C. Structural and kinetic studies of the pyruvate-ferredoxin oxidoreductase/ferredoxin complex from *Desulfovibrio africanus. Eur. J. Biochem.* **1999**, *264*, 500–508.

107. Pieulle, L.; Chabriere, E.; Hatchikian, C.; Fontecilla-Camps, J.C.; Charon, M.-H. Crystallization and preliminary crystallographic analysis of the pyruvate-ferredoxin oxidoreductase from *Desulfovibrio africanus. Acta Crystallogr. D Biol. Crystallogr.* **1999**, *55*, 329–331.

108. Blamey, J.M.; Adams, M.W. Characterization of an ancestral type of pyruvate ferredoxin oxidoreductase from the hyperthermophilic bacterium, *Thermotoga maritima. Biochemistry (Mosc.)* **1994**, *33*, 1000–1007.

109. Blamey, J.M.; Adams, M.W.W. Purification and characterization of pyruvate ferredoxin oxidoreductase from the hyperthermophilic archaeon *Pyrococcus furiosus. Biochim. Biophys. Acta* **1993**, *1161*, 19–27.

110. Kunow, J.; Linder, D.; Thauer, R.K. Pyruvate: Ferredoxin oxidoreductase from the sulfate-reducing *Archaeoglobus fulgidus*: Molecular composition, catalytic properties, and sequence alignments. *Arch. Microbiol.* **1995**, *163*, 21–28.

111. Bock, A.-K.; Prieger-Kraft, A.; Schönheit, P. Pyruvate a novel substrate for growth and methane formation in *Methanosarcina barkeri. Arch. Microbiol.* **1994**, *161*, 33–46.

112. Bock, A.K.; Kunow, J.; Glasemacher, J.; Schönheit, P. Catalytic properties, molecular composition and sequence alignments of pyruvate: Ferredoxin oxidoreductase from the methanogenic archaeon *Methanosarcina Barkeri* (Strain Fusaro). *Eur. J. Biochem.* **1996**, *237*, 35–44.

113. Tersteegen, A.; Dietmar, L.R.K.; Thauer, R.H. Structures and functions of four anabolic 2-oxoacid oxidoreductases in *Methanobacterium thermoautotrophicum. Eur. J. Biochem.* **1997**, *244*, 862–868.

114. Chabrière, E.; Vernede, X.; Guigliarelli, B.; Charon, M.-H.; Hatchikian, E.C.; Fontecilla-Camps, J.C. Crystal structure of the free radical intermediate of pyruvate:ferredoxin oxidoreductase. *Science* **2001**, *294*, 2559–2563.

115. Chabrière, E.; Charon, M.-H.; Volbeda, A.; Pieulle, L.; Hatchikian, E.C.; Fontecilla-Camps, J.-C. Crystal structures of the key anaerobic enzyme pyruvate: Ferredoxin oxidoreductase, free and in complex with pyruvate. *Nat. Struct. Mol. Biol.* **1999**, *6*, 182–190.

116. Garczarek, F.; Dong, M.; Typke, D.; Witkowska, H.E.; Hazen, T.C.; Nogales, E.; Biggin, M.D.; Glaeser, R.M. Octomeric pyruvate-ferredoxin oxidoreductase from *Desulfovibrio vulgaris*. *J. Struct. Biol.* **2007**, *159*, 9–18.

117. Bock, A.-K.; Schönheit, P.; Teixeira, M. The iron-sulfur centers of the pyruvate:ferredoxin oxidoreductase from *Methanosarcina barkeri* (Fusaro). *FEBS Lett.* **1997**, *414*, 209–212.

118. Charon, M.-H.; Volbeda, A.; Chabriere, E.; Pieulle, L.; Fontecilla-Camps, J.C. Structure and electron transfer mechanism of pyruvate: Ferredoxin oxidoreductase. *Curr. Opin. Struct. Biol.* **1999**, *9*, 663–669.

119. Shiba, H.; Kawasumi, T.; Igarashi, Y.; Kodama, T.; Minoda, Y. The CO_2 assimilation via. the reductive tricarboxylic acid cycle in an obligately autotrophic, aerobic hydrogen-oxidizing bacterium, *Hydrogenobacter thermophilus*. *Arch. Microbiol.* **1985**, *141*, 198–203.

120. Ikeda, T.; Ochiai, T.; Morita, S.; Nishiyama, A.; Yamada, E.; Arai, H.; Ishii, M.; Igarashi, Y. Anabolic five subunit-type pyruvate: Ferredoxin oxidoreductase from *Hydrogenobacter thermophilus* TK-6. *Biochem. Biophys. Res. Commun.* **2006**, *340*, 76–82.

121. Ikeda, T.; Yamamoto, M.; Arai, H.; Ohmori, D.; Ishii, M.; Igarashi, Y. Enzymatic and electron paramagnetic resonance studies of anabolic pyruvate synthesis by pyruvate: Ferredoxin oxidoreductase from *Hydrogenobacter thermophilus*. *FEBS J.* **2010**, *277*, 501–510.

122. Yamamoto, M.; Ikeda, T.; Arai, H.; Ishii, M.; Igarashi, Y. Carboxylation reaction catalyzed by 2-oxoglutarate: Ferredoxin oxidoreductases from *Hydrogenobacter thermophilus*. *Extremophiles* **2010**, *14*, 79–85.

123. Lin, W.C.; Yang, Y.-L.; Whitman, W.B. The anabolic pyruvate oxidoreductase from *Methanococcus maripaludis*. *Arch. Microbiol.* **2003**, *179*, 444–456.

124. Lin, W.; Whitman, W. The importance of *por*E and *por*F in the anabolic pyruvate oxidoreductase of *Methanococcus maripaludis*. *Arch. Microbiol.* **2004**, *181*, 68–73.

125. Imlay, A.J. Iron-sulphur clusters and the problem with oxygen. *Mol. Microbiol.* **2006**, *59*, 1073–1082.

126. Linn, T.C.; Pettit, F.H.; Reed, L.J. α-Keto acid dehydrogenase complexes, X. Regulation of the activity of the pyruvate dehydrogenase complex from beef kidney mitochondria by phosphorylation and dephosphorylation. *Proc. Natl. Acad. Sci. USA* **1969**, *62*, 234–241.

127. Patel, M.S.; Roche, T.E. Molecular biology and biochemistry of pyruvate dehydrogenase complexes. *FASEB J.* **1990**, *4*, 3224–3233.

128. Witzmann, S.; Bisswanger, H. The pyruvate dehydrogenase complex from thermophilic organisms: Thermal stability and re-association from the enzyme components. *Biochim. Biophys. Acta* **1998**, *1385*, 341–352.

129. Potter, S.; Fothergill-Gilmore, L.A. Purification and properties of pyruvate kinase from *Thermoplasma acidophilum*. *FEMS Microbiol. Lett.* **1992**, *94*, 235–239.

130. Heath, C.; Jeffries, A.C.; Hough, D.W.; Danson, M.J. Discovery of the catalytic function of a putative 2-oxoacid dehydrogenase multienzyme complex in the thermophilic archaeon *Thermoplasma acidophilum*. *FEBS Lett.* **2004**, *577*, 523–527.

131. Selig, M.; Schönheit, P. Oxidation of organic compounds to CO_2 with sulfur or thiosulfate as electron acceptor in the anaerobic hyperthermophilic archaea *Thermoproteus tenax* and *Pyrobaculum islandicum* proceeds via. the citric acid cycle. *Arch. Microbiol.* **1994**, *162*, 286–294.

132. Ma, K.; Weiss, R.; Adams, M.W.W. Characterization of hydrogenase II from the hyperthermophilic archaeon *Pyrococcus furiosus* and assessment of its role in sulfur reduction. *J. Bacteriol.* **2000**, *182*, 1864–1871.

133. Jenney, F.E.; Adams, M.W.W. Hydrogenases of the model hyperthermophiles. *Ann. NY Acad. Sci.* **2008**, *1125*, 252–266.

134. Rudolph, F.B.; Purich, D.L.; Fromm, H.J. Coenzyme A-linked aldehyde dehydrogenase from *Escherichia coli. J. Biol. Chem.* **1968**, *243*, 5539–5545.

135. Lurz, R.; Mayer, F.; Gottschalk, G. Electron microscopic study on the quaternary structure of the isolated particulate alcohol-acetaldehyde dehydrogenase complex and on its identity with the polygonal bodies of *Clostridium kluyveri. Arch. Microbiol.* **1979**, *120*, 255–262.

136. Nair, R.V.; Bennett, G.N.; Papoutsakis, E.T. Molecular characterization of an aldehyde/alcohol dehydrogenase gene from *Clostridium acetobutylicum* ATCC 824. *J. Bacteriol.* **1994**, *176*, 871–885.

137. Tóth, J.; Ismaiel, A.A.; Chen, J.-S. The *ald* gene, encoding a coenzyme A-acylating aldehyde dehydrogenase, distinguishes *Clostridium beijerinckii* and two other solvent-producing clostridia from *Clostridium acetobutylicum. Appl. Environ. Microbiol.* **1999**, *65*, 4973–4980.

138. Sánchez, L.B. Aldehyde dehydrogenase (CoA-acetylating) and the mechanism of ethanol formation in the amitochondriate protist, *Giardia lamblia. Arch. Biochem. Biophys.* **1998**, *354*, 57–64.

139. Bruchhaus, I.; Tannich, E. Purification and molecular characterization of the NAD(+)-dependent acetaldehyde/alcohol dehydrogenase from *Entamoeba histolytica. Biochem. J.* **1994**, *303*, 743–748.

140. Burdette, D.; Zeikus, J.G. Purification of acetaldehyde dehydrogenase and alcohol dehydrogenases from *Thermoanaerobacter ethanolicus* 39E and characterization of the secondary-alcohol dehydrogenase (2 degrees Adh) as a bifunctional alcohol dehydrogenase--acetyl-CoA reductive thioesterase. *Biochem. J.* **1994**, *302*, 163–170.

141. Brown, S.D.; Guss, A.M.; Karpinets, T.V.; Parks, J.M.; Smolin, N.; Yang, S.; Land, M.L.; Klingeman, D.M.; Bhandiwad, A.; Rodriguez, M. Mutant alcohol dehydrogenase leads to improved ethanol tolerance in *Clostridium thermocellum. Proc. Natl. Acad. Sci. USA* **2011**, *108*, 13752–13757.

152

Microbial Enzymes with Special Characteristics for Biotechnological Applications

Poonam Singh Nigam

Abstract: This article overviews the enzymes produced by microorganisms, which have been extensively studied worldwide for their isolation, purification and characterization of their specific properties. Researchers have isolated specific microorganisms from extreme sources under extreme culture conditions, with the objective that such isolated microbes would possess the capability to bio-synthesize special enzymes. Various Bio-industries require enzymes possessing special characteristics for their applications in processing of substrates and raw materials. The microbial enzymes act as bio-catalysts to perform reactions in bio-processes in an economical and environmentally-friendly way as opposed to the use of chemical catalysts. The special characteristics of enzymes are exploited for their commercial interest and industrial applications, which include: thermotolerance, thermophilic nature, tolerance to a varied range of pH, stability of enzyme activity over a range of temperature and pH, and other harsh reaction conditions. Such enzymes have proven their utility in bio-industries such as food, leather, textiles, animal feed, and in bio-conversions and bio-remediations.

Reprinted from *Biomolecules*. Cite as: Nigam, P.S. Microbial Enzymes with Special Characteristics for Biotechnological Applications. *Biomolecules* **2013**, *3*, 597-611.

1. Enzymes from Microbial Sources

Enzymes are the bio-catalysts playing an important role in all stages of metabolism and biochemical reactions. Certain enzymes are of special interest and are utilized as organic catalysts in numerous processes on an industrial scale. Microbial enzymes are known to be superior enzymes obtained from different microorganisms, particularly for applications in industries on commercial scales. Though the enzymes were discovered from microorganisms in the 20th century, studies on their isolation, characterization of properties, production on bench-scale to pilot-scale and their application in bio-industry have continuously progressed, and the knowledge has regularly been updated. Many enzymes from microbial sources are already being used in various commercial processes. Selected microorganisms including bacteria, fungi and yeasts have been globally studied for the bio-synthesis of economically viable preparations of various enzymes for commercial applications [1].

In conventional catalytic reactions using biocatalysts the use of enzymes, either in free or in immobilized forms, is dependent on the specificity of enzyme. In recent advances of biotechnology, according to the requirements of a process, various enzymes have been and are being designed or purposely engineered. Various established classes of enzymes are specific to perform specialized catalytic reactions and have established their uses in selected bio-processes. A large number of new enzymes have been designed with the input of protein-engineering, biochemical-reaction engineering and metagenomics. Various molecular techniques have also been applied to improve the quality and performance of microbial enzymes for their wider applications in many industries [2]. As a result, many added-value products are being synthesized in global market with the use of established bioprocess-technology employing purposely engineered biocatalyst-enzymes.

Most of the commercially applicable proteases are alkaline and are bio-synthesized mainly by bacteria such as *Pseudomonas*, *Bacillus*, and *Clostridium*, and some fungi are also reported to produce these enzymes [3]. The xylanases with significant applications in bio-industries are produced by the fungal species belonging to genera *Trichoderma*, *Penicillium* and *Aspergillus*; the xylanases produced by these microorganisms have been found to possess high activity over a wide range of temperatures (40–60 °C) [4].

2. Enzymes with Special Characteristics

Special characteristics of microbial enzymes include their capability and appreciable activity under abnormal conditions, mainly of temperature and pH. Hence, certain microbial enzymes are categorized as thermophilic, acidophilic or alkalophilic. Microorganisms with systems of thermostable enzymes that can function at higher than normal reaction temperatures would decrease the possibility of microbial contamination in large scale industrial reactions of prolonged durations [5–7]. The quality of thermostability in enzymes promotes the breakdown and digestion of raw materials; also the higher reaction temperature enhances the penetration of enzymes [8]. The complete saccharification and hydrolysis of polysaccharides containing agricultural residues requires a longer reaction time, which is often associated with the contamination risks over a period of time. Therefore, the hydrolytic enzymes are well sought after, being active at higher temperatures as well as retaining stability over a prolonged period of processing at a range of temperatures. The high temperature enzymes also help in enhancing the mass-transfer and reduction of the substrate viscosity [9,10] during the progress of hydrolysis of substrates or raw materials in industrial processes. Thermophilic xylanase are considered to be of commercial interest in many industries particularly in the mashing process of brewing. The thermostable plant xerophytic isoforms of laccase enzyme are considered to be useful for their applications in textile, dyeing, pulping and bioremediation [1,4].

3. Enzymes with Special Characteristics in Biotechnology

3.1. Protease

Though the hydrolytic enzymes belong to the largest group of enzymes and are the most commercially-applicable enzymes, among the enzymes within this group the microbial proteases have been extensively studied [11–16]. Proteases prepared from microbial systems are of three types: acidic, neutral and alkaline. Alkaline proteases are efficient under alkaline pH conditions and consist of a serine residue at their active site [15]. Alkaline serine proteases have the largest applications in bio-industry. Alkaline proteases are of particular interest being more suitable for a wide range of applications, since these possess high activity and stability in abnormal conditions of extreme physiological parameters. Alkaline proteases have shown their capability to work under high pH, temperature and in presence of inhibitory compounds [15–18].

Vijayalakshmi *et al.* [16] have optimized and characterized the cultural conditions for the production of alkalophilic as well as a thermophilic extracellular protease enzyme from *Bacillus*. This bacteria named *Bacillus* RV.B2.90 was found to be capable of producing an enzyme preparation possessing special characteristics such as being highly alkalophilic, moderately halophilic, thermophilic, and exhibiting the quality of a thermostable protease enzyme. Alkaline proteases possess the property of a great stability in their enzyme activity when used in detergents [16,18,19]. The alkaline protease produced from *Bacilli* and proteases from other microorganisms have found more applications overall in bio-industries such as: washing powders, tannery, food-industry, leather processing, pharmaceuticals, for studies in molecular biology and in peptide synthesis [1,3].

3.2. Keratinases

Keratin is an insoluble and fibrous structural protein that is a constituent of feathers and wool. The protein is abundantly available as a by-product from keratinous wastes, representing a valuable source of proteins and amino acids that could be useful for animal feeds or as a source of nitrogen for plants [20]. However, the keratin-containing substrates and materials have high mechanical stability and hence are difficult to be degraded by common proteases. Keratinases are specific proteolytic enzymes which are capable of degrading insoluble keratins. The importance of these enzymes is being increasingly recognized in fields as diverse as animal feed production, textile processing, detergent formulation, leather manufacture, and medicine. Proteolytic enzymes with specialized keratinase activity are required to degrade keratins and for this purpose the keratinases have been isolated and purified from certain bacteria, actinomycetes, and fungi [20,21].

Keratinases have been classified as serine- or metallo-proteases. Cloning and expression of keratinase genes in a variety of expression systems have also been reported [22]. A higher operation temperature is required in the degradation of materials like feathers and wool, which would be possible using a thermostable keratinase. This aspect is of added advantage in achieving a higher reactivity due to lower diffusional restrictions and hence a higher reaction rate would be established. The enhanced stability of keratinase would increase the overall process yield due to the increased solubility of keratin and favorable equilibrium displacement in endothermic reactions.

Baihong *et al.* [23] have reported the enhanced thermostability of a preparation of keratinase by computational design and empirical mutation. The quadruple mutant of *Bacillus subtilis* has been characterised to exhibit the synergistic and additive effects at 60 °C with an increase of 8.6-fold in the t1/2 value. The N122Y substitution also led to an approximately 5.6-fold increase in catalytic efficiency compared to that of the wild-type keratinase.

An alkalophilic strain of *Streptomyces albidoflavus* has been reported to produce extracellular proteases [24]. This particular type of protease was capable of hydrolyzing keratin. The biosynthesis of this specific enzyme was optimized in submerged batch cultures at highly alkaline pH 10.5 and the enzyme yield was stimulated by using an inducer substrate containing keratin in the form of white chicken feathers. An enhanced (six-fold) protease production could be achieved with modified composition of culture-medium containing inducer at the concentration of 0.8% in the fermentation medium. The novelty of this crude enzyme has been reported to be its activity and stability in neutral and alkaline conditions. The maximum activity has been obtained at pH 9.0 and in the temperature range of 60–70 °C. This type of protease (keratinase- hydrolyzing keratins) is of particular significance for its application in industries since the crude enzyme showed its tolerance to the detergents and solvents tested [24]. Liu *et al.* [25] have studied the expression of extreme alkaline, oxidation-resistant keratinase from *Bacillus licheniformis* into the recombinant *Bacillus subtilis* WB600 expression system. The alkaline keratinase was characterized for its application in the processing of wool fibers.

3.3. Amylase

Amylases are significant enzymes for their specific use in the industrial starch conversion process [26]. Amylolytic enzymes act on starch and related oligo- and polysaccharides [27]. The global research on starch hydrolyzing enzymes based on the DNA sequence, structural analysis and catalytic mechanism has led to the concept of one enzyme family—the alpha amylase. The amylolytic and related enzymes have been classified as glycoside hydrolases. The enzymes have been produced by a wide range of microorganisms and substrates [28–30] and categorized as exo-, endo-, de-branching and cyclodextrin producing enzyme. The application of these enzymes has been established in starch liquefaction, paper, food, sugar and pharmaceutical industries. In the food industry amylolytic enzymes have a large scale of applications, such as the production of glucose syrups, high fructose corn syrups, maltose syrup, reduction of viscosity of sugar syrups, reduction of turbidity to produce clarified fruit juice for longer shelf-life, solubilisation and saccharification of starch in the brewing industry [31]. The baking industry uses amylases to delay the staling of bread and other baked products; the paper industry uses amylases for the reduction of starch viscosity to achieve the appropriate coating of paper. Amylase enzyme is used in the textile industry for warp sizing of textile fibers, and used as a digestive aid in the pharmaceutical industry [28].

Li *et al.* [32] have recently isolated, characterized and cloned a themotolerant isoamylase. For this purpose the enzyme was bio-synthesized using a thermophilic bacterium *Bacillus* sp. This novel enzyme has been reported to display its optimal activity at a remarkably high temperature of 70 °C, as well as being active in the alkaline range. This thermophilic enzyme has also been found to be thermo-stable between 30 and 70 °C, and its activity has been reported to be stable within a pH range of 5.5 to 9.0.

Gurumurthy *et al.* [33] completed the molecular characterization of an extremely thermostable alpha-amylase for industrial applications. This novel enzyme was produced by a bacterium *Geobacillus* sp. which was isolated from the thermal water of a geothermal spring. This isolated bacterium showed the characteristics of thermo-tolerance and alkali-resistance. A purified preparation of amylase suitable for application was obtained using a DEAE-cellulose column and Sephadex G-150 gel filtration chromatography. The enzyme is a novel alpha-amylase due to its optimum activity at a very high temperature of 90 °C and an alkaline pH 8.0. However, this purified preparation enzyme was found to be stable only for 10 min at 90 °C.

3.4. Xylanase

Hemicellulose is one of main constituents of agricultural residues and plants along with cellulose, lignin and pectin [34]. Xylan is the major component of hemicellulose consisting of β-1,4-linked D-xylopyranosyl residues. The hydrolysis of xylan in plant materials is achieved by the use of a mixture of hydrolytic enzymes including endo-β-1,4-xylanase and β-D-xylosidase [35]. The importance of xylanase has tremendously increased due to its biotechnological applications for pentose production, fruit-juice clarification, improving rumen digestion and the bioconversion of lignocellulosic agricultural residues to fuels and chemicals [34]. Collins *et al.* [36] have extensively studied the xylanase enzyme and its families as well as the special xylanases possessing extremophilic characteristics. Xylanases have established their uses in the food, pulp, paper and textile industries, agri-industrial residues utilization, and ethanol and animal feed production [37,38].

The enzyme used for the purpose of bio-bleaching of wood pulp should be active in the conditions of alkaline pH, high temperature and at the same time it is desirable that this enzyme is stable at high reaction temperatures. Xylanase preparations used for wood processing in the paper industry should be free of cellulose activity. Cellulase-free xylanase preparations have applications in the paper industry to provide brightness to the paper due to their preferential solubilisation of xylans in plant materials and selective removal of hemicelluloses from the kraft-pulp. Kohli *et al.* [39] have studied the production of a c cellulase free extracellular endo-1,4-β-xylanase at a higher temperature of 50 °C and at pH 8.5 employing a selected microorganism: *Thermoactinomyces thalophilus*. The enzyme preparation was found to be thermostable at 65 °C, retaining its activity at 50% after 125 min of incubation at 65 °C. The crude enzyme preparation showed no cellulase activity and the optimum temperature and pH for maximum xylanase activity was found to be 65 °C and 8.5–9.0, respectively. A thermotolerant and alkalotolerant xylanase has been reported to be produced by *Bacillus* sp. [40]. To make the applications of xylanase viable on commercial scales, heterologous systems of *Escherichis coli*, *Pichia pastoris* and *Bacillus* sp. have been used to express xylanase activity [41,42]. The thermophilic microorganism *Humicola* spp. has been studied for its capability of bio-synthesising an alkali-tolerant β-mannase xylanase [43]. Acidophilic xylanases stable under acidic conditions of reaction are reported to be produced by an acidophilic fungus *Bispora* [44], in contrast a xylanase active under conditions of alkaline pH has been studied by Mamo *et al.* [45] for the mechanism of their high pH catalytic adaptation.

Recently three novel xylanases thermophilic in nature (XynA,B,C) have been characterized by Yanlong *et al.* [46], these were produced by *Humicola* sp. for their potential applications in the brewing industry. One xylanase gene, XynA, has been found to adapt to alkaline conditions and stability at higher temperatures. This XynA also possessed higher catalytic efficiency and specificity for a range of substrates. Yanlong *et al.* [46] have reported the application of three xylanases, XynA-C, in simulated mashing conditions in the brewing industry and found the better performance of 37% on filtration acceleration and 13% reduction in viscosity of substrate in comparison to the performance of a commercial trade enzyme, Ultraflo, a product from Novozyme.

3.5. Laccase/Ligninase

Ligninolytic enzymes are applicable in the hydrolysis of lignocellulosic agricultural residues, particularly for the degradation of the complex and recalcitrant constituent lignin. This group of enzymes is a mixture of synergistic enzymes, hence they are highly versatile in nature and can be used in a range of industrial processes [47–49]. The complex enzyme system consists of three oxidative enzymes: lignin peroxidase (LiP), manganese peroxidase (MnP) and laccase. These enzymes have established their applications in bio-remediation, pollution control and in the treatment of industrial effluents containing recalcitrant and hazardous chemicals such as textile dyes, phenols and other xenobiotics [50–53].

The paper and pulp industry requires a step of separation and degradation of lignin from plant material, where the pretreatment of wood pulp using ligninolytic enzymes is important for a milder and cleaner strategy of lignin removal compared to chemical bleaching. Bleach enhancement of mixed wood pulp has been achieved using co-culture strategies, through the combined activity of xylanase and laccase [54]. The ligninolytic enzyme system is used in bio-bleaching of craft pulp and in other industries such as for the stabilization of wine and fruit juices, denim washing [49], the cosmetic industry and biosensors [1,34]. Fungi are the most potent producers of lignin degrading enzymes. White rot fungi have been specifically studied for the production of these enzymes by Robinson *et al.* [50–52]. For the economical production of ligninolytic enzymes, agricultural residues have been used as the substrate in microbial production of lignin degrading enzymes [34].

Thermophilic laccase enzyme is of particular use in the pulping industry. Recently, Gali and Kotteazeth [55] reported the biophysical characterization of thermophilic laccase isoforms. These were initially isolated from the xerophytic plant species *Cereus pterogonus* and *Opuntia vulgaris* and showed thermophilic property [56–58]. In order to prepare laccase enzymes with special characteristics, several studies have been conducted to provide a scientific basis for the employment of laccases in biotechnological processes [59–62]. Forms of laccase with unusual properties have been isolated from the basidiomycetes culture of *Steccherinum ochraceum* [63], *Polyporus versicolor* [64] and a microbial consortium [65].

3.6. Cellulase

Cellulase enzymes are the third most important enzyme for industrial uses: world-wide research has been focused on the commercial potential of cellulolytic enzymes for the commercial production of glucose feedstock from the agricultural cellulosic materials [1]. The significance of cellulose hydrolyzing thermophilic enzymes in various industries includes the production of bio-ethanol and value-added organic compounds from renewable agricultural residues [66]. Cellulose is the most abundant natural resource available globally for bioconversion into numerous products in bio-industry on a commercial scale. For efficient bioconversion a strategy of efficient saccharification using cellulolytic enzymes is required. Hardiman *et al.* [66] used the approach of thermophilc directed evolution of a thermophilic β-glucosidase.

Cellulase is complex of three important enzymes which work synergistically owing to the crystalline and amorphous complex structure of cellulose. These enzymes, acting synergistically, hydrolyse cellulose to cello-biose, glucose and oligo-saccharides. Endoglucanase enzyme is the first one acting on amorphous cellulose fibers, attacking the glucose-polymer chain randomly, which releases small fibers consisting of free-reducing and non-reducing ends. The free-ends of the chain are then exposed to the activity of exoglucanase enzyme, which produces cellobiose. The third component of cellulase is β-glucosidase, which hydrolyses the cellobiose, producing the glucose as the final product of cellulose sacharification.

Thermostability is an important technical property for cellulases: since the saccharification of cellulose is faster at higher temperatures, the stability of enzyme activity is necessary to be maintained for the completion of the process. Though the enzymes have been prepared using thermophilic microorganisms, these enzyme preparations are not necessarily heat-stable. The activity profile for the thermal activation and stability of cellulases derived from two *Basidiomycetes* cultures was studied by Nigam and Prabhu [67]. The results proved that the prior heat-treatment of enzyme preparation caused activation of exo- and endo-glucanase activities, and improved the stability of enzymes over a period of reaction time. Therefore, the efficiency of cellulolytic enzymes may be increased by heat-treatment, by incubating buffered enzyme preparations without cellulose or substrates prior to the saccharification process [67].

Cellulolytic enzymes have been produced by a range of microorganisms including bacteria and fungi. The studies have been performed for the biosynthesis of a high-activity preparation in high yields [68–70]. Researchers have cultivated microorganisms to achieve cellulases of desired quality under submerged and solid state fermentation conditions for the economical production of enzyme using waste agricultural residues [1].

3.7. Miscellaneous Enzymes in Biotechnology

Various enzymes other than those described above have a significant place in the list of microbial enzymes, which have established their applications in bio-industries. Lipases have been widely studied for their properties and utilization in many industries [71–75]. Pectinases have established their role in the fruit and juice industries [76]. Certain enzymes are specifically required in pharmaceutical industry for diagnostic kits and analytical assays [77–80].

Bornscheuer et al. [81] have currently mentioned that in all the research and developments so far in the field of biocatalysis, the researchers have contributed in three waves of outcomes. These innovations have played an important role in the establishment of current commercially successful level of bio-industries. As a result recent bioprocess-technology is capable of meeting future challenges and the requirements of conventional and modern industries, for example Trincone [82] has reviewed the options for unique enzymatic preparation of glycosides. Earlier enzymatic process were performed within the limitations of an enzyme, whereas currently with the knowledge of modern techniques, the enzyme can be engineered to be a suitable biocatalyst to meet the process requirement. Riva [83] has identified the scope of a long-term research in biocatalysis, since there are underlying problems in the shift from classical processes to bio-based processes for commercial market.

Table 1 summarizes some enzymes produced by microorganisms possessing special characteristics useful in various bio-processes. There is a tremendous scope for research and development to meet the challenges of third generation biorefeneries [83], for the production of numerous chemicals and bio-products from renewable biomasses [34]; or by the new glycoside hydrolases [82]; or new enzymes found in marine environments [84]. Although the research for the hemicellulases as important biorefining enzymes has not well established, biocatalysis for xylan processing is slowly progressing and a wide range of hemicellulases have been isolated and characterized [85]. Specifically about the biobased glycosynthesis, Trincone [82] has mentioned that the new prospects are open for the use of pentose sugars as main building blocks for engineered pentosides to be used as non-ionic surfactants or as the ingredients for prebiotic food and feed preparations.

Table 1. A summarized overview of some microbial enzymes with special characteristics of industrial importance.

Enzyme	Properties	Producer Microbes-	Applications	Reference
PROTEASE (Proteolytic activity)	Acidic, Neutral, Alkaline, Thermophilic, Active in presence of inhibitory compounds	*Bacilli*; *Pseudomonas*; *Clostridium*; *Rhizopus*; *Penicillium*; *Aspergillus*	Washing Powders; Detergents; Tannery; Food Industry; Leather processing; Pharmaceuticals; Molecular Biology; Peptide synthesis	[1,3,11–19,34]
KERATINASE (Keratin-hydrolysing activity)	Specific Proteolytic Activity for Insoluble & Fibrous Proteins in furs, feathers, wool, hair; Thermophilic; Alkalophilic; Oxidation-Resistant	Bacteria; Actinomycetes; Fungi	Animal Feed Production; Textile Processing; Detergent Formulation; Leather Manufacturing; Medicine	[1,20–25,34]
AMYLASE (Starch-hydrolyzing activity)	Thermotolerant, Thermostable, Alkali-resistant-Exo-, endo-, de-branching, cyclodextrin-producing enzymes	*Bacillus* sp.; *Geobacillus*	Starch industry (for liquefaction); Paper, Food industry (Glucose & Maltose syrups, High Fructose Corn syrups, clarified fruit-juices); Pharmaceutical industries (Digestive aid); Brewing Industry (Starch-processing); Textile industry (Warp-sizing of fibers); Baking industry (delayed staling)	[1,26–34]

160

Table 1. *Cont.*

Enzyme	Properties	Producer Microbes-	Applications	Reference
XYLANASE (Xylan–Pentose polymer hydrolyzing activity)	Extremophilic characteristics– Alkalophilic, Thermophilic & Thermostable	*Thermoactinomy ces thalophilus*; *Bacillus* sp.; *Humicola insolens. Bispora* (acidophilic fungus)	Pentose production - Bioconversion of hemicellulose for fuel & Chemicals; Fruit-juice clarification; Improving rumen digestion; Paper industry- selective removals of xylans from kraft-pulp; Brewing industry	[1,34–46]
LIGNINASE (Ligninolytic-Complex-enzyme)	Oxidative properties in Lignin peroxidase, Manganese peroxidase & Laccase; Thermophilic	Basidiomycetes strains—*Stecche rinum ochraceum, Polyporus versicolor, Panus tigrinus*	Denim washing; Bio-sensors; Bio-bleaching of Kraft-pulp; Bioremediation; Pollution-control; Treatment of recalcitrant chemicals in Textile and Industrial effluents	[1,34,47–65]
CELLULASE (Cellulolytic-complex enzyme)	Saccahrification of crystalline & amorphous cellulose; Thermophilic; Thermostable	Basidiomycetes strains *Polyporus* sp.; *Pleurotus* sp.; *Trichoderma* sp.; *Aspergillus* sp.	Glucose feedstock from cellulose; Bio-refinery; Bio-ethanol; Paper-pulp industry	[1,34,66–70]
LIPASE (Lipolytic activity)	Fat- splitting; Stereoselectivity; Racemic-Resolution activity; Solvents-resistant; Thermotolerant	Yeasts and Fungal strains-*Candida* sp., *Aspergillus* sp, *Penicillium* sp., *Rhizopus, Mucor*	Detergents; Dairy Industry-oils, fats, Butter, Cream, Fat-Spreads; Feed supplement; Therapeutic agent	[1,34,71–75]

4. Conclusions

Biotechnology is utilizing a wide range of enzymes synthesized on a commercial scale employing purposely screened microorganisms. Selected microorganisms have been characterized, purposely designed and optimized to produce a high-quality enzyme preparation on large scales for industrial applications. Different industries require enzymes for different purposes; hence microbial enzymes have been studied for their special characteristics applicable in various bio-processes. Recent molecular biology techniques have allowed to tailor a specific microorganism, to produce not only the high yields of an enzyme, but also enzyme with desired special characteristics such as thermostability, tolerance at high temperature and its stability in acidic or alkaline environment, and retaining the enzyme activity under severe reaction conditions such as in presence of other metals and compounds.

Conflicts of Interest

The author declares no conflict of interest.

References

1. Pandey, A.; Selvakumar, P.; Soccol, C.R.; Nigam, P. Solid-state fermentation for the production of industrial enzymes. *Curr. Sci.* **1999**, *77*, 149–162.
2. Chirumamilla, R.R.; Muralidhar, R.; Marchant, R.; Nigam, P. Improving the quality of industrially important enzymes by directed evolution. *Mol. Cell. Biochem.* **2001**, *224*, 159–168.
3. Kumar, C.G.; Takagi, H. Microbial alkaline proteases: From a bioindustrial viewpoint. *Biotechnol. Adv.* **1999**, *17*, 561–594.
4. Ahmed, S.; Riaz, S.; Jamil, A. Molecular cloning of fungal xylanases: An overview. *Appl. Microbiol. Biotechnol.* **2009**, *84*, 19–35.
5. Wang, X.; Li, D.; Watanabe, T.; Shigemori, Y.; Mikawa, T.; Okajima, T.; Mao, L.Q.; Ohsaka, T. A glucose/o-2 biofuel cell using recombinant thermophilic enzymes. *Int. J. Electrochem. Sci.* **2012**, *7*, 1071–1078.
6. Banat, I.M.; Nigam, P.; Marchant, R. Isolation of a thermotolerant, fermentative yeasts growing at 52 °C and producing ethanol at 45 °C & 50 °C. *World J. Microbiol. Biotechnol.* **1992**, *8*, 259-263.
7. Wati, L.; Dhamija, S.S.; Singh, D.; Nigam, P.; Marchant, R. Characterisation of genetic control of thermotolerance in mutants of *Saccharomyces cerevisiae*. *Genet. Eng. Biotechnol.* **1996**, *16*, 19–26.
8. Zhang, S.B.; Wu, Z.L. Identification of amino acid residuesresponsible for increased thermostability of feruloyl esterase A from *Aspergillus niger* using the PoPMuSiC algorithm. *Bioresour. Technol.* **2011**, *102*, 2093–2096.
9. Berka, R.M.; Grigoriev, I.V.; Otillar, R.; Salamov, A.; Grimwood, J.; Reid, I.; Ishmael, N.; John, T.; Darmond, C.; Moisan, M.C.; *et al.* Comparative genomic analysis of the thermophilic biomass-degrading fungi. *Myceliophthora thermophila* and *Thielavia terrestris. Nat. Biotechnol.* **2011**, *29*, 922–927.
10. Cai, H.; Shi, P.; Bai, Y.; Huang, H.; Yuan, T.; Yang, P.; Luo, H.; Meng, K.; Yao, B. A novel thermoacidophilic family 10 xylanase from *Penicillium pinophilum* C1. *Process Biochem.* **2011**, *46*, 2341–2346.
11. Mukherjee, A.K.; Adhikari, H.; Rai, S.K. Production of alkaline protease by a thermophilic *Bacillus subtilis* under solid-state fermentation (SSF) condition using *Imperata* cylindrical grass and potato peel as low-cost medium: Characterization and application of enzyme in detergent formulation. *J. Biochem. Eng.* **2008**, *39*, 353–361.

12. Rahman, R.N.Z.R.A.; Basri, M.; Salleh, A.B. Thermostable alkaline protease from *Bacillus stearothermophilus* F1; Nutritional factors affecting protease production. *Ann. Microbiol.* **2003**, *53*, 199–210.

13. Chudasama, C.J.; Jani, S.A.; Jajda, H.M.; Pate, H.N. Optimization and production of alkaline protease from *Bacillus thuringiensis* CC7. *J. Cell Tissue Res.* **2010**, *10*, 2257–2262.

14. Genckal, H.; Tari, C. Alkaline protease production from alkalophilic *Bacillus* sp. isolated from natural habitats. *Enzym. Microb. Technol.* **2006**, *39*, 703–710.

15. Gupta, R.; Beg, Q.K.; Lorenz, P. Bacterial alkaline proteases: Molecular approaches and Industrial Applications. *Appl. Microbiol. Biotechnol.* **2002**, *59*, 15–32.

16. Vijayalakshmi, S.; Venkat Kumar, S.; Thankamani, V. Optimization and cultural characterization of *Bacillus* RV.B2.90 producing alkalophilic thermophilic protease. *Res. J. Biotechnol.* **2011**, *6*, 26–32.

17. Gupta, A.; Joseph, B.; Mani, A.; Thomas, G. Biosynthesis and properties of an extracellular thermostable serine alkaline protease from *Virgibacillus pantothenticus*. *World J. Microbiol. Biotechnol.* **2008**, *24*, 237–243.

18. Johnvesly, B.; Naik, G.K. Studies on production of thermostable alkaline protease from thermophilic and alkaliphilic *Bacillus* sp. JB-99 in a chemical defined medium. *Process Biochem.* **2001**, *37*, 139–144.

19. Hadj-Ali, N.E.; Rym, A.; Basma, G.F.; Alya, S.K.; Safia, K.; Moncef, N. Biochemical and molecular characterization of a detergent stable alkaline serineprotease from a newly isolated *Bacillus licheniformis* NH1. *Enzym. Microb. Technol.* **2007**, *40*, 515–523.

20. Gushterova, A.; Vasileva-Tonkova, E.; Dimova, E.; Nedkov, P.; Haertle, T. Keratinase production by newly isolated Antarctic actinomycete strains. *World J. Microbiol. Biotechnol.* **2005**, *21*, 831–834.

21. Brandelli, A.; Daroit, D.J.; Riffel, A. Biochemical features of microbial keratinases and their production and applications. *Appl. Microbiol. Biotechnol.* **2010**, *85*, 1735–1750.

22. Gupta, R.; Sharma, R.; Beg, Q.K. Revisiting microbial keratinases: Next generation proteases for sustainable biotechnology. *Crit. Rev. Biotechnol.* **2013**, *33*, 216–228.

23. Baihong, L.; Juan, Z.; Zhen, F.; Lei, G.; Xiangru, L.; Guocheng, D.; Jian, C. Enhanced thermostability of keratinase by computational design and empirical mutation. *J. Ind. Microbiol. Biotechnol.* **2013**, *40*, 697–704.

24. Indhuja, S.; Shiburaj, S.; Pradeep, N.S.; Thankamani, V.; Abraham, T.K. Extracellular keratinolytic proteases from an Alkalophilic *Streptomyces albidoflavus* TBG-S13A5: Enhanced production and characterization. *J. Pure Appl. Microbiol.* **2012**, *6*, 1599–1607.

25. Liu, B.; Zhang, J.; Li, B.; Liao, X.; Du, G.; Chen, J. Expression and characterization of extreme alkaline, oxidation-resistant keratinase from *Bacillus licheniformis* in recombinant *Bacillus subtilis* WB600 expression system and its application in wool fiber processing. *World J. Microbiol. Biotechnol.* **2013**, *29*, 825–832.

26. Nigam, P.; Singh, D. Enzyme and microbial systems involved in starch processing. *Enzym. Microb. Technol.* **1995**, *17*, 770–778.

27. Pandey, A.; Soccol, C.R.; Nigam, P. Biotechnological potential of agro-industrial residues, II-Cassava Bagasse. *Bioresour. Technol.* **2000**, *74*, 81–87.

28. Sivaramakrishnan, S.; Gangadharan, D.; Nampoothiri, K.M.; Soccol, C.R.; Pandey, A. α-amylases from microbial sources—An overview on recent developments. *Food Technol. Biotechnol.* **2006**, *44*, 173–184.

29. Kumar, J.; Dahiya, J.S.; Singh, D.; Nigam, P. Production of endo-1, 4- β-glucanase by a biocontrol fungus *Cladorrhinum foecundissimum*. *Bioresour. Technol.* **2000**, *75*, 95–97.

30. Singh, D.; Dahiya, J.S.; Nigam, P. Simultaneous raw starch hydrolysis and ethanol fermentation by glucoamylase from *Rhizoctonia solani* and *Saccharomyces cerevisiae*. *J. Basic Microbiol.* **1995**, *35*, 117–121.

31. Pandey, A.; Nigam, P.; Soccol, C.R.; Soccol, V.T.; Singh, D.; Mohan, R. Advances in Microbial Amylases. *Biotechnol. Appl. Biochem.* **2000**, *31*, 135–152.

32. Li, Y.; Niu, D.; Zhang, L.; Wang, Z.; Shi, G. Purification, characterization and cloning of a thermotolerant isoamylase produced from Bacillus sp. CICIM 304. *J. Ind. Microbiol. Biotechnol.* **2013**, *40*, 437–446.

33. Gurumurthy, D.M.; Neelagund, S.E. Molecular characterization of industrially viable extreme thermostable novel alpha-amylase of geobacillus sp. Iso5 Isolated from geothermal spring. *J. Pure Appl. Microbiol.* **2012**, *6*, 1759–1773.

34. Nigam, P.; Pandey, A. *Biotechnology for Agro-Industrial Residues Utilisation*; Nigam, P., Pandey, A., Eds.; Publisher Springer Science Business Media B.V.: Berlin/Heidelberg, Germany, 2009; pp. 1–466.

35. Polizeli, M.L.; Rizzatti, A.C.; Monti, R.; Terenzi, H.F.; Jorge, J.A.; Amorim, D.S. Xylanases from fungi: Properties and industrial applications. *Appl. Microbiol. Biotechnol.* **2005**, *67*, 577–591.

36. Collins, T.; Gerday, C.; Feller, G. Xylanases, xylanase families and extremophilic xylanases. *FEMS Microbiol. Rev.* **2005**, *29*, 3–23.

37. Srinivasan, M.C.; Rele, M.V. Cellulase free xylanase from microorganisms and their applications to pulp and paper biotechnology: An overview. *Indian J. Microbiol.* **1995**, *35*, 93–101.

38. Garg, A.P.; Roberts, J.C.; McCarthy, A. Bleach boosting effect of cellulase free xylanase of *Streptomyces thermoviolaceus* and its comparison with two commercial enzyme preparations on birchwood Kraft pulp. *Enzym. Microb. Biotechnol.* **1998**, *22*, 594–598.

39. Kohli, U.; Nigam, P.; Singh, D.; Chaudhary, K. Thermostable, alkalophilic and cellulase free xylanase production by *Thermonoactinomyces* thalophilus subgroup C. *Enzym. Microb. Technol.* **2001**, *28*, 606–610.

40. Marques, S.; Alves, L.; Ribeiro, S.; Girio, F.M.; Amaralcollaco, M.T. Characterisation of a thermotolerant and alkalotolerant xylanase from a *Bacillus* sp. *Appl. Biochem. Biotechnol. A* **1998**, *73*, 159–172.

41. Jhamb, K.; Sahoo, D.K. Production of soluble recombinant proteins in *Escherichia coli*: Effects of process conditions and chaperone co-expression on cell growth and production of xylanase. *Bioresour. Technol.* **2012**, *123*, 135–143.

42. Prade, R.A. Xylanases: From biology to biotechnology. *Biotechnol. Genet. Eng. Rev.* **1996**, *13*, 100–131.

43. Luo, H.; Wang, K.; Huang, H.; Shi, P.; Yang, P.; Yao, B. Gene cloning, expression and biochemical characterization of an alkali-tolerant b-mannanase from *Humicola insolens* Y1. *J. Ind. Microbiol. Biotechnol.* **2012**, *39*, 547–555.

44. Luo, H.; Li, J.; Yang, J.; Wang, H.; Yang, Y.; Huang, H.; Shi, P.; Yuan, T.; Fan, Y.; Yao, B. A thermophilic and acid stable family-10 xylanase from the acidophilic fungus *Bispora* sp. MEY-1. *Extremophiles* **2009**, *13*, 849–857.

45. Mamo, G.; Thunnissen, M.; Hatti-Kaul, R.; Mattiasson, B. An alkaline active xylanase: Insights into mechanisms of high pH catalytic adaptation. *Biochimie* **2009**, *91*, 1187–1196.

46. Du, Y.; Shi, P.; Huang, H.; Zhang, X.; Luo, H.; Wang, Y.; Yao, B. Characterization of three novel thermophilic xylanases from Humicola insolens Y1 with application potentials in the brewing industry. *Bioresour. Technol.* **2013**, *130*, 161–167.

47. Nigam, P.; Pandey, A.; Prabhu, K.A. Cellulase and ligninase production by Basidiomycetes culture in solid-state fermentation. *Biol. Wastes* **1987a**, *20*, 1–9.

48. Nigam, P.; Pandey, A.; Prabhu, K.A. Ligninolytic activity of two Basidiomycetes moulds in the decomposition of bagasse. *Biol. Wastes* **1987b**, *21*, 1–10._

49. Dahiya, J.S.; Singh, D.; Nigam, P. Characterisation of laccase produced by *Coniotherium minitans*. *J. Basic Microbiol.* **1998**, *38*, 349–359.

50. Robinson, T.; Chandran, B.; Nigam, P. Studies on the production of enzymes by white-rot fungi for the decolourisation of textile dyes. *Enzym. Microb. Technol.* **2001**, *29*, 575–579.

51. Robinson, T.; Chandran, B.; Nigam, P. Studies on the decolourisation of an artificial effluent through lignolytic enzyme production by white-rot fungi in *N*-rich and *N*-limited media. *Appl. Microbiol. Biotechnol.* **2001b**, *57*, 810–813.

52. Robinson, T.; Nigam, P. Remediation of textile dye-waste water using a white rot fungus *Bjerkandera adusta* through solid state fermentation (SSF). *Appl. Biochem. Biotechnol.* **2008**, *151*, 618-628.

53. Dahiya, J.; Singh, D.; Nigam, P. Decolourisation of synthetic and spentwash-melanoidins using the white-rot fungus *Phanerochaete chrysosporium* JAG-40. *Bioresour. Technol.* **2001**, *78*, 95–98.

54. Dwivedi, P.; Vivikanand, V.; Pareek, N.; Sharma, A.; Singh, R.P. Bleach enhancement of mixed wood pulp by xylanase-laccase concoction derived through co-culture strategy. *Appl. Biochem. Biotechnol.* **2010**, *160*, 255–268.

55. Gali, N.K.; Kotteazeth, S. Biophysical characterization of thermophilic laccase from the xerophytes: *Cereus pterogonus* and *Opuntia vulgaris*. *Cellulose* **2013**, *20*, 115–125.

56. Gali, N.K.; Kotteazeth, S. Isolation, purification and characterization of thermophilic laccase from xerophyte *Cereus pterogonus*. *Chem. Nat. Compd.* **2012**, *48*, 451–456.

57. Kumar, G.N.; Srikumar, K. Thermophilic laccase from xerophyte species *Opuntia vulgaris*. *Biomed. Chromatogr.* **2011**, *25*, 707–711.

58. Kumar, G.N.; Srikumar, K. Characterization of xerophytic thermophilic laccase exhibiting metal ion-dependent dye decolorization potential. *Appl. Biochem. Biotechnol.* **2012**, *167*, 662–676.

59. Quaratino, D.; Federici, F.; Petruccioli, M.; Fenice, M.; D'Annibale, A. Production, purification and partial characterisation of a novel laccase from the white-rot fungus *Panus tigrinus* CBS 577.79. *Anton. Leeuw. Int. J.G.* **2007**, *91*, 57–69.

60. Uthandi, S.; Saad, B.; Humbard, M.A.; Maupin-Furlow, J.A. LccA, an archaeal laccase secreted as a highly stable glycoprotein into the extracellular medium by *Haloferax volcanii*. *Appl. Environ. Microbiol.* **2010**, *76*, 733–743.

61. Papinutti, L.; Dimitriu, P.; Forchiassin, F. Stabilization studies of *Fomes sclerodermeus* laccases. *Bioresour. Technol.* **2008**, *99*, 419–424.

62. Mishra, A.; Kumar, S. Kinetic studies of laccase enzyme of *Coriolus versicolor* MTCC 138 in an inexpensive culture medium. *Biochem. Eng. J.* **2009**, *46*, 252–256.

63. Chernykh, A.; Myasoedova, N.; Kolomytseva, M.; Ferraroni, M.; Briganti, F.; Scozzafava, A.; Golovleva, L. Laccase isoforms with unusual properties from the basidiomycete Steccherinum ochraceum strain 1833. *J. Appl. Microbiol.* **2008**, *105*, 2065–2075.

64. Nigam, P.; Prabhu, K.A. The effects of some added carbohydrates on cellulases and ligninase and decomposition of bagasse. *Agric. Wastes* **1986**, *17*, 293–299.

65. Wongwilaiwalin, S.; Rattanachomsri, U.; Laothanachareon, T.; Eurwilaichitr, L.; Igarashi, Y.; Champreda, V. Analysis of a thermophilic lignocellulose degrading microbial consortium and multi-species lignocellulolytic enzyme system. *Enzym. Microb. Technol.* **2010**, *47*, 283–290.

66. Hardiman, E.; Gibbs, M.; Reeves, R.; Bergquist, P. Directed Evolution of a thermophilic beta-glucosidase for Cellulosic Bioethanol Production. *Appl. Biochem. Biotechnol.* **2010**, *161*, 301–312.

67. Nigam, P.; Prabhu, K.A. Thermal activation and stability of cellulases derived from two Basidiomycetes. *Biotechnol. Lett.* **1988**, *10*, 919–920.

68. Nigam, P.; Prabhu, K.A. Effect of cultural factors on cellulase biosynthesis in submerged bagasse fermentation by basidiomycetes cultures. *J. Basic Microbiol.* **1991**, *31*, 285–292.

69. Nigam, P.; Prabhu, K.A. Isolation and recovery of cellulase and ligninase from crude enzymes produced by two basidiomycetes cultures in submerged bagasse fermentation. *Sharkara* **1988**, *27*, 40–46.

70. Nigam, P.; Prabhu, K.A. Microbial degradation of bagasse: Isolation and cellulolytic properties of Basidiomycetes spp. from biomanure from a biogas plant. *Agric. Wastes* **1985**, *12*, 273–285.

71. Reddivari, M.; Chirumamilla, R.; Nigam, P. Understanding lipase stereoselectivity. *World J. Microbiol. Biotechnol.* **2002**, *18*, 81–97.

72. Muralidhar, R.; Chirumamilla, R.R.; Nigam, P. Resolution of proglumide using lipase from *Candida cylindraceae*. *Bioorg. Med. Chem.* **2002**, *10*, 1471–1475.

73. Muralidhar, R.; Chirumamilla, R.R.; Marchant, R.; Nigam, P. A response surface approach for the comparison of lipase production by *Candida cylindraceae* using two different carbon sources. *Biochem. Eng. J.* **2001**, *9*, 17–23.

74. Pandey, A.; Benzamin, S.; Soccol, C.R.; Nigam, P.; Krieger, N.; Soccol, V.T. The realm of microbial lipases in biotechnology. *Biotechnol. Appl. Biochem.* **1999**, *29*, 119–131.

75. Muralidhar, R.; Chirumamilla, C.; Marchant, R.; Nigam, P. Lipases in racemic resolutions. *J. Chem. Technol. Biotechnol.* **2001**, *76*, 3–8.

76. Sunnotel, O.; Nigam, P. Pectinolytic activity of bacteria isolated from soil and two fungal strains during submerged fermentation. *World J. Microbiol. Biotechnol.* **2002**, *18*, 835–839.

77. Zhou, D.M.; Nigam, P.; Marchant, R.; Jones, J. Production of salicylate hydroxylase from Pseudomonas putida UUC-1 and its application in the construction of biosensor. *J. Chem. Technol. Biotechnol.* **1995**, *64*, 331–338.

78. Banat, I.M.; Marchant, A.; Nigam, P.; Gaston, S.J.S.; Kelly, B.; Marchant, R. Production, partial characterization and potential diagnostic use of salicylate hydroxylase from Pseudomonas putida UUC-1. *Enzym. Microb. Technol.* **1994**, *16*, 665–670._

79. Nigam, P.; Marchant, R. Production of enzyme dihydrofolate reductase by methotrexate-resistant bacteria isolated from soil. *J. Chem. Technol. Biotechnol.* **1993**, *56*, 35–40.

80. Nigam, P.; Banat, I.M.; Kelly, B.; Marchant, R. Dihydrofolate reductase synthesis in continuous culture using methotrexate-resistant *Escherichia coli*. *Enzym. Microb. Technol.* **1993**, *15*, 652–656.

81. Bornscheuer, U.T.; Huisman, G.W.; Kazlausaks, R.J.; Lutz, S.; Moore, J.C.; Robins, K. Engineering the third wave of biocatalysis. *Nature* **2012**, *485*, 185–194.

82. Trincone, A. Angling for uniqueness in enzymatic preparation of glycosides. *Biomolecules* **2013**, *3*, 334–350.

83. Riva, S. 1983–2013: The long wave of biocatalysis. *Trends Biotechnol.* **2013**, *31*, 120–121.

84. Trincone, A. Potential biocatalysts originating from sea environments. *J. Mol. Catal. B-Enzym.* **2010**, *66*, 241–256.

85. Dumon, C.; Songa, L.; Bozonneta, S.; Fauréa, R.; O'Donohue, M.J. Progress and future prospects for pentose-specific biocatalysts in biorefining. *Proc. Biochem.* **2012**, *47*, 346–357.

Fungal Beta-Glucosidases: A Bottleneck in Industrial Use of Lignocellulosic Materials

Annette Sørensen, Mette Lübeck, Peter S. Lübeck and Birgitte K. Ahring

Abstract: Profitable biomass conversion processes are highly dependent on the use of efficient enzymes for lignocellulose degradation. Among the cellulose degrading enzymes, beta-glucosidases are essential for efficient hydrolysis of cellulosic biomass as they relieve the inhibition of the cellobiohydrolases and endoglucanases by reducing cellobiose accumulation. In this review, we discuss the important role beta-glucosidases play in complex biomass hydrolysis and how they create a bottleneck in industrial use of lignocellulosic materials. An efficient beta-glucosidase facilitates hydrolysis at specified process conditions, and key points to consider in this respect are hydrolysis rate, inhibitors, and stability. Product inhibition impairing yields, thermal inactivation of enzymes, and the high cost of enzyme production are the main obstacles to commercial cellulose hydrolysis. Therefore, this sets the stage in the search for better alternatives to the currently available enzyme preparations either by improving known or screening for new beta-glucosidases.

Reprinted from *Biomolecules*. Cite as: Sørensen, A.; Lübeck, M.; Lübeck, P.S.; Ahring, B.K. Fungal Beta-Glucosidases: A Bottleneck in Industrial Use of Lignocellulosic Materials. *Biomolecules* **2013**, *3*, 612-631.

1. Introduction

The ever-increasing energy consumption and the depletion of fossil resources have laid the foundation for a shift towards sustainable production of biofuels and bioproducts in biorefineries from renewable sources. Oil is currently the primary source of energy for the transportation sector and for production of chemicals and plastics. However, biorefineries are in the coming decades expected to supplement or replace oil refineries by maximizing biomass value, producing fuels and platform molecules for use as building blocks in the synthesis of chemicals and polymeric materials [1]. Biorefineries rely on the use of plant biomass in the form of dedicated energy crops or lignocellulosic agricultural residues as an abundant and inexpensive renewable energy resource [2]. Most biorefineries focus on production of a sugar platform of simple sugars that are released from biomass [1]. These sugars can then biologically or chemically be converted into fuels (e.g., ethanol, butanol and hydrocarbons), building block chemicals (e.g., different organic acids), as well as other high value bioproducts [3].

Plant biomasses are rich in lignocellulose which consists mainly of polysaccharides such as cellulose and hemicelluloses that together with the phenolic lignin polymer form a complex and rigid structure. The biomass composition depends on the plant/crop type, with cellulose being the most abundant component [4]. Cellulose is a long homogenous linear polymer of beta-D-glucosyl units linked by 1,4-beta-D-glucosidic bonds. The cellulose chains are assembled in larger rigid units held together by hydrogen bonds and weak van der Wall's forces. Through parallel orientation, the chains form a highly ordered crystalline structure, but are interspersed with amorphous regions of more disordered structure [5–7].

The complex structure of the cellulose fibrils embedded in an amorphous matrix of lignin and hemicellulose strengthen the plant cell wall and give plants a natural recalcitrance to biological degradation. Pretreatment is crucial as a first step for increasing the accessibility of the biomass polymers for the following enzyme hydrolysis. The different pretreatment methods available are plentiful—including alkali-, acid-, or organic—solvent pretreatment, steam-, ammonia fiber- or CO_2 explosion, and wet-oxidation [8–10]. The type of plant material as well as the severity of the pretreatment method applied will influence the characteristics of the lignocellulosic substrate for enzyme hydrolysis with regard to cellulose accessibility, degree of polymerization, hemicellulose content, lignin content, and other potential interfering compounds [11–13]. Such variation in biomass characteristics will influence the composition requirements for an optimal enzyme cocktail for the breakdown of different types of lignocellulosic biomasses [14]. Balanced enzyme cocktails and tailoring of enzymes for increased performance is of major importance for obtaining high yields of sugar monomers from hydrolysis, and especially the complete hydrolysis of cellulose is the main challenge that must be overcome. Among the cellulolytic enzyme complex, beta-glucosidases play a key role for the final conversion of cellobiose into glucose.

This review provides an overview of fungal beta-glucosidases in relation to industrial use of lignocellulosic materials. We discuss the significance of beta-glucosidases, how they represent the bottleneck in biomass conversion and the challenges in biomass hydrolysis in biorefineries.

2. Hydrolysis of Cellulose

The general biochemistry of cellulosic enzymatic hydrolysis has been reviewed extensively in previous literature [5,11,15,16] and will only be briefly discussed here.

The classical scheme for cellulose hydrolysis involves three main categories of enzymes: endo-1,4-beta-glucanases (EC 3.2.1.4), cellobiohydrolases (or exo-1,4-beta-glucanases) (EC 3.2.1.91), and beta-glucosidases (EC 3.2.1.21). Cellulose polymers are, through sequential and synergistic actions of these enzymes, degraded to glucose. The general consensus is that endo-glucanases randomly hydrolyze the internal 1,4-beta-linkages in primarily the amorphous regions of cellulose, rapidly decreasing the degree of polymerization. Cellobiohydrolases hydrolyze the cellulose polymer from the free ends, releasing cellobiose as product in a processive fashion, and finally, beta-glucosidases hydrolyze the cellobiose to glucose. Several fungal beta-glucosidases have furthermore been shown to produce glucose from larger cellodextrins, thus having the potential to increase the reaction rate and extent of cellulose hydrolysis [5,11,15,16].

The classical concept of cellulose hydrolysis described above has been agreed on for decades, but more recently, attention has been paid to accessory enzymes that are co-regulated or co-expressed by microbes during growth on cellulosic substrates. The crystalline chains in cellulose are tightly packed and additional factors are needed in order to make the substrate more accessible for the hydrolytic enzymes. Among such accessory enzymes are the GH61 proteins and the bacterial family 33 Carbohydrate Binding Modules (CBM33), which lack measurable hydrolytic activity, yet they are able to significantly enhance the activity of cellulases on pretreated biomass. Both proteins have flat substrate-binding surfaces and are capable of cleaving polysaccharide chains by oxidative reactions to disrupt the polymer packing, thereby increasing its accessibility [17–20].

The commercial viability of biorefineries has been burdened by the use of expensive enzymes needed to hydrolyze the biomass material after pretreatment [21,22]. It has been well established that producing higher concentration of sugars is an absolute necessity in an industrial setting as it lowers the heating requirements (lowering operating costs) and increases the volumetric efficiency (lowering capital costs) of the equipment [23]. Therefore, lowering the enzyme input and increasing the dry matter content during enzyme hydrolysis for higher cellulose conversion would be one of the most significant steps towards the direction of bioethanol production cost reduction and eventually leading to the commercialization of second generation biorefineries based on the lignocellulosic feedstock.

Several researchers have worked on using corn stover for the bioethanol production. Karr *et al.* used lime pretreatment followed by enzymatic hydrolysis at 5% solids concentration (SC) and 20 FPU (Spezyme CP and Novozym 188) and obtained 60% cellulose conversion [24]. Kim *et al.* introduced ammonia recycle percolation pretreatment followed by enzyme hydrolysis at 1% SC and 10 FPU (Spezyme CP and β-glucosidase (Sigma-Aldrich, St Louis, MO, USA)) and obtained 92% cellulose conversion [25,26]. This concentration of solids will, however, be far from an industrial process. Bura *et al.* used SO_2 catalyzed pretreatment followed by enzyme hydrolysis at 8% SC and 10 FPU (Spezyme CP, Novozym 188 and Multifect® Xylanase) and obtained 100% cellulose conversion [27]. However, again the solid concentration was far lower than needed for operating any industrial process. Using chemicals such as sulfur could further affect the down-stream processing of products, and for instance, sulfur will be attached to the solid fraction remaining after sugar extraction [28]. Recently, Yang *et al.* used steam explosion pretreatment followed by enzyme hydrolysis at 25% SC and 20 FPU (Celluclast) and obtained 85% cellulose conversion [29]. Even though this study achieved high glucose concentrations, the amount of enzymes used was higher, affecting the applicability of the process.

Cellobiohydrolases and endoglucanases are often inhibited by cellobiose [30], making beta-glucosidases important for avoiding product inhibition through conversion of cellobiose to glucose, and thereby, avoiding decreased hydrolysis rates of cellulose over time. However, beta-glucosidases are often themselves inhibited by their product glucose [31,32] making beta-glucosidase the rate-limiting enzyme. Maintaining a high hydrolysis rate of cellulose ultimately requires highly efficient beta-glucosidases that tolerate glucose at high levels.

3. Enzymes: Past to Present

Trichoderma reesei is one of the most widely used species of filamentous fungi for the production of cellulolytic enzymes. The fungus was originally isolated during the Second World War where it was found to thrive on the US Army's tent canvas (cellulose). Since the 1950s, the original strain of *T. reesei* has been subjected to multiple rounds of strain improvement for enhanced cellulase production, including increasing enzyme titers and reducing the catabolite repression effect as well as protease activity [33]. The fungal enzyme product, however, lacks sufficient beta-glucosidase activity for complete and efficient industrial cellulose hydrolysis [5,34].

Enhancement of the beta-glucosidase activity of the *T. reesei* enzyme product has been achieved through displacement of the native promoter by homologous recombination with xylanase and cellulase promoters obtaining a 4–7.5-fold increase in beta-glucosidase activity [35]. Other ways of increasing the beta-glucosidase activity of *T. reesei* include heterologous expression of beta-glucosidase from other fungi [36–39] thus creating a single expression host for the production of all relevant enzymes for converting cellulosic biomass into monomeric sugars.

Beta-glucosidases are widely produced by different genera and species of the fungal kingdom including Ascomycetes and Basidiomycetes, where especially the ascomycete genus *Aspergillus* has been widely studied for beta-glucosidase production. *A. niger* has been setting the standard in commercial beta-glucosidase production [40], but within the last few years more research papers have been published on efficient beta-glucosidases e.g., from other *Aspergillus* species and from the *Penicillium* genus [38,41,42].

Commercial enzyme preparations for cellulosic biomass hydrolysis were initially prepared as separate fungal fermentation products that needed to be combined for efficient hydrolysis, e.g., Celluclast (a *T. reesei* cellobiohydrolase and endo-glucanase product) and Novozym188 (an *A. niger* beta-glucosidase product) by Novozymes. More recently, the enzyme companies, Novozymes and Genencor, have replaced these two preparations with single products that contain the full array of enzymes for cellulosic biomass hydrolysis. Whether the products originate from strain improvement of the production strain to express all enzymes or if the products are mixes based on two or more fermentations is not disclosed by the companies. The optimal hydrolysis conditions of most commercial cellulosic enzymes are temperatures around 50 °C and a pH around 5. The enzyme loading must be optimized based on the biomass.

The current trend for the major enzyme companies is to team up with cellulosic biorefinery companies to specifically meet their needs in hydrolysis, working on optimizing the enzymes for a particular biomass and pretreatment method. Recently, Genencor has partnered with DuPont (http://biosciences.dupont.com), DSM with Poet (www.poetdsm.com), and Novozymes with Mossi & Ghisolfi Group (www.novozymes.com/en/news/news-archive/Pages/novozymes-partner-to-open-largest-cellulosic-ethanol-plant-in-2012.aspx), building the world's first commercial-scale cellulosic ethanol plant in Crescentino, Italy.

With enzymes being an expensive part of biomass processing, it would be of great interest to make enzyme production part of the processes within the biorefinery. Other research therefore looks at producing enzymes on-site to cut away the profit enzyme companies include in their pricing. By efficiently implementing enzyme production within the biorefinery, completing the value chain can be achieved by using streams within the biorefinery as fungal growth medium for enzyme production, and directly using this product (enzymes, fungus, and medium) in hydrolysis of biomass. This has already been shown for different fungi, e.g., *T. reesei* cultured on pretreated wheat straw [43], *A. niger* and *A. saccharolyticus* [44] cultured on the fiber waste fraction left after hydrolysis and fermentation, and *A. japonicus* cultured on castor bean meal waste for the biodiesel production [45].

Evaluating the overall production cost, the price of enzymes typically contributes to a large part of the total cost [37]. Efficient enzymes for lignocellulose degradation are, therefore, of high demand. As most of the currently used pretreatment methods remove lignin from the sugar polymers and in many cases also hydrolyze most of the hemicellulose, the main target for enzyme treatment is cellulose decomposition into glucose with beta-glucosidases being key enzymes in terms of complete cellulose hydrolysis.

4. The Bottleneck Enzyme: Beta-Glucosidase

Beta-glucosidases are most commonly classified based on either substrate specificity or nucleotide sequence identity. Beta-glucosidases hydrolyze the *O*-glycosyl linkage of terminal, non-reducing beta-D-glucosyl residues with release of beta-D-glucose, e.g., the bond in cellobiose. A wide specificity for beta-D-glucosides is found and there are examples of beta-glucosidases hydrolyzing beta-D-galactosides, alpha-L-arabinosides, beta-D-xylosides, or beta-D-fucosides [46]. Based on substrate specificity, beta-glucosidases have traditionally been divided into cellobiases (high specificity towards cellobiose), aryl- beta-glucosidases (high specificity towards substrates such as *p*-nitrophenyl-beta-D-glucopyranoside (pNPG)), or broad specificity beta-glucosidases [31,47]. Most beta-glucosidases are placed in the last category.

A classification based on substrate specificity cannot sufficiently accommodate enzymes that act on several substrates; the best accommodation for this is the classification system proposed by Henrissat (1991) which is based on sequence and structural features [48]. The strength of this system especially lies in the investigation of the active site of the enzymes, with significant similarity of sequences being a strong indication of similarity in the fold of the structure, and analysis of the primary structure can thereby assign potential conserved active-site residues. Fungal beta-glucosidases are primarily placed in the family 3 glycosyl hydrolases with the active site signature pattern defined as written below, where the aspartate (D) is the active site residue involved in catalysis (underlined) [46,49].

GH3 active site signature:

[LIVM](2) – [KR] – X – [EQKRD] – X(4) – G – [LIVMFTC] – [LIVT] – [LIVMF] – [ST] – D̲ – X(2) – [SGADNIT]

Structural information is valuable for protein engineering purposes to improve enzyme activity and stability. Only a few GH3 beta-glucosidase structures have been solved and published: *Hordeum vulgare* (barley) [50], *Kluyveromyces marxianus* (a yeast) [51], *Thermotoga neapolitana* (a hyperthermophilic bacterium) [52], *Pseudoalteromonas* sp. (a marine bacterium) [53], a compost microbial community [54], and only recently, one crystal structure from a filamentous fungus: the *Aspergillus aculeatus* beta-glucosidase BGL1 [55]. Furthermore, the BGL1 of *T. reesei* is in the protein database PDB, but the accompanying research article has not been published. Homology modeling has been the method of choice for obtaining structural information from fungal beta-glucosidases which have no available crystal structures. The beta-glucosidases from *Aspergillus saccharolyticus* and *Penicillium purpugenum* were modeled prior to the availability of other fungal beta-glucosidase crystal structures, and even though the sequence identity was relatively low to the template structures used, it was obvious that the residues important for substrate binding and catalysis were conserved and that the distance between the catalytic residues is similar to that of other solved beta-glucosidases [38,56].

The solved structure of the fungal *A. aculeatus* BGL1 consists of three domains: a catalytic TIM (triosephosphateisomerase) barrel-like domain, an α/β sandwich domain, and a FnIII (fibronectin type III) domain. These domains are connected with two linker regions. The active site and the catalytic residues of AaBGL1 are located at the domain interface between the barrel and the α/β sandwich domains [55]. Hydrolysis of beta-1,4-glycosidic bonds by beta-glucosidases is carried out by an overall retaining double-displacement mechanism [57]. Two catalytic carboxylic acid residues at the active site facilitate the reaction with one carboxylic acid acting as a nucleophile and the other as an acid/base catalyst [58]. The catalytic nucleophile of GH3 family enzymes is always present at a specific structural location just after the $\beta7$ strand of the TIM barrel domain, however, the position and identities for the acid/base catalyst are not completely conserved but are rather phylogenetically variable, and thus, less readily divined [55,59]. The topology of the active sites of all glycoside hydrolases falls into three general classes: (i) pocket or crater; (ii) cleft or groove; and (iii) tunnel. Beta-glucosidases and non-processive exo-acting enzymes have a pocket or crater topology that is well suited for recognition of a saccharide non-reducing extremity [60], with the depth and shape of the pocket or crater reflecting the number of sub-sites that contribute to substrate binding and the length of the leaving group [61]. Hydrolytic activity towards cellodextrins is commonly reported for fungal beta-glucosidases [11], and compared to other beta-glucosidases, the structure of the *A. aculeatus* BGL1 active site has a long cleft extending from sub-site +1 which appears to be a more suitable binding pocket for cellooligosaccharides [55]. Meanwhile, the catalytic pocket of *A. saccharolyticus* BGL1 is wider than other beta-glucosidases as it is missing a loop structure by the active site. Amino acids at this loop have been described to have weak H-bonds with glucose at the -1 sub-site, thus the deletion of this loop may plan an important role in altering substrate accessibility as well as rapid release of the product from the enzymes [38].

Based on genomic data, fungal beta-glucosidases are often reported to have several putative glycosylation sites based on their predicted amino acid sequence. The crystal structure of the *A. aculeatus* BGL1 was found to be highly glycosylated by many large N-glycan chains, which is believed to facilitate increased resistance to proteolytic attack and contributes to protein stability [55].

5. Beta-Glucosidases in Biomass Hydrolysis: The Challenges

In relation to industrial biomass conversion, a good beta-glucosidase facilitates efficient hydrolysis at specified operating conditions. Key points to consider when evaluating a beta-glucosidase are hydrolysis rate, inhibitors, and stability, with product inhibition and thermal instability often being a restriction for maintaining high conversion rates throughout the hydrolysis. It is obvious that activity and stability varies among different beta-glucosidases. Previous papers have listed beta-glucosidases and their properties [47,62]; as an addition to this, in Table 1 we here present a list of some more recently characterized fungal beta-glucosidases.

Table 1. Beta-glucosidases and their properties.

Microorganism	Substrate	Activity Km (mM)	Vmax (U/mg)	Temp. Opt. (°C)	pH Opt.	Inhibition Substrate	Inhibitor	Ki (mM)	Ref.
Aspergillus fumigatus Z5	pNPG			60	6.0				[42]
Aspergillus niger NRRL 599	pNPG	3.11	20.83	60	4.8				[63]
Aspergillus saccharolyticus	pNPG	1.9	45	58	4.2				[38]
Aspergillus terreus NRRL 265	pNPG	2.5		60	5.0	pNPG	Glucose	13.6	[64]
	Cellobiose	3.7							
Daldinia eschscholzii	pNPG	1.52	3.21	50	5.0	pNPG	Glucose	0.79	[65]
Fomitopsis palustris FFPRI 0507	pNPG	0.117		70	4.5	pNPG	Glucose	0.35	[66]
	Cellobiose	4.81							
Fusarium solani	pNPG	1	55.6	65	4.5				[67]
Humicola insolens	pNPG	0.16	18.1		6.2				[68]
	Cellobiose	0.51	86.0						
Neosartorya ficheri NRRL181	pNPG	68	886	40	6.0				[69]
Peniclillium funiculosum NCL1	pNPG	0.057	1920	60	4.0–5.0	pNPG	Glucose	1.5	[70]
Phoma sp. KCTC11825BP	pNPG	0.3		60	4.5	pNPG	Glucose	1.7	[71]
	Cellobiose	3.2							
Tolypocladium cylinndrosporum	pNPG	0.85	85.23	60	2.4	pNPG	Glucose	39.5	[72]
Trichoderma koningii AS3.2774	pNPG	2.67		50	5.0				[73]
Trichoderma reesei	pNPG			70	5.0				[74]

Fungi naturally produce a broad array of lignocellulosic enzymes, and with more and more full genome sequences available, it becomes evident just how many different enzymes their genome encode for. However, the genetic code itself does not necessarily imply that the fungus is optimally expressing the needed enzymes for efficient biomass hydrolysis. For example, the amount and types of cellulases (GH5, 6, 7, 12, 45, 61) and associated hemicellulase activities (GH10, 11, 26, 29, 39, 62, 67, 74, 93) are relatively small in the genome of T. reesei compared with other ascomycetes, even though the fungus is one of the most efficient cellulose degraders known [75]. Function can be predicted from the genetic code, but profound expertise does not yet exist in linking gene sequence to the actual activity and efficiency of the encoded enzyme [76]. The pathway to this has been initiated through homology modeling based on known 3D enzyme structures. Structures of most enzyme families have been resolved, including beta-glucosidases as mentioned previously, and with more templates becoming available, homology modeling can predict the folds and activity of gene sequences. This knowledge is useful for enzyme optimization using protein engineering methods such as site-directed mutagenesis, e.g., for higher thermal stability [22]. However, most current research has focused on testing the performance of individual enzymes heterologously expressed and purified, free from contaminating activities, against each other, and studies on optimally balanced enzyme cocktails have been undertaken to identify the best combination and ratio of de novo enzyme mixtures for biomass hydrolysis [22,77]. However, among the difficulties in expressing the enzymes heterologously for studying their activities are that different hosts might alter the original glycosylation pattern in the enzyme, thereby seriously altering their activity and/or stability [78].

One area of focus that must be addressed is how to perform such enzyme screenings in high through-put systems on actual biomass samples [79]. In practical terms, when studying the activity and kinetics of beta-glucosidases, it is important to consider the substrate that is being used, as substrate specificity of beta-glucosidases varies [47,62,80–82] and the choice of substrate will influence the kinetic data obtained. Several different substrates with varying sensitivity and ease of use can be applied for the determination of beta-glucosidase activity. Some enzyme testing is currently done on artificial or purified substrates rather than complex biomasses. However, data obtained using synthetic biomass substrates or single purified components have little value and limited applicability in predicting and modeling real biomass hydrolysis [11]. Those substrates can be valuable in terms of studying specific activities, but conclusions should never be extended to actual biomass hydrolysis as it is often the case that activities are found to be lower due to reduced substrate accessibility as well as enzyme inhibitors.

High conversion rates are essential for efficient conversion of biomass. Accumulation of glucose during hydrolysis can significantly lower the rate of cellulose hydrolysis through inhibition by blocking the active site or preventing the hydrolyzed substrate from leaving [83]. In case of product inhibition (glucose), the effect is naturally increased during the course of the reaction as more and more glucose is formed, and for beta-glucosidases the end-product is generally not removed during hydrolysis so the actual reaction rate will differ more and more from maximum reaction rate. High tolerance of beta-glucosidases towards glucose accumulation is, therefore, of great importance. A broad range of data on inhibition by glucose is described in the literature, with several of the published K_i values collected in a table in the Handbook of Carbohydrate Engineering [47]. The K_i values reported range from below one to thousands. Even within the same fungal species, there is great variation in the extent of product inhibition reported for different beta-glucosidases [47]. Compounds other than glucose are potentially present in biomass that can be inhibitory and influence the activity of beta-glucosidases, including (but not exclusively) other simple sugars, sugar derivatives, amines, and phenols [84].

A decrease in the rate of glucose formation can also be caused by transglycosylation events as the enzyme reaction is a reversible process. Other than inhibiting the reaction by occupying the active site, glucose can also be considered to take part in transglycosylation, thus using the active site capacity in non-hydrolyzing action which will decrease the overall rate of hydrolysis. Transglycosylation is obviously an unwanted event in biomass hydrolysis, but it is frequently reported for beta-glucosidases [62]; especially at high substrate concentrations, the transglycosylation is observed [85]. Targeted mutagenesis aiming at displacing essential amino acids involved in transglycosylation could potentially reduce this mechanism [86].

Enzyme performance in actual biomass hydrolysis is affected by several factors including temperature, pH, and solids loading. First of all, the condition of the biomass is defined by the pretreatment method applied. Many pretreatment methods rely on high temperatures and acidic conditions to make the biomass accessible for enzyme hydrolysis. Enzymes will, depending on extremity and time of exposure be inactivated by pH and temperature variations. Ionic groups are involved in enzyme catalysis, such as the acid-base catalyst in the beta-glucosidase active site, and the protonation state of the carboxylic acid residue catalyst and the carboxylate nucleophile is essential for the enzymatic reaction, therefore, a pH change could impair the catalytic mechanism [87]. Beta-glucosidases perform well at pH 4–5 [47,62], but at pH much lower than that, a significant decrease in activity is found. Therefore, in most cases, the pretreated biomass must be pH adjusted to some degree as the acidity is usually beyond this. Regarding temperature, according to the van't Hoff rule, reaction rates double with every 10 degrees Celsius increase of temperature, which applies to all chemical reactions including enzyme catalyzed reactions. However, when reaching high temperatures, protein stability will be affected, leading to denaturation, and thus irreversible inactivation of the enzyme. Mesophilic fungi that typically grow at 24–27 degrees Celsius are often times reported to produce beta-glucosidases with temperature optima around 60–75 degrees Celsius, and only moderate increases in thermal stability are seen in enzymes derived from thermophilic fungi [88]. Temperature and pH optimum for microbial beta-glucosidases have been reported in different reviews [47,62,88], but for biomass hydrolysis processes that typically run for the duration of several hours or even days, the stability of the enzyme at specified temperatures is important. Several papers claim to have discovered thermostable beta-glucosidases, however, often the activity was only verified at the high temperature for a short duration of time [88].

In industrial biofuel production, the pretreatment of biomass needs to be performed at very high dry matter content, above 20% (w/w), in order to increase product concentrations and decrease reactor volumes and distillation costs [23]. Most studies have, however, shown that hydrolysis rates decrease with increasing dry matter content in biomass hydrolysis. Suggested explanations for this are inefficient means of mixing, product inhibition, lignin or hemicellulose derivatives, or inhibition by adsorption of the enzymes to the biomass surface. Based on different correlation studies, it has been found that the adsorption effect best describes the decrease in hydrolysis with increase in solids' loading [23]. It has further been recognized that enzyme performance is reduced by interaction with lignin or lignin–carbohydrate complex; however, of the cellulase and xylanase enzymes tested, beta-glucosidase was the least affected by lignin [89]. Attempts have been made to deal with this issue by adding non-enzyme proteins to the hydrolysis that will be absorbed by the biomass instead of the active enzymes [90]. Another more advanced solution would be to engineer the hydrophobicity of the surface amino acids on the enzymes to make them less prone to adsorption by the biomass.

Beta-glucosidases act on soluble substrates and are with regards to biomass hydrolysis highly dependent on the action of cellobiohydrolases and endoglucanases to provide substrate, as the beta-glucosidases cannot access the insoluble cellulose fibers. Meanwhile, cellobiohydrolases and endoglucanases are highly dependent on beta-glucosidases to maintain efficient hydrolysis by relieving product inhibition. Therefore, a balanced enzyme cocktail is essential for efficient hydrolysis of biomass. The optimal ratio of the enzymes will depend on the specific activity of the enzymes used, the condition of the biomass substrate (sugar accessibility) as well as physical reaction conditions [91]. The total amount of enzyme required directly reflects on cost. Economics of enzymatic hydrolysis has long been a topic of discussion and concern for the feasibility of lignocellulosic biomass conversion. Properties of new enzymes are continuously reported in literature as well as research on optimizing the enzyme cocktails for biomass hydrolysis with emphasis on using reduced enzyme loadings yet obtaining same hydrolysis efficiency. One strategy for resolving this is the minimal enzyme cocktail concept which concerns identification of the minimal number, the minimal levels, and the optimal combination of the best performing mono-active enzymatic activities to achieve degradation to monomeric sugar units [14]. Ideally, based on minimal enzyme cocktail concept studies, rather than using purified enzymes, a selected enzyme producing microorganism should be genetically modified with distinct promoters for each enzyme gene to facilitate optimal expression of each enzyme component. It should be ensured that the enzymes are correctly post-processed by such host microorganisms so that they are correctly folded and have optimal activity, stability, *etc*. Furthermore, such microorganisms should not have intra- or extracellular proteolytic activity that would affect enzyme expression.

6. New and Improved Beta-Glucosidases

In order to optimize the use of different biomasses, it is important to identify new beta-glucosidases with improved abilities on the specific biomasses as well as with improved abilities such as stability and high conversion rates. As already discussed, product inhibition impairing yields, thermal inactivation of enzymes, and high cost of enzyme production are main obstacles of commercial cellulose hydrolysis and therefore set the stage in the search for better alternatives to the currently available enzyme preparations. The choice stands between screening for new beta-glucosidases and improving known beta-glucosidases.

The number of fungal species on earth is estimated to 1.5 million of which as little as approximately 5% are known [92,93], a statement that calls for a more directed effort for unraveling the potential of unknown species found in nature. The identification and characterization of new fungal species are often encountered in literature. Within the black Aspergilli, to which several efficient beta-glucosidase products belong, several new species have been identified within recent years [94–102]. Screening for new enzymes can be performed at the genomic as well as the proteomic level—in either case, it can be a mixed gene or protein pool or a sample representing a specific species. The number of organisms being fully genome-sequenced is constantly increasing, and along with it, the sequences for new genes. Comparative searches in databases can reveal new beta-glucosidase sequences, but to know if they are better than current standard, they must be cloned, expressed, and assayed. Using a metagenomics approach, environmental DNA has been screened for beta-glucosidase activity with the findings of novel beta-glucosidases [103–105]. As another approach, screening secreted fungal proteins for new and improved beta-glucosidases has been reported with success, generally finding black Aspergilli to be superior [106,107].

Through genetic changes, enzymes can be tailored to obtain improved abilities. The changes can either be random by classical methods of mutagenesis or specifically targeted improvements aided by the solved crystal structures.

The increased activity obtained from classical mutagenesis is most often due to changes at the regulatory level of enzyme expression leading to increased production of the gene of interest or decreased expression of conflicting genes and is therefore minded on production strain improvements, rather than changes to the enzyme itself for improved activity. One good example was the use of a combination of UV irradiation and nitrosomethyl guanidine treatment to develop the *T. reesei* strain RutC30 with improved total protein production and activity; one of the best existing *T. reesei* cellulase mutants [108].

Mutation, recombination, and selection set the stage for functional evolution in nature. Directed evolution mimics natural evolution by combining reiterative random mutagenesis and recombination with screening or selection for enzyme variants with improved properties [109–111]. Compared to classical mutagenesis, directed evolution targets a specific gene of choice with random changes being performed delimited to the gene of choice, followed by evaluation of the mutants [112]. Several publications exist on such strategy for non-fungal beta-glucosidases. For example, several single amino acid substitutions generated through error prone PCR were found to contribute to increased thermal resistance of *Paenibacillus polymyxa* beta-glucosidase that were then further recombined by gene shuffling [113]. The improvements of the final best clone were attributed to three mutations leading to formation of salt bridges and amino acids less prone to oxidation [114]. A similar approach of combining error prone PCR and gene shuffling was performed on *Pyrococcus furiosus* beta-glucosidase, generating an improvement of low temperature cellobiose hydrolysis [115]. More recently, gene shuffling of beta-glucosidases from *Thermobifida fusca* and *Paebibacillus polymxyxa* resulted in a mutant with increased thermostability compared to both parental enzymes, reported as a 144-fold increase in half-life of inactivation, and a 94% increase in k_{cat} towards cellobiose [116].

To perform more advanced mutagenesis, such as rational design, bioinformatics is a prerequisite. Protein structure can guide the fine-tuning of e.g., the active site by rational design by only a few specific mutations. A great amount of knowledge is available on the protein engineering possibilities for improving activity as well as stability [117]. With only a few filamentous fungal beta-glucosidase structures recently having been solved, most rational design has been performed on non-fungal beta-glucosidases. However, in a recent study, specific amino acids were mutated in the outer channel of the active site of a *T. reesei* beta-glucosidase to significantly improve activity as well as increase the thermostability [118].

7. Conclusions

Fungal beta-glucosidases are important enzymes in efficient hydrolysis of cellulosic biomass, as they relieve the inhibition of the cellobiohydrolases and endoglucanases by reducing cellobiose accumulation. They are key enzymes in the final part of biomass hydrolysis for producing the monomer sugars for the production of biofuels and platform molecules that can serve as building blocks in the synthesis of chemicals and polymeric materials. They are often the bottleneck in the process, and the most important challenge to overcome is product inhibition. To have a profitable biomass conversion process, the hydrolysis must yield high glucose concentrations and the beta-glucosidases must, therefore, not be inhibited by their product but maintain high conversion rates at high glucose concentrations.

178

Conflicts of Interest

The authors declare no conflict of interest.

References

1. Cherubini, F. The biorefinery concept: Using biomass instead of oil for producing energy and chemicals. *Energy Conver. Manag.* **2010**, *51*, 1412–1421.
2. Knauf, M.; Moniruzzaman, M. Lignocellulosic biomass processing: A perspective. *Int. Sugar J.* **2004**, *106*, 147–150.
3. Werpy, T.; Petersen, G.; Aden, A.; Bozell, J.; Holladay, J.; White, J.; Manheim, A. *Top Value added Chemicals from Biomass, Volume 1: Results of screening for potential candidates from sugars and synthesis gas*; U.S. Department of Energy, Oak Ridge, TN, USA, **2004**; available at heep://www.eere.energy.gov/biomass/pdfs/35523.pdf (access on 2 September 2013).
4. U.S. Department of Energy. *Biomass Feedstock Composition and Property Database*; Available online at: http://www.afdc.energy.gov/biomass/progs/search1.cgi (access on 30 August 2013).
5. Lynd, L.R.; Weimer, P.J.; van Zyl, W.H.; Pretorius, I.S. Microbial cellulose utilization: Fundamentals and biotechnology. *Microbiol. Mol. Biol. Rev.* **2002**, *66*, 506–577.
6. Beguin, P.; Aubert, J.P. The biological degradation of cellulose. *FEMS Microbiol. Rev.* **1994**, *13*, 25–58.
7. Berg, J.M.; Tymoczko, J.L.; Stryer, L. *Biochemistry*, 5th ed.; W.H. Freeman and Company: New York, NY, USA, 2002.
8. Alvira, P.; Tomas-Pejo, E.; Ballesteros, M.; Negro, M.J. Pretreatment technologies for an efficient bioethanol production process based on enzymatic hydrolysis: A review. *Bioresour. Technol.* **2010**, *101*, 4851–4861.
9. Mosier, N.; Wyman, C.; Dale, B.; Elander, R.; Lee, Y.Y.; Holtzapple, M.; Ladisch, M. Features of promising technologies for pretreatment of lignocellulosic biomass. *Bioresour. Technol.* **2005**, *96*, 673–686.
10. Sun, Y.; Cheng, J.Y. Hydrolysis of lignocellulosic materials for ethanol production: A review. *Bioresour. Technol.* **2002**, *83*, 1–11.
11. Zhang, Y.-P.; Himmel, M.E.; Mielenz, J.R. Outlook for cellulase improvement: Screening and selection strategies. *Biotechnol. Adv.* **2006**, *24*, 452–481.
12. Kabel, M.A.; Bos, G.; Zeevalking, J.; Voragen, A.G.J.; Schols, H.A. Effect of pretreatment severity on xylan solubility and enzymatic breakdown of the remaining cellulose from wheat straw. *Bioresour. Technol.* **2007**, *98*, 2034–2042.
13. Chang, V.S.; Holtzapple, M.T. Fundamental factors affecting biomass enzymatic reactivity. *Appl. Biochem. Biotechnol.* **2000**, *84–86*, 5–37.
14. Meyer, A.S.; Rosgaard, L.; Sorensen, H.R. The minimal enzyme cocktail concept for biomass processing. *J. Cereal. Sci.* **2009**, *50*, 337–344.
15. Zhang, Y.-P.; Lynd, L.R. Toward an aggregated understanding of enzymatic hydrolysis of cellulose: Noncomplexed cellulase systems. *Biotechnol. Bioeng.* **2004**, *88*, 797–824.

16. Wang, M.; Liu, K.; Dai, L.; Zhang, J.; Fang, X. The structural and biochemical basis for cellulose biodegradation. *J. Chem. Technol. Biotechnol.* **2013**, *88*, 491–500.

17. Harris, P.V.; Welner, D.; McFarland, K.C.; Re, E.; Poulsen, J.N.; Brown, K.; Salbo, R.; Ding, H.; Vlasenko, E.; Merino, S.; *et al.* Stimulation of lignocellulosic biomass hydrolysis by proteins of glycoside hydrolase family 61: Structure and function of a large, enigmatic family. *Biochemistry (N Y)* **2010**, *49*, 3305–3316.

18. Langston, J.A.; Shaghasi, T.; Abbate, E.; Xu, F.; Vlasenko, E.; Sweeney, M.D. Oxidoreductive cellulose depolymerization by the enzymes cellobiose dehydrogenase and glycoside hydrolase 61. *Appl. Environ. Microbiol.* **2011**, *77*, 7007–7015.

19. Quinlan, R.J.; Sweeney, M.D.; lo Leggio, L.; Otten, H.; Poulsen, J.N.; Johansen, K.S.; Krogh, K.B.R.M.; Jørgensen, C.I.; Tovborg, M.; Anthonsen, A.; *et al.* Insights into the oxidative degradation of cellulose by a copper metalloenzyme that exploits biomass components. *Proc. Natl. Acad. Sci. USA* **2011**, *108*, 15079–15084.

20. Vaaje-Kolstad, G.; Westereng, B.; Horn, S.J.; Liu, Z.; Zhai, H.; Sorlie, M.; Eijsink, V.G.H. An oxidative enzyme boosting the enzymatic conversion of recalcitrant polysaccharides. *Science* **2010**, *330*, 219–222.

21. Lynd, L.R.; Laser, M.S.; Bransby, D.; Dale, B.E.; Davison, B.; Hamilton, R.; Himmel, M.; Keller, M.; McMillan, J.D.; Sheehan, J.; *et al.* How biotech can transform biofuels. *Nat. Biotechnol.* **2008**, *26*, 169–172.

22. Banerjee, G.; Scott-Craig, J.S.; Walton, J.D. Improving enzymes for biomass conversion: A basic research perspective. *Bioenergy Res.* **2010**, *3*, 82–92.

23. Kristensen, J.B.; Felby, C.; Jorgensen, H. Yield-determining factors in high-solids enzymatic hydrolysis of lignocellulose. *Biotechnol. Biofuels* **2009**, *2*, 11.

24. Kaar, W.; Holtzapple, M. Using lime pretreatment to facilitate the enzymic hydrolysis of corn stover. *Biomass Bioenergy* **2000**, *18*, 189–199.

25. Kim, S.; Holtzapple, M. Lime pretreatment and enzymatic hydrolysis of corn stover. *Bioresour. Technol.* **2005**, *96*, 1994–2006.

26. Kim, T.; Lee, Y. Pretreatment of corn stover by soaking in aqueous ammonia. *Appl. Biochem. Biotechnol.* **2005**, *124*, 1119–1131.

27. Bura, R.; Chandra, R.; Saddler, J. Influence of xylan on the enzymatic hydrolysis of steam-pretreated corn stover and hybrid poplar. *Biotechnol. Prog.* **2009**, *25*, 315–322.

28. Zhu, J.Y.; Zhu, W.; OBryan, P.; Dien, B.S.; Tian, S.; Gleisner, R.; Pan, X.J. Ethanol production from SPORL-pretreated lodgepole pine: Preliminary evaluation of mass balance and process energy efficiency. *Appl. Microbiol. Biotechnol.* **2010**, *86*, 1355–1365.

29. Yang, J.; Zhang, X.; Yong, Q.; Yu, S. Three-stage enzymatic hydrolysis of steam-exploded corn stover at high substrate concentration. *Bioresour. Technol.* **2011**, *102*, 4905–4908.

30. Murphy, L.; Bohlin, C.; Baumann, M.J.; Olsen, S.N.; Sorensen, T.H.; Anderson, L.; Borch, K.; Westh, P. Product inhibition of five *Hypocrea jecorina* cellulases. *Enzyme Microb. Technol.* **2013**, *52*, 163–169.

31. Shewale, J.G. Beta-Glucosidase—Its role in cellulase synthesis and hydrolysis of cellulose. *Int. J. Biochem.* **1982**, *14*, 435–443.

32. Xiao, Z.Z.; Zhang, X.; Gregg, D.J.; Saddler, J.N. Effects of sugar inhibition on cellulases and beta-glucosidase during enzymatic hydrolysis of softwood substrates. *Appl. Biochem. Biotechnol.* **2004**, *113–116*, 1115–1126.

33. Peterson, R.; Nevalainen, H. *Trichoderma reesei* RUT-C30—Thirty years of strain improvement. *Microbiology* **2012**, *158*, 58–68.

34. Reczey, K.; Brumbauer, A.; Bollok, M.; Szengyel, Z.; Zacchi, G. Use of hemicellulose hydrolysate for beta-glucosidase fermentation. *Appl. Biochem. Biotechnol.* **1998**, *70–72*, 225–235.

35. Rahman, Z.; Shida, Y.; Furukawa, T.; Suzuki, Y.; Okada, H.; Ogasawara, W.; Morikawa, Y. Application of *Trichoderma reesei* cellulase and xylanase promoters through homologous recombination for enhanced production of extracellular beta-glucosidase I. *Biosci. Biotechnol. Biochem.* **2009**, *73*, 1083–1089.

36. Murray, P.; Aro, N.; Collins, C.; Grassick, A.; Penttila, M.; Saloheimo, M.; Tuohy, M. Expression in *Trichoderma reesei* and characterisation of a thermostable family 3 beta-glucosidase from the moderately thermophilic fungus *Talaromyces emersonii*. *Protein Expr. Purif.* **2004**, *38*, 248–257.

37. Merino, S.T.; Cherry, J. Progress and challenges in enzyme development for Biomass utilization. *Biofuels* **2007**, *108*, 95–120.

38. Sørensen, A.; Ahring, B.K.; Lübeck, M.; Ubhayasekera, W.; Bruno, K.S.; Culley, D.E.; Lübeck, P.S. Identifying and characterizing the most significant beta-glucosidase of the novel species *Aspergillus saccharolyticus*. *Can. J. Microbiol.* **2012**, *58*, 1035–1046.

39. Nakazawa, H.; Kawai, T.; Ida, N.; Shida, Y.; Kobayashi, Y.; Okada, H.; Tani, S.; Sumitani, J. Kawaguchi, T.; Morikawa, Y.; Ogasawara, W. Construction of a recombinant *Trichoderma reesei* strain expressing *Aspergillus aculeatus* beta-glucosidase 1 for efficient biomass conversion. *Biotechnol. Bioeng.* **2012**, *109*, 92–99.

40. Dekker, R.F.H. Kinetic, inhibition, and stability properties of a commercial beta-D-glucosidase (cellobiase) preparation from *Aspergillus niger* and its suitability in the hydrolysis of lignocellulose. *Biotechnol. Bioeng.* **1986**, *28*, 1438–1442.

41. Krogh, K.B.R.; Morkeberg, A.; Jorgensen, H.; Frisvad, J.C.; Olsson, L. Screening genus *Penicillium* for producers of cellulolytic and xylanolytic enzymes. *Appl. Biochem. Biotechnol.* **2004**, *113–116*, 389–401.

42. Liu, D.; Zhang, R.; Yang, X.; Zhang, Z.; Song, S.; Miao, Y.; Shen, Q. Characterization of a thermostable beta-glucosidase from *Aspergillus fumigatus* Z5, and its functional expression in *Pichia pastoris* X33. *Microb. Cell Factories* **2012**, *11*, 25.

43. Gyalai-Korpos, M.; Mangel, R.; Alvira, P.; Dienes, D.; Ballesteros, M.; Reczey, K. Cellulase production using different streams of wheat grain- and wheat straw-based ethanol processes. *J. Ind. Microbiol. Biotechnol.* **2011**, *38*, 791–802.

44. Sørensen, A.; Teller, P.J.; Lübeck, P.S.; Ahring, B.K. Onsite enzyme production during bioethanol production from biomass: Screening for suitable fungal strains. *Appl. Biochem. Biotechnol.* **2011**, *164*, 1058–1070.

45. Herculano, P.N.; Porto, T.S.; Moreira, K.A.; Pinto, G.A.S.; Souza-Motta, C.M.; Porto, A.L.F. Cellulase production by *Aspergillus japonicus* URM5620 Using Waste from Castor Bean (Ricinus communis L.) Under Solid-State Fermentation. *Appl. Biochem. Biotechnol.* **2011**, *165*, 1057–1067.

46. Bairoch, A. The ENZYME database in 2000. *Nucleic Acids Res.* **2000**, *28*, 304–305.

47. Eyzaguirre, J.; Hidalgo, M.; Leschot, A. Beta-Glucosidases from Filamentous Fungi: Properties, Structure, and Applications. In *Handbook of Carbohydrate Engineering*; Taylor and Francis Group, LLC: Boca Raton, FL 33487, USA, 2005; pp. 645–685.

48. Henrissat, B. A classification of glycosyl hydrolases based on amino-acid-sequence similarities. *Biochem. J.* **1991**, *280*, 309–316.

49. Bairoch, A. Prosite—A dictionary of sites and patterns in proteins. *Nucleic Acids Res.* **1992**, *20*, 2013–2018.

50. Varghese, J.N.; Hrmova, M.; Fincher, G.B. Three-dimensional structure of a barley beta-D-glucan exohydrolase, a family 3 glycosyl hydrolase. *Structure* **1999**, *7*, 179–190.

51. Yoshida, E.; Hidaka, M.; Fushinobu, S.; Koyanagi, T.; Minami, H.; Tamaki, H.; Kitaoka, M.; Katayama, T.; Kumagai, H. Purification, crystallization and preliminary X-ray analysis of beta-glucosidase from *Kluyveromyces marxianus* NBRC1777. *Acta Crystallogr. Sect. F-Struct. Biol. Cryst. Commun.* **2009**, *65*, 1190–1192.

52. Pozzo, T.; Pasten, J.L.; Karlsson, E.N.; Logan, D.T. Structural and functional analyses of beta-glucosidase 3B from *Thermotoga neapolitana*: A thermostable three-domain representative of glycoside hydrolase 3. *J. Mol. Biol.* **2010**, *397*, 724–739.

53. Nakatani, Y.; Cutfield, S.M.; Cowieson, N.P.; Cutfield, J.F. Structure and activity of exo-1,3/1,4- beta-glucanase from marine bacterium *Pseudoalteromonas* sp. BB1 showing a novel *C*-terminal domain. *Febs. J.* **2012**, *279*, 464–478.

54. McAndrew, R.P.; Park, J.I.; Heins, R.A.; Reindl, W.; Friedland, G.D.; D'haeseleer, P.; Northen, T.; Sale, K.L.; Simmons, B.A.; Adams, P.D. From soil to structure, a novel dimeric beta-glucosidase belonging to the glycoside hydrolase family 3 isolated from compost using metagenomic analysis. *J. Biol. Chem.* **2013**, *288*, 14985–14992.

55. Suzuki, K.; Sumitani, J.; Nam, Y.; Nishimaki, T.; Tani, S.; Wakagi, T.; Kawaguchi, T.; Fushinobu, S. Crystal structures of glycoside hydrolase family 3 β-glucosidase 1 from *Aspergillus aculeatus*. *Biochem. J.* **2013**, *452*, 211–221.

56. Jeya, M.; Joo, A.; Lee, K.; Tiwari, M.K.; Lee, K.; Kim, S.; Lee, J. Characterization of beta-glucosidase from a strain of *Penicillium purpurogenum* KJS506. *Appl. Microbiol. Biotechnol.* **2010**, *86*, 1473–1484.

57. Sinnott, M.L. Catalytic mechanisms of enzymatic glycosyl transfer. *Chem. Rev.* **1990**, 90, 1171–1202.

58. McCarter, J.D.; Withers, S.G. Mechanisms of enzymatic glycoside hydrolysis. *Curr. Opin. Struct. Biol.* **1994**, *4*, 885–892.

59. Thongpoo, P.; McKee, L.S.; Araujo, A.C.; Kongsaeree, P.T.; Brumer, H. Identification of the acid/base catalyst of a glycoside hydrolase family 3 (GH3) beta-glucosidase from *Aspergillus niger* ASKU28. *Biochim. Biophys. Acta-Gen.* **2013**, *1830*, 2739–2749.

60. Davies, G.; Henrissat, B. Structures and mechanisms of glycosyl hydrolases. *Structure* **1995**, *3*, 853–859.

61. Davies, G.J.; Wilson, K.S.; Henrissat, B. Nomenclature for sugar-binding subsites in glycosyl hydrolases. *Biochem. J.* **1997**, *321*, 557–559.

62. Bhatia, Y.; Mishra, S.; Bisaria, V.S. Microbial beta-glucosidases: Cloning, properties, and applications. *Crit. Rev. Biotechnol.* **2002**, *22*, 375–407.

63. Zahoor, S.; Javed, M.M.; Aftab, S.; Latif, F.; Ikram-ul-Haq. Metabolic engineering and thermodynamic characterization of an extracellular beta-glucosidase produced by *Aspergillus niger*. *Afr. J. Biotechnol.* **2011**, *10*, 8107–8116.

64. Elshafei, A.M.; Hassan, M.M.; Morsi, N.M.; Elghonamy, D.H. Purification and some kinetic properties of beta-glucosidase from *Aspergillus terreus* NRRL 265. *Afr. J. Biotechnol.* **2011**, *10*, 19556–19569.

65. Karnchanatat, A.; Petsom, A.; Sangvanich, P.; Piaphukiew, J.; Whalley, A.J.S.; Reynolds, C.D.; Sihanonth, P. Purification and biochemical characterization of an extracellular beta glucosidase from the wood-decaying fungus *Daldinia eschscholzii* (Ehrenb.: Fr.) Rehm. *FEMS Microbiol. Lett.* 2007, *270*, 162–170.

66. Yoon, J.; Kim, K.; Cha, C. Purification and characterization of thermostable beta-glucosidase from the brown-rot basidiomycete *Fomitopsis palustris* grown on microcrystalline cellulose. *J. Microbiol.* **2008**, *46*, 51–55.

67. Bhatti, H.N.; Batool, S.; Afzal, N. Production and characterization of a novel beta-glucosidase from *Fusarium solani*. *Int. J. Agric. Biol.* **2013**, *15*, 140–144.

68. Kalyani, D.; Lee, K.; Tiwari, M.K.; Ramachandran, P.; Kim, H.; Kim, I.; Jeya, M.; Lee, J. Characterization of a recombinant aryl beta-glucosidase from *Neosartorya fischeri* NRRL181. *Appl. Microbiol. Biotechnol.* **2012**, *94*, 413–423.

69. Moreira Souza, F.H.; Nascimento, C.V.; Rosa, J.C.; Masui, D.C.; Leone, F.A.; Jorge, J.A.; Furriel, R.P.M. Purification and biochemical characterization of a mycelial glucose- and xylose-stimulated beta-glucosidase from the thermophilic fungus *Humicola insolens*. *Process Biochem.* 2010, *45*, 272–278.

70. Ramani, G.; Meera, B.; Vanitha, C.; Rao, M.; Gunasekaran, P. Production, purification, and characterization of a beta-glucosidase of *Penicillium funiculosum* NCL1. *Appl. Biochem. Biotechnol.* **2012**, *167*, 959–972.

71. Choi, J.; Park, A.; Kim, Y.J.; Kim, J.; Cha, C.; Yoon, J. Purification and characterization of an extracellular beta-glucosidase produced by *Phoma* sp. KCTC11825BP isolated from rotten mandarin peel. *J. Microbiol. Biotechnol.* **2011**, *21*, 503–508.

72. Zhang, Y.B.; Yuan, L.J.; Chen, Z.J.; Fu, L.; Lu, J.H.; Meng, Q.F.; He, H.; Yu, X.X.; Lin, F.; Teng, L.R. Purification and characterization of beta-glucosidase from a newly isolated strain *Tolypocladium cylindrosporum* Syzx4. *Chem. Res. Chin. Univ.* **2011**, *27*, 557–561.

73. Lin, J.; Pillay, B.; Singh, S. Purification and biochemical characteristics of beta-D-glucosidase from a thermophilic fungus, *Thermomyces lanuginosus* SSBP. *Biotechnol. Appl. Biochem.* **1999**, *30*, 81–87.

74. Chen, P.; Fu, X.Y.; Ng, T.B.; Ye, X.Y. Expression of a secretory beta-glucosidase from *Trichoderma reesei* in *Pichia pastoris* and its characterization. *Biotechnol. Lett.* **2011**, *33*, 2475–2479.

75. Kubicek, C.P.; Herrera-Estrella, A.; Seidl-Seiboth, V.; Martinez, D.A.; Druzhinina, I.S.; Thon, M.; Zeilinger, S.; Casas-Flores, S.; Horwitz, B.A.; Mukherjee, P.K; *et al.* Comparative genome sequence analysis underscores mycoparasitism as the ancestral life style of *Trichoderma*. *Genome Biol.* **2011**, *12*, R40.

76. Yan, S.; Wu, G. Prediction of optimal pH in hydrolytic reaction of beta-glucosidase. *Appl. Biochem. Biotechnol.* **2013**, *169*, 1884–1894.

77. Banerjee, S.; Mudliar, S.; Sen, R.; Giri, B.; Satpute, D.; Chakrabarti, T.; Pandey, R.A. Commercializing lignocellulosic bioethanol: Technology bottlenecks and possible remedies. *Biofuels Bioprod. Bioref.* **2010**, *4*, 77–93.

78. Jeoh, T.; Michener, W.; Himmel, M.E.; Decker, S.R.; Adney, W.S. Implications of cellobiohydrolase glycosylation for use in biomass conversion. *Biotechnol. Biofuels* **2008**, *1*, 10.

79. Banerjee, G.; Car, S.; Scott-Craig, J.S.; Borrusch, M.S.; Bongers, M.; Walton, J.D. Synthetic multi-component enzyme mixtures for deconstruction of lignocellulosic biomass. *Bioresour. Technol.* **2010**, *101*, 9097–9105.

80. Riou, C.; Salmon, J.M.; Vallier, M.J.; Gunata, Z.; Barre, P. Purification, characterization, and substrate specificity of a novel highly glucose-tolerant beta-glucosidase from *Aspergillus oryzae*. *Appl. Environ. Microbiol.* **1998**, *64*, 3607–3614.

81. Langston, J.; Sheehy, N.; Xu, F. Substrate specificity of *Aspergillus oryzae* family 3 beta-glucosidase. *Biochim. Biophys. Acta-Proteins Proteomics* **2006**, *1764*, 972–978.

82. Korotkova, O.G.; Semenova, M.V.; Morozova, V.V.; Zorov, I.N.; Sokolova, L.M.; Bubnova, T.M.; Okunev, O.N.; Sinitsyn, A.P. Isolation and properties of fungal beta-glucosidases. *Biochemistry (Mosc.)* **2009**, *74*, 569–577.

83. Andric, P.; Meyer, A.S.; Jensen, P.A.; Dam-Johansen, K. Reactor design for minimizing product inhibition during enzymatic lignocellulose hydrolysis: I. Significance and mechanism of cellobiose and glucose inhibition on cellulolytic enzymes. *Biotechnol. Adv.* **2010**, *28*, 308–324.

84. Dale, M.P.; Ensley, H.E.; Kern, K.; Sastry, K.A.R.; Byers, L.D. Reversible inhibitors of beta-glucosidase. *Biochemistry (N Y)* **1985**, *24*, 3530–3539.

85. Bohlin, C.; Praestgaard, E.; Baumann, M.J.; Borch, K.; Praestgaard, J.; Monrad, R.N.; Westh, P. A comparative study of hydrolysis and transglycosylation activities of fungal beta-glucosidases. *Appl. Microbiol. Biotechnol.* **2013**, *97*, 159–169.

86. Frutuoso, M.A.; Marana, S.R. A single amino acid residue determines the ratio of hydrolysis to transglycosylation catalyzed by beta-glucosidases. *Protein Peptide Lett.* **2013**, *20*, 102–106.

87. McIntosh, L.P.; Hand, G.; Johnson, P.E.; Joshi, M.D.; Korner, M.; Plesniak, L.A.; Ziser, L.; Wakarchuk, W.W.; Withers, S.G. The pK_a of the general acid/base carboxyl group of a glycosidase cycles during catalysis: A C-13-NMR study of *Bacillus circulans* xylanase. *Biochemistry (N Y)* **1996**, *35*, 9958–9966.

88. Yeoman, C.J.; Han, Y.; Dodd, D.; Schroeder, C.M.; Mackie, R.I.; Cann, I.K.O. Thermostable enzymes as biocatalysts in the biofuel industry. *Adv. Appl. Microbiol.* **2010**, *70*, 1–55.
89. Berlin, A.; Balakshin, M.; Gilkes, N.; Kadla, J.; Maximenko, V.; Kubo, S.; Saddler, J. Inhibition of cellulase, xylanase and beta-glucosidase activities by softwood lignin preparations. *J. Biotechnol.* **2006**, *125*, 198–209.
90. Yang, B.; Wyman, C.E. BSA treatment to enhance enzymatic hydrolysis of cellulose in lignin containing substrates. *Biotechnol. Bioeng.* **2006**, *94*, 611–617.
91. Selig, M.J.; Hsieh, C.C.; Thygesen, L.G.; Himmel, M.E.; Felby, C.; Decker, S.R. Considering water availability and the effect of solute concentration on high solids saccharification of lignocellulosic biomass. *Biotechnol. Prog.* **2012**, *28*, 1478–1490.
92. Hawksworth, D.L. The fungal dimension of biodiversity—Magnitude, significance, and conservation. *Mycol. Res.* **1991**, *95*, 641–655.
93. Hawksworth, D.L. The magnitude of fungal diversity: The 1.5 million species estimate revisited. *Mycol. Res.* **2001**, *105*, 1422–1432.
94. Mares, D.; Andreotti, E.; Maldonado, M.E.; Pedrini, P.; Colalongo, C.; Romagnoli, C. Three new species of *Aspergillus* from Amazonian forest soil (Ecuador). *Curr. Microbiol.* **2008**, 57, 222–229.
95. De Vries, R.P.; Frisvad, J.C.; van de Vondervoort, P.J.I.; Burgers, K.; Kuijpers, A.F.A.; Samson, R.A.; Visser, J. *Aspergillus vadensis*, a new species of the group of black Aspergilli. *Antonie Leeuwenhoek* **2005**, *87*, 195–203.
96. Samson, R.A.; Houbraken, J.A.M.P.; Kuijpers, A.F.A.; Frank, J.M.; Frisvad, J.C. New ochratoxin A or sclerotium producing species in *Aspergillus* section *Nigri*. *Stud. Mycol.* **2004**, *50*, 45–61.
97. Perrone, G.; Varga, J.; Susca, A.; Frisvad, J.C.; Stea, G.; Kocsube, S.; Tóth, B.; Kozakiewicz, Z.; Samson, R.A. *Aspergillus uvarum* sp. nov., an uniseriate black Aspergillus species isolated from grapes in Europe. *Int. J. Syst. Evol. Microbiol.* **2008**, *58*, 1032–1039.
98. Noonim, P.; Mahakarnchanakul, W.; Varga, J.; Frisvad, J.C.; Samson, R.A. Two novel species of *Aspergillus* section *Nigri* from Thai coffee beans. *Int. J. Syst. Evol. Microbiol.* **2008**, *58*, 1727–1734.
99. Noonim, P.; Mahakarnchanakul, W.; Nielsen, K.F.; Frisvad, J.C.; Samson, R.A. Isolation, identification and toxigenic potential of ochratoxin A-producing *Aspergillus* species from coffee beans grown in two regions of Thailand. *Int. J. Food Microbiol.* **2008**, *128*, 197–202.
100. Varga, J.; Kocsube, S.; Toth, B.; Frisvad, J.C.; Perrone, G.; Susca, A.; Meijer, M.; Samson, R.A. *Aspergillus brasiliensis* sp. nov., a biseriate black *Aspergillus* species with world-wide distribution. *Int. J. Syst. Evol. Microbiol.* **2007**, *57*, 1925–1932.
101. Serra, R.; Cabanes, F.J.; Perrone, G.; Castella, G.; Venancio, A.; Mule, G.; Kozakiewicz, Z. *Aspergillus ibericus*: A new species of section *Nigri* isolated from grapes. *Mycologia* **2006**, *98*, 295–306.
102. Sørensen, A.; Lubeck, P.S.; Lubeck, M.; Nielsen, K.F.; Ahring, B.K.; Teller, P.J.; Frisvad, J.C. *Aspergillus saccharolyticus* sp. nov., a black *Aspergillus* species isolated in Denmark. *Int. J. Syst. Evol. Microbiol.* **2011**, *61*, 3077–3083.

103. Kim, S.; Lee, C.; Kim, M.; Yeo, Y.; Yoon, S.; Kang, H.; Koo, B. Screening and characterization of an enzyme with beta-glucosidase activity from environmental DNA. *J. Microbiol. Biotechnol.* **2007**, *17*, 905–912.

104. Jiang, C.; Ma, G.; Li, S.; Hu, T.; Che, Z.; Shen, P.; Yan, B.; Wu, B. Characterization of a novel beta-glucosidase-like activity from a soil metagenome. *J. Microbiol.* **2009**, *47*, 542–548.

105. Jiang, C.; Hao, Z.; Jin, K.; Li, S.; Che, Z.; Ma, G.; Wu, B. Identification of a metagenome-derived beta-glucosidase from bioreactor contents. *J. Mol. Catal. B-Enzym.* **2010**, *63*, 11–16.

106. Sternberg, D.; Vijayakumar, P.; Reese, E.T. Beta-glucosidase—microbial-production and effect on enzymatic-hydrolysis of cellulose. *Can. J. Microbiol.* **1977**, *23*, 139–147.

107. Sørensen, A.; Lübeck, P.S.; Lübeck, M.; Teller, P.J.; Ahring, B.K. Beta-Glucosidases from a new *Aspergillus* species can substitute commercial beta-glucosidases for saccharification of lignocellulosic biomass. *Can. J. Microbiol.* **2011**, *57*, 638–650.

108. Montenecourt, B.S.; Eveleigh, D.E. Selective screening methods for the isolation of high yielding cellulase mutants of *Trichoderma reesei*. In *Hydrolysis of Cellulose: Mechanisms of Enzymic and Acid Catalysis*; Brown, R.D., Jurasek, L., Eds.; American Chemical Society: Washington, DC, USA, 1979; pp. 289–301.

109. Chirumamilla, R.R.; Muralidhar, R.; Marchant, R.; Nigam, P. Improving the quality of industrially important enzymes by directed evolution. *Mol. Cell. Biochem.* **2001**, *224*, 159–168.

110. Cherry, J.R.; Fidantsef, A.L. Directed evolution of industrial enzymes: An update. *Curr. Opin. Biotechnol.* **2003**, *14*, 438–443.

111. Tobin, M.B.; Gustafsson, C.; Huisman, G.W. Directed evolution: The "rational" basis for "irrational" design. *Curr. Opin. Struct. Biol.* **2000**, *10*, 421–427.

112. Antikainen, N.M.; Martin, S.F. Altering protein specificity: Techniques and applications. *Bioorg. Med. Chem.* **2005**, *13*, 2701–2716.

113. Gonzalez-Blasco, G.; Sanz-Aparicio, J.; Gonzalez, B.; Hermoso, J.A.; Polaina, J. Directed evolution of beta-glucosidase A from *Paenibacillus polymyxa* to thermal resistance. *J. Biol. Chem.* **2000**, *275*, 13708–13712.

114. Arrizubieta, M.J.; Polaina, J. Increased thermal resistance and modification of the catalytic properties of a beta-glucosidase by random mutagenesis and *in vitro* recombination. *J. Biol. Chem.* **2000**, *275*, 28843–28848.

115. Lebbink, J.H.G.; Kaper, T.; Bron, P.; van der Oost, J.; de Vos, W.M. Improving low-temperature catalysis in the hyperthermostable *Pyrococcus furiosus* beta-glucosidase CelB by directed evolution. *Biochemistry (N Y)* **2000**, *39*, 3656–3665.

116. Pei, X.; Yi, Z.; Tang, C.; Wu, Z. Three amino acid changes contribute markedly to the thermostability of beta-glucosidase BglC from *Thermobifida fusca*. *Bioresour. Technol.* **2011**, *102*, 3337–3342.

117. Steiner, K.; Schwab, H. Recent Advances in rational approaches for enzyme engineering. *Comput. Struct. Biotechnol. J.* **2012**, *2*, doi:10.5936/csbj.201209010.

118. Lee, H.; Chang, C.; Jeng, W.; Wang, A.H.-J.; Liang, P. Mutations in the substrate entrance region of beta-glucosidase from *Trichoderma reesei* improve enzyme activity and thermostability. *Protein Eng. Des. Sel.* **2012**, *25*, 733–740.

Arming Technology in Yeast—Novel Strategy for Whole-Cell Biocatalyst and Protein Engineering

Kouichi Kuroda and Mitsuyoshi Ueda

Abstract: Cell surface display of proteins/peptides, in contrast to the conventional intracellular expression, has many attractive features. This arming technology is especially effective when yeasts are used as a host, because eukaryotic modifications that are often required for functional use can be added to the surface-displayed proteins/peptides. A part of various cell wall or plasma membrane proteins can be genetically fused to the proteins/peptides of interest to be displayed. This technology, leading to the generation of so-called "arming technology", can be employed for basic and applied research purposes. In this article, we describe various strategies for the construction of arming yeasts, and outline the diverse applications of this technology to industrial processes such as biofuel and chemical productions, pollutant removal, and health-related processes, including oral vaccines. In addition, arming technology is suitable for protein engineering and directed evolution through high-throughput screening that is made possible by the feature that proteins/peptides displayed on cell surface can be directly analyzed using intact cells without concentration and purification. Actually, novel proteins/peptides with improved or developed functions have been created, and development of diagnostic/therapeutic antibodies are likely to benefit from this powerful approach.

Reprinted from *Biomolecules*. Cite as: Kuroda, K.; Ueda, M. Arming Technology in Yeast—Novel Strategy for Whole-cell Biocatalyst and Protein Engineering. *Biomolecules* **2013**, *3*, 632-650.

1. Introduction

Arming technology in yeast using the cell surface display system is an innovative technology for the construction of whole-cell biocatalysts and protein engineering through high-throughput screening of protein libraries. Although intracellular expression and extracellular secretion have been employed in conventional strategies for molecular breeding, the cell surface (including the cell wall and plasma membrane) is an attractive location for heterologous gene expression. Proteins localized at the cell surface play an important role in signal transduction, recognition and transport of environmental substances, morphology formation, and various other reactions. In arming technology, functional heterologous proteins/peptides are genetically immobilized on the cell surface by fusion with the domain for cell wall- or plasma membrane-anchoring domains. Cell surface-engineered yeasts constructed using the arming technology, have been termed "arming yeasts" [1–3]. Arming technology has advantages that are not found in conventional intracellular expression and extracellular secretion approaches. Immobilization on the cell surface itself retains the features of immobilized enzymes, and increases the thermal stability of the displayed proteins/peptides [4,5]. Preparation of protein/peptide-displaying cells can be achieved only by cell cultivation, in which the two processes of production of proteins/peptides and immobilization on cell surface are simultaneously undertaken, leading to cost effectiveness. Furthermore, the displayed proteins/peptides can interact with environmental substances with high molecular mass that cannot be imported into a cell. Surface-engineered cells prepared by cell cultivation are ready to use as microparticles covered by proteins/peptides, whereas troublesome protein purification and concentration procedures are required for the analysis and subsequent application of proteins produced by intracellular expression and extracellular secretion. Therefore, arming technology is also suitable for high-throughput screening of proteins/peptides from the mutant library at the single-cell level, and amino acid sequences of the screened proteins/peptides can be easily determined by DNA sequencing of the introduced plasmid [6–10]. Therefore, arming technology has been applied to wide range of targets such as whole-cell biocatalysts, bioremediation, biosensors, live vaccines, high-throughput screening of ligand peptides for receptors, and protein engineering [2,3,11–14].

The cell surface display system has also been established in gram-negative bacteria, gram-positive bacteria, and phages [11,15–18]. So far, many proteins/peptides have been successfully displayed with maintenance of their functions. In contrast to bacteria and phages, yeasts are equipped with the quality control and modification systems of eukaryotic secretory pathways. Therefore, in the case of target proteins that have a high molecular mass or require glycosylation modification, yeasts are suitable hosts for cell surface display. In addition, simultaneous display of multiple kinds of proteins/peptides on the same cell surface can be performed in yeasts by using different auxotrophic markers, leading to the enhanced potential of surface-engineered yeasts. Recently, the cell surface display system has also been developed in *Aspergillus oryzae* as a eukaryote except yeasts [19,20]. Here, we review the advances of molecular breeding of novel cells and protein engineering by arming technology in yeasts such as *Saccharomyces cerevisiae*, *Pichia pastoris*, and *Yarrowia lipolytica*.

2. Cell Surface Display System in Yeast

Among yeasts, arming technology was first developed in *S. cerevisiae*. Subsequently, based on the success of this approach using full length or cell wall-anchoring domains of cell wall proteins from *S. cerevisiae*, similar display systems have been transferred into other yeasts, including *P. pastoris* and *Y. lipolytica*. The cell surface display systems (Figure 1) are classified into two systems. One is the *N*-terminus free display in which target proteins/peptides are produced as fusions with the secretion signal sequence at the *N*-terminus and the cell wall-anchoring domain at the *C*-terminus. The other is the *C*-terminus free display, in which secretion signal sequence, cell wall-anchoring domain, and target proteins/peptides are fused in this order. The effect of the orientation on the display efficiency and on the functional properties depends on the kinds of target proteins/peptides to be displayed. Therefore, the fusion order itself, namely whether the *N*- or *C*-terminus of target proteins/peptides is fused with cell wall-anchoring domain, is important. In addition, the length of spacer peptides between target proteins/peptides and the cell wall-anchoring domain is also important. By optimizing the spacer length, there are cases in which the function of displayed proteins/peptides has been improved [21,22].

Figure 1. Cell surface display system in *S. cerevisiae* (**a**) α-agglutinin-based display system; (**b**) **a**-agglutinin-based display system; (**c**) Flo1p-based display system; (**d**) Membrane display system by anchoring domain of Yps1p.

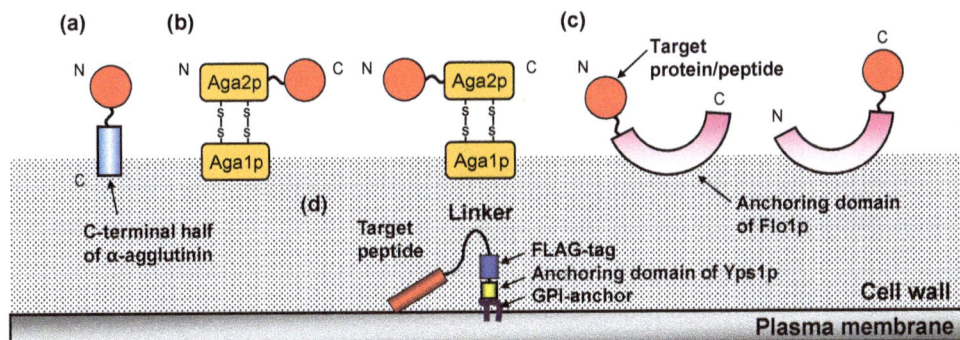

2.1. Cell Surface Display System in S. cerevisiae

S. cerevisiae has the "generally regarded as safe" (GRAS) approval of the Food and Drug Administration, and thus is suitable for industrial use. Among the cell wall proteins that are linked to the glucan layer by a covalent bond in yeast, α-agglutinin and **a**-agglutinin are representatives of cell wall-anchoring proteins used for cell surface display of target proteins/peptides. These proteins are involved in sexual adhesion of mating type α and **a** cells, and have characteristics specific to cell wall proteins. Specifically, they possess an *N*-terminal secretion signal sequence for transportation to the cell surface and *C*-terminal glycosylphosphatidylinositol (GPI) anchor attachment signal sequence for transient anchoring in the plasma membrane [23]. GPI-anchored proteins in the plasma membrane are released via cleavage by phosphatidylinositol-specific phospholipase C (PI-PLC), and then bind to the cell wall with a covalent bond by cell wall-anchoring domain. For the *N*-terminus free display system, α-agglutinin is the most frequently used approach (Figure 1a). Many proteins/peptides, including those with relatively large molecular masses and glycosylation requirements, have been successfully displayed on the yeast cell surface using the cell wall-anchoring domain of α-agglutinin [3,13,14,24]. In the α-agglutinin-based display system, target proteins/peptides are fused to the secretion signal sequence at the *N*-terminus and to the cell wall-anchoring domain (including the GPI anchor attachment signal sequence) at the *C*-terminus. In addition, Flo1p, which is a GPI-anchored cell wall protein involved in flocculation, is available for the *N*-terminal free display in a similar manner (Figure 1c) [25]. Other GPI-anchored cell wall proteins (Cwp1p, Cwp2p, Tip1p, Sed1p, YCR89w, and Tir1p) have the potential as cell wall-anchoring domains, although they are less frequently used because of the past successful performance of α- and **a**-agglutinin-based display system [26].

On the other hand, **a**-agglutinin has been used in the *C*-terminus free display system (Figure 1b). **a**-Agglutinin consists of Aga1p and Aga2p subunits [7]. The secreted Aga2p subunit is linked to the Aga1p subunit via two disulfide bonds, which are incorporated in the cell wall. Therefore, in the **a**-agglutinin-based display system, target proteins/peptides are fused with the *C*-terminus of Aga2p. In addition, this system has also been used in the *N*-terminal free display by fusing target proteins/peptides with the *N*-terminus of Aga2p [27]. Flo1p is also available for the *C*-terminus free display, in which truncated Flo1p without GPI anchor attachment signal sequence is used as an adhesive region (Figure 1c) [28]. Pir proteins (Pir1–4p) have been used as anchoring proteins in the *C*-terminus free display, and this permits extraction of displayed proteins/peptides from the cell wall by alkali treatment [29].

Several strategies have been employed to improve the efficiency of cell surface display in *S. cerevisiae*. Vector engineering by high copy number plasmid and the improvement of host strain enhanced the efficiency in the α-agglutinin-based display system [30]. Additionally, screening from a cDNA library identified five genes whose overexpression improved the efficiency of the **a**-agglutinin-based display system [31].

2.2. Cell Surface Display System in P. pastoris

The methylotrophic strain *P. pastoris* can grow on an economical carbon source and allows high-density culture. Therefore, it is also a suitable host for use in large-scale fermentation cultures of surface-engineered cells. In *P. pastoris*, both the *N*- and *C*-terminus-free display systems have been established using cell wall proteins (α-agglutinin, **a**-agglutinin, Flo1p, Pir1p, Sed1p, and Tip1p) from *S. cerevisiae* in the same strategy as outlined above [32–34].

2.3. Cell Surface Display System in Y. lipolytica

The oleaginous yeast *Y. lipolytica* is a heterothallic and dimorphic yeast, and has the high potential for secreting heterologous proteins, which is a preferred feature in industrial uses. Several cell wall proteins in *Y. lipolytica* have been identified. YlCWP1 and YlPIR1 from *Y. lipolytica*, which are GPI-anchored cell wall proteins, allow *N*-terminus free display and *C*-terminus free display, respectively [35].

2.4. Membrane Display System in S. cerevisiae

Almost all displayed proteins/peptides in yeasts are localized to the cell wall as described above. However, the display of proteins/peptides on the plasma membrane is desirable when there is a requirement for interaction with membrane proteins such as receptors. Membrane display of proteins/peptides is performed using the anchoring domain of Yps1p, a GPI-anchored plasma membrane protein. The fusion of this domain with the *C*-terminus of the peptide ligand allows the display on the plasma membrane and activation of either endogenous or heterologous G protein-coupled receptors (GPCRs) in *S. cerevisiae* [36,37].

3. Whole-Cell Biocatalyst by Arming Technology

3.1. Biofuel Production

Development of whole-cell biocatalysts to produce biofuel from biomass such as grain or cellulosic biomass has attracted attention as a means of creating a sustainable society based on biomass resources. Especially, consolidated bioprocessing (CBP) of lignocellulose to ethanol is an ideal system combining all processes such as enzyme production, hydrolytic degradation, and fermentation of sugar [38]. The arming technology has been applied to yeasts for the construction of whole-cell biocatalysts that can perform saccharification and fermentation. Starch and cellulose are major components in grain and cellulosic biomass, respectively. Therefore, the cell surface display of enzymes for hydrolytic degradation of these components was attempted in order to achieve CBP (Figure 2). As a starch-degrading enzyme, an exotype glucoamylase from *Rhizopus oryzae* was displayed on *S. cerevisiae* using the α-agglutinin-based display system, which allowed the direct production of ethanol from starch through the saccharification of starch on the cell surface and the subsequent fermentation of released glucose [39]. In addition to glucoamylase, an endotype α-amylase from *Bacillus stearothermophilus* was co-displayed with glucoamylase, leading to an improved production efficiency of ethanol from starch [40]. In the same way, α-amylase from *Streptococcus bovis* was also displayed using the Flo1p-based display system on glucoamylase-displaying yeast constructed by the α-agglutinin-based display system [41]. The arming yeasts described above show improved ethanol production and faster growth in the medium including starch as the sole carbon source.

Figure 2. Whole-cell biocatalyst constructed by arming technology and their applications.

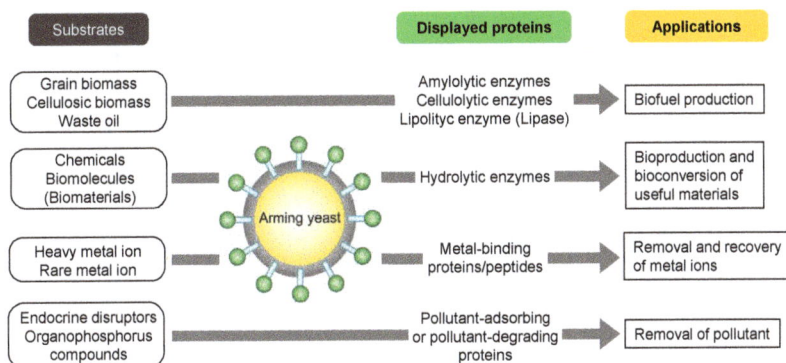

For degradation of cellulose, various enzymes including endoglucanases (EGs), cellobiohydrolases (CBHs), and β-glucosidases (BGLs) are necessary. Therefore, the potential of co-display on the same cell surface is an important feature in yeast, which is suitable for the reaction by multiple enzymes. Actually, the co-display of carboxymethylcellulase (CMCase) and BGL1 from *Aspergillus aculeatus* on *S. cerevisiae* enabled assimilation of cellobiose or oligosaccharide and growth in medium containing these materials as the sole carbon source [42]. EG acts randomly against the amorphous region of the cellulose chain to produce reducing and nonreducing ends, and CBH releases cellobiose from both ends. Therefore, efficient degradation of cellulose to cellobiose and cellooligosaccharides is achieved by the endo-exo synergism of EG and CBH. Finally, BGL hydrolyzes the generated cello-oligosaccharides to glucose. The arming yeast constructed by co-display of endoglucanase II (EG II) and cellobiohydrolase II (CBH II) from *Trichoderma reesei* and BGL1 from *A. aculeatus* can produce ethanol directly from phosphoric-acid-swollen cellulose due to the combined activities of these three cell surface enzymes [43]. In sake yeast, ethanol production from β-glucan can be achieved by cell surface display of EG and BGL from *A. oryzae* [44]. Furthermore, in arming yeast co-displaying EG II, CBH II, and BGL1, four non-conserved amino acids in the carbohydrate-binding module (CBM) of EG II were comprehensively mutated. In the case of co-displaying multiple kinds of enzymes on the same cell surface, the control or design of the display ratio of enzymes is a next challenge in arming technology. Recently, some approaches to this challenge were performed for optimized synergistic effects of displayed enzymes [45,46]. The optimal combination of yeasts displaying EG II with mutated CBMs was determined by inoculating a yeast library into selection liquid medium that included newspaper as the sole carbon source. The selected yeast mixture showed the improved ethanol production from newspaper, suggesting that this strategy is useful for the selection of the optimal combination of CBMs for each type of biomass [47].

The cellulosome, which is a multi-enzyme complex composed of scaffolding proteins and various cellulosomal enzymes, is produced by some clostridia and plays an important role in efficient degradation of polysaccharides in the plant cell wall. The complex is constructed through the interaction between a cohesin module in the scaffolding protein and a dockerin module in cellulosomal enzymes. Recently, reconstruction of mini-cellulosome on the yeast cell surface has been attempted. The engineered scaffolding protein consisting of three cohesin domains derived from *Clostridium thermocellum*, *Clostridium cellulolyticum*, and *Ruminococcus flavefaciens* was displayed on the *S. cerevisiae* cell surface using the a-agglutinin-based display system. The incubation of the scaffolding protein-displaying yeast with three recombinant cellulases (EG, CBH, and BGL) fused with a dockerin domain produced by *Escherichia coli* led to the synergistic hydrolytic degradation of cellulose [48]. Furthermore, a yeast consortium system has been developed, in which four kinds of engineered yeasts are co-cultivated [49]. In this system, construction of the mini-cellulosome was achieved by co-cultivation of a yeast displaying scaffolding protein and yeasts secreting three kinds of dockerin-fused enzymes.

Hemicellulose, including xylan, is also a major component of cellulosic biomass, Furthermore, ethanol production from hemicellulose is important for full utilization of cellulosic biomass. Xylan is hydrolyzed to xylo-oligosaccharides by endo-β-xylanase, and the produced xylo-oligosaccharides are hydrolyzed to D-xylose by β-xylosidase. *S. cerevisiae* co-displaying xylanase II (XYN II) from *T. reesei* and β-xylosidase (XylA) from *A. oryzae* was constructed using the α-agglutinin-based display system, and shown to hydrolyze xylan to xylose [50]. In a further development for ethanol production from xylan, xylose reductase (XR) and xylitol dehydrogenase (XDH) from *Pichia stipitis* and xylulokinase (XK) from *S. cerevisiae* were produced in the XYN II- and XylA-co-displaying yeast. The arming yeast catalyzes simultaneous saccharification and fermentation of xylan [50,51]. In addition to the two-step isomerization of xylose into xylulose, xylose isomerase (XI) is an alternative enzyme that shows great promise, as it is not associated with a cofactor imbalance. Recently, XI from *Clostridium cellulovorans* was successfully displayed and retained activity on *S. cerevisiae*. The constructed XI-displaying yeast could grow in medium containing xylose as the sole carbon source and directly produce ethanol from xylose [52].

Lignin is also a major component of cellulosic biomass, and inhibits cellulose degradation by cellulases, because of its physiological recalcitrancy and its masking the cellulose fibers. Therefore, the removal of lignin from cellulosic biomass is required for efficient degradation. Laccase from white-rot fungus, which participates in several biological pathways including lignin degradation, was displayed on *S. cerevisiae* via the α-agglutinin-based display system. By pretreatment of hydrothermally processed rice straw with laccase-displaying yeast, ethanol production by yeast co-displaying EG II, CBH II, and BGL1 was improved [53].

3.2. Bioproduction of Chemicals

Lipase is one of the most applied enzymes in cell surface display on yeast because lipases are used in wide range of industries and the display of lipase is an attractive approach for creating a whole-cell biocatalyst (Figure 2). *R. oryzae* lipase (ROL) and *Candida antarctica* lipase B (CALB) have been extensively studied and are one of the most widely used lipases. ROL was displayed on *S. cerevisiae* by the α-agglutinin-based display system, and the activity of displayed ROL was improved by inserting a spacer peptide with a Gly/Ser repeat between ROL and the cell wall-anchoring domain of α-agglutinin [21,22]. ROL displayed on *S. cerevisiae* showed higher activity than commercially available free and immobilized lipases in organic solvents because the displayed lipase is stabilized by the cell wall [54]. ROL-displaying *S. cerevisiae*, constructed by the Flo1p-based display system, could synthesize methylesters from triglyceride and methanol [28]. In addition, yeast displaying ROL could be used for the optical resolution of (*R,S*)-1-benzyloxy-3-chloro-2-propyl monosuccinate [55]. CALB has also been displayed on *S. cerevisiae* in several studies. Mutated CALB displayed on yeast using the α-agglutinin-based display system has higher thermal stability [56]. Furthermore, CALB-displaying yeasts constructed using the α-agglutinin- or Flo1p-display systems have been used for several ester syntheses with reduced amount of by-products [57–60]. With regard to lipases, several cell surface display strategies have been attempted in yeasts other than *S. cerevisiae*. In *P. pastoris*, CALB was displayed on the cell surface using the *S. cerevisiae* α-agglutinin-based display system. Compared to CALB-displaying *S. cerevisiae*, the engineered *P. pastoris* showed higher activity, and the ability to synthesize ethyl hexanoate was enhanced [61]. CALB was also displayed on *P. pastoris* via the Sed1p-based display system, and exhibited improved thermal stability [4]. ROL, *Y. lipolytica* lipases, and *Pseudomonas fluorescens* lipase were displayed on *P. pastoris* using the Flo1p-based display system [32,62,63]. Furthermore, *Y. lipolytica* lipase was displayed on *Y. lipolytica* by using the Flo1p-based display system [35].

Isoflavone aglycones, which are bioactive and easily adsorbed by human cells, are hydrolysates of isoflavone glycosides by β-glucosidase. Three kinds of β-glucosidases were independently displayed on *S. cerevisiae* using the α-agglutinin-based display system. Among them, BGL1-displaying yeast could convert isoflavone glycosides into isoflavone aglycones most efficiently [64]. Carnosine and chitosan oligosaccharides also show bioactivities such as antioxidant, antiglycation, cytoplasmic buffering, antitumor, and anticancer properties. The synthesis of carnosine from β-alanine and histidine was achieved through a reverse reaction catalyzed by human carnosinase (CN1)-displaying *S. cerevisiae* in organic solvents and ionic liquids [65]. Cell surface display of chitosanase from *Paenibacillus fukuinensis* enabled the production of chitosan oligosaccharides from chitosan [66]. In *Y. lipolytica*, alginate lyase from *Vibrio* sp. was displayed by fusion with the cell wall-anchoring domain of YlCWP1. The *Y. lipolytica* displaying alginate lyase could hydrolyze poly-β-D-mannuronate, poly-α-L-guluronate, and sodium alginate to produce oligosaccharides [67].

3.3. Bioadsorption

Arming technology has been applied to bioadsorption of toxic metal ions and rare-metal ions, leading to bioremediation and resource recovery (Figure 2) [12,13]. The cell surface display of metal-binding proteins/peptides enables the enhanced adsorption and recovery of metal ions on the cell surface. Cell surface adsorption has advantages that are lacking in intracellular accumulation; (i) no requirement for cell disruption for recovery of the adsorbed metal ions; (ii) repeated use of arming yeasts for the further adsorption of metal ions; (iii) rapid and selective adsorption of target metal ions. For the construction of bioadsorbents for bioremediation, toxic metal-binding proteins/peptides such as hexa-His, NP peptides (harboring the CXXEE metal fixation motif of the bacterial Pb^{2+}-transporting P1-type ATPases), and metallothionein were displayed on *S. cerevisiae* using the α-agglutinin-based display system [68–71]. The bioadsorbents constructed by arming technology showed enhanced adsorption of heavy metal ions. Furthermore, cell surface adsorption of metal ions improved cellular tolerance to heavy metal ions [69,71].

Bioadsorption to the cell surface has also been used for adsorption and recovery of rare metal ions. Some of these ions are essential trace metals that play an important role in living cells. For the specific binding and recovery of target metal ions, metal-responsive transcription factors that can bind and dissociate metal ions are displayed and repurposed as cell surface metal-binding proteins. Uptake of molybdenum, one of the rare metals, is regulated by transcription factor ModE that binds molybdate and controls the expression of downstream operon in *E. coli* [72]. Therefore, the full length or *C*-terminal domain of ModE from *E. coli* has been displayed on *S. cerevisiae* via the α-agglutinin-based display system. Molybdate adsorption was achieved using yeast displaying the *C*-terminal domain of ModE, and more than 50% of the molybdate adsorbed on the cell surface could be recovered by papain treatment [73]. Furthermore, a single amino acid mutation (T163Y) of the metal-binding pocket of ModE was efficient to convert it to a selective binder of tungstate, in contrast to the wild-type protein, which binds both tungstate and molybdate. Arming yeast displaying this mutant ModE was shown to selectively uptake tungstate [74].

3.4. Bioremediation

To remove or degrade environmental pollutants other than heavy metal ions, arming yeasts for bioremediation have been constructed (Figure 2). For example, to antagonize endocrine disruptors, which are environmental pollutants that perturb natural endocrine function, the ligand-binding domain of the rat estrogen receptor (ERLBD) has been displayed on *S. cerevisiae* using the α-agglutinin-based display system. The ERLBD-displaying yeast was able to bind estrogen-like compounds with an affinity comparable to the native receptor, suggesting the possible application in screening, adsorption, and removal of endocrine disruptor-like chemicals from the environment [75].

Organophosphorus compounds (OPs) are one of the most widely used pesticides, but discharge to the environment is a problem to be solved due to significant threat to public health. Therefore, to degrade OPs using a cell-based system, organophosphorus hydrolase (OPH) from *Flavobacterium* spp. was displayed on *S. cerevisiae* using the α-agglutinin- and Flo1p-based display systems. OPH-displaying yeasts showed hydrolase activity against paraoxon; the activity in the Flo1p-based display system was higher than that in the α-agglutinin-based display system because the active center is located near the *C*-terminal of OPH [76,77]. Furthermore, the development of a biosensor for the sensitive and rapid detection of OPs was achieved by detecting the protons generated by OPs hydrolysis. In this system, additional display of EGFP was performed in OPH-displaying yeast to evaluate the proton generation by the change in fluorescence intensity of EGFP. Together with OPH-dependent hydrolysis, the fluorescence intensity of EGFP was decreased [78]. In another system for OP sensing, the concentration of *p*-nitrophenol produced by OP hydrolysis in OPH-displaying yeast was examined [79].

3.5. Other Applications

Other applications of arming technology include biosensors, oral vaccines, antibodies, and stress tolerance. For the non-invasive sensing of environmental changes or monitoring of heterologous protein production, the cell surface display of fluorescent proteins on *S. cerevisiae* was used as a reporter system. The strategy for biosensor construction is that different fluorescent protein variants under the control of different promoters are displayed on the cell surface. GFP display has been placed under the control of the *GAPDH* promoter that is induced in the presence of glucose, whereas BFP was displayed under the control of the *UPR-ICL* promoter from *Candida tropicalis*, which is activated upon the exhaustion of glucose. Therefore, the concentration of intra- or extracellular glucose could be estimated by measuring the fluorescence intensities of GFP and BFP [80]. In addition, monitoring of intra- and extracellular concentrations of phosphate and ammonium ions has been performed by arming yeasts in which the *PHO5* and *MEP2* promoters regulate the genes for cell surface display of ECFP and EYFP, respectively [81]. By using the same *GAL1* promoter for the production of heterologous proteins and cell surface display of EGFP, protein production could be monitored by measuring the fluorescence intensity of EGFP [82].

Construction of an oral vaccine was attempted by displaying antigen on the cell surface of *S. cerevisiae*. 380R antigen from the red sea bream iridovirus (RSIV) was displayed for oral vaccination of cultured marine fish using the α-agglutinin-based display system [83]. In *P. pastoris*, hemagglutinin protein from a highly pathogenic avian influenza (HPAI), subtype H5N1, was displayed with the α-agglutinin-based display system. Oral vaccination of chickens with the hemagglutinin-displaying *P. pastoris* caused the production of virus neutralizing antibodies in the serum [84]. For diagnostics and therapeutics, antibodies and related molecules are attractive targets to be displayed. As a feature of cell surface display system in yeast, produced proteins undergo post-translational modification and efficient disulfide isomerization in a manner that is mechanistically similar to that in mammalian cells. Therefore, hetero-oligomeric proteins such as Fab fragments of catalytic antibodies have been successfully displayed on *S. cerevisiae*, in which the light chain (Lc fragment) of a Fab fragment was displayed on cell surface and the heavy chain (Fd fragment) of a Fab fragment was produced by secretion. As one example, the arming yeast displaying the Fab fragment of hydrolytic antibody 6D9 could catalyze the hydrolysis of a chloramphenicol monoester derivative and showed high stability in binding with a transition-state analog (TSA) [85,86]. In a similar strategy, an engineered Fab fragment, in which mutations were introduced into the Lc fragment to form a catalytic triad, was displayed on *S. cerevisiae*, leading to a higher catalytic activity compared to the wild type Fab fragment [87]. The ZZ domain of protein A from *Staphylococcus aureus* is a repeat of the Z domain that binds to the Fc fragment of human or rabbit IgG. Arming yeast displaying the ZZ domain could be applied to the detection of IgG by enzyme-linked immunosorbent assay (ELISA) and repeated affinity purification of IgG from serum [88].

Arming technology has been also used in molecular breeding of stress-tolerant *S. cerevisiae*. The yeast cell surface was modified by displaying combinatorial random peptides, and acid-tolerant yeast from a yeast library displaying random peptides was successfully selected by culture in acidic conditions. As a result, Scr35 peptide (25 a.a.) was found to enhance the acid tolerance of yeast when displayed on the cell surface [89]. In addition, a combinatorial random protein library was constructed from cDNA of *S. cerevisiae*, and this library was displayed on the yeast cell surface. From the yeast library, nonane-tolerant yeast has been obtained by screening on nonane-overlaid culture medium [90,91]. Cell surface display of leucine-rich peptides has also allowed the creation of yeasts with increased resistance to salt, ethanol, and acetonitrile [92].

4. Protein Engineering and Directed Evolution by Arming Technology

4.1. Engineering of Enzymes

The advantages of arming technology, including direct analysis of target proteins/peptides using intact cells without concentration and purification, are suitable for high-throughput screening of protein/peptide libraries containing random or comprehensive mutations. Therefore, protein engineering has been performed by display of randomly and/or comprehensively mutated proteins/peptides and subsequent high-throughput screening (Figure 3). A combinatorial library of the lid domain of ROL was displayed on the *S. cerevisiae* cell surface. Using a halo assay on soybean oil-containing plates and a assay using fluorescent substrates, lipase mutants with a high substrate specificity toward short-chain substrates and a unique oxyanion hole have been identified from the library [93]. Neurolysin is a metalloendopeptidase that cleaves the bioactive peptide neurotensin. A mutant library of neurolysin constructed by semirational mutagenesis was displayed, and screening was performed using two fluorescence-quenching peptides, the matrix metalloproteinases-2/9- (MMPs-2/9) and MMP-3-specific substrates. As a result, the Y610L mutant of neurolysin was found to show the altered substrate specificity [94]. In addition, the protease inhibitory activity of matrix metalloproteinase-2/9 was improved by arming technology and an automatic single-cell pickup system [6]. Luciferase is also an interesting target for protein engineering, as it plays an important role in the pyrosequencing system of next-generation DNA sequencers. A mutant luciferase library was constructed by arming technology, and interesting mutant luciferases with improved specific activity and dATP discrimination were obtained through only three step-wise screenings [95]. The further technological innovation of the system for single cell analysis and isolation would lead to more efficient protein engineering and directed evolution by arming technology.

Figure 3. Creation of novel proteins/peptides with improved or developed function by arming technology.

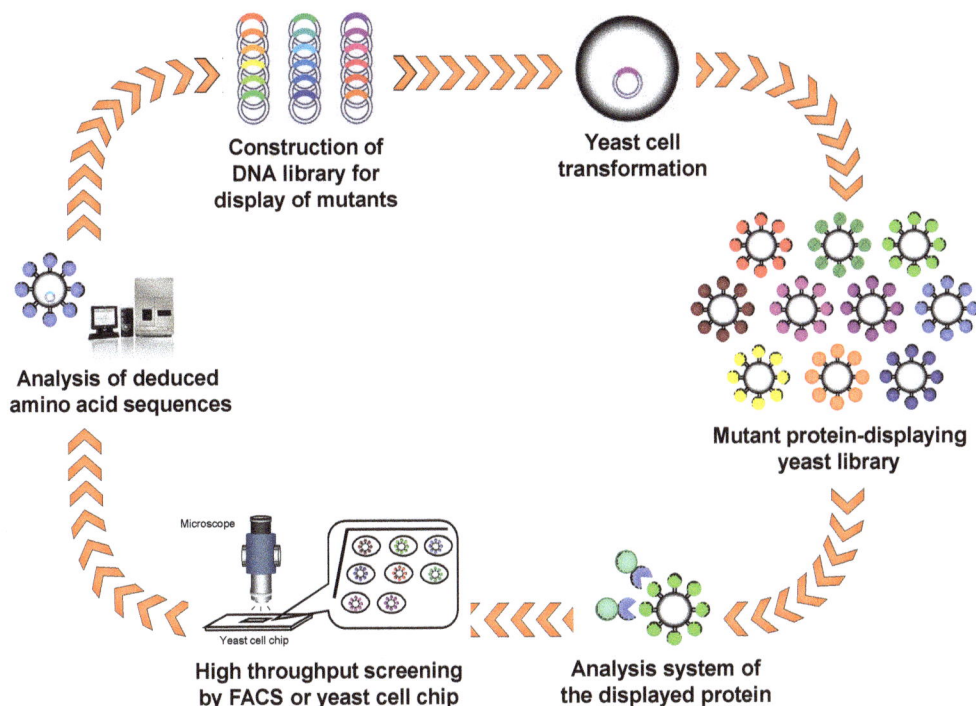

Construction of DNA library for display of mutants

Yeast cell transformation

Mutant protein-displaying yeast library

Analysis of deduced amino acid sequences

Microscope

Yeast cell chip

High throughput screening by FACS or yeast cell chip

Analysis system of the displayed protein

4.2. Antibody Engineering

Improvement of the affinity of antibodies for target biomolecules is an important and essential challenge in diagnostic and therapeutic development. Single-chain variable fragments (scFv) are those in which the light and heavy chains are linked by a flexible linker. A scFv library was displayed on *S. cerevisiae* by using the **a**-agglutinin-based display system, and the display efficiency was monitored using *N*-terminal or *C*-terminal epitope tags. scFv clones with improved properties could be efficiently isolated from the library through the incubation of scFv-displaying yeast library with fluorescently labeled antigen and the subsequent screening by fluorescently activated cell sorting (FACS) [7]. Furthermore, antibodies to botulinum neurotoxins, carcinoembryonic antigen, CD3 diphtheria toxin, lysozyme, and streptavidin have been improved or developed using the similar strategies based on arming technology [96–101]. Thus, arming technology is an attractive methodology for the isolation of antibodies with high affinity and other specific biological functions.

4.3. Ligand Screening for Activation of GPCRs

G protein-coupled receptors (GPCRs) are seven transmembrane-domain proteins with the ability to mediate rapid responses to extracellular signals, and they play an important role in many aspects of cellular physiology. Therefore, the design and identification of peptide-ligands for GPCRs are an attractive research area contributing to diagnostics. In the study of ligand-GPCR interactions and identification of ligands against orphan GPCRs, display of peptide ligands specifically on the plasma membrane is important, because ligands displayed only on the cell wall would be unable to access GPCRs on the plasma membrane. Hara *et al.* [36] have developed a display system of peptide-ligand on the yeast plasma membrane for activation of GPCR signaling. First, this system was applied to activation of Ste2 signaling in *S. cerevisiae*, where activation was detected using a Ste2-responsive *FUS1* promoter driving EGFP reporter expression. The α-factor displayed on the plasma membrane was shown to functionally activate the pheromone response pathway. Furthermore, this system has been applied to the activation of human GPCR signaling as well as the yeast pheromone response pathway using chimeric Gα protein. Somatostatin is a naturally occurring gastrointestinal hormone that regulates various endocrine and exocrine processes. After the construction of yeast producing human somatostatin receptor subtype-2 (SSTR2) and chimeric Gα protein, somatostatin was displayed on plasma membrane. The somatostatin displayed on the plasma membrane could activate human SSTR2 in *S. cerevisiae* [37]. This technological platform, namely "PepDisplay" is useful for identification of novel peptide-ligands for heterologously produced GPCRs by membrane display of peptides with random and/or comprehensive sequences and screening based on the activation of reporter genes.

5. Conclusions

Arming technology is well established and has been applied to a wide range of research areas, owing to the advantages that are absent in the conventional expression systems. In the construction of whole-cell biocatalysts, cell surface display of enzymes enables bioconversion of the substrate with high-molecular mass that can not enter in the cells, and multistep and synergistic reactions can be achieved on the cell surface by co-displaying multiple kinds of enzymes on the cell surface. Bioadsorption on the cell surface is advantageous in that it does not affect intracellular biological mechanisms, and the adsorbed materials such as metal ions can be easily concentrated and rapidly recovered. Furthermore, arming technology is an innovative molecular tool for protein engineering and directed evolution. The fact that proteins/peptides displayed on the cell surface can be directly, speedily, and conveniently analyzed using intact cells without concentration and purification is suitable for high-throughput screening of a protein/peptide library carrying random and/or comprehensive mutations. Therefore, arming technology is a powerful technology that will facilitate the development of a wide range of biotechnologies and contribute to the production of various kinds of materials for a sustainable society in the future.

Conflicts of Interest

The authors declare no conflict of interest.

References

1. Anonymous. Arming yeast with cell-surface catalysts. *Chem. Eng. News* **1997**, *75*, 32.
2. Ueda, M.; Tanaka, A. Genetic immobilization of proteins on the yeast cell surface. *Biotechnol. Adv.* **2000**, *18*, 121–140.
3. Ueda, M.; Tanaka, A. Cell surface engineering of yeast: Construction of arming yeast with biocatalyst. *J. Biosci. Bioeng.* **2000**, *90*, 125–136.
4. Su, G.D.; Zhang, X.; Lin, Y. Surface display of active lipase in *Pichia pastoris* using Sed1 as an anchor protein. *Biotechnol. Lett.* **2010**, *32*, 1131–1136.
5. Chen, Y.P.; Hwang, I.E.; Lin, C.J.; Wang, H.J.; Tseng, C.P. Enhancing the stability of xylanase from *Cellulomonas fimi* by cell-surface display on *Escherichia coli. J. Appl. Microbiol.* **2012**, *112*, 455–463.
6. Aoki, W.; Yoshino, Y.; Morisaka, H.; Tsunetomo, K.; Koyo, H.; Kamiya, S.; Kawata, N.; Kuroda, K.; Ueda, M. High-throughput screening of improved protease inhibitors using a yeast cell surface display system and a yeast cell chip. *J. Biosci. Bioeng.* **2011**, *111*, 16–18.
7. Boder, E.T.; Wittrup, K.D. Yeast surface display for screening combinatorial polypeptide libraries. *Nat. Biotechnol.* **1997**, *15*, 553–557.
8. Chen, W.; Georgiou, G. Cell-Surface display of heterologous proteins: From high-throughput screening to environmental applications. *Biotechnol. Bioeng.* **2002**, *79*, 496–503.
9. Fukuda, T.; Kato-Murai, M.; Kadonosono, T.; Sahara, H.; Hata, Y.; Suye, S.; Ueda, M. Enhancement of substrate recognition ability by combinatorial mutation of β-glucosidase displayed on the yeast cell surface. *Appl. Microbiol. Biotechnol.* **2007**, *76*, 1027–1033.
10. Yeung, Y.A.; Wittrup, K.D. Quantitative screening of yeast surface-displayed polypeptide libraries by magnetic bead capture. *Biotechnol. Prog.* **2002**, *18*, 212–220.
11. Georgiou, G.; Poetschke, H.L.; Stathopoulos, C.; Francisco, J.A. Practical applications of engineering gram-negative bacterial cell surfaces. *Trends Biotechnol.* **1993**, *11*, 6–10.
12. Kuroda, K.; Ueda, M. Engineering of microorganisms towards recovery of rare metal ions. *Appl. Microbiol. Biotechnol.* **2010**, *87*, 53–60.
13. Kuroda, K.; Ueda, M. Molecular design of the microbial cell surface toward the recovery of metal ions. *Curr. Opin. Biotechnol.* **2011**, *22*, 427–433.
14. Kuroda, K.; Ueda, M. Cell surface engineering of yeast for applications in white biotechnology. *Biotechnol. Lett.* **2011**, *33*, 1–9.
15. Samuelson, P.; Gunneriusson, E.; Nygren, P.A.; Ståhl, S. Display of proteins on bacteria. *J. Biotechnol.* **2002**, *96*, 129–154.
16. Ståhl, S.; Uhlén, M. Bacterial surface display: Trends and progress. *Trends Biotechnol.* **1997**, *15*, 185–192.
17. Smith, G.P. Filamentous fusion phage: Novel expression vectors that display cloned antigens on the virion surface. *Science* **1985**, *228*, 1315–1317.
18. Smith, G.P. Surface presentation of protein epitopes using bacteriophage expression systems. *Curr. Opin. Biotechnol.* **1991**, *2*, 668–673.

19. Tabuchi, S.; Ito, J.; Adachi, T.; Ishida, H.; Hata, Y.; Okazaki, F.; Tanaka, T.; Ogino, C.; Kondo, A. Display of both *N*- and *C*-terminal target fusion proteins on the *Aspergillus oryzae* cell surface using a chitin-binding module. *Appl. Microbiol. Biotechnol.* **2010**, *87*, 1783–1789.

20. Adachi, T.; Ito, J.; Kawata, K.; Kaya, M.; Ishida, H.; Sahara, H.; Hata, Y.; Ogino, C.; Fukuda, H.; Kondo, A. Construction of an *Aspergillus oryzae* cell-surface display system using a putative GPI-anchored protein. *Appl. Microbiol. Biotechnol.* **2008**, *81*, 711–719.

21. Breinig, F.; Schmitt, M.J. Spacer-elongated cell wall fusion proteins improve cell surface expression in the yeast *Saccharomyces cerevisiae*. *Appl. Microbiol. Biotechnol.* **2002**, *58*, 637–644.

22. Washida, M.; Takahashi, S.; Ueda, M.; Tanaka, A. Spacer-mediated display of active lipase on the yeast cell surface. *Appl. Microbiol. Biotechnol.* **2001**, *56*, 681–686.

23. Lipke, P.N.; Kurjan, J. Sexual agglutination in budding yeasts: Structure, function, and regulation of adhesion glycoproteins. *Microbiol. Rev.* **1992**, *56*, 180–194.

24. Kuroda, K.; Ueda, M. Generation of arming yeasts with active proeins and peptides via cell surface display system—Cell surface engineering, bio-arming technology. *Methods Mol. Biol.* **2013**, in press.

25. Sato, N.; Matsumoto, T.; Ueda, M.; Tanaka, A.; Fukuda, H.; Kondo, A. Long anchor using Flo1 protein enhances reactivity of cell surface-displayed glucoamylase to polymer substrates. *Appl. Microbiol. Biotechnol.* **2002**, *60*, 469–474.

26. Van der Vaart, J.M.; te Biesebeke, R.; Chapman, J.W.; Toschka, H.Y.; Klis, F.M.; Verrips, C.T. Comparison of cell wall proteins of *Saccharomyces cerevisiae* as anchors for cell surface expression of heterologous proteins. *Appl. Environ. Microbiol.* **1997**, *63*, 615–620.

27. Wang, Z.; Mathias, A.; Stavrou, S.; Neville, D.M., Jr. A new yeast display vector permitting free scFv amino termini can augment ligand binding affinities. *Protein Eng. Des. Sel.* **2005**, *18*, 337–343.

28. Matsumoto, T.; Fukuda, H.; Ueda, M.; Tanaka, A.; Kondo, A. Construction of yeast strains with high cell surface lipase activity by using novel display systems based on the Flo1p flocculation functional domain. *Appl. Environ. Microbiol.* **2002**, *68*, 4517–4522.

29. Abe, H.; Ohba, M.; Shimma, Y.; Jigami, Y. Yeast cells harboring human α-1,3-fucosyltransferase at the cell surface engineered using Pir, a cell wall-anchored protein. *FEMS Yeast Res.* **2004**, *4*, 417–425.

30. Kuroda, K.; Matsui, K.; Higuchi, S.; Kotaka, A.; Sahara, H.; Hata, Y.; Ueda, M. Enhancement of display efficiency in yeast display system by vector engineering and gene disruption. *Appl. Microbiol. Biotechnol.* **2009**, *82*, 713–719.

31. Wentz, A.E.; Shusta, E.V. A novel high-throughput screen reveals yeast genes that increase secretion of heterologous proteins. *Appl. Environ. Microbiol.* **2007**, *73*, 1189–1198.

32. Tanino, T.; Fukuda, H.; Kondo, A. Construction of a *Pichia pastoris* cell-surface display system using Flo1p anchor system. *Biotechnol. Prog.* **2006**, *22*, 989–993.

33. Wang, Q.; Li, L.; Chen, M.; Qi, Q.; Wang, P.G. Construction of a novel system for cell surface display of heterologous proteins on *Pichia pastoris*. *Biotechnol. Lett.* **2007**, *29*, 1561–1566.

34. Wang, Q.; Li, L.; Chen, M.; Qi, Q.; Wang, P.G. Construction of a novel *Pichia pastoris* cell-surface display system based on the cell wall protein Pir1. *Curr. Microbiol.* **2008**, *56*, 352–357.

35. Yuzbasheva, E.Y.; Yuzbashev, T.V.; Laptev, I.A.; Konstantinova, T.K.; Sineoky, S.P. Efficient cell surface display of Lip2 lipase using C-domains of glycosylphosphatidylinositol-anchored cell wall proteins of *Yarrowia lipolytica*. *Appl. Microbiol. Biotechnol.* **2011**, *91*, 645–654.

36. Hara, K.; Ono, T.; Kuroda, K.; Ueda, M. Membrane-displayed peptide ligand activates the pheromone response pathway in *Saccharomyces cerevisiae*. *J. Biochem.* **2012**, *151*, 551–557.

37. Hara, K.; Shigemori, T.; Kuroda, K.; Ueda, M. Membrane-displayed somatostatin activates somatostatin receptor subtype-2 heterologously produced in *Saccharomyces cerevisiae*. *AMB Express* **2012**, *2*, e63.

38. Lynd, L.R.; van Zyl, W.H.; McBride, J.E.; Laser, M. Consolidated bioprocessing of cellulosic biomass: An update. *Curr. Opin. Biotechnol.* **2005**, *16*, 577–583.

39. Murai, T.; Ueda, M.; Yamamura, M.; Atomi, H.; Shibasaki, Y.; Kamasawa, N.; Osumi, M.; Amachi, T.; Tanaka, A. Construction of a starch-utilizing yeast by cell surface engineering. *Appl. Environ. Microbiol.* **1997**, *63*, 1362–1366.

40. Murai, T.; Ueda, M.; Shibasaki, Y.; Kamasawa, N.; Osumi, M.; Imanaka, T.; Tanaka, A. Development of an arming yeast strain for efficient utilization of starch by co-display of sequential amylolytic enzymes on the cell surface. *Appl. Microbiol. Biotechnol.* **1999**, *51*, 65–70.

41. Shigechi, H.; Koh, J.; Fujita, Y.; Matsumoto, T.; Bito, Y.; Ueda, M.; Satoh, E.; Fukuda, H.; Kondo, A. Direct production of ethanol from raw corn starch via fermentation by use of a novel surface-engineered yeast strain codisplaying glucoamylase and α-amylase. *Appl. Environ. Microbiol.* **2004**, *70*, 5037–5040.

42. Murai, T.; Ueda, M.; Kawaguchi, T.; Arai, M.; Tanaka, A. Assimilation of cellooligosaccharides by a cell surface-engineered yeast expressing β-glucosidase and carboxymethylcellulase from *Aspergillus aculeatus*. *Appl. Environ. Microbiol.* **1998**, *64*, 4857–4861.

43. Fujita, Y.; Ito, J.; Ueda, M.; Fukuda, H.; Kondo, A. Synergistic saccharification, and direct fermentation to ethanol, of amorphous cellulose by use of an engineered yeast strain codisplaying three types of cellulolytic enzyme. *Appl. Environ. Microbiol.* **2004**, *70*, 1207–1212.

44. Kotaka, A.; Bando, H.; Kaya, M.; Kato-Murai, M.; Kuroda, K.; Sahara, H.; Hata, Y.; Kondo, A.; Ueda, M. Direct ethanol production from barley β-glucan by sake yeast displaying *Aspergillus oryzae* β-glucosidase and endoglucanase. *J. Biosci. Bioeng.* **2008**, *105*, 622–627.

45. Ito, J.; Kosugi, A.; Tanaka, T.; Kuroda, K.; Shibasaki, S.; Ogino, C.; Ueda, M.; Fukuda, H.; Doi, R.H.; Kondo, A. Regulation of the display ratio of enzymes on the *Saccharomyces cerevisiae* cell surface by the immunoglobulin G and cellulosomal enzyme binding domains. *Appl. Environ. Microbiol.* **2009**, *75*, 4149–4154.

46. Yamada, R.; Taniguchi, N.; Tanaka, T.; Ogino, C.; Fukuda, H.; Kondo, A. Cocktail δ-integration: A novel method to construct cellulolytic enzyme expression ratio-optimized yeast strains. *Microb. Cell Fact.* **2010**, *9*, e32.

47. Nakanishi, A.; Bae, J.; Kuroda, K.; Ueda, M. Construction of a novel selection system for endoglucanases exhibiting carbohydrate-binding modules optimized for biomass using yeast cell-surface engineering. *AMB Express* **2012**, *2*, e56.

48. Tsai, S.L.; Oh, J.; Singh, S.; Chen, R.; Chen, W. Functional assembly of minicellulosomes on the *Saccharomyces cerevisiae* cell surface for cellulose hydrolysis and ethanol production. *Appl. Environ. Microbiol.* **2009**, *75*, 6087–6093.

49. Goyal, G.; Tsai, S.L.; Madan, B.; DaSilva, N.A.; Chen, W. Simultaneous cell growth and ethanol production from cellulose by an engineered yeast consortium displaying a functional mini-cellulosome. *Microb. Cell Fact.* **2011**, *10*, e89.

50. Katahira, S.; Fujita, Y.; Mizuike, A.; Fukuda, H.; Kondo, A. Construction of a xylan-fermenting yeast strain through codisplay of xylanolytic enzymes on the surface of xylose-utilizing *Saccharomyces cerevisiae* cells. *Appl. Environ. Microbiol.* **2004**, *70*, 5407–5414.

51. Katahira, S.; Mizuike, A.; Fukuda, H.; Kondo, A. Ethanol fermentation from lignocellulosic hydrolysate by a recombinant xylose- and cellooligosaccharide-assimilating yeast strain. *Appl. Microbiol. Biotechnol.* **2006**, *72*, 1136–1143.

52. Ota, M.; Sakuragi, H.; Morisaka, H.; Kuroda, K.; Miyake, H.; Tamaru, Y.; Ueda, M. Display of *Clostridium cellulovorans* xylose isomerase on the cell surface of *Saccharomyces cerevisiae* and its direct application to xylose fermentation. *Biotechnol. Prog.* **2013**, *29*, 346–351.

53. Nakanishi, A.; Bae, J.G.; Fukai, K.; Tokumoto, N.; Kuroda, K.; Ogawa, J.; Nakatani, M.; Shimizu, S.; Ueda, M. Effect of pretreatment of hydrothermally processed rice straw with laccase-displaying yeast on ethanol fermentation. *Appl. Microbiol. Biotechnol.* **2012**, *94*, 939–948.

54. Shiraga, S.; Kawakami, M.; Ishiguro, M.; Ueda, M. Enhanced reactivity of *Rhizopus oryzae* lipase displayed on yeast cell surfaces in organic solvents: Potential as a whole-cell biocatalyst in organic solvents. *Appl. Environ. Microbiol.* **2005**, *71*, 4335–4338.

55. Nakamura, Y.; Matsumoto, T.; Nomoto, F.; Ueda, M.; Fukuda, H.; Kondo, A. Enhancement of activity of lipase-displaying yeast cells and their application to optical resolution of (*R*,*S*)-1-benzyloxy-3-chloro-2-propyl monosuccinate. *Biotechnol. Prog.* **2006**, *22*, 998–1002.

56. Kato, M.; Fuchimoto, J.; Tanino, T.; Kondo, A.; Fukuda, H.; Ueda, M. Preparation of a whole-cell biocatalyst of mutated *Candida antarctica* lipase B (mCALB) by a yeast molecular display system and its practical properties. *Appl. Microbiol. Biotechnol.* **2007**, *75*, 549–555.

57. Inaba, C.; Maekawa, K.; Morisaka, H.; Kuroda, K.; Ueda, M. Efficient synthesis of enantiomeric ethyl lactate by *Candida antarctica* lipase B (CALB)-displaying yeasts. *Appl. Microbiol. Biotechnol.* **2009**, *83*, 859–864.

58. Tanino, T.; Aoki, T.; Chung, W.Y.; Watanabe, Y.; Ogino, C.; Fukuda, H.; Kondo, A. Improvement of a *Candida antarctica* lipase B-displaying yeast whole-cell biocatalyst and its application to the polyester synthesis reaction. *Appl. Microbiol. Biotechnol.* **2009**, *82*, 59–66.

59. Tanino, T.; Ohno, T.; Aoki, T.; Fukuda, H.; Kondo, A. Development of yeast cells displaying *Candida antarctica* lipase B and their application to ester synthesis reaction. *Appl. Microbiol. Biotechnol.* **2007**, *75*, 1319–1325.

60. Han, S.Y.; Pan, Z.Y.; Huang, D.F.; Ueda, M.; Wang, X.N.; Lin, Y. Highly efficient synthesis of ethyl hexanoate catalyzed by CALB-displaying *Saccharomyces cerevisiae* whole-cells in non-aqueous phase. *J. Mol. Catal. B* **2009**, *59*, 168–172.

61. Su, G.D.; Huang, D.F.; Han, S.Y.; Zheng, S.P.; Lin, Y. Display of *Candida antarctica* lipase B on *Pichia pastoris* and its application to flavor ester synthesis. *Appl. Microbiol. Biotechnol.* **2010**, *86*, 1493–1501.

62. Jiang, Z.; Gao, B.; Ren, R.; Tao, X.; Ma, Y.; Wei, D. Efficient display of active lipase LipB52 with a *Pichia pastoris* cell surface display system and comparison with the LipB52 displayed on *Saccharomyces cerevisiae* cell surface. *BMC Biotechnol.* **2008**, *8*, e4.

63. Jiang, Z.B.; Song, H.T.; Gupta, N.; Ma, L.X.; Wu, Z.B. Cell surface display of functionally active lipases from *Yarrowia lipolytica* in *Pichia pastoris*. *Protein Expr. Purif.* **2007**, *56*, 35–39.

64. Kaya, M.; Ito, J.; Kotaka, A.; Matsumura, K.; Bando, H.; Sahara, H.; Ogino, C.; Shibasaki, S.; Kuroda, K.; Ueda, M.; *et al.* Isoflavone aglycones production from isoflavone glycosides by display of β-glucosidase from *Aspergillus oryzae* on yeast cell surface. *Appl. Microbiol. Biotechnol.* **2008**, *79*, 51–60.

65. Inaba, C.; Higuchi, S.; Morisaka, H.; Kuroda, K.; Ueda, M. Synthesis of functional dipeptide carnosine from nonprotected amino acids using carnosinase-displaying yeast cells. *Appl. Microbiol. Biotechnol.* **2010**, *86*, 1895–1902.

66. Fukuda, T.; Isogawa, D.; Takagi, M.; Kato-Murai, M.; Kimoto, H.; Kusaoke, H.; Ueda, M.; Suye, S. Yeast cell-surface expression of chitosanase from *Paenibacillus fukuinensis*. *Biosci. Biotechnol. Biochem.* **2007**, *71*, 2845–2847.

67. Liu, G.; Yue, L.; Chi, Z.; Yu, W.; Chi, Z.; Madzak, C. The surface display of the alginate lyase on the cells of *Yarrowia lipolytica* for hydrolysis of alginate. *Mar. Biotechnol. (NY)* **2009**, *11*, 619–626.

68. Kotrba, P.; Ruml, T. Surface display of metal fixation motifs of bacterial P1-type ATPases specifically promotes biosorption of Pb^{2+} by *Saccharomyces cerevisiae*. *Appl. Environ. Microbiol.* **2010**, *76*, 2615–2622.

69. Kuroda, K.; Shibasaki, S.; Ueda, M.; Tanaka, A. Cell surface-engineered yeast displaying a histidine oligopeptide (hexa-His) has enhanced adsorption of and tolerance to heavy metal ions. *Appl. Microbiol. Biotechnol.* **2001**, *57*, 697–701.

70. Kuroda, K.; Ueda, M. Bioadsorption of cadmium ion by cell surface-engineered yeasts displaying metallothionein and hexa-His. *Appl. Microbiol. Biotechnol.* **2003**, *63*, 182–186.

71. Kuroda, K.; Ueda, M. Effective display of metallothionein tandem repeats on the bioadsorption of cadmium ion. *Appl. Microbiol. Biotechnol.* **2006**, *70*, 458–463.

72. Grunden, A.M.; Ray, R.M.; Rosentel, J.K.; Healy, F.G.; Shanmugam, K.T. Repression of the *Escherichia coli* modABCD (molybdate transport) operon by ModE. *J. Bacteriol.* **1996**, *178*, 735–744.

73. Nishitani, T.; Shimada, M.; Kuroda, K.; Ueda, M. Molecular design of yeast cell surface for adsorption and recovery of molybdenum, one of rare metals. *Appl. Microbiol. Biotechnol.* **2010**, *86*, 641–648.

74. Kuroda, K.; Nishitani, T.; Ueda, M. Specific adsorption of tungstate by cell surface display of the newly designed ModE mutant. *Appl. Microbiol. Biotechnol.* **2012**, *96*, 153–159.

75. Yasui, M.; Shibasaki, S.; Kuroda, K.; Ueda, M.; Kawada, N.; Nishikawa, J.; Nishihara, T.; Tanaka, A. An arming yeast with the ability to entrap fluorescent 17β-estradiol on the cell surface. *Appl. Microbiol. Biotechnol.* **2002**, *59*, 329–331.

76. Fukuda, T.; Tsuchiyama, K.; Makishima, H.; Takayama, K.; Mulchandani, A.; Kuroda, K.; Ueda, M.; Suye, S. Improvement in organophosphorus hydrolase activity of cell surface-engineered yeast strain using Flo1p anchor system. *Biotechnol. Lett.* **2010**, *32*, 655–659.

77. Takayama, K.; Suye, S.; Kuroda, K.; Ueda, M.; Kitaguchi, T.; Tsuchiyama, K.; Fukuda, T.; Chen, W.; Mulchandani, A. Surface display of organophosphorus hydrolase on *Saccharomyces cerevisiae*. *Biotechnol. Prog.* **2006**, *22*, 939–943.

78. Fukuda, T.; Tsuchiya, K.; Makishima, H.; Tsuchiyama, K.; Mulchandani, A.; Kuroda, K.; Ueda, M.; Suye, S. Organophosphorus compound detection on a cell chip with yeast coexpressing hydrolase and eGFP. *Biotechnol. J.* **2010**, *5*, 515–519.

79. Takayama, K.; Suye, S.; Tanaka, Y.; Mulchandani, A.; Kuroda, K.; Ueda, M. Estimation of enzyme kinetic parameters of cell surface-displayed organophosphorus hydrolase and construction of a biosensing system for organophosphorus compounds. *Anal. Sci.* **2011**, *27*, 823–826.

80. Shibasaki, S.; Ueda, M.; Ye, K.; Shimizu, K.; Kamasawa, N.; Osumi, M.; Tanaka, A. Creation of cell surface-engineered yeast that display different fluorescent proteins in response to the glucose concentration. *Appl. Microbiol. Biotechnol.* **2001**, *57*, 528–533.

81. Shibasaki, S.; Ninomiya, Y.; Ueda, M.; Iwahashi, M.; Katsuragi, T.; Tani, Y.; Harashima, S.; Tanaka, A. Intelligent yeast strains with the ability to self-monitor the concentrations of intra- and extracellular phosphate or ammonium ion by emission of fluorescence from the cell surface. *Appl. Microbiol. Biotechnol.* **2001**, *57*, 702–707.

82. Shibasaki, S.; Tanaka, A.; Ueda, M. Development of combinatorial bioengineering using yeast cell surface display—Order-made design of cell and protein for bio-monitoring. *Biosens. Bioelectron.* **2003**, *19*, 123–130.

83. Tamaru, Y.; Ohtsuka, M.; Kato, K.; Manabe, S.; Kuroda, K.; Sanada, M.; Ueda, M. Application of the arming system for the expression of the 380R antigen from red sea bream iridovirus (RSIV) on the surface of yeast cells: A first step for the development of an oral vaccine. *Biotechnol. Prog.* **2006**, *22*, 949–953.

84. Wasilenko, J.L.; Sarmento, L.; Spatz, S.; Pantin-Jackwood, M. Cell surface display of highly pathogenic avian influenza virus hemagglutinin on the surface of *Pichia pastoris* cells using α-agglutinin for production of oral vaccines. *Biotechnol. Prog.* **2010**, *26*, 542–547.

85. Lin, Y.; Shiraga, S.; Tsumuraya, T.; Matsumoto, T.; Kondo, A.; Fujii, I.; Ueda, M. Comparison of two forms of catalytic antibody displayed on yeast-cell surface. *J. Mol. Catal. B* **2004**, *28*, 241–246.

86. Lin, Y.; Tsumuraya, T.; Wakabayashi, T.; Shiraga, S.; Fujii, I.; Kondo, A.; Ueda, M. Display of a functional hetero-oligomeric catalytic antibody on the yeast cell surface. *Appl. Microbiol. Biotechnol.* **2003**, *62*, 226–232.

87. Okochi, N.; Kato-Murai, M.; Kadonosono, T.; Ueda, M. Design of a serine protease-like catalytic triad on an antibody light chain displayed on the yeast cell surface. *Appl. Microbiol. Biotechnol.* **2007**, *77*, 597–603.

88. Nakamura, Y.; Shibasaki, S.; Ueda, M.; Tanaka, A.; Fukuda, H.; Kondo, A. Development of novel whole-cell immunoadsorbents by yeast surface display of the IgG-binding domain. *Appl. Microbiol. Biotechnol.* **2001**, *57*, 500–505.

89. Matsui, K.; Kuroda, K.; Ueda, M. Creation of a novel peptide endowing yeasts with acid tolerance using yeast cell-surface engineering. *Appl. Microbiol. Biotechnol.* **2009**, *82*, 105–113.

90. Zou, W.; Ueda, M.; Tanaka, A. Screening of a molecule endowing *Saccharomyces cerevisiae* with *n*-nonane-tolerance from a combinatorial random protein library. *Appl. Microbiol. Biotechnol.* **2002**, *58*, 806–812.

91. Zou, W.; Ueda, M.; Yamanaka, H.; Tanaka, A. Construction of a combinatorial protein library displayed on yeast cell surface using DNA random priming method. *J. Biosci. Bioeng.* **2001**, *92*, 393–396.

92. Andreu, C.; del Olmo, M. Yeast arming by the Aga2p system: Effect of growth conditions in galactose on the efficiency of the display and influence of expressing leucine-containing peptides. *Appl. Microbiol. Biotechnol.* **2013**, doi:10.1007/s00253-013-5086-4.

93. Shiraga, S.; Ishiguro, M.; Fukami, H.; Nakao, M.; Ueda, M. Creation of *Rhizopus oryzae* lipase having a unique oxyanion hole by combinatorial mutagenesis in the lid domain. *Appl. Microbiol. Biotechnol.* **2005**, *68*, 779–785.

94. Kadonosono, T.; Kato-Murai, M.; Ueda, M. Alteration of substrate specificity of rat neurolysin from matrix metalloproteinase-2/9-type to -3-type specificity by comprehensive mutation. *Protein Eng. Des. Sel.* **2008**, *21*, 507–513.

95. Fushimi, T.; Miura, N.; Shintani, H.; Tsunoda, H.; Kuroda, K.; Ueda, M. Mutant firefly luciferases with improved specific activity and dATP discrimination constructed by yeast cell surface engineering. *Appl. Microbiol. Biotechnol.* **2013**, *97*, 4003–4011.

96. Van den Beucken, T.; Pieters, H.; Steukers, M.; van der Vaart, M.; Ladner, R.C.; Hoogenboom, H.R.; Hufton, S.E. Affinity maturation of Fab antibody fragments by fluorescent-activated cell sorting of yeast-displayed libraries. *FEBS Lett.* **2003**, *546*, 288–294.

97. Rajpal, A.; Beyaz, N.; Haber, L.; Cappuccilli, G.; Yee, H.; Bhatt, R.R.; Takeuchi, T.; Lerner, R.A.; Crea, R. A general method for greatly improving the affinity of antibodies by using combinatorial libraries. *Proc. Natl. Acad. Sci. USA* **2005**, *102*, 8466–8471.

98. Graff, C.P.; Chester, K.; Begent, R.; Wittrup, K.D. Directed evolution of an anti-carcinoembryonic antigen scFv with a 4-day monovalent dissociation half-time at 37 °C. *Protein Eng. Des. Sel.* **2004**, *17*, 293–304.

99. Razai, A.; Garcia-Rodriguez, C.; Lou, J.; Geren, I.N.; Forsyth, C.M.; Robles, Y.; Tsai, R.; Smith, T.J.; Smith, L.A.; Siegel, R.W.; *et al.* Molecular evolution of antibody affinity for sensitive detection of botulinum neurotoxin type A. *J. Mol. Biol.* **2005**, *351*, 158–169.

100. VanAntwerp, J.J.; Wittrup, K.D. Thermodynamic characterization of affinity maturation: The D1.3 antibody and a higher-affinity mutant. *J. Mol. Recognit.* **1998**, *11*, 10–13.

101. Wang, Z.; Kim, G.B.; Woo, J.H.; Liu, Y.Y.; Mathias, A.; Stavrou, S.; Neville, D.M., Jr. Improvement of a recombinant anti-monkey anti-CD3 diphtheria toxin based immunotoxin by yeast display affinity maturation of the scFv. *Bioconjug. Chem.* **2007**, *18*, 947–955.

Production of Fungal Glucoamylase for Glucose Production from Food Waste

Wan Chi Lam, Daniel Pleissner and Carol Sze Ki Lin

Abstract: The feasibility of using pastry waste as resource for glucoamylase (GA) production via solid state fermentation (SSF) was studied. The crude GA extract obtained was used for glucose production from mixed food waste. Our results showed that pastry waste could be used as a sole substrate for GA production. A maximal GA activity of 76.1 ± 6.1 U/mL was obtained at Day 10. The optimal pH and reaction temperature for the crude GA extract for hydrolysis were pH 5.5 and 55 °C, respectively. Under this condition, the half-life of the GA extract was 315.0 minutes with a deactivation constant (k_d) $2.20 \times 10^{-3} min^{-1}$. The application of the crude GA extract for mixed food waste hydrolysis and glucose production was successfully demonstrated. Approximately 53 g glucose was recovered from 100 g of mixed food waste in 1 h under the optimal digestion conditions, highlighting the potential of this approach as an alternative strategy for waste management and sustainable production of glucose applicable as carbon source in many biotechnological processes.

Reprinted from *Biomolecules*. Cite as: Lam, W.C.; Pleissner, D.; Ki Lin, C.S. Production of Fungal Glucoamylase for Glucose Production from Food Waste. *Biomolecules* **2013**, *3*, 651-661.

1. Introduction

Food waste is a serious global problem, especially in many developed countries. In Hong Kong, over 3500 tons of food wastes are generated every day [1]. Currently, landfilling and incineration are the major practices for managing these wastes in many countries. These practices, however, may cause severe environmental pollutions and adds burden to the economy. Due to its high contents of carbohydrates and proteins, food wastes may serve as feedstock in biorefineries for production of fungal enzymes, e.g., glucoamylase (GA) and offers an innovative approach to waste management.

GA is a family of amylolytic enzymes that catalyze the cleavage of α-(1,4) glycosidic bonds in starch and release glucose as end product [2,3]. Glucose is the principle carbon source in many biotechnological processes and of great importance for fermentative chemicals and fuel production such as succinic acid, bio-plastic and ethanol. Starch is usually the major component of mixed food waste from restaurants [4–6], application of GA for food waste hydrolysis to recover glucose from starch, therefore, may not only offer a solution for managing food waste but also help to save precious resources.

Aspergillus awamori is a known secretor of GA with beneficial properties for industrial bioprocesses such as high productivity and enzyme activity at high temperatures [3,7]. Therefore, *Aspergillus awamori* is employed in this study for GA production through solid state fermentation (SSF). SSF is a fermentation process conducted in the absence of free water, thus it is desirable for industrial enzymes production since the enzymes produced at the end are not diluted by the amount water added in comparison to submerge fermentation. Consequently, the enzymes produced are at a

208

much higher concentration. Pastry waste collected from local Starbucks contains 44.6% of starch and 7% of protein [8]. Starch has been shown as an inducer for GA synthesis by some *Aspergillus* producers [9–11]; thus, the significant amount of starch in pastry waste could be desirable for GA production. The smaller amount of protein, 7%, on the other hand could provide a source of nitrogen to promote the fungal growth and facilitate GA production. Therefore, pastry waste was selected in this study for GA production. The crude GA extract obtained without further purification was characterized in terms of optimal pH and reaction temperature, as well as thermo-stability. Additionally, application of the crude GA extract was studied for hydrolysis of mixed food waste collected from a local restaurant to produce high glucose solution.

2. Results and Discussion

2.1. Glucoamylase Production from Pastry Waste

To demonstrate the feasibility of pastry waste as the sole substrate for GA production, SSF was conducted with *Aspergillus awamori* without addition of any other nitrogen or carbon sources. GA production from pastry waste over time is shown in Figure 1. Production of GA reached maximal activity at Day 10. Approximately, 253.7 ± 20.4 U of GA was produced from one gram of pastry waste on dry basis (d.b.); the GA activity of the crude GA extract was 76.1 ± 6.1 U/mL. The result demonstrates that pastry waste can be used solely for GA production.

Figure 1. Glucoamylase (GA) production from pastry waste with *Aspergillus awamori* during solid state fermentation (SSF) for 11 days at 30 °C. Experiments were duplicated. The mean values are plotted and the standard errors are reported.

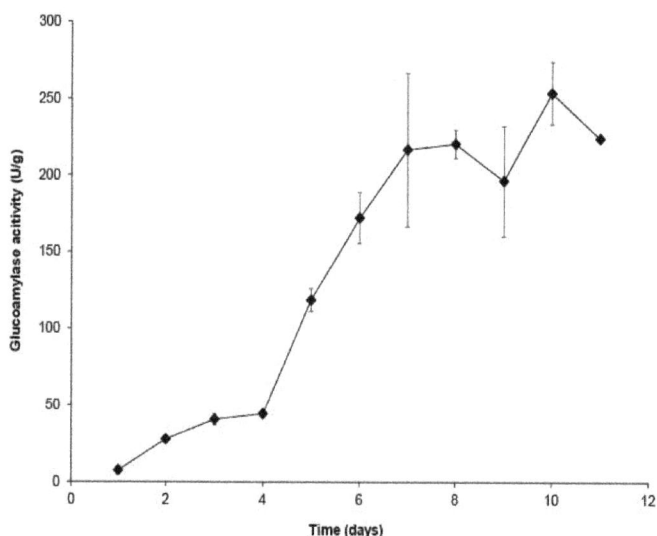

GA production with different wastes as substrates have been studied and the results are summarized in Table 1. In some studies, nitrogen in form of ammonium, urea and yeast extract was supplemented to substrates to facilitate fungal growth and GA production [4,12–14]. In contrast, nitrogen supplement was not involved in this study, but the GA activity of enzyme extract appears higher than in earlier studies with nitrogen supplement most likely due to a good balance of carbon (C) to nitrogen (N) and phosphorus (P) ratios. The data suggests that pastry waste is a promising substrate for GA production.

Table 1. GA production and yields from different studied substrates with or without nitrogen supplement through solid state fermentation.

Substrate	Crude GA Concentration (U/mL)	Yield (U/g)	Fungus	Nitrogen Supplement	References
Rice powder	N/A	71.3 ± 2.34 [a]	*Aspergillus niger*	+	[12]
Wheat bran	N/A	110 ± 1.32 [a]	*Aspergillus niger*	+	[12]
Mixed food waste	137	N/A	*Aspergillus niger*	+	[13]
Cowpea waste	970	N/A	*Aspergillus oryzae*	-	[14]
Wheat bran	4.4	48	*Aspergillus awamori*	-	[15]
Wheat pieces	3.32	81.3	*Aspergillus awamori*	-	[16]
Waste bread	3.94	78.4	*Aspergillus awamori*	-	[16]
Waste bread	N/A	114	*Aspergillus awamori*	-	[17]
Pastry waste	76.1 ± 6.1 [a]	253.7 ± 20.4 [a]	*Aspergillus awamori*	-	This study

[a] Values indicate means ± standard errors.

2.2. Characterization of Optimal Reaction Temperature and pH of the Crude Glucoamylase Extract

Optimal pH and reaction temperature of the crude GA extract were determined. The results are shown in Figure 2. In order to determine the optimal reaction pH of the crude GA extract, assays were carried out at various pHs from 3.5 to 7.5 and the results are indicated in Figure 2A. The maximal enzyme activity was obtained at pH 5.5, indicating it was the optimal pH for starch hydrolysis. Fungal GAs from *Aspergillus* strains are usually active at acidic pH, their enzyme activities vary from pH 3.5 to 7 depending on the strains and amino acid sequences (isoform) [3]. Similarly, GA assay was conducted at different temperatures as indicated in Figure 2B from 40–75 °C with 5 °C increment at pH 5.5 in order to determine the optimal reaction temperature for the crude GA extract and assuming that the pH factor is independent of the temperature factor. A significant increase in enzyme activity was observed as temperature increases from 40 to 55 °C. Maximal GA activity was observed from 55 to 65 °C suggesting the range for optimal reaction temperature of the crude GA extract and in accordance with optimal reaction temperatures in the range of 50 to 60 °C usually found for GAs from *Aspergillus* [3]. Further increase in reaction temperature greatly reduced the enzyme activity most likely due to enzyme denaturation.

Figure 2. Effect of (**A**) pH at 55 °C and (**B**) temperature at pH 5.5 on crude GA extract activity. Experiments were duplicated. The mean values are plotted and the standard errors are reported.

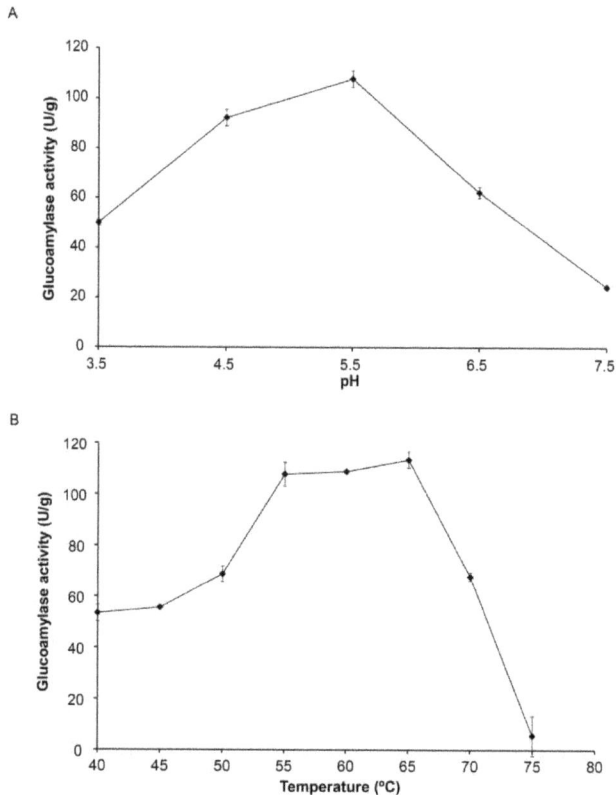

2.3. Thermo-Stability of the Crude Glucoamylase Extract at Optimal Reaction Temperatures

Since high GA activity was observed at 55, 60 and 65 °C, thermo-stability of the crude GA extract at these temperatures was further investigated in order to determine the optimal digestion temperature for the subsequent food waste hydrolysis experiment. The residual enzyme activity after heated at 55, 60 and 65 °C for over 90 min is shown in Figure 3. The rate constant (k_d, min^{-1}) for the first-order thermal deactivation was determined from the slope of the deactivation time course as shown in Figure 3 using Equation (1) [18], where E_t is the residual GA activity after heat treatment for time t. E_0 is the initial enzyme activity before heat treatment. The half-life of thermal deactivation ($t_{1/2}$) was determined according to Equation (2) [19]. The thermal deactivation of the crude GA extract exhibited a linear relationship showing that it followed first-order kinetics as reported [20]. The thermal deactivation rate constant k_d (min^{-1}) of the crude GA extract at 55 °C was found approximately 10 times slower than the rates at 60 and 65 °C, suggesting the crude GA is more thermo-stable at 55 °C. The k_d of the crude GA extract at 55 °C was 2.20×10^{-3} in comparison with 2.13×10^{-2} and 2.17×10^{-2} at 60 and 65 °C, respectively. The half-life ($t_{1/2}$) of the enzyme extract at 55 °C was 315 min in comparison with 32.5 and 31.9 min for 60 and 65 °C, respectively (Table 2). Since the enzymatic activity of the crude GA extract at 55 °C was close to the activity at 60 and 65 °C, but more stable, it was adopted as the optimal digestion temperature for the subsequent food hydrolysis experiment.

$$\ln (E_t/E_0) = -k_d t \qquad (1)$$

$$t_{1/2} = \ln(2)/k_d \qquad (2)$$

Figure 3. Thermal deactivation of crude GA extract at ($\blacklozenge$) 55 °C, ($\blacksquare$) 60 °C and ($\blacktriangle$) 65 °C over 90 min at pH 5.5. Experiments were duplicated. The mean values are plotted and the standard errors were reported.

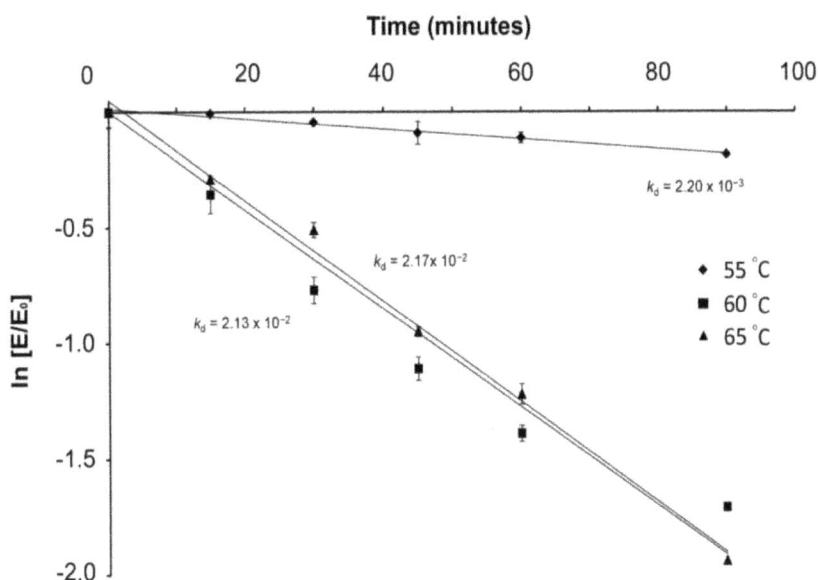

Table 2. Deactivation constant (k_d) and half-lives ($t_{1/2}$) of the crude GA extract at 55, 60 and 65 °C at pH 5.5.

Temperature (°C)	k_d (min^{-1})	$t_{1/2}$ (min)
55	2.20×10^{-3}	315.0
60	2.13×10^{-2}	32.5
65	2.17×10^{-2}	31.9

2.4. Application of Crude Glucoamylase Extract on Mixed Food Waste Hydrolysis for Glucose Production

In the reality, mixed food waste is rich in salt [21] that may inhibit the enzymatic hydrolysis. To verify if the crude GA extract produced was applicable to food waste digestion for glucose production, it was used to hydrolyse the food waste which was collected from a local restaurant, under its optimal digestion conditions (at pH 5.5 and 55 °C). Increasing concentration of enzyme was added to the food waste and the time required for hydrolysis to produce glucose was determined (Figure 4). Significant difference in glucose concentration was only observed for the first hour but not after. In all cases, the food waste hydrolysis by the enzyme extracts was completed in 1 h. At the end of the hydrolysis, approximately 12 g/L glucose was produced and that was corresponding to approximately 53 g glucose produced from 100 g of mixed food waste (d.b.), while no production of glucose occurred in a control without crude GA extract. The amount of glucose produced from 100 g of mixed food waste hydrolysis was consistent with our previous study using a different hydrolysis approach [5].

Figure 4. Hydrolysis of mixed food waste for glucose production in the presence of crude GA extract with (●) no enzyme, (◆) 7.1 U/mL, (■) 14.2 U/mL and (▲) 28.4 U/mL at pH 5.5 and 55 °C for 3 h. Experiments were duplicated. The mean values are plotted and the standard errors are reported.

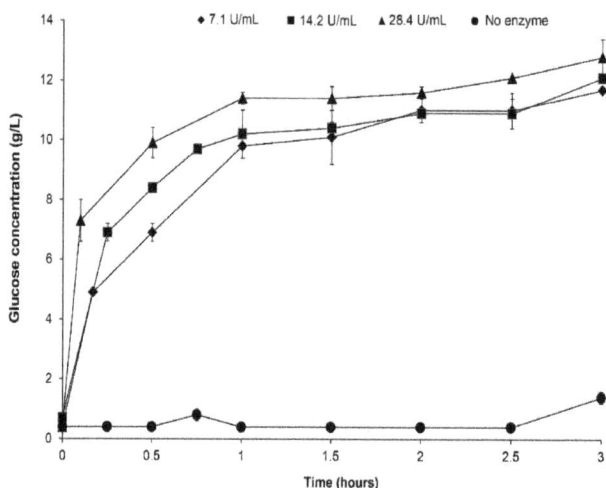

The two commonly used approaches for cereal-based waste and food waste hydrolysis to produce glucose rich solution, include simultaneous fungus culturing and hydrolysis with the enzymes actively secreted [5,8,16,22,23] or direct addition of enzyme solution to digest the substrate [24]. In the first case, food waste hydrolysis is usually completed after 24 h [5,8,16,22,23]. In this study, the latter approach was adopted. Food waste hydrolysis by the crude GA extract was completed in 1 h under optimal conditions found. Similar experiment has been reported by *Yan et al.* using commercial GA for food waste hydrolysis. In their studies, food waste hydrolysis was completed in 2.5 h when GA to substrate ratio reached 80–140 U/g food waste [24]. When the GA to substrate ratio in the solution is reduced to 7.4 U/g substrate, 24 h was needed for complete substrate hydrolysis [16]. The higher efficiency for food waste hydrolysis (in 1 h) in this study was likely due to the higher initial GA to substrate ratio.

2.5. Material Balance for Glucose Production from 1 kg Mixed Food Waste with Crude Glucoamylase Extract

Scheme I shows the material balance of the studied process for crude GA production from pastry waste and glucose recovery from 1 kg mixed food waste (d.b.). All the calculations are provided in the supplementary information. According to our study, hydrolysis of 1 kg mixed food waste (d.b.) could lead to 0.53 kg glucose production. Approximately, 1.4 kg pastry waste (d.b.) is required to produce sufficient amount of crude GA extract for 1 kg mixed food waste hydrolysis. Furthermore, the material balance only presents the theoretical values of the up-scaled process based on our laboratory-scale experimental data. However, upscale study is needed in order to demonstrate the process can be applied at industrial scale.

Scheme I. Material balance of the process in this study for processing 1 kg mixed food waste to produce glucose using crude GA extract produced from pastry waste based on the laboratory-scale experimental data.

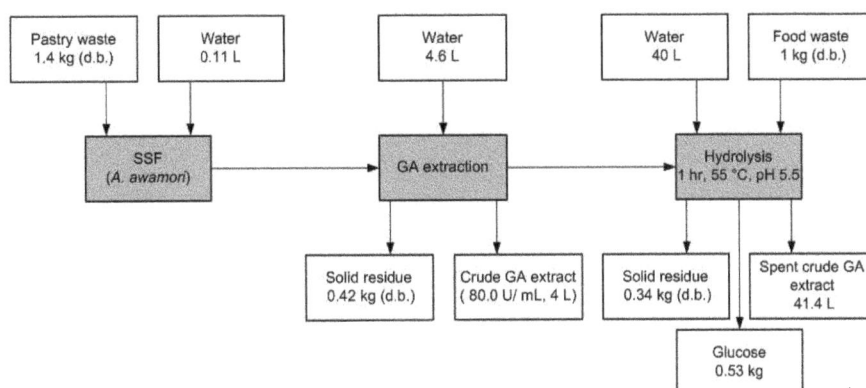

3. Experimental Section

3.1. Microorganism

Frozen spores of the fungus *Aspergillus awamori* (ATCC 14331), were used for SSF. Spores were suspended in demineralized water and loaded into conical flasks containing cornmeal agar and incubated at 30 °C for 7 days. Harvesting of fresh spores was carried out using 10% glycerol and the number of spores was counted using a haemocytometer. Fresh spore suspension of 1 mL was diluted to the required concentration with sterile demineralized water and used immediately for SSF.

3.2. Food Wastes Preparation

Pastry waste and mixed food waste were obtained from a local Starbucks store and canteen for SSFs and enzymatic hydrolysis experiments, respectively. Once the pastry waste was collected, it was homogenized with a kitchen blender and stored at −20 °C. Pastry waste was autoclaved before subjected to SSF and mixed food waste was lyophilized before enzymatic hydrolysis.

3.3. Solid State Fermentation for Glucoamylase Production

Sterilized pastry waste of 20 g was placed in a petri dish and inoculated with 1 mL of fresh spore suspension of *Aspergillus awamori* loaded onto the surface of the substrate. For each g of substrate, 5×10^5 spores were used. The plates were incubated under static condition at 30 °C for 11 days. Whole plate content was withdrawn regularly and analyzed for GA production.

3.4. Glucoamylase Extraction

Whole content of the fermented solid in the petri dish was mixed thoroughly in a kitchen blender containing 20 mL demineralized water and the mixture was transferred into a 500 mL Duran bottle. The kitchen blender was rinsed with another portion of 20 mL demineralized water and pooled with the previously obtained mixture. The suspension was then mixed for 30 min with a magnetic stirrer at 30 °C, followed by centrifugation at 22,000 × g for 10 min. The supernatant was collected and filtered with Whitman no. 1 filter paper. The solution obtained refers to crude GA extract.

3.5. Food Waste Hydrolysis for Glucose Production

Food waste hydrolysis was conducted by adding increasing amount of crude GA extract to test tubes containing 50 mg dried food waste in 2.2 mL of 0.2 M sodium acetate (pH 5.5). The reaction mixture was incubated at 55 °C for 3 h and mixed by pipetting for every 30 min. Aliquots of samples were withdrawn regularly from the reaction mixture and mixed with 10% (w/v) trichloroacetic acid prior to glucose determination.

3.6. Glucoamylase Activity

Activity of the crude GA extract was determined using the method described by Melikoglu *et al.* [17]. Wheat flour solution of 6% (w/v) was used as substrate and it was prepared in sodium acetate (pH 5.5) and gelatinized at 80 °C for 15 min before usage. The assay was conducted by mixing 0.25 mL of 5 times diluted crude GA extract and 0.5 mL of gelatinized wheat flour solution, and incubated at 55 °C. The reaction was terminated after 10 min by adding 0.25 mL 10% (w/v) trichloroacetic acid solution to the reaction mixture. The reaction mixture was centrifuged and the glucose concentration in the supernatant was analyzed using the Analox GL6 glucose analyzer. One unit (U) of GA activity is defined as the amount of enzyme that releases 1 µmol of glucose per minute under assay conditions and is expressed as U/g of dry substrate as described [12].

For determination of optimal reaction pH, the crude GA extract and the gelatinized wheat flour solutions were prepared in sodium acetate buffer from pH 3.5 to 7.5. Optimal reaction temperature determination of the crude GA extract was carried out at temperature range of 40–75 °C with 5 °C increment at optimal pH. Thermo-stability of the crude GA extract was investigated at different temperatures (55–65 °C) at optimal pH. Experiments were performed in duplicate and the standard errors were reported.

4. Conclusions

In this work, we have demonstrated the feasibility of pastry waste as feedstock for GA production. High GA yield (253.7 ± 20.4 U/g) of the crude enzyme extract was obtained without addition of nitrogen in comparison to other reported waste substrates, highlighting its potential as a feedstock for GA production in industrial scale. Under the optimal digestion conditions (pH 5.5 and 55 °C), the crude GA extract could hydrolyze mixed food waste in 1 h and generate around 53 g glucose from 100 g of mixed food waste. The work is of great significance as it shows sustainable GA production from food waste for potential municipal food waste treatment and sustainable chemicals production.

Acknowledgments

The authors acknowledge the Biomass funding from the Ability R&D Energy Research Centre (AERC) at the School of Energy and Environment in the City University of Hong Kong. We are also grateful to the donation from the Coffee Concept (Hong Kong) Ltd. For the "Care for Our Planet" campaign, as well as a grant from the City University of Hong Kong (Project No. 7200248). Authors acknowledge the Industrial Technology Funding from the Innovation and Technology Commission (ITS/323/11) in Hong Kong.

Conflicts of Interest

The authors declare no conflict of interest.

References

1. Hong Kong SAR Environmental Protection Department. Monitoring of solid waste in Hong Kong—Waste statistics for 2011, in Hong Kong 2011. Available online: https://www.wastereduction.gov.hk/en/materials/info/msw2011.pdf (accessed on 21 June 2013).
2. Sauer, J.; Sigurskjold, B.W.; Christensen, U.; Frandsen, T.P.; Mirgorodskaya, E.; Harrison, M.; Roepstorff, P.; Svensson, B. Glucoamylase: Structure/Function relationships, and protein engineering. *Biochim. Biophys. Acta* **2000**, *1543*, 275–293.
3. Norouzian, D.; Akbarzadeh, A.; Scharer, J.M.; Young, M.M. Fungal glucoamylases. *Biotechnol. Adv.* **2006**, *24*, 80–85.
4. Wang, X.Q.; Wang, Q.H.; Liu, Y.Y.; Ma, H.Z., On-Site production of crude glucoamylase for kitchen waste hydrolysis. *Waste Manag. Res.* **2010**, *28*, 539–544.
5. Pleissner, D.; Lam, W.C.; Sun, Z.; Lin, C.S.K. Food waste as nutrient source in heterotrophic microalgae cultivation. *Bioresour. Technol.* **2013**, *137*, 139–146.
6. Sayeki, M.; Kitagawa, T.; Matsumoto, M.; Nishiyama, A.; Miyoshi, K.; Mochizuki, M.; Takasu, A.; Abe, A. Chemical composition and energy value of dried meal from food waste as feedstuff in swine and cattle. *Anim. Sci. J.* **2001**, *72*, 34–40.

7. Koutinas, A.A.; Wang, R.; Webb, C. Estimation of fungal growth in complex, heterogeneous culture. *Biochem. Eng. J.* **2003**, *14*, 93–100.

8. Zhang, A.Y.-Z.; Sun, Z.; Leung, C.C.J.; Han, W.; Lau, K.Y.; Li, M.; Lin, C.S.K. Valorisation of bakery waste for succinic acid production. *Green Chem.* **2013**, *15*, 690–695.

9. Zambare, V. Solid state fermentation of *Aspergillus. oryzae* for glucoamylase production on agro residues. *Int. J. Life Sci.* **2010**, *4*, 16–25.

10. Ganzlin, M.; Rinas, U. In-Depth analysis of the *Aspergillus. niger* glucoamylase (glaA) promoter performance using high-throughput screening and controlled bioreactor cultivation techniques. *J. Biotechnol.* **2008**, *135*, 266–271.

11. Ventura, L.; González-Candelas, L.; Pérez-Gonzáez, J.A.; Ramón, D. Molecular cloning and transcriptional analysis of the *Aspergillus. terreus* gla1 gene encoding a glucoamylase. *Appl. Environ. Microbiol.* **1995**, *61*, 399–402.

12. Anto, H.; Trivedi, U.B.; Patel, K.C. Glucoamylase production by solid-state fermentation using rice flake manufacturing waste products as substrate. *Bioresour. Technol.* **2006**, *97*, 1161–1166.

13. Wang, Q.; Wang, X.; Wang, X.; Ma, H. Glucoamylase production from food waste by *Aspergillus. niger* under submerged fermentation. *Process. Biochem.* **2008**, *43*, 280–286.

14. Kareem, S.O.; Akpan, I.; Oduntan, S.B. Cowpea waste: A novel substrate for solid state production of amylase by *Aspergillus. oryzae. Afr. J. Microbiol. Res.* **2009**, *3*, 974–977.

15. Du, C.; Lin, S.K.C.; Koutinas, A.; Wang, R.; Dorado, P.; Webb, C. A wheat biorefining strategy based on solid-state fermentation for fermentative production of succinic acid. *Bioresour. Technol.* **2008**, *99*, 8310–8315.

16. Wang, R.; Godoy, L.C.; Shaarani, S.M.; Melikoglu, M.; Koutinas, A.; Webb, C. Improving wheat flour hydrolysis by an enzyme mixture from solid state fungal fermentation. *Enzyme Microb. Technol.* **2009**, *44*, 223–228.

17. Melikoglu, M.; Lin, C.S.K.; Webb, C. Stepwise optimisation of enzyme production in solid state fermentation of waste bread pieces. *Food Bioprod. Process.* **2013**, in press.

18. Lawton, J.M.; Doonan, S. Thermal inactivation and chaperonin-mediated renaturation of mitochondrial aspartate aminotransferase. *Biochem. J.* **1998**, *334*, 219–224.

19. Johannes, T.W.; Woodyer, R.D.; Zhao, H. Directed evolution of a thermostable phosphite dehydrogenase for NAD(P)H regeneration. *Appl. Environ. Microbiol.* **2005**, *71*, 5728–5734.

20. Allen, M.J.; Coutinho, P.M.; Ford, C.F. Stabilization of *Aspergillus. awamori* glucoamylase by proline substitution and combining stabilizing mutations. *Protein Eng.* **1998**, *11*, 783–788.

21. Myer, R.O.; Brendemuhl, J.H.; Johnson, D.D. Evaluation of dehydrated restaurant food waste products as feedstuffs for finishing pigs. *J. Anim. Sci.* **1999**, *77*, 685–692.

22. Leung, C.C.J.; Cheung, A.S.Y.; Zhang, A.Y.-Z.; Lam, K.F.; Lin, C.S.K. Utilisation of waste bread for fermentative succinic acid production. *Biochem. Eng. J.* **2012**, *65*, 10–15.

23. Dorado, M.P.; Lin, S.K.C.; Koutinas, A.; Du, C.; Wang, R.; Webb, C. Cereal-Based biorefinery development: Utilisation of wheat milling by-products for the production of succinic acid. *J. Biotechnol.* **2009**, *143*, 51–59.
24. Yan, S.; Yao, J.; Yao, L.; Zhi, Z.; Chen, X.; Wu, J. Fed batch enzymatic saccharification of food waste improves the sugar concentration in the hydrolysates and eventually the ethanol fermentation by *Saccharomyces. Cerevisiae* H058. *Braz. Arch. Biol. Technol.* **2012**, *55*, 183–192.

Quantum Mechanical Modeling: A Tool for the Understanding of Enzyme Reactions

Gábor Náray-Szabó, Julianna Oláh and Balázs Krámos

Abstract: Most enzyme reactions involve formation and cleavage of covalent bonds, while electrostatic effects, as well as dynamics of the active site and surrounding protein regions, may also be crucial. Accordingly, special computational methods are needed to provide an adequate description, which combine quantum mechanics for the reactive region with molecular mechanics and molecular dynamics describing the environment and dynamic effects, respectively. In this review we intend to give an overview to non-specialists on various enzyme models as well as established computational methods and describe applications to some specific cases. For the treatment of various enzyme mechanisms, special approaches are often needed to obtain results, which adequately refer to experimental data. As a result of the spectacular progress in the last two decades, most enzyme reactions can be quite precisely treated by various computational methods.

Reprinted from *Biomolecules*. Cite as: Náray-Szabó, G.; Oláh, J.; Krámos, B. Quantum Mechanical Modeling: A Tool for the Understanding of Enzyme Reactions. *Biomolecules* **2013**, *3*, 662-702.

1. Introduction

Enzyme reactions are extremely complicated processes involving directly or indirectly a large number of atoms in the chemical rearrangement of the reacting species. Accordingly, their understanding in atomic details is also very difficult and needs combined application of a variety of experimental and molecular modeling techniques. Rate and binding constants, as well as inhibitory power provide direct information on energetic aspects; however, they are bulk descriptors of the reaction and give information on subtleties only in cases when they can be associated with a single step. A direct method, X-ray diffraction, helps in constructing three-dimensional models at the atomic resolution but does not allow drawing conclusions on energetic aspects of the process. Detailed and precise elucidation of an enzymatic reaction is therefore not possible using present-day experimental methods alone; application of molecular modeling seems to be a must in order to clarify subtle details.

Because of the very large number of atoms involved in the reaction enzymatic processes, in general, cannot be modeled as accurately as interactions between small molecules with a few atoms. Though in some specific cases, by the application of high-level quantum mechanical methods quantitative agreement with experiment could be achieved [1], this is presently not routine. A promising way to obtain a detailed and adequate description of the process is to combine experimental evidence with modeling techniques. The reliability of a model can be checked by comparing calculated and experimental data and if an appropriate agreement is achieved, one may be confident on its validity.

With the spectacular development of computer hardware and software a substantial progress has been made in the development of quantum chemical methods. High-performance models of solvation, as well as combination of *a priori* quantum mechanical and empirical molecular mechanical approaches have become an integral part of commercial molecular modeling program packages. Along with the dramatic increase of the computer performance to price ratio, computational chemistry became suitable even for predictions, and thus it complements experimental findings. It seems that direct mapping between calculated and experimentally observed properties, as well as molecular structures represents a major advantage of quantum chemical modeling since this type of information is very difficult to obtain experimentally. If the observed properties, related to enzyme reactions, can be quantitatively reproduced by calculations we may consider reaction profiles and other calculated parameters to be reliable, too. Agreement between theory and experiment may imply that the reaction mechanism of the studied enzyme can be considered as clarified.

In this review we give an overview first on models, which can be used for the understanding of an enzyme reaction. Then, up-to-date and popular methods of calculation will be surveyed without laying emphasis on their mathematical background and technical details, rather focusing on their performance. The main part of the paper is written on case studies on some enzyme reactions, either involving special effects or dealing with a widely studied class of processes. First we discuss serine proteases, an important enzyme family for which three-dimensional structures have been available very early [2]. While the key reaction, general base assisted catalysis, is well-known in organic chemistry, a variety of factors contributing to rate enhancement has to be considered, and it seems that by now most of them are understood in detail [3]. Next we treat biological phosphate ester hydrolysis, which is a key step e.g., in the transfer of the phosphoryl group from a phosphate ester or anhydride to a nucleophile [4]. Understanding of this process is closely linked to the elucidation of mechanisms for the corresponding non-enzymatic reactions in solution. A wide variety of experimental data is available; however, it is difficult to summarize indirect conclusions in the absence of explicit molecular models. Accordingly, quantum mechanical calculations provide an important option to obtain a reasonable guess for the reaction energy profile. An interesting process is long-range electron transfer in heme peroxidases, its understanding in detail involves special experimental techniques. Therefore, to study enzyme-catalyzed electron transfer reactions we need to perform sophisticated quantum mechanical calculations, classical molecular mechanics alone is not appropriate (*cf.* Section 4.3). Cytochrome P450 enzymes form a very large superfamily of heme enzymes, their regioselectivity, oxidizing power and reactivity are therefore of outstanding interest, we treat them in Section 4.4. At last we deal with a special case, xylose isomerase catalysis [5], where quantum effects, namely proton tunneling, play a certain role in determining the reaction rate. Tunneling could be relatively precisely reproduced by direct calculations on other enzyme reactions, too.

2. Models

An enzyme has thousands of atoms, therefore the whole molecule and its transformations cannot be treated by direct quantum mechanical methods. Instead of striving for complete models, including all atoms of the enzyme and its surroundings, the system is better partitioned into various regions, which can be described at various levels of sophistication. The active site (**A**) is embedded in the amino-acid residues of the protein core (**P**) with ionizable surface, eventually buried, side chains and the whole protein is dissolved in the bulk (**B**). For most enzymes studied, this latter contains, beside water molecules, counter ions, partly or fully shielding the electrostatic field of the positively or negatively charged side chains. However, in some specific cases, the bulk is not necessarily aqueous, it can be formed by e.g., the atoms of a membrane, where the enzyme is located. The above three regions, schematically depicted in Figure 1, can be calculated at different levels of sophistication.

Figure 1. Hierarchical composition of a full enzyme system. Active site or quantum mechanical region (**A**); protein core or molecular mechanical region (**P**); bulk or dielectric continuum shell (**B**) (figure drawn on the basis of the crystal structure of human aromatase, 3EQM).

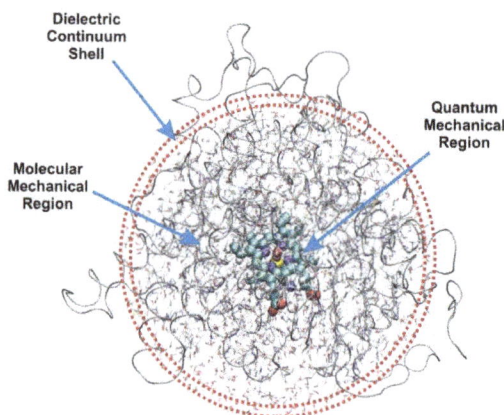

For most enzymes **A** includes the catalytic machinery, *i.e.*, key amino-acid side chains, one or more water molecules and substrate, these fragments are directly involved in catalysis. The minimum number of non-hydrogen atoms in this model may range from 10 to 200, which should be extended by a further number of atoms belonging to essential prosthetic groups, if present. Up-to-date quantum mechanical methods are available even for the high-level treatment of such systems, even if these contain one or more third or higher row atoms, e.g., sulfur, phosphorus or some transition metal. Special electronic effects, like excitation or transfer can be accounted for using sophisticated computational methods, which make use of high-performance software and hardware. The basic reason, why quantum mechanics is indispensable for the adequate description of these models, is that bond fission and formation taking place during the vast majority of enzymatic processes needs such an exact treatment. We may obtain structural parameters for **A** mainly from the Protein Data Bank [6], in some specific cases from other sources. If geometry optimization is necessary, atoms at the boundary of **A** must be fixed in order to avoid artificial distortions from the experimental, chemically relevant structure, which may essentially influence final results and lead to artifacts in the modeling procedure. The atoms of the active site must be kept within the geometric frame of the protein core, which is absent from **A**, therefore sometimes spurious effects may arise as a result of geometry optimization potentially leading to lethal distortion of the active-site structure. In a concrete model covalent bonds linking side chains or other groups of the active site to atoms in **P** must be split, while the resulting dangling bonds can be saturated by hydrogen atoms, eventually methyl groups. This is quite feasible for apolar single C–C bonds, but for polar links, like C–N or C–O replacement of an atom with another, for which the electronegativity is essentially different from that of hydrogen, it causes spurious charge accumulation at the boundary. Similar effects may occur if multiple bonds are cut. Most preferably, the active site should be constructed by cutting C^α–C^β bonds of the amino-acid residues. A further problem is that hydrogen atoms, used for the saturation of dangling bonds emerging after cutting, may be in steric conflict with some atoms of **P** and this may even lead to convergence problems in quantum mechanical calculations as well as spurious terms in the energy expression within a force field applied in the molecular mechanical calculation. In case of some electron transfer reactions it is very difficult to define the active site atoms appropriately, since localization of an unpaired electron may be uncertain. In these cases, results are very sensitive to the definition of the model, adding or dropping one or two atoms may considerably influence, e.g., the calculated spin density distribution. In such cases, the gradual extension of the size of the model may bring certain saturation in calculated sensitive properties, like charge or spin distribution. In a series of calculations on models with gradually increasing size, the smallest model for which these properties do not change, as compared to previous one, may be appropriate.

Enzymatic mechanisms cannot be understood quantitatively on the basis of active-site models alone. Even in cases, like phosphoryl transfer (*cf.* Section 4.2), where the basic reaction step seems to be determined by covalent bond fission and formation within the active site, electrostatic, steric and hydration effects influence the formation, structure and protonation state of the active site, which may have some or even basic importance. At least two important phenomena, electrostatics and protein fluctuation cannot be reduced solely to the active site; distant protein residues may and quite often do play a role. In case of electrostatics incorporation of atomic monopoles in the model provides often quite good results; however, sophisticated non-quantum mechanical methods are available for the consideration of such effects. Atomic monopoles can be treated as transferable from one protein to the other; this means, however, that mutual polarization between the active site and protein residues is neglected. This approach is quite feasible; but even semi-quantitative agreement with experiment is rarely achieved. Backbone and side-chain fluctuation can be treated on the basis of molecular dynamics (see Section 3); restriction of the number of protein atoms in the model is allowed only, if local effects (e.g., separated side-chain fluctuation) are investigated.

In most cases the overwhelming majority of the bulk, **B**, is water; however, dissolved inorganic ions and eventually other components are quite important when estimating its effect on the reaction process. The dielectric constant of water is large; therefore the effect of **B** on electrostatic factors, influencing the reaction, may be quite important. In a precise model it is not sufficient to consider only **A** and **P**, the influence of **B** must also be estimated some way. Water molecules may influence the outcome of the enzyme reaction by three different ways. One or more molecules may act as proton donor or proton acceptor during reaction, these have to be explicitly included in **A**. Structural water molecules bind quite strongly to the protein core or the surface, because of their reduced mobility they have to be explicitly included in **P**. Locations can be obtained from X-ray diffraction studies, for which results are deposited in the Protein Data Bank. Like for other atoms, belonging to the protein core, electrostatic effect of structural water molecules can be considered by including appropriate point charges in the Hamiltonian. In case of a molecular dynamics study **P** must include all structural water molecules explicitly. The most complicated type of water in biological systems is bulk, for which a manifold of models with varying adequacy is available. It is possible to model the bulk by a finite set of point charges, however, their electrostatic effect converges very slowly, thus a very large number of molecules has to be included. An implicit way is to use an empirically selected dielectric constant in the force field. Because of the strong effect, *i.e.*, the large dielectric constant of bulk water on protein electrostatics, energy differences for various intermediates and transition states of the reaction are reduced to a quite large extent as compared to the corresponding reaction in the gas phase. Accordingly, great care is needed when comparing quantum mechanically computed values to experimental ones. The bulk may contain small inorganic ions (e.g., Na^+, K^+, Ca^{2+}, Cl^-, HO^-), which partly shield the charge of surface side chains, their concentration is characterized by the ionic strength. Counter ions are not fixed; rather they form a loose distribution of charges. Their effect can be best simulated by high-performance methods like the Poisson-Boltzmann equation, to be discussed in the next section. In some cases when the enzyme reaction is diffusion-controlled the process can be described by Brownian dynamics simulation techniques. These are developed to estimate the rate at which the reactant molecules would collide with the active site in the appropriate orientation [7].

The role of protein dynamics in enzyme catalysis is a controversial question in computational enzymology. Some claim that protein dynamics are essential in understanding enzymatic processes, while others state that dynamics is not an important contribution to catalysis. However computer simulations demonstrate the importance of structural fluctuations and the need to include them in the modeling of certain enzyme reactions [8,9]. In some cases, e.g., in processes with significant changes in solvation it is even impossible to correctly predict activation energies if the dynamics of the protein and its active site is not considered in the calculation. In other reactions fluctuations have only a slight effect on the reaction path (see trypsin in Section 4.1).

It is often supposed that entropy effects play an important role in enzyme catalysis by fixing the reaction partners in the proper orientation and thus reducing translational and rotational entropy in the transition state. This means that an "entropy trap" may contribute very much to rate acceleration. However, these effects may be smaller than anticipated since enzyme molecules are quite flexible. For example in case of serine proteases entropic contribution to rate acceleration is relatively small, rather preorganization of the active site to ensure maximum interaction between reacting partners is the basis of rate enhancement [10]. As we will show in Section 4.1 electrostatic stabilization of the active-site complex plays here a prominent role, while in other cases the liberation of water molecules from the active site into bulk solvent may be also crucial.

3. Methods

In this section we give an overview on some popular methods for the quantum mechanical treatment of enzyme reactions, more details can be found in recent reviews [11,12]. It must be stressed that presently available methods cannot be considered as black-box applications, those who apply them must have some experience in judging the reliability of some of their special features. Otherwise, potential artefacts may appear, which become especially dangerous, if remain hidden. For example, in case of an ill-defined model of the boundary between **A** and **P** iteration, needed to reach the quantum mechanical result, may diverge. This is easily detectable, however, if the iteration converges to a false value, the mistake may remain hidden.

Depending on the size of the active site (**A**) and the required accuracy various quantum mechanical methods can be selected for a calculation on the restricted model, **A**, which contains some dozens of atoms. Several software packages are available for the application of these methods at higher or lower accuracy, like the latest version of the GAUSSIAN program package [13], which incorporates several specific applications. In case of enzyme reactions it is a very appealing feature that it allows to compute the reaction path and the activation energy and to determine the structure of reactants and products, which are connected by a given transition structure. Basically, either the *ab initio* molecular orbital [14] or the density functional [15] method can be applied, as far as the size of **A** allows it. If the size of **A** allows, electron correlation can be accounted for in the calculation, which is highly recommended if a covalent bond is formed or cleaved during the enzymatic process. The quantum chemical treatment of transition metal atoms, which are in a number of enzymes essential parts of **A**, is a notoriously difficult task. The metal-ligand interactions are often highly directional and the selection of the appropriate quantum mechanical method is not always straightforward. The problem is even more difficult if the system may exist in several energetically close-lying spin states which are all characterized by different coordination numbers and local geometries. If **A** is very large with more than 200 non-hydrogen atoms, semiempirical methods can be applied which may provide a rough description of the mechanism and pave the way toward a more precise treatment.

Like in case of partitioning of the whole enzyme system into active site, protein core and surrounding bulk, a layering of the quantum region is also possible. It is the ONIOM method, available within the Gaussian package that allows this [16]. The molecular system under investigation is partitioned into three layers, which are described at successively more accurate levels. The innermost one, where bond formation and breaking takes place, is treated with the most accurate method, referring to electron correlation, if necessary. The outermost layer corresponds to **P** + **B** and is treated with molecular mechanics, a semi-empirical or an *ab initio*, small basis set Hartree-Fock method. The middle layer, which is sometimes dropped from the model, is treated with a method of intermediate accuracy between those applied to the high and low-level layers. It is necessary if electronic effects play a role in **P**, which cannot be treated by any molecular force field.

If the size of **P** is too large for a quantum mechanical method molecular mechanics can be applied for the calculation of various hypothetical or real structures and their energies [17]. In this approximation molecular systems are considered in the frame of the classic Newtonian mechanics approach. The energy is expressed as a sum of bond stretching, bending, torsional, non-bonding and cross terms. These contributions are estimated using mathematically very simple expressions; therefore, calculation of energy changes is very fast, several orders of magnitude faster than in the case of quantum mechanical methods. In earlier versions, the parameters of these simple expressions are fitted either to experimentally determined structural quantities, like bond lengths, bond angles, equilibrium torsional angles, vibration spectra, thermochemical and other data. Up-to-date methods of parameterization refer to high-precision quantum mechanical calculations, which is a better approach since direct correspondence between calculated and estimated parameters can be achieved. It is supposed that parameters are transferable within a relatively large set of molecules, which are constructed of similar fragments. Bonded parameters can be approximated quite precisely; bond lengths and angles, as calculated by molecular mechanics, reproduce experimental values very precisely. Determination of non-bonding parameters often means a problem. Van der Waals parameters can be obtained relatively accurately; however, definition and derivation of atomic point charges is not straightforward, even in modern force fields. The basic problem is that the charge distribution of an atom is not perfectly defined by the simple Coulomb monopole expression, dipole and higher moments. Furthermore, polarization and electron delocalization should be considered, too. In some cases the two-atom term additivity does not hold perfectly, three-body and higher interactions may be essential.

For a wide class of biomolecules, including proteins and nucleic acids the AMBER parameterization and software package became very popular. Since its first publication in 1981 it has been further developed several times until it reached its present version [18]. The original AMBER force field and program package was used for the search for energy minima of separate molecular systems in the gas phase. The current versions are aimed more at the simulation of biomolecules in water solution. Both explicit and implicit models for water as well as for some organic solvents are accounted for. Beside AMBER, several other force fields are available in the literature. For example, GROMOS force fields do not consider aliphatic hydrogen atoms. In contrast to most other ones, this parameterization aims primarily at reproducing the free enthalpies of hydration and apolar solvation for a range of organic compounds [19]. A versatile software GROMACS was developed at the University of Groningen, starting twenty years ago [20]. This is a fast program for molecular dynamics simulation, which does not have a force field of its own, but is compatible with several parameterizations. It was developed and optimized for use on PC-clusters. The CHARMM software is also widely used; it has been developed with focus on biomolecules, like proteins. With its newest parameter set it can be used with various energy functions and models, e.g., combined quantum mechanical-molecular mechanical methods, all-atom classical potentials, explicit and implicit solvent models, as well as various boundary conditions [21]. The OPLS force field is also often applied to elucidate enzyme mechanisms [22].

For the treatment of time-dependent phenomena molecular dynamics methods can be used [23]. The term molecular dynamics (MD) typically refers to the propagation of atoms or groups combining several atoms according to the laws of classical mechanics. The forces acting on the particles are calculated only at discrete points along the trajectory. This method allows computer simulation of local or global molecular movements. The atoms of a molecular system are allowed to interact and the trajectories describing their movement can be calculated by solving Newton's equations of motion. Forces between the particles and the potential energy of the system are obtained by expressions from molecular mechanics. For a large number of atoms within most systems investigated, it is impossible to solve these equations analytically; numerical methods are needed. Long simulations are often mathematically ill-conditioned thus errors may accumulate, which can be minimized using appropriate algorithms. Molecular dynamics simulations may be used to determine macroscopic thermodynamic properties by calculating statistical averages.

If quantum effects play a substantive role in the enzymatic process, the *ab initio* molecular dynamics approach can be applied [24]. In this method the quantum mechanical effect of the electrons is included in the calculation of the energy and forces for the classical motion of the atomic nuclei, explicitly including the electrons as active degrees of freedom in the calculation. This is a first principles molecular dynamics approach, which usually employs periodic boundary conditions, plane-wave basis sets, and density functional theory. Application of this method ranges from the thermodynamics of solids and liquids to the study of chemical reactions in solution and quantum mechanical design of enzymes [25]. Referring to the present-day computer capacity, the size of the system studied is limited to about 250 atoms.

Application of classical force fields to enzyme reactions is problematic if covalent bonds are formed or broken during the process. In such cases quantum mechanical (QM) and molecular mechanical (MM) approaches are combined in a variety of hybrid, quantum classical methods denoted by the acronym QM/MM [11,12]. The active site, $\mathbf{A}$, is treated by a quantum mechanical method, while its environment, $\mathbf{P} + \mathbf{B}$, can be described by molecular mechanics. Both Hartee-Fock and density functional methods can be applied in various QM/MM schemes; the latter allows us to include dispersion effects, which is an important feature. The basic assumption in the QM/MM approach is that the system can be partitioned in four regions; accordingly, the Hamiltonian becomes a sum of four terms. Two of them are the QM and MM terms, while the interaction between them (*i.e.*, interaction between $\mathbf{A}$ and $\mathbf{P} + \mathbf{B}$ and their mutual polarization), as well as the boundary between QM and MM regions are treated separately. In most versions polarization of $\mathbf{P}$ by $\mathbf{A}$ (the response) is neglected, thus the mathematical procedure becomes much simpler. The boundary, introduced to mimic the rest of the system, is formed of saturated dangling bonds, which remain after cutting the quantum region out of its environment. Several boundary atom schemes have been developed to avoid the artifacts due to them. Thus, the saturation may be done by hydrogen atoms, dummy centers or special, strictly localized molecular orbitals [26]. A boundary center appears as a normal atom in the molecular mechanical calculation.

In order to provide an accurate thermodynamic description of reaction processes in solution and in enzymes free energy perturbation schemes can be combined with QM/MM calculations [27]. The smooth connection between the QM and MM regions in the boundary is crucial to avoid instabilities during the iterative optimization as well as in the free energy calculations. The basic idea is to sample only the molecular mechanics degrees of freedom while the quantum mechanically related atoms are kept fixed. This allows a significant reduction of the computational effort. Warshel and co-workers proposed that the sampling is based on the empirical valence bond (EVB) scheme [28,29], where parameters are fitted to *ab initio* data [30].

A variety of enzyme processes is determined, or at least influenced, by the electrostatic field of the protein core and the bulk. Quite often, the polarity of transition-state structures is different from those of the initial or final ones, which means that their electrostatic interaction with the environment is also different. Protonation and deprotonation, almost always determined by electrostatics, are also important part of the enzymatic reaction process. Thus, for a precise description of the energetic aspects of the reaction, considering the electrostatic effect of the environment on the various steps of the reaction is crucial. One of the most effective and popular methods for the adequate estimation of protein electrostatics is the solution of the Poisson-Boltzmann equation for the whole system containing $\mathbf{A}$, $\mathbf{P}$ and $\mathbf{B}$, as well [31]. The method is based on the Poisson equation, which relates the spatial variation of the electrostatic potential as a function of the charge density and the dielectric polarizability. In case of a uniform polarizability, represented by a single dielectric constant, and a point charge distribution the Poisson equation is reduced to the simple Coulomb's law. If the polarizability is not uniform, the dielectric constant is a function of spatial co-ordinates. It is possible to consider the effect of ions dissolved in the bulk via representing the mobile ions by a mean-field approximation. The ionic concentration is determined by the Boltzmann equation and replacing the charge density in the Poisson equation by the sum of densities due to dissolved ions and the protein a combination, the Poisson-Boltzmann equation is obtained. This equation can be applied to systems including **A**, **P** and **B**, which is described by a non-uniform dielectric constant. If the protein does not accumulate a high amount of charges, the equation can be linearized allowing a numeric solution. Advanced finite difference methods can be applied with success and a commercial software is available, which can be applied even by the non-specialist [32].

The combined effect of the **P** and **B** regions is recently more and more frequently treated by the Polarizable Continuum Model (PCM) developed by Tomasi and coworkers [33]. This calculates the molecular free energy in solution as the sum of electrostatic and dispersion-repulsion contributions extended by the cavitation energy, which is needed to form the solvent cavity embedding the solute. The electrostatic energy is calculated from point charges located on the molecular surface, which is constructed from spheres representing non-hydrogen atoms with appropriate van der Waals-radii. The dispersion-repulsion contribution is calculated using the solvent accessible surface. The PCM is clearly less precise than the sophisticated Poisson-Boltzmann method; however, it allows much faster calculations. Its use may be amended in cases where the protein core surrounding the active site can be considered as uniform to at least a certain extent. In cases if **P** consists of several ionizable side chains and ionic strength effects in **B** are thought to be important, the Poisson-Boltzmann method is recommended.

4. Case Studies

4.1. Electrostatic Catalysis: Serine Proteases

Over one third of known proteolytic enzymes are serine proteases [34]. They are found both in prokaryotes as well as in eukaryotes and cleave covalent peptide bonds of proteins. At the molecular level this is a very important event in case of several life processes. For example, serine proteases digest food for bacteria and help viruses to infect cells. These enzymes co-ordinate various physiological functions in humans, e.g., digestion, immune response, blood coagulation as well as reproduction. They were given this name because their active site includes a highly reactive serine side chain, which is crucial for catalytic activity and is part of a Ser-His-Asp triad, which is buried in the protein core. The mechanism of action is identical in the various members of the serine protease family; they differ only in substrate specificity. The spatial arrangement of amino acids in the triad is optimized for catalysis by convergent evolution at the molecular level [35].

Serine protease-catalyzed hydrolysis of the peptide bond is a reaction involving a tetrahedral intermediate (see Figure 2). During catalysis a nucleophilic attack by the serine hydroxyl group on the carbonyl carbon atom of the substrate is helped by the histidine imidazole group as a general base. This leads to formation of a tetrahedral intermediate and an imidazolium ion. In a subsequent step the tetrahedral intermediate is broken down by general acid catalysis to an acyl-enzyme, an imidazole base and an amine product. During the acylation step, the imidazole group transfers the proton of the serine hydroxyl to the amine leaving group. The acyl-enzyme is then deacylated through the reverse reaction pathway of acylation, but in the second addition-elimination reaction a water molecule instead of the serine residue is the attacking nucleophile.

Figure 2. Reaction steps during serine protease catalyzed cleavage of the peptide bond (**left**). The acyl-enzyme intermediate hydrolyses via the reverse route (**right**).

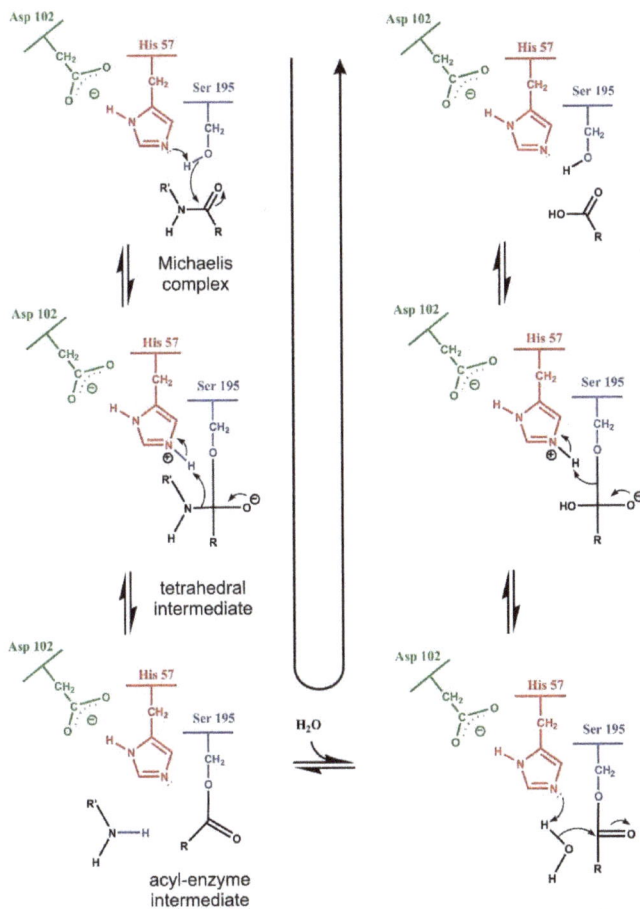

Crucial step of the reaction is the formation of the tetrahedral intermediate, facilitated by the surrounding oxyanion hole, stabilizing the intermediate by hydrogen bonds (see Figure 3). Backbone amide groups form hydrogen bonds with the strongly polarized oxygen atom, keeping the carbonyl bond in the right position for a nucleophilic attack and stabilizing the intermediate structure. Formation of the oxyanion hole is a general feature of serine proteases and it is precisely tailored for the oxygen atom. Thionoester substrates, containing sulfur with a somewhat larger atomic radius than the oxygen atom, are not hydrolyzed by chymotrypsin and subtilisin, although they do not differ significantly from esters in reactivity [36]. The contribution of the oxyanion binding site to the catalytic rate acceleration was estimated by replacing the hydrogen-bond donor Asn155 of subtilisin with a neutral glycine residue. This lowered k_{cat} for a specific substrate by a factor of 150 to 300, however, did not alter the Michaelis constant, K_M at all. Thus, it can be concluded that the binding site contributes only to transition-state stabilization and leaves the binding power unaffected [37].

Figure 3. The oxyanion hole stabilizing the tetrahedral intermediate in α-chymotrypsin. Backbone amide NH groups of Gly193 and Ser195 form hydrogen bonds with the amide oxygen atom of the substrate.

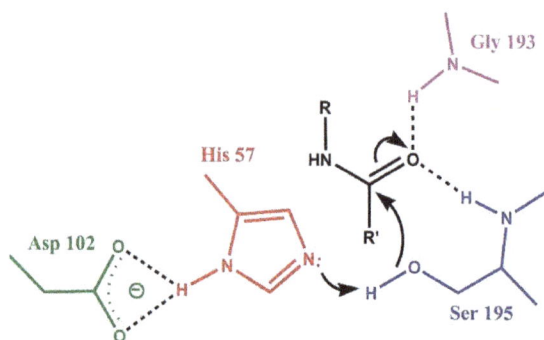

X-ray diffraction studies have shown that catalysis is assisted by a hydrogen-bonded triad of amino-acid side chains. A buried aspartate is linked to the imidazole moiety of histidine, which binds to the catalytic serine hydroxyl group (see Figure 2) [38]. The geometric relation of the Asp, His and Ser side chains allows assuming that histidine serves for transferring the proton from Ser to Asp in a mechanism called charge relay. However, since proton transfer from the highly basic serine hydroxyl group to the acidic carboxylate side chain of aspartate is unlikely, it was supposed that the role of the buried aspartate is the stabilization of the ion-pair formed by the positive imidazoliun ion and the negatively charged-tetrahedral intermediate [39]. Nuclear magnetic resonance [40] and neutron diffraction [41] studies have confirmed that it is the imidazole and not the aspartate that is protonated.

The stabilizing role of the buried aspartate is also supported by site-directed mutagenesis. Replacement of Asp102 of trypsin with a neutral Ala residue results in a reduction of four orders of magnitude in the rate constant. It is evident from the three-dimensional structure of the mutant enzyme that the catalytic His57 is unable to accept proton from Ser195 [42]. Studies on the D641A mutant of prolyl oligopeptidase, belonging to another family of serine proteases, also indicate the importance of the negative charge of the buried aspartate [43]. It is thus quite clear that it electrostatically stabilizes the ion pair formed in the transition state. This has been shown by empirical valence bond free energy calculations, too [44]. It has been found that in trypsin and subtilisin the buried aspartate contributes to the stabilization of the transition state by 26 (25) and 17 (25) kJ/mol, respectively (experimental values are in parentheses). These calculations clarified the role of the buried aspartate side chain, which is electrostatic stabilization of the ion pair formed between the positive imidazolium side chain and the negative tetrahedral intermediate rather than proton transfer to its carboxylate.

It is interesting to note that mutation of all three members of the catalytic triad to alanine does not reduce activity to zero. This implies that the catalytic triad is not the sole source of the enzyme activity since even in its absence the mutant enzyme hydrolyzes substrates three orders of magnitude faster relative to the reaction in water. This remaining activity may arise from the contribution of stabilization by the preorganized binding pocket and the oxyanion hole. Calculations by Warshel and coworkers provide ample evidence for the crucial role of electrostatic effects due to the preorganization of active sites, which strongly stabilize the transition states of enzymatic reactions [45,46]. Such a preorganization could happen via convergent evolution organizing the hydrogen-bond network around the catalytic triad in such a way that it stabilizes the (- + -) charge distribution. Poisson-Boltzmann electrostatic calculations provided relative stabilization energies, calculated as the electrostatic interaction energy of atoms of the catalytic triad with the protein environment. These numbers reflect changes in relative experimental enzyme activities, proportional to log k_{cat}/k_M for the same substrate, correctly (*cf.* Table 1) [47].

Table 1. Calculated relative electrostatic interaction energies, *vs.* relative experimental enzyme activities (kJ/mol) of the catalytic triad in some serine proteases.

Enzyme	Calculated	Experimental
subtilisin Carlsberg	−102.6	−36.5
α-chymotrypsin	−71.9	−34.2
subtilisin NOVO	−62.1	−31.6
β-trypsin	−40.7	−26.7
α-lytic protease	9.3	0.3

On the basis of the above and other calculations we may say that enzymes, acting as a "supersolvent", can strongly stabilize polar structures, like ion pairs or the charge distribution located in their active sites. Stabilization in enzymes is stronger than in water, since preorganized and fixed protein dipoles are almost optimally oriented at the active site. The enzyme, therefore, provides a preoriented environment that stabilizes the transition state of the reaction. In contrary, water dipoles are distributed randomly and have to reorient in order to stabilize transition states. Reduction of the preorganization free energy in the enzyme is due to its folding into its final configuration, which precedes the catalytic process and takes place independently, during protein synthesis.

Even if we have diverse experimental evidence for the elucidation of the mechanism of action, direct information, especially on energetic aspects, can be obtained only from molecular modeling. Results should be in line with experimental observation, furthermore, providing subtle details, which cannot be obtained from experiments. For serine proteases, the crucial role of protein electrostatics in enzymatic rate acceleration can be discussed in appropriate detail only by calculation [48]. Early quantum mechanical approaches were based on gas-phase models containing the catalytic triad and the minimum-size substrate [49]. Such models could be extended by consideration of protein electrostatic effects on the reaction process [50]. It was shown by *ab initio* calculations that the electrostatic interaction originating from the hydrogen bond network involving residues around the buried aspartate plays a significant role in lowering the barrier height of the proton transfer. Later on, the basic statements of the above calculations were supported by further studies. Ishida and Kato [51] performed calculations on the entire reaction path of the acylation step catalyzed by trypsin using *ab initio* QM/MM methods combined with molecular dynamics. It was found that the rate-determining step is the formation of the tetrahedral intermediate, while breakdown of the intermediate has a small energy barrier. Their calculated activation free energy is 75 kJ/mol. It was shown that the proton transfer from Ser to His and the nucleophilic attack of Ser to the carbonyl carbon of the scissile bond are concerted. The most important catalytic factor of stabilizing the tetrahedral intermediate is the electrostatic interaction between the active site and the protein core. Topf and Richards [52] studied the deacylation step of serine protease catalysis using extended quantum mechanical calculations on a model containing all protein atoms and the bulk as a continuum. The calculations show that in the enzyme the tetrahedral intermediate is a relatively stable species lying 30 kJ/mol lower in energy than the transition state. The stabilization is mainly due to the electrostatic effect provided by the oxyanion hole and the buried aspartate. The rate-determining step of the reaction is proton transfer from the attacking water molecule to the histidine side chain; the activation energy is about 92 kJ/mol, 21 kJ/mol, less than for the reference reaction in water, and close to the value obtained by Ishida and Kato.

Hudáky and Perczel [53] built a model of the catalytic triad of chymotrypsin containing 18 amino acid residues of the enzyme and its substrate. They found that this model forms a molecule ensemble, which is stable in itself. They obtained an activation barrier of 85 kJ/mol, just between those obtained by the above two groups. Calculations allowed locating elements of the catalytic machinery, which are responsible for the stabilization of the transition state. Most important of these are the catalytic aspartate (by 27 kJ/mol) and the oxyanion hole (by 57 kJ/mol). The full reaction path is displayed in Figure 4. The acylation mechanism of trypsin and its complete free energy reaction profile have been determined also by Born-Oppenheimer *ab initio* QM/MM molecular dynamics simulations with umbrella sampling [54].

Figure 4. Reaction energy profile of the chymotrypsin-catalyzed cleavage of a model substrate (after Hudáky and Perczel [53]). Note that the tetrahedral intermediates as well as the acyl enzyme represent local minima.

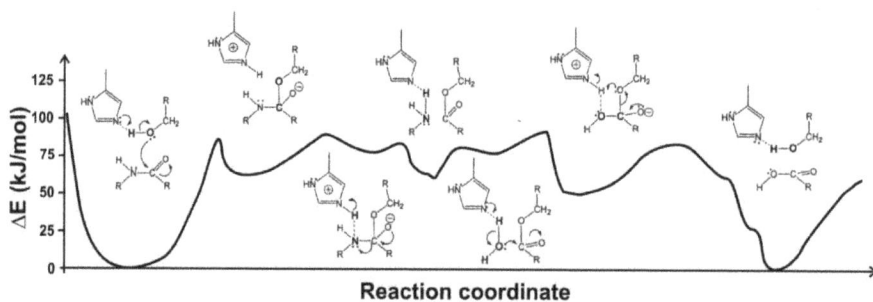

4.2. Phosphoryl Transfer

Phosphoryl transfer belongs to the most important molecular reactions in living systems. These are involved in DNA replication, signal transduction, metabolism and transcription, furthermore they ensure the production of chemical energy, which is required as a driving force for important processes within living cells [4]. Phosphoryl transfer may be catalyzed by kinases, mutases, phosphatases or endonucleases. Along such reactions enormous, even as large as 10^{27}-fold, rate acceleration is observed as compared to the corresponding non-enzymatic process. Despite their central importance, because of the complicated structure of the catalyst, no final information is available about the details of the process although intensive research has been conducted since decades.

Three different types of reaction paths can be considered for enzymatic and non-enzymatic phosphoryl transfer reactions, these are outlined in Figure 5. In the dissociative mechanism (Figure 5, top) a stepwise displacement takes place via a solvated planar metaphosphate intermediate, while in the associative mechanism (Figure 5, bottom) the reaction proceeds via a trigonal bipyramidal phosphorane intermediate. In both cases the intermediates are locally stable; they represent a local minimum on the reaction energy path. In contrast, in case of the S_N2-type concerted displacement the pentacoordinated phosphorane structure represents a transition state represented by a maximum on the reaction energy profile.

Figure 5. Reaction paths for phosphoryl transfer reactions. (a) Dissociative (top); (b) associative (middle); (c) S_N2-type (bottom) mechanism. Square brackets represent the transition state.

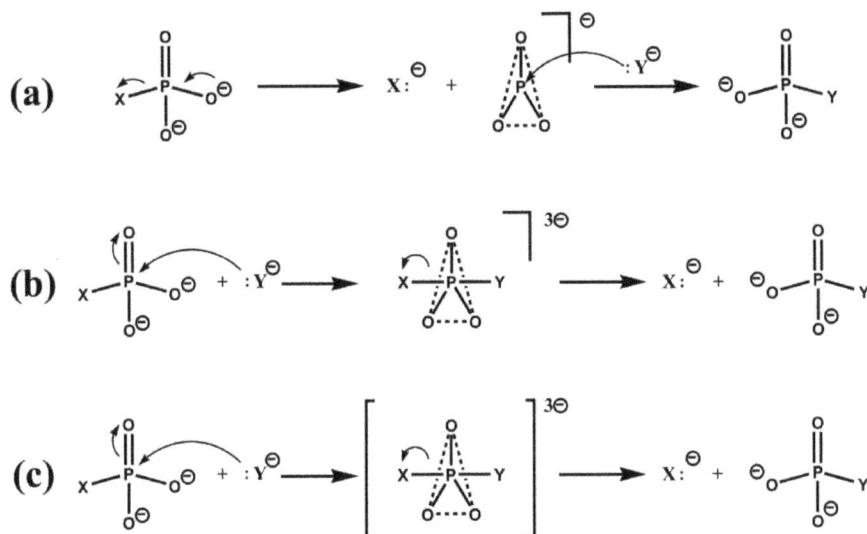

According to Florián and Warshel [55] both associative and dissociative mechanisms may be operative in the aqueous phase. On the other hand, as stated by Herschlag et al. [4] for phosphate monoesters considerable experimental evidence supports a concerted reaction mechanism, where no stable intermediate, rather a transition state can be located on the reaction path. Furthermore, they state that enzymatic catalysis generally does not influence the structure of transition states as compared to those in solution. While this might be true in some cases, we found on the basis of density functional calculations on a model of HIV integrase that metal ions, located at the active site, as well as the electrostatic effect of the protein core considerably reduces the activation energy [56]. The high (295 kJ/mol) reaction barrier in the gas-phase reduces to less than the half, 141 kJ/mol, within the enzyme. This means that the protein environment has an important impact on the reaction, which is partly due to the fact that electrostatic repulsion is reduced in the active site due to a diffuse charge distribution. The nucleophile is only partially charged in the transition state. A further effect is that of the doubly positively charged magnesium ion at the active site, which reduces the barrier height by 42 kJ/mol. A similar result using the density functional theory was obtained for the hydrolysis of guanosine triphosphate [57]. Accordingly, combined geometric and electrostatic effects may play an important role in rate acceleration, like in case of hydrolytic reactions catalyzed by serine proteases (see Section 4.1).

While several experimental arguments can be mentioned strengthening the hypothesis that the concerted mechanism may be operative in enzymes, two different X-ray studies seemed to support the associative mechanism, *i.e.*, the formation of a relatively stable phosphorane intermediate during the catalytic process. Lahiri and coworkers thought to locate such a pentacovalent structure (an XPO_3Y moiety) in the phosphoryl transfer reaction catalyzed by β-phosphoglucomutase [58]. However, their results have been questioned by Blackburn *et al.* [59] who suggested that this structure represents an MgF_3^- transition-state analogue, which is hydrogen-bonded to ligands at the binding site. Subsequent evidence from ^{19}F and ^{31}P nuclear magnetic resonance, further X-ray experiments, and kinetic data [60] as well as quantum mechanical calculations [61,62] provided strong support for this latter assignment. A second example of a potentially trapped high-energy intermediate has been published by Barabás *et al.* [63]. Crystal structure of the complex with a special substrate, α,β-imino-dUTP, was determined. In this case the catalytic process slowed down considerably; therefore the reaction path could be followed by localizing snapshot structures. A relatively stable intermediate was thought to be trapped, for which the crystal structure is available. However, the resolution of the active site structure was not enough to present a convincing argument, so the final proof that the associative mechanism is operative in these enzymes is not yet available.

Quantum mechanical studies on various enzymes catalyzing phosphoryl transfer support different mechanisms. Our early calculations for HIV integrase [56] indicate that an S_N2-type mechanism may be effective. We calculated the reaction path carefully and found a very shallow minimum, rather a shoulder on the reactant side (*cf.* Figure 6). This means that if environmental effects, mainly electrostatics, influences the stability of the transition-state complex, under certain circumstances a locally stable phosphorane intermediate can be formed. Thus, the associative reaction route may be realized. Studies for the DNA repair enzyme endonuclease IV [64] as well as for cyclin-dependent kinase [65,66], DNA polymerase [67] and phosphodiesterase [68] support S_N2-type concerted mechanisms, too. A recent study stresses that a water mediated and substrate assisted mechanism is followed in DNA polymerase, and provides an asymmetric intermediate, which is stabilized by nearby amino-acid residues [69]. This intermediate transforms to the product via a pentacovalent phosphorane transition state, which remains stable for over a nanosecond of MD simulation. This study provides further support for the concerted mechanism because the lifetime of a true phosphorane intermediate should be much longer.

Figure 6. Quantum mechanically calculated reaction profile for the phosphoryl transfer reaction catalyzed by HIV integrase (figure drawn on the basis of Ref. 56).

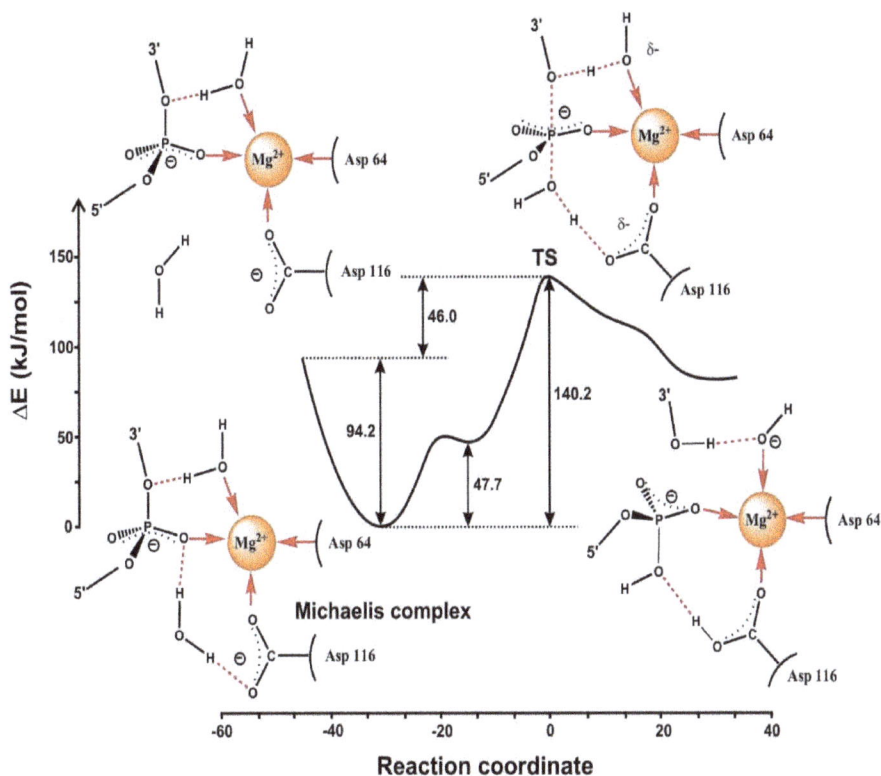

Ab initio QM/MM studies on phoshoenol-pyruvate (PEP) mutase suggest that the catalytic reaction follows a concerted mechanism with a planar trigonal transition state representing metaphosphate (see Figure 7) [70]. This mechanism is consistent with the failure in detecting the putative intermediate in rapid quench experiments and is in line with the statement of Herschlag and coworkers, who call for a concerted reaction mechanism in case of phosphate monoesters [4]. It is interesting to note that the transition state is planar trigonal, in contrast to other cases, where it is thought to be trigonal bipyramidal. Making a distinction between potentially existing structures of transition states complicates appropriate selection of a given mechanism, since it often leaves out of consideration, whether the given structure represents a local minimum or a maximum on the reaction energy profile. At present it is not possible to collect direct experimental evidence for the existence of a given structure in the transition state, since its lifetime is practically zero. Quantum mechanical calculations can provide concrete models, like in Figure 6; however, these may not reproduce experimental data sufficiently accurately, and therefore conclusions on such basis are often questioned. York and coworkers studied the uncatalyzed conversion of PEP to phosphonopyruvate and they have found that due to the large negative charge located at the active site, solvation has a crucial effect on the reaction pathway [71].

Figure 7. Molecular graphics model of the transition state in the reaction catalyzed by phoshoenol-pyruvate (PEP) mutase (on the basis of Figure 3 by Xu and Guo [70]). Note the planar metaphosphate intermediate stabilized by hydrogen bonds to amino-acid residues of the active site.

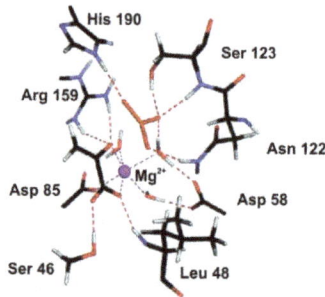

Figure 8. Two possible reaction routes for the hydrolysis of ribonuclease H. Top: schematic structure of the active site, bottom: blue line: attack by a water molecule, red line: attack by a hydroxyl group (figure drawn on the basis of Figure 3 of Ref. 72).

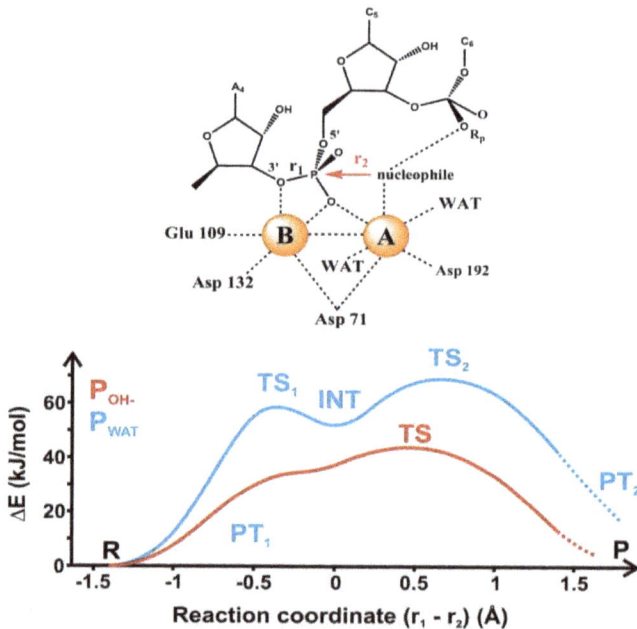

Two recent sophisticated quantum mechanical studies indicate that in ribonuclease H the phosphodiester cleavage occurs via an associative mechanism [72,73]. These calculations indicate that as the reaction approaches the barrier, one of the protons of the attacking water molecule transfers to one of the oxygen atoms of the phosphate group and a penta-coordinated phosphorane intermediate is formed. The calculated energy barrier is consistent with the experimental rate found for the human enzyme. *De vivo* and coworkers made a distinction between the attack of a neutral water molecule and a negatively charged hydroxyl group [72]. They have found that in both cases an in-line S_N2-like nucleophilic attack takes place on the central phosphorus atom. This results in an associative mechanism with phosphorane-like transition states, in agreement with crystal structures of transition- state analogues [74]. It is interesting that the attack of a water molecule leads to the formation of a meta-stable pentavalent phosphorane intermediate, as depicted in Figure 8. This is a unique characteristic of the energy profile of the reaction, which has not been observed in previous computational studies. Like in e.g., xylose isomerase (see below), one or more structural water molecules near the active site may facilitate the reaction [75,76].

Warshel and coworkers [77] compared the associative and dissociative mechanisms of phosphate monoester hydrolysis on the example of the methyl phosphate dianion and the methyl pyrophosphate trianion in aqueous solution. They have found that, in good agreement with experimental findings, both associative and dissociative transition states have near-zero entropies of activation. This means that near-zero activation entropy is not indicative of a dissociative pathway, as supposed earlier.

4.3. Long-Range Electron Transfer in Heme Peroxidases

Peroxidases oxidize a variety of substrates by reacting with hydrogen peroxide. In most cases the typical substrates are small aromatic molecules, however, in case of cytochrome c peroxidase (CCP) a protein, cytochrome c, is the redox partner. The overall reaction mechanism is given in Scheme 1. Several peroxidase structures were determined by X-ray diffraction (e.g., yeast cytochrome c peroxidase [78], lignin peroxidase (LIP) [79], pea cytosolic ascorbate peroxidase (APX) [80], and horseradish peroxidase (HRP) [81]. On this basis it is possible to construct a model of the active site (see Figure 9). A histidine and an aspartic acid side chain are present in the proximal heme pocket in all these structures, whereas the proximal tryptophan is only present in CCP and APX.

Scheme 1. Reaction mechanism of heme peroxidases. P is the porphyrin group of the enzyme whose heme iron is indicated, S is the substrate.

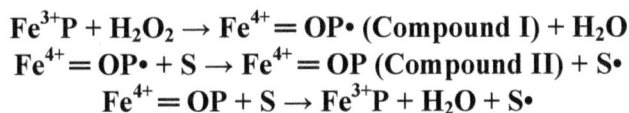

$$Fe^{3+}P + H_2O_2 \rightarrow Fe^{4+} = OP\bullet \text{ (Compound I)} + H_2O$$
$$Fe^{4+} = OP\bullet + S \rightarrow Fe^{4+} = OP \text{ (Compound II)} + S\bullet$$
$$Fe^{4+} = OP + S \rightarrow Fe^{3+}P + H_2O + S\bullet$$

In the first step of the catalytic process (*cf.* Scheme 1 and Figure 10) the peroxide removes two electrons from the enzyme and the so-called Compound I is formed. During this process the peroxide O–O bond is broken, water is produced and the second oxygen atom of the peroxide remains coordinated to the metal, which loses one electron to give an oxy-ferryl intermediate ($Fe^{4+} = O$). A second electron is removed from the heme providing a cation radical. In the next step, P• is reduced and a substrate radical, S• is formed. Finally, in the last step Compound II is reduced by a second substrate molecule.

236

Figure 9. Schematic active-site models of cytochrome *c* peroxidase (CCP) (**left**) and ascorbate peroxidase (APX) (**right**). Top: distal position, bottom: proximal position, a separated red dot represents a water molecule (figure drawn on the basis of the crystal structures 1ZBZ and 2XI6).

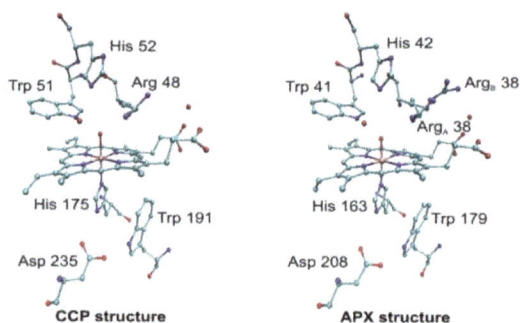

Figure 10. Catalytic mechanism of the formation of Compound I. The distal His assists in removing a proton from the incoming peroxide and delivering it to the peroxide O_2 atom.

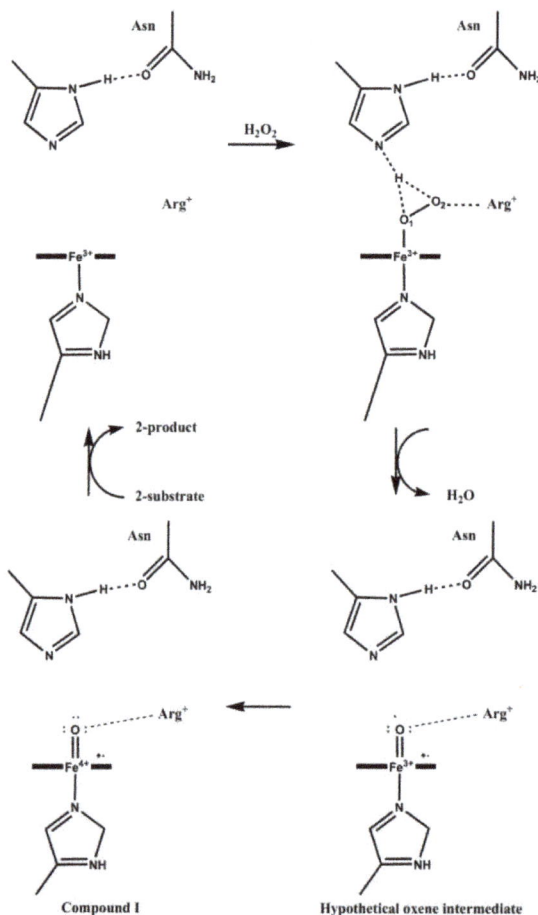

Discussing the mechanism at the computational level an interesting problem arises. APX shares 33% global sequence identity with CCP and has a very similar active site structure [82]. Despite very similar protein structures, APX and CCP stabilize different radical species during enzyme turnover. At variance with CCP, in APX the free electron is shifted to the porphyrin ring of the active site during reaction. This difference is thought to contribute to the different substrate specificities of the two proteins. Earlier, we suggested, on the basis of *ab inito*, minimal basis set molecular orbital and Poisson-Boltzmann electrostatic potential calculations that both in APX and CCP proton transfer involving the proximal histidine (His163 or His175), the radical-forming tryptophan (Trp179 and Trp191), and a nearby aspartic acid (Asp208 and Asp235) side chains may control the location of the radical state [83]. Both molecular orbital and electrostatic potential calculations suggest that the spin distribution depends on the protonation state of the proximal His...Asp...Trp triad. If the transferable proton is shifted from the Trp side chain to Asp, the free electron is localized on the indole group, while if it remains on Trp the unpaired electron transfers to the heme group. Therefore, in Compound I of CCP Trp is supposed to be deprotonated, while in case of APX it is supposed to be protonated and neutral. Protonation state of the side chains is influenced by the electrostatic effect of the protein environment, which differs in these enzymes, especially in the immediate vicinity of the Asp side chain.

The above hypothesis is not supported by some other calculations. Warshel and coworkers applied the empirical Protein Dipoles Langevin Dipoles method and found that the electrostatic effect of the protein environment of CCP stabilizes the tryptophan cation radical by 330 mV relative to that in APX. They proposed that mainly the cation binding site contributes to radical stabilization, but is not the sole cause [84]. The study by Siegbahn and coworkers [85] supports the mechanism, which has been proposed on the basis of X-ray diffraction studies. They have found that if the proximal His-Asp-Trp triad of both enzymes is included in the computational model the free electron of the cationic radical is shared between the porphyrin ring and the protonated histidine side chain. The difference in ionization potential between tryptophan and porphyrin ring in the oxyferryl form of APX and CCP seems to be small. This strengthens the statement that location of the free electron depends on subtle differences of the protein environment in both enzymes. It has been shown that location of the protein radical in APX is most probably Trp179 [86]. Quantum mechanical optimization of the crystal structure of the active site in CCP show that the geometric differences of the two states are quite small and it cannot be decided where the proton is in the crystal structure [87]. QM/MM calculations indicate that the proton is located on the His ligand in all states in the reaction mechanism. According to de Visser [88] the quartet-doublet energy splitting is strongly dependent on local perturbations. Even a point charge far away from the tryptophan radical can transfer the system from a mixed porphyrin-tryptophan radical into a pure porphyrin or tryptophan radical. These perturbations cause varying quartet-doublet energy splitting, which eventually may influence reactivity. Calculations by Mulholland and coworkers [89] reproduced the observed difference in electronic structure, and called the attention to the subtle electrostatic effects which may affect the ionization state of both the tryptophan and porphyrin groups. Their calculations did not support the deprotonation of the tryptophan group, or protonation of the oxoferryl oxygen atom. The remarkable difference in electronic structure between the compound I intermediates in CCP and APX seems to be due to differences in the electrostatic potential around the key groups in the two enzymes.

On the basis of their QM/MM calculations Thiel and coworkers concluded that in another heme peroxidase, horseradish peroxidase the proximal ligand is imidazole and not imidazolate [90].Similar conclusions were drawn by Jensen and Ryde for reduced models of heme proteins [91]. A recent review on QM/MM calculations for heme proteins is also available [92], while the catalase activity of heme peroxidases is treated by Vlasitsa et al. [93]. Harris and Loew [94] performed density functional calculations and showed that the imidazolate/Asp-H and imidazole/Asp⁻ tautomers are very close in energy (the difference is 4 kJ/mol), but only the first representation reproduces the observed shift in the Soret band of Compound I in horseradish peroxidase as compared to chloroperoxidase.

4.4. Cytochrome P450 Enzymes

Cytochrome P450 enzymes (P450s) form a huge superfamily of thiolate-ligated heme enzymes with more than 10,000 members sequenced up-to date. They can be found in almost all living organisms, in bacteria and archaea, in fungi, plants and animals indicating the ancient nature of these enzymes. The great variety of P450s can be attributed to their vital role: they defend the organisms from xenobiotics by oxidizing them to products that can be excreted more easily. As the structure and properties of xenobiotics may differ almost indefinitely, during evolution a very large number of P450s have evolved [95], in some cases acquiring new functions as well. P450s also play a vital role in hormone biosynthesis in mammals, e.g., in man they are responsible for the aromatization of androstenedione and testosterone to estrone and estradiol [96]. In the following we present three case studies, which may shed light on some interesting issues related to P450s.

4.4.1. Is the Oxidizing Power of Active Species of Various P450 Isoforms the Same?

The catalytic cycle of P450s consists of many electron or proton transfer steps [97], which leads to the formation of Compound I, the ultimate oxidizing species carrying out the oxidation reaction. The species is very reactive and elusive that has only been recently observed [98]. Compound I has low-lying quartet and doublet spin states, which differ in energy by less than 4 kJ/mol. In both states there are two electrons in the Fe–O π^* antibonding orbitals which can be coupled via an anti- or ferromagnetic scheme to the porphyrin a_{2u} orbital with significant contribution from the sulfur p orbital giving rise to the doublet and quartet states. (Figure 11). As several P450 isoforms are responsible for the metabolism of drugs taken by man several crucial questions have been raised: (1) does the reactivity of the different isoforms depend on the oxidizing power of the isoform; (2) is the oxidizing power of Compound I of the different isoforms very similar? As the active site of the different isoforms shows great variability it may tune the reactivity of the oxidizing species and influence the regioselectivity of the enzyme [99,100], which has been called "chameleon" behavior [101]. Therefore, a systematic study involving three human P450 isoforms (P450 2D6, P450 2C9, P450 3A4) and a bacterial enzyme (P450$_{cam}$) has been conducted in the presence and absence of substrate in the active site in order to reveal the similarities and differences between the active species of these isoforms [102]. Dextromethorphan was used as a substrate of P450 2D6 and P450 3A4, warfarin as the substrate of P450 2C9, and propene as the substrate of P450$_{cam}$. 5ns long molecular dynamics simulations were run on the ligand-free and ligand bound enzymes and every 200 ps a snapshot has been taken (altogether 26 for each system) that was subjected to QM/MM optimization, in the quartet spin state. After the QM/MM optimization of each snapshot, the oxo group bonded to the iron was deleted and a single point calculation was carried out to estimate the energy of the resting state of the enzyme.

Figure 11. Singly occupied molecular orbitals of Compound I.

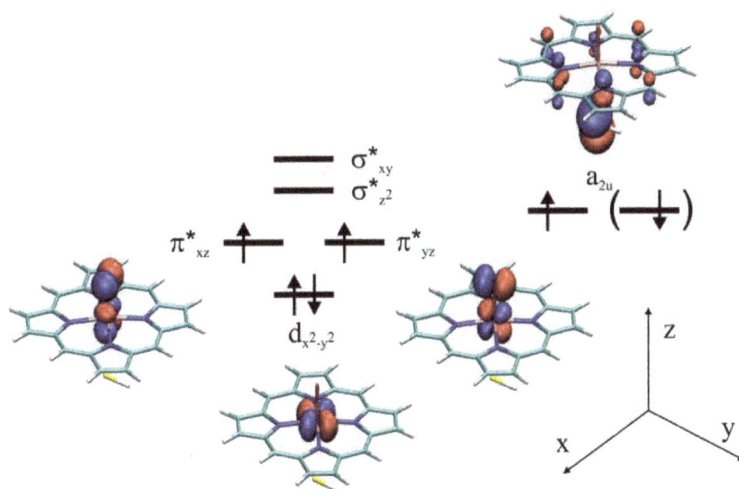

The thermodynamic cycle, shown in Figure 12, depicts the importance of the Fe–O bond enthalpy (ΔE_2) calculated in the study. ΔE_1 includes the energy of oxidation of the substrate by Compound I to form the product and the resting state of the heme. Its value is dependent on the substrate, and could be expressed as $\Delta E_1 = \Delta E_2 + \Delta E_3$, where ΔE_2 is the energy required to break the Fe–O bond in Compound I, and ΔE_3 is the energy released upon addition of the oxygen atom to the substrate to yield the product. ΔE_2 is independent of the substrate, and smaller values correspond to a more reactive and oxidizing state of Compound I. In our study ΔE_2 was estimated as $\Delta E_2 = E_{QM}(O) + E_{QM}(Fe) - E_{QM}(Fe^*) + E_{QM/MM}(Fe^*) - E_{QM/MM}(FeO)$, where $E_{QM}(O)$ is the energy of oxygen *in vacuo* in the triplet state, $E_{QM}(Fe) - E_{QM}(Fe^*)$ accounts for the relaxation energy of the resting state of the heme complex compared to the structure in Compound I and for the energy difference between the sextet and doublet states of the resting state (103 kJ/mol). $E_{QM/MM}(Fe^*)$ was obtained by a single-point calculation on the QM/MM optimized geometry of Compound I by deleting the oxygen atom from it $E_{QM/MM}(FeO)$ is the QM/MM energy of Compound I. The last two quantities were calculated for each snapshot and averaged over each system.

Figure 12. Thermodynamic cycle showing the relationship between ΔE_1, ΔE_2, (Fe-O bond enthalpy) and ΔE_3.

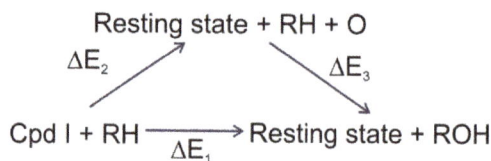

$$\text{Resting state + RH + O}$$

$$\Delta E_2 \nearrow \qquad \searrow \Delta E_3$$

$$\text{Cpd I + RH} \xrightarrow[\Delta E_1]{} \text{Resting state + ROH}$$

In order to assess the electronic configuration of the oxidizing species, structural data (especially the Fe–S bond length), and charge and spin density data (on the Fe, O, S atoms and the porphyrin ring) have been collected and compared. All these data indicated that Compound I of the P450s is very similar in the studied human isoforms, as variation of the data for the different snapshots taken for a given isoform was larger than the variation between isoforms. However, the bacterial P450$_{cam}$ isoform showed an increased spin density on sulfur compared to the human isoforms. It has been suggested that the different hydrogen bonding environment of the sulfur atom could be the main reason behind it. In P450s the axial cysteinate ligand of the heme is hydrogen bonded to the amide groups of the three consecutive amino acids of the protein chain as depicted for P450 2D6 in Figure 13, and one of the hydrogen bonds to sulfur was found to be much stronger in P450$_{cam}$ than in the human isoforms. Upon substrate binding a slight decrease in the spin density of sulfur was observed in all cases, which was attributed to the displacement of water molecules from the active site, thereby changing its polarity. These results imply that the properties of Compound I are sensitive to changes in the hydrogen bonding environment and also to polarization effects exerted by the active site.

Figure 13. Quantum mechanical/molecular mechanical (QM/MM) optimized snapshot of Compound I with residues hydrogen-bonded to the axial cysteinate in P450 2D6.

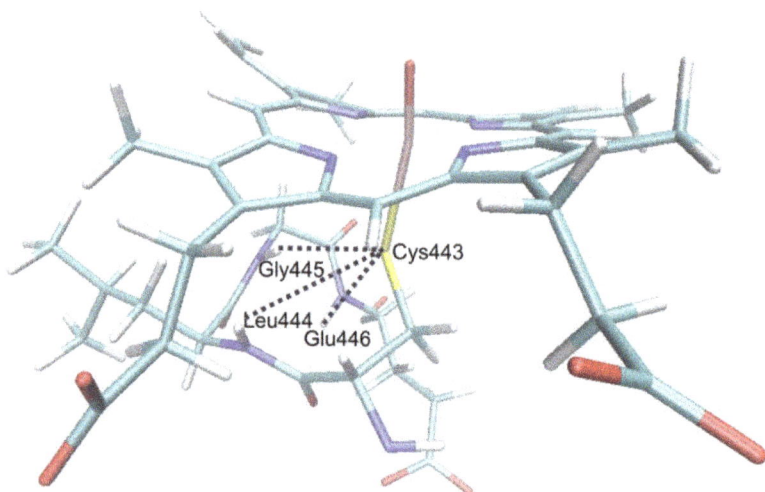

The Fe–O bond enthalpy does not show great variability over the various isoforms either, as its variation is on the order of the same magnitude for the different snapshots of a given isoform as those between the various isoforms. This result suggests a similar oxidizing power for the different isoforms, which is slightly lowered in the presence of the substrate in the active site. This latter effect is most likely due to the fact that the substrate expels the water out of the active site and decreases the number of hydrogen bonds to the ferryl oxygen. As a consequence the spin density on oxygen increases and the charge associated to it decreases. It was also shown that structures with largest spin density on oxygen have the lowest Fe–O bond enthalpy.

The overall conclusion of this study is that active species of the studied P450 isoforms exhibited very similar properties; therefore, it is reasonable to assume that the reactivity of Compounds I of different isoforms will be very similar. However, it was also shown that the electronic structure of Compound I varies with thermal fluctuations, therefore conclusions drawn on a single QM/MM optimized snapshot may not be necessarily reliable and it could be more appropriate to average the data over a number of structures.

4.4.2. Metabolism of Dextromethorphan by P450 2D6: What Drives the Regioselectivity of the Enzymes?

Most P450s are promiscuous enzymes: a substrate molecule may be metabolized by various P450 isoforms leading to different products. A good example of this is the case of dextromethorphan, a common antitussive compound, which is even frequently used in various experimental studies of the P450 2D6 enzyme. In the human body, dextromethorphan is metabolized by P450 3A4 yielding an *N*-demethylated product (see Figure 14), while *O*-demethylation is catalyzed by P450 2D6 [103]. In contrast, the aromatic ring of this compound is not oxidized, despite the fact that aromatic oxidation of other aromatic ethers have been observed in rat [104] and rabbit [105]. The interesting metabolic properties of dextromethorphan make it a good candidate for the computational study of the factors influencing the regioselectivity of P450 isoforms. Earlier computation studies showed that in general the barrier of *N*-demethylation is lower than that of O-demethylation [106], therefore it is not astonishing that P450 3A4, which has a large active site capable of accommodating two substrate molecules and in which the substrate may be oriented in any position catalyzes the thermodynamically favored *N*-demethylation. However, it is more surprising that P450 2D6 only catalyzes the *O*-demethylation despite that fact that the aromatic ring is located close to the heme iron as well.

In order to clarify this problem, we conducted a study to investigate the factors influencing the regioselectivity of P450 2D6 [107]. First we carried out gas-phase quantum mechanical calculations on a model system (shown in Figure 15) to get an idea about the relative energy barriers of hydrogen abstraction from the methoxy group. This is the rate-determining step of *O*-demethylation, and of aromatic oxidation. Both reactions have a lower barrier in the doublet spin state than in the quartet spin state, 50.2 kJ/mol for hydrogen abstraction and 64.0 kJ/mol for aromatic oxidation. Although the barrier for *O*-demethylation is lower, the difference between the barriers of the two reaction channels does not explain why only *O*-demethylation is observed.

Figure 14. Metabolic routes of dextromethorphan in man as indicated by arrows.

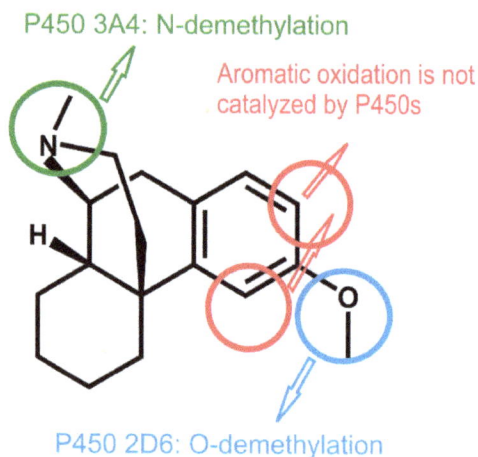

Figure 15. (a) QM region used in the calculations (b) Barriers of *O*-demethylation and aromatic carbon oxidation obtained from quantum mechanical and QM/MM calculations.

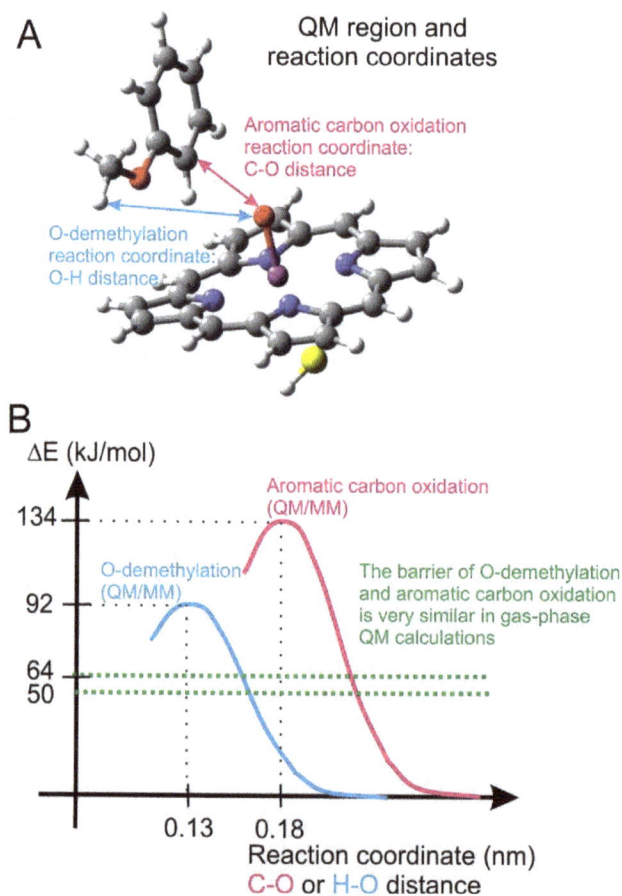

The above result indicates that the regioselectivity of P450 2D6 might be also modified by its active site architecture. For this reason we turned our attention towards docking, molecular dynamics and QM/MM methods which are capable of taking into account the enzymatic structure. There are two important pharmacophores of the ligands of P450 2D6: all of them contain basic nitrogen and an aromatic ring [108]. Therefore the N-protonated form of dextromethorphan was used throughout together with the crystallographic structure (PDB code 2F9Q) [109] of P450 2D6.

First, the ligand was docked into the active site of P450 2D6 in five different orientations, two of which seemed to be allowing for the O-demethylation reaction. In one of these two positions the protonated nitrogen of dextromethorphan interacts with the acidic Glu216 residue, and in the other one with Asp301, both of which have been implicated as important for catalysis [110]. In both structures the aromatic ring of the ligand participates in a π–π interaction with Phe120 whose mutation also leads to altered regioselectivity [111]. The structure in which interaction with Glu-216 was observed was chosen for further MD simulations and QM/MM calculations. During the course of a 2ns MD simulation, the docked structure maintained its major interactions with the active site residues, and it was observed that both the methoxy group and the aromatic ring of dextromethorphan remained in the close proximity of the heme iron during the whole time span of the simulation, indicating the possibility to be oxidized, in contrast to the fact that experimentally only the former one is known to occur.

As neither gas-phase quantum mechanical calculations nor docking alone could explain the experimental regioselectivity, it seemed to be essential to combine in the calculations the accuracy of quantum mechanical calculations with the steric restraints exerted by the protein structure in the frame of QM/MM calculations. The trajectory of the MD run was thoroughly analyzed and 3–3 suitable starting structures were chosen to model the two reaction channels. The QM region in the QM/MM calculations consisted of the same atoms as in the quantum mechanical calculations (Figure 15), but the axial thiolate ligand was modeled by an SCH_3^- moiety. Dangling bonds were saturated by hydrogen-type link atoms. Using adiabatic mapping, which gives an estimate of the enthalpy component of the Gibbs-free energy of the reaction, we obtained 92 kJ/mol for the barrier of hydrogen abstraction (O-demethylation) and 134 kJ/mol for the barrier of aromatic carbon oxidation. The difference between the activation energies of the two reaction channels increased to about 40 kJ/mol in contrast to the 14 kJ/mol calculated for the gas-phase (see the green dotted lines in Figure 15). The reason for the great increase of the barrier of the aromatic carbon oxidation is that the active site of P450 2D6 is relatively tight and the movement of dextromethorphan is hindered by several non-polar active site residues, e.g., Phe120, Ala305, Val308 (see Figure 16). Therefore the favorable transition state structure for aromatic oxidation cannot be formed in the active site, and its barrier considerably increases. The most important conclusion of the study was that gas-phase calculations or docking studies alone or even when they are combined are not enough to predict the regioselectivity of the P450 2D6 enzyme and more sophisticated models are needed. It was suggested that the metabolite predicting algorithms might be improved by docking the approximate transition state structures into the active site of the enzyme and assessing the feasibility of its formation [101].

244

Figure 16. Active site of P450 2D6 with dextromethorphan. The movement of dextromethorphan in the active site is hindered by its salt bridge to Glu216 and by the steric hindrance of the bulky amino acid side-chains.

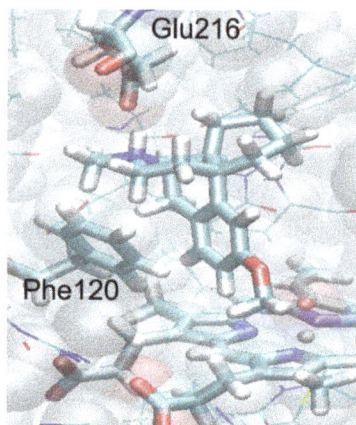

For a comprehensive study of the oxidation of further three pharmacologically important molecules see Lonsdale *et al.* [112].

4.4.3. Reactivity of the P450$_{nor}$ Enzyme

Nitric oxide reductase (P450$_{nor}$) is a very special member of the superfamily of P450s. Instead of the most generally catalyzed oxidation reactions of P450s, it catalyzes the reduction of nitric oxide to dinitrogen oxide and for its proper functioning it does not require a redox mediator, but contains its own NADH binding site [113]. P450$_{nor}$ is a soluble protein found in the cytosol of the fungus *Fusarium oxysporum*, a denitrifying organism, which can generate N_2O from NO_3^- ions in three main steps using three different enzymes. The last step of the conversion is nitric oxide reduction to N_2O by nitric oxide reductase. Since N_2O has a 300 times larger greenhouse effect than carbon dioxide [114], it should be taken into account in chemically fertilized nitrate abundant area [115]. Nitric oxide plays an important role in mammals for instance as a neurotransmitter or as part of the immune response against pathogens [116]. *Histoplasma capsulatum* is a human pathogen, which can avoid damage using the Nor1p enzyme, which shows great similarity to P450$_{nor}$ (61% sequence identity, 79% similarity) [117], and a similar mode of action can be assumed for converting NO.

The conversion catalyzed by P450$_{nor}$ takes place in three main steps (see Scheme 2). The first step is the binding of nitric oxide in the active site of P450$_{nor}$, which is followed by hydride transfer to (Fe^{III}P450$_{nor}$)NO from NADH to form the intermediate (**I** in Scheme 2). After the binding of a second molecule of nitric oxide, the final product, N_2O, is generated and the resting state of the enzyme is restored. Several suggestions have been put forward for the structure for the intermediate based on experimental and theoretical investigations [118–123]. According to the most accepted and experimentally proven mechanism direct hydride transfer occurs from the NADH co-factor to the oxygen or nitrogen atom of nitric oxide. DFT calculations performed by Lehnert *et al.* suggested that the hydride is most likely transferred to the nitrogen atom of nitric oxide in the key step, and intermediate (**I**) is the doubly protonated [Fe(Porph)(CH$_3$S)(NHOH)] species [123]. Based on the calculated relative energies at the B3LYP/LanL2DZ* and BP86/TZVP levels the [Fe(P)(CH$_3$S)(NHO)]$^-$ species is 109.7 kJ/mol more stable than the [Fe(P)(CH$_3$S)(NOH)]$^-$ species, and the protonation of [Fe(P)(CH$_3$S)(NHO)]$^-$ is a slightly exothermic process ($\Delta G = -36.0$ kJ/mol).

Scheme 2. Conversion reaction catalyzed by P450$_{nor}$.

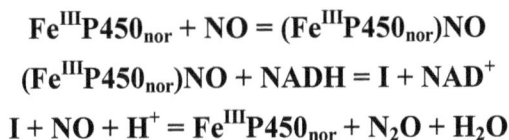

$$\text{Fe}^{III}\text{P450}_{nor} + \text{NO} = (\text{Fe}^{III}\text{P450}_{nor})\text{NO}$$

$$(\text{Fe}^{III}\text{P450}_{nor})\text{NO} + \text{NADH} = \text{I} + \text{NAD}^+$$

$$\text{I} + \text{NO} + \text{H}^+ = \text{Fe}^{III}\text{P450}_{nor} + \text{N}_2\text{O} + \text{H}_2\text{O}$$

In the previous sections it was shown that steric and electronic factors significantly influence the reactivity of enzymes, and that QM/MM calculations may provide a better description of enzymatic processes than gas phase calculations alone. Two QM/MM studies addressing the reactivity of P450$_{nor}$ were published recently, however dealing with partially different aspects of its reactivity. Our study focused on two key questions, (1) to which atom of nitric oxide will the hydride be transferred; and (2) how does the origin (docked or co-crystallized) influence the outcome of QM/MM calculations [124]. To answer the questions we used quantum mechanical and QM/MM methods, and based on experimental findings we assumed that the spin multiplicity of the system is singlet [125,126] and applied a closed-shell formalism in the calculations.

The results suggest that in the active site pocket of P450$_{nor}$ hydride transfer from NADH occurs to the nitrogen end of nitric oxide. In this respect all of our calculations (quantum mechanical or QM/MM) provided the same result, but the barriers were significantly higher in the QM/MM calculations. For instance the calculated barrier for hydride transfer from NADH to the nitrogen atom of nitric oxide is 37.3 kJ/mol in quantum mechanical and 113.5 kJ/mol in QM/MM calculations including zero-point energy correction in contrast to the 139.0 kJ/mol (quantum mechanical) and 161.2 kJ/mol (QM/MM) values obtained for the hydride transfer to the oxygen end of nitric oxide. The obtained high QM/MM barriers were most likely due to the incomplete sampling of initial complexes, and the chosen complexes did not provide an ideal starting structure for the reaction to occur. Nevertheless, the relative energy of the barriers convincingly showed that the hydride transfer will occur to the nitrogen of nitric oxide.

Comparing QM/MM calculations on two different structures of NADH bound P450$_{nor}$ brought also interesting results. Two structures were used. In structure **A** NADH has been docked to the active site of the NO-bound P450$_{nor}$ enzyme (Protein Data Bank code: 1CL6) [127], while structure **B** was obtained from the crystal structure of P450$_{nor}$ in complex with NAAD (nicotinic acid adenine dinucleotide), an analogue of NADH (Protein Data Bank code: 1XQD) [128]. In the latter structure nitric oxide was manually inserted. The position of the ligand and its interaction with active site residues was significantly different in the two models (see Figure 17). In structure **A** the pro-S hydrogen, while in structure **B** the pro-R hydrogen atom of NADH could be transferred as hydride to nitric oxide. We obtained significantly lower barriers using structure **B**, in accordance with the results of experimental kinetic isotope effect measurements, which also suggested the transfer of the pro-R hydrogen [121]. Therefore our results imply that the selection of docked structures as models should be avoided, since upon ligand binding a major rearrangement of the active site may take place. Unfortunately, present docking methods cannot take these rearrangements into account, and therefore the obtained results on the regioselectivity of the enzyme may contradict to experiments, furthermore, barrier heights may also be considerably influenced.

Figure 17. The position of the NADH ligand in the docked structure (structure **A**) and in the crystal structure (structure **B**).

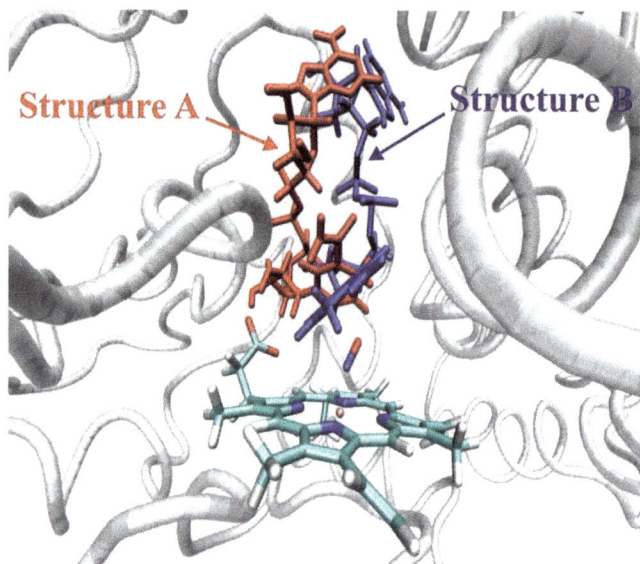

In another QM/MM study hydride shift directed to the nitrogen atom of nitric oxide was investigated [129]. This study resulted in considerably lower energy barriers: 38.9 kJ/mol for a closed-shell system at the DFT(RIJCOSX-B3LYP)/MM(OPLS-AA) level including zero-point energy correction. The lower barrier could be explained by the presence of a stabilizing hydrogen bond interaction between the amide group of the NADH molecule and the Ser286, Thr243 and Ala239 residues (see Figure 18), which are responsible for stabilization of the transition state. These were absent in models used in the work discussed above. When the authors applied an unrestricted formalism to obtain the wave function of the broken-symmetry singlet state, the calculated barrier further dropped to 27.2 kJ/mol, and showed that that the open-shell singlet state of the [Fe(Porph)(Met)(NHO)]$^-$ species is by about 16.7 kJ/mol more stable than the closed-shell one. The study also suggested that the N–N bond of N$_2$O is formed in a spin-recoupling process, followed by the release and spontaneous decomposition of the N$_2$O$_2$H$_2$ ligand to N$_2$O and H$_2$O.

Figure 18. Energy profiles for closed-shell and open-shell singlet pathways for hydride transfer in the P450$_{nor}$ and the schematic structure of the transition state.

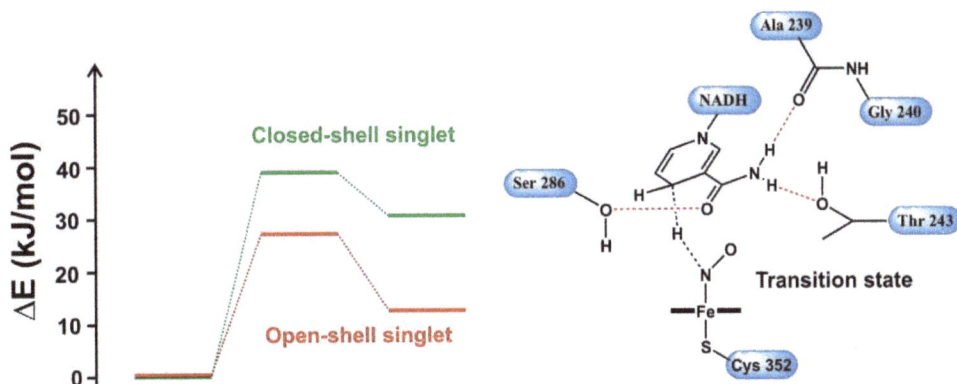

4.5. Xylose Isomerase

D-Xylose isomerase catalyzes the conversion of D-xylose to D-xylulose and the transformation of other sugars from aldose to ketose. It is widely used in industry for the conversion of D-glucose to D-fructose. The enzyme is activated by divalent metal cations (Mg^{2+}, Co^{2+} or Mn^{2+}), whereas other cations (e.g., Ca^{2+}, Ba^{2+} and Al^{3+}) inhibit the reaction [130]. The 3D structures of xylose isomerases isolated from different species have been extensively investigated by X-ray diffraction techniques [131–133]. On this basis the following mechanism of action has been proposed (see Figure 19 and Ref. 5). Binding the ring form of the sugar substrate to the structural metal ion is followed by a ring-opening step in which the hydrogen atom of the hydroxyl group on C1 is transferred to O5. This step is accompanied by the formation of a (– + –) charge distribution, involving the substrate hydroxide; His54 and Asp57, similar to those found in serine proteases (see Section 4.1). In the extended conformation, O2 and O4 of the sugar substrate are bound to the structural metal ion (M$_{str}$), while the catalytic metal ion (M$_{cat}$) is not in direct contact with the substrate. A structural water molecule coordinated to M$_{cat}$ removes the OH2 proton of the substrate. Isomerization takes place via hydride-shift, in which the C2 hydrogen is transferred to C1 via an anionic transition state, assisted by M$_{cat}$. This is the rate-limiting step of the reaction.

Extended calculations have been done on the validity of the above mechanism by Hu, Shiu and Li [134]. Their results indicate that in the enzyme M$_{cat}$ moves from one site to another, which is close to the substrate and stays there. M$_{cat}$ acts as a Lewis acid, polarizes the substrate and catalyzes the hydride shift step. Calculations showed that Lys183 plays an important role in the isomerization reaction, because its protonated terminal ammonium group provides a proton to the carboxide ion of the substrate to form a hydroxyl group after the hydride shift step. If this side chain is dropped from the active-site, model proton transfer instead of hydride shift is found to be rate limiting [135]. The calculated activation energies for ring opening and hydride shift steps were found to be 42 and 71 kJ/mol. respectively. If the activating metal cation, Mg^{2+}, was replaced by an inhibiting one, Zn^{2+}, calculated activation energies increased to 63 and 138 kJ/mol, respectively.

248

Figure 19. Catalytic mechanism of xylose isomerase. Top: ring opening, middle: substrate deprotonation, bottom: hydride shift.

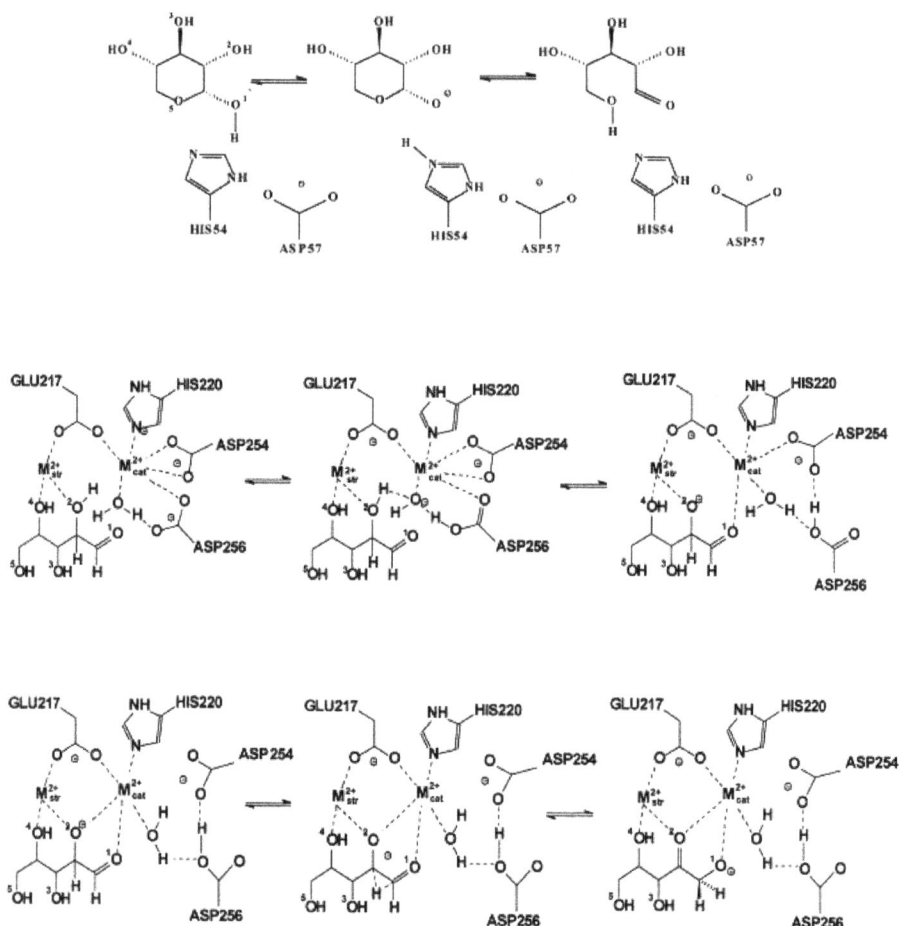

Our early calculations [136] indicated that the sugar ring opens only after the proton becomes shared between NE2 of His54 and O5 of the sugar. Ring opening is initiated by the approach of Asp57 towards His54 enhancing the basicity of the imidazole side chain of the latter. After the transition state has been reached, the movement in the opposite direction has been predicted by the calculations. The hypothesis that the charge-relay mechanism may be effective in catalysis, like in case of serine proteases, could be ruled out, because the electrostatic potential pattern provided by the protein environment and the bound metal cation (M_{str}) stabilizes the ion-pair form of the Asp57...NE2^{+}...O1^{-} triad. The negatively charged side chains of Asp57, as well as two bound structural water molecules assist in stabilizing the polar transition states. As it is seen in Figure 20, the activation energies of the proton transfer from O1 to NE2, as well as from NE2 to O5 become quite high if we do calculations on a small model, excluding Asp57 and the structural water molecules.

Figure 20. Initial, transition and final structures in the proton transfer steps of the ring opening reaction (relative energies are given in kJ/mol).

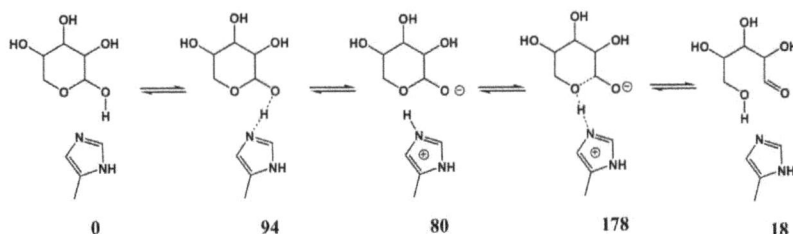

0	94	80	178	18

The anomeric specificity of the enzyme was also accounted for, since only the α-anomer is properly positioned for a proton transfer. Similarly, Lambeir *et al.* found that it is the His54 residue, which is responsible for the conformational specificity of xylose isomerases [137]. After abstracting a proton from the structural water by Asp256 the hydroxyl ion formed binds to the O_2H moiety of the substrate, the structural water breaks the M_{cat}…Asp256 link and a hydrogen-bond forms between them.

A specific effect, hydrogen tunneling takes place in xylose isomerases. This is especially interesting, since it cannot be described by other methods; specific quantum mechanics is needed. Gao and coworkers combined molecular dynamics with quantum mechanics including consideration of hydrogen tunneling to calculate the reaction rate of the transformation of xylose catalyzed by xylose isomerase in the presence of two divalent magnesium cations. Their model includes more than 25,000 explicit atoms. The simulation confirms the essential features of a mechanism involving a rate-determining 1,2-hydride shift with prior and post proton transfers. They have found that inclusion of quantum mechanical vibrational energy is important for computing the free energy of activation, and quantum mechanical tunneling effects are essential for computing kinetic isotope effects. It is predicted that 85% of the hydride shift reaction proceeds by tunneling. The computed kinetic isotope effect was found to be in good agreement with experimental results. The molecular dynamics simulations reveal that proton and hydride transfer reactions are assisted by breathing motions of the mobile Mg^{2+} ion in the active site during the hydride transfer step [138,139].

Further studies have been reported on tunneling in various other enzymes, too. The reaction pathway for tryptamine oxidation by aromatic amine dehydrogenase was studied by Masgrau *et al.* [140]. It has been shown by combining experiment and computer simulation, that proton transfer occurs in a reaction, which is dominated by tunneling. In this enzyme system instead of long-range coupled motions tunneling is promoted by a short-range motion modulating the proton-acceptor distance. Hydrogen tunneling was studied in a model system that represents the active site of soybean lipoxygenase-1. Calculations showed that the tunneling process has a three-dimensional nature [141].

5. Conclusions

Enzyme reactions involve a large number of atoms, of which some, belonging to the active site, are crucial in understanding the process, while others are of less, however, not negligible importance. Owing to this special situation, special models and computational methods are needed for an adequate description. The active site can be modeled by small organic structures and some basic

250

features of the reaction mechanisms can be elucidated by these. Calculations on this region must be at the quantum mechanical (Hartree-Fock, density functional or Empirical Valence Bond) level since bonds are broken and formed during the reaction, this needs a special treatment. More distant regions may be also of some importance, especially if the electrostatic field induced by them at the active site is strong. This is the case in point mutants where an ionizable side chain, which is close to the active site becomes charged or neutral by mutation. Those reactions, which involve a change in the polarity of the active site during transformation to the transition state, are strongly influenced, in most cases accelerated by the protein electrostatic field. In some cases subtle changes in the structure of the protein core may trigger essential changes in the mechanism. X-ray diffraction studies provide adequate models for the calculations.

Acknowledgments

This work was supported by grants from the Hungarian Scientific Research Fund (OTKA NK101072). J.O. and B. K. thank the financial support of the New Széchenyi Plan (TÁMOP-4.2.2/B-10/1-2010-0009).

Conflicts of Interest

The authors declare no conflict of interest.

References

1. Claeyssens, F.; Harvey, J.N.; Manby, F.R.; Mata, R.A.; Mulholland, A.J.; Ranaghan, K.E.; Schütz, M.; Thiel, S.; Thiel, W.; Werner, H.J. High-accuracy computation of reaction barriers in enzymes. *Angew. Chem.* **2006**, *118*, 7010–7013.
2. Matthews, B.W.; Sigler, P.B.; Henderson, R.; Blow, D.M. Three-Dimensional structure of tosyl α-chymotrypsin. *Nature* **1967**, *214*, 652–656.
3. Hedström, L. Serine protease mechanism and specificity. *Chem. Rev.* **2002**, *102*, 4501–4523.
4. Lassila, J.K.; Zalatan, J.G.; Herschlag, D. Biological phosphoryl-transfer reactions: Understanding mechanism and catalysis. *Annu. Rev. Biochem.* **2011**, *80*, 669–702.
5. Asbóth, B.; Náray-Szabó, G. Mechanism of action of d-xylose isomerase. *Curr. Protein Pept. Sci.* **2000**, *1*, 237–254.
6. Berman, H.M.; Westbrook, J.; Feng, Z.; Gilliland, G.; Bhat, T.N.; Weissig, H.; Shindyalov, I.N.; Bourne, P.E. The protein data bank. *Nucleic Acids Res.* **2000**, *28*, 235–242.
7. Wade, R.C.; Luty, B.A.; Demchuk, E.; Madura, J.D.; Davis, M.E.; Briggs, J.M.; McCammon, J.A. Simulation of enzyme-substrate encounter with gated active sites. *Nat. Struct. Biol.* **1994**, *1*, 65–69.
8. Hammes-Schiffer, S.; Benkovic, S.J. Relating protein motion to catalysis. *Annu. Rev. Biochem.* **2006**, *75*, 519–541.
9. McGeagh, J.D.; Ranaghan, K.E.; Mulholland, A.J. Protein dynamics and enzyme catalysis: Insights from simulations. *Biochim. Biophys. Acta* **2011**, *1814*, 1077–1092.

10. Warshel, A. *Computer Modeling of Chemical Reactions in Enzymes and Solutions*; Wiley: New York, NY, USA, 1991.

11. Ranaghan, K.E.; Mulholland, A.J. Investigations of enzyme-catalysed reactions with combined quantum mechanics/molecular mechanics (QM/MM) methods. *Int. Rev. Phys. Chem.* **2010**, *29*, 65–133.

12. Senn, H.M.; Thiel, W. QM/MM methods for biomolecular systems. *Angew. Chem. Int. Ed.* **2009**, *48*, 1198–1229.

13. Frisch, M.J.; Trucks, G.W.; Schlegel, H.B.; Scuseria, G.E.; Robb, M.A.; Cheeseman, J.R.; Scalmani, G.; Barone, V.; Mennucci, B.; Petersson, G.A. *et al. Gaussian 09*; Revision B.01; Gaussian, Inc.: Wallingford, CT, USA, 2010.

14. Szabo, A.; Ostlund, N.S. *Modern Quantum Chemistry: Introduction to Advanced Electronic Structure Theory*; Dover Publications: Mineola, NY, USA, 1996.

15. Jacobsen, H.; Cavallo, L. Directions for Use of Density Functional Theory: A Short Introduction Manual for Chemists. In *Handbook of Computational Chemistry*; Leszczynski, J., Ed.; Springer: Berlin, Germany, 2011; pp. 97–133.

16. Vreven, T.; Morokuma, K. Hybrid methods: ONIOM(QM:MM) and QM/MM. *Annu. Repts Comput. Chem.* **2006**, *2*, 35–51.

17. Poltev, V. Molecular Mechanics: Method and Applications. In *Handbook of Computational Chemisry*; Leszczynski, J., Ed.; Springer: Berlin, Germany, 2011; pp. 260–291.

18. Case, D.A.; Darden, T.A.; Cheatham, T.E., III; Simmerling, C.L.; Wang, J.; Duke, R.E.; Luo, R.; Walker, R.C.; Zhang, W.; Merz, K.M.; *et al. AMBER 11, 2010*; University of California: San Francisco, CA, USA.

19. Christen, M.; Hunenberger, P.H.; Bakowies, D.; Baron, R.; Bürgi, R.; Geerke, D.P.; Heinz, T.N.; Kastenholz, M.A.; Krautler, V.; Oostenbrink, C.; *et al.* The gromos software for biomolecular simulation: Gromos05. *J. Comp. Chem.* **2005**, *26*, 1719–1751.

20. Available online: http://www.gromacs.org/ (accessed on 6 August 2013).

21. Brooks, B.R.; Brooks, C.L., III; Mackerell, A.D.; Nilsson, L.; Petrella, R.J.; Roux, B.; Won, Y.; Archontis, G.; Bartels, C.; Boresch, S.; *et al.* CHARMM: The biomolecular simulation program. *J. Comp. Chem.* **2009**, *30*, 1545–1615.

22. Jorgensen, W.L.; Tirado-Rives, J. Potential energy functions for atomic-level simulations of water and organic and biomolecular systems. *Proc. Natl. Acad. Sci. USA* **2005**, *102*, 6665–6670.

23. Nowak, W. Applications of Computational Methods to Simulations of Proteins Dynamics. In *Handbook of Computational Chemistry*; Leszczynski, J., Ed.; Springer: Berlin, Germany, 2011; pp. 1129–1155.

24. Marx, D.; Hutter, J. *Ab Initio Molecular Dynamics: Basic Theory and Advanced Methods*; Cambridge University Press: Cambridge, UK, 2009.

25. Röthlisberger, D.; Khersonsky, O.; Wollacott, A.M.; Jiang, J.; DeChancie, J.; Betker, J.; Gallaher, J.L.; Althoff, E.A.; Zanghellini, A.; Dym, O.; *et al.* Kemp elimination catalysts by computational enzyme design. *Nature* **2008**, *453*, 190–195.

26. Náray-Szabó, G.; Surján, P.R. Bond orbital framework for rapid calculation of environmental effects on molecular potential energy surfaces. *Chem. Phys. Lett.* **1983**, *96*, 499–501.

27. Hu, H.; Yang, W. Free energies of chemical reactions in solution and in enzymes with ab initio quantum mechanics/molecular mechanics methods. *Annu. Rev. Phys. Chem.* **2008**, *59*, 573–560.

28. Warshel, A.; Florian, J. *Empirical Valence Bond and Related Approaches*; Wiley: New York, NY, USA, 2004.

29. Kamerlin, S.C.L.; Cao, J.; Rosta, E.; Warshel, A. On unjustifiably misrepresenting the EVB approach while simultaneously adopting it. *J. Phys. Chem. B* **2009**, *113*, 10905–10915.

30. Bentzien, J.; Muller, R.P.; Florián, J.; Warshel, A. Hybrid ab initio quantum mechanics/molecular mechanics calculations of free energy surfaces for enzymatic reactions: The nucleophilic attack in subtilisin. *J. Phys. Chem B* **1998**, *102*, 2293–2301.

31. Rocchia, W.; Alexov, E.; Honig, B. Extending the applicability of the nonlinear poisson-boltzmann equation: Multiple dielectric constants and multivalent ions. *J. Phys. Chem. B* **2001**, *105*, 6507–6514.

32. Sarkar, S.; Witham, S.; Zhang, J.; Zhenirovskyy, M.; Rocchia, W.; Alexov, E. DelPhi Web Server: A comprehensive online suite for electrostatic calculations of biological macromolecules and their complexes. *Comm. Comp. Phys.* **2013**, *13*, 269–284.

33. Tomasi, J.; Mennucci, B.; Cammi, R. Quantum mechanical continuum solvation models. *Chem. Rev.* **2005**, *105*, 2999–3094.

34. Polgár, L. *Mechanisms of Protease Action*; CRC Press: Boca Raton, FL, USA, 1989.

35. Brenner, S. The molecular evolution of genes and proteins: A tale of two serines. *Nature* **1988**, *334*, 528–530.

36. Asbóth, B.; Polgár, L. Transition-state stabilization at the oxyanion binding sites of serine and thiol proteinases: Hydrolyses of thiono and oxygen esters. *Biochemistry* **1983**, *22*, 117–122.

37. Carter, P.; Wells, J.A. Functional interaction among catalytic residues in subtilisin BPN'. *Proteins Struct. Funct. Genet.* **1990**, *7*, 335–342.

38. Blow, D.M.; Birktoft, J.J.; Hartley, B.S. Role of a buried acid group in the mechanism of action of chymotrypsin. *Nature* **1969**, *221*, 337–340.

39. Polgár, L.; Bender, M.L. The nature of general base-general acid catalysis in serine proteases. *Proc. Natl. Acad. Sci. USA* **1969**, *64*, 1335–1342.

40. Bachovchin, W.W. Confirmation of the assignment of the low-field proton resonance of serine proteases by using specifically nitrogen-15 labeled enzyme. *Proc. Natl. Acad. Sci. USA* **1985**, *82*, 7948–7951.

41. Kossiakoff, A.A.; Spencer, S.A. Direct determination of the protonation states of aspartic acid-102 and histidine-57 in the tetrahedral intermediate of the serine proteases: Neutron structure of trypsin. *Biochemistry* **1981**, *20*, 6462–6474.

42. Sprang, S.; Standing, T.; Fletterick, R.J.; Stroud, R.M.; Finer-Moore, J.; Xuong, N.H.; Hamlin, R.; Rutter, W.J.; Craik, C.S. The Three-dimensional structure of Asn102 mutant of trypsin: Role of Asp102 in serine protease catalysis. *Science* **1987**, *237*, 905–909.

43. Szeltner, Z.; Rea, D.; Renner, V.; Fülöp, V.; Polgár, L. Electrostatic effects and binding determinants in the catalysis of prolyl oligopeptidase. Site specific mutagenesis at the oxyanion binding site. *J. Biol. Chem.* **2002**, *277*, 42613–42622.

44. Warshel, A.; Náray-Szabó, G.; Sussman, F.; Hwang, J.K. How do serine proteases really work? *Biochemistry* **1989**, *28*, 3629–3637.

45. Warshel, A. Electrostatic origin of the catalytic power of enzymes and the role of preorganized active sites. *J. Biol. Chem.* **1998**, *273*, 27035–27038.

46. Kamerlin, S.C.L.; Sharma, P.K.; Chu, Z.T.; Warshel, A. Ketosteroid isomerase provides further support for the idea that enzymes work by electrostatic preorganization. *Proc. Natl. Acad. Sci. USA* **2010**, *107*, 4075–4080.

47. Gérczei, T.; Asbóth, B.; Náray-Szabó, G. Conservative electrostatic potential patterns at enzyme active sites. The anion-cation-anion triad. *J. Chem. Inf. Comput. Sci.* **1999**, *39*, 310–315.

48. Náray-Szabó, G.; Fuxreiter, M.; Warshel, A. Electrostatic Basis of Enzyme Catalysis. In *Computational Approaches to Biochemical Reactivity*; Warshel, A., Náray-Szabó, G., Eds.; Kluwer: Dordrecht, The Netherlands, 1997; pp. 237–293.

49. Umeyama, H.; Nakagawa, S.; Kudo, T. Role of Asp102 in the enzymatic reaction of bovine beta-trypsin. A molecular orbital study. *J. Mol. Biol.* **1981**, *150*, 409–421.

50. Náray-Szabó, G. Electrostatic effect on catalytic rate enhancement in serine proteinases. *Int. J. Quant. Chem.* **1982**, *22*, 575–582.

51. Ishida, T.; Kato, S. Theoretical perspectives on the reaction mechanism of serine proteases: The reaction free energy profiles of the acylation process. *J. Am. Chem. Soc.* **2003**, *125*, 12035–12048.

52. Topf, M.; Richards, W.G. Theoretical studies on the deacylation step of serine protease catalysis in the gas phase, in solution, and in elastase. *J. Am. Chem. Soc.* **2004**, *126*, 14631–14641.

53. Hudáky, P.; Perczel, A. A self-stabilized model of the chymotrypsin catalytic pocket. The energy profile of the overall catalytic cycle. *Proteins Struct. Funct. Bioinf.* **2006**, *62*, 749–759.

54. Zhou, Y.; Zhang, Y. Serine protease acylation proceeds with a subtle re-orientation of the histidine ring at the tetrahedral intermediate. *Chem. Commun.* **2011**, *47*, 1577–1579.

55. Florián, J.; Warshel, A. Phosphate ester hydrolysis in aqueous solution: Associative versus dissociative mechanisms. *J. Phys. Chem. B* **1998**, *102*, 719–734.

56. Bernardi, F.; Bottoni, A.; de Vivo, M.; Garavelli, M.; Keserű, G.; Náray-Szabó, G. A hypothetical mechanism for HIV-1 integrase catalytic action: DFT modelling of a bio-mimetic environment. *Chem. Phys. Lett.* **2002**, *362*, 1–7.

57. Franzini, E.; Fantucci, P.; de Gioia, L. Density functional theory investigation of guanosine triphosphate models. Catalytic role of Mg^{2+} ions in phosphate ester hydrolysis. *J. Mol. Catal. A* **2003**, *204*, 409–417.

58. Lahiri, S.D.; Zhang, G.; Dunaway-Mariano, D.; Allen, K.N. The pentacovalent phosphorus intermediate of a phosphoryl transfer reaction. *Science* **2003**, *299*, 2067–2071.

59. Blackburn, G.M.; Williams, N.H.; Gamblin, S.J.; Smerdon, S.J. The pentacovalent phosphorus intermediate of a phosphoryl transfer reaction. *Science* **2003**, *301*, 1184c.

60. Baxter, N.J.; Bowler, M.W.; Alizadeh, T.; Cliff, M.J.; Hounslow, A.M.; Wu, B.; Berkowitz, D.B.; Williams, N.H.; Blackburn, G.M.; Waltho, J.P. Atomic details of near-transition state conformers for enzyme phosphoryl transfer revealed by MgF3- rather than by phosphoranes. *Proc. Natl. Acad. Sci. USA* **2010**, *107*, 4555–4560.

61. Webster, C.E. High-energy intermediate or stable transition state analogue: Theoretical perspective of the active site and mechanism of β-phosphoglucomutase. *J. Am. Chem. Soc.* **2004**, *126*, 6840–6841.

62. Berente, I.; Beke, T.; Náray-Szabó, G. Quantum mechanical studies on the existence of a trigonal bipyramidal phosphorane intermediate in enzymatic phosphate ester hydrolysis. *Theor. Chem. Acc.* **2007**, *118*, 129–134.

63. Barabás, O.; Pongrácz, V.; Kovári, J.; Wilmanns, M.; Vértessy, B.G. Structural insights into the catalytic mechanism of phosphate ester hydrolysis by dUTPase. *J. Biol. Chem.* **2004**, *279*, 42907–42915.

64. Ivanov, I.; Tainer, J.A.; McCammon, J.A. Unraveling the three-metal-ion catalytic mechanism of the DNA repair enzyme endonuclease IV. *Proc. Natl. Acad. Sci. USA* **2007**, *104*, 1465–1470.

65. Cavalli, A.; de Vivo, M.; Recanatini, M. Computational study of the phosphoryl transfer catalyzed by a cyclin-dependent kinase. *Chem. Eur. J.* **2007**, *13*, 8437–8444.

66. Smith, G.K.; Ke, Z.; Guo, H. Insights into the phosphoryl transfer mechanism of cyclin-dependent protein kinases from ab initio QM/MM free-energy studies. *J. Phys. Chem. B* **2011**, *115*, 13713–13722.

67. Kamerlin, S.C.L.; McKenna, C.E.; Goodman, M.F.; Warshel, A. A computational study of the hydrolysis of dGTP analogues with halomethylene-modified leaving groups in solution: Implications for the mechanism of DNA polymerases. *Biochemistry* **2009**, *48*, 5963–5971.

68. Wong, K.-Y. Gao, J. Insight into the phosphodiesterase mechanism from combined QM/MM free energy simulations. *FEBS J.* **2011**, *278*, 2579–2595.

69. Lior-Hoffmann, L.; Wang, L.; Wang, S.; Geacintov, N.E.; Broyde, S.; Zhang, Y. Preferred WMSA catalytic mechanism of the nucleotidyl transfer reaction in human DNA polymerase κ elucidates error-free bypass of a bulky DNA lesion. *Nucleic Acids Res.* **2012**, *40*, 9193–9205.

70. Xu, D.; Guo, H. Ab initio QM/MM studies of the phosphoryl transfer reaction catalyzed by PEP Mutase suggest a dissociative metaphosphate transition state. *J. Phys. Chem. B* **2008**, *112*, 4102–4108.

71. Xu, D.; Guo, H.; Liu, Y.; York, D.M. Theoretical studies of dissociative phosphoryl transfer in interconversion of phosphoenolpyruvate to phosphonopyruvate: Solvent effects, thio effects, and implications for enzymatic reactions. *J. Phys. Chem. B* **2005**, *109*, 13827–13834.

72. De Vivo, M.; Dal Peraro, M.; Klein, M.L. Phosphodiester cleavage in ribonuclease H occurs via an associative two-metal-aided catalytic mechanism. *J. Am. Chem. Soc.* **2008**, *130*, 10955–10962.

73. Rosta, E.; Woodcock, H.L.; Brooks, B.R.; Hummer, G. Artificial reaction coordinate "Tunneling" in free-energy calculations: The catalytic reaction of RNase H. *J. Comput. Chem.* **2009**, *30*, 1634–1641.

74. Schlichting, I.; Reinstein, J. pH influences fluoride coordination number of the AlFx phosphoryl transfer transition state analog. *Nat. Struct. Biol.* **1999**, *6*, 721–723.

75. De Vivo, M.; Ensing, B.; Dal Peraro, M.; Gomez, G.A.; Christianson, D.W.; Klein, M.L. Proton shuttles and phosphatase activity in soluble epoxide hydrolase. *J. Am. Chem. Soc.* **2007**, *129*, 387–394.

76. Ram Prasad, B.; Plotnikov, N.V.; Warshel, A. Addressing open questions about phosphate hydrolysis pathways by careful free energy mapping. *J. Phys. Chem. B* **2013**, *117*, 153–163.

77. Kamerlin, S.C.L.; Florián, J.; Warshel A. Associative versus dissociative mechanisms of phosphate monoester hydrolysis: On the interpretation of activation entropies. *ChemPhysChem* **2008**, *9*, 1767–1773.

78. Finzel, B.C.; Poulos, T.L.; Kraut, J. Crystal structure of yeast cytochrome c peroxidase refined at 1.7 Å resolution. *J. Biol. Chem.* **1984**, *269*, 32759–32767.

79. Poulos, T.L.; Edwards, S.L.; Wariishi, H.; Gold, M.H. Crystallographic Refinement of lignin peroxidase at 2 Å. *J. Biol. Chem.* **1993**, *268*, 4429–4440.

80. Patterson, W.R.; Poulos, T.L.; Goodin, D.B. Identification of a porphyrin Pi cation radical in ascorbate peroxidase compound I. *Biochemistry* **1995**, *34*, 4342–4345.

81. Gajhede, M.; Schuller, D.J.; Henriksen, A.; Smith, A.T.; Poulos, T.L. Crystal structure of horseradish peroxidase C at 2.15 Å resolution. *Nat. Struct. Biol.* **1997**, *4*, 1032–1038.

82. Patterson, W.R.; Poulos, T.L. Crystal structure of recombinant pea cytosolic ascorbate peroxidase. *Biochemistry* **1995**, *34*, 4331–4341.

83. Menyhárd, D.K.; Náray-Szabó, G. Electrostatic effect on electron transfer at the active site of heme peroxidases: A comparative molecular orbital study on Cytochrome C peroxidase and ascorbate peroxidase. *J. Phys. Chem. B* **1999**, *103*, 227–233.

84. Jensen, G.M.; Bunte, S.W.; Warshel, A.; Goodin, D.B. Energetics of cation radical formation at the proximal active site tryptophan of cytochrome *c* peroxidase and ascorbate peroxidase. *J. Phys. Chem.* **1998**, *102*, 8221–8228.

85. Wirstam, M.; Blomberg, M.R.A.; Siegbahn, P.E.M. Reaction mechanism of compound I formation in heme peroxidases: A density functional theory study. *J. Am. Chem. Soc.* **1999**, *121*, 10178–10185.

86. Hiner, A.N.; Martínez, J.I.; Arnao, M.B.; Acosta, M.; Turner, D.D.; Lloyd Raven, E.; Rodríguez-López, J.N. Detection of a tryptophan radical in the reaction of ascorbate peroxidase with hydrogen peroxide. *Eur. J. Biochem.* **2001**, *268*, 3091–3098.

87. Heimdal, J.; Rydberg, P.; Ryde, U. Protonation of the proximal histidine ligand in heme peroxidases. *J. Phys. Chem. B* **2008**, *112*, 2501–2510.

88. De Visser, S.P. What affects the quartet-doublet energy splitting in peroxidase enzymes? *J. Phys. Chem. A* **2005**, *109*, 11050–11057.

89. Bathelt, C.M.; Mulholland, A.J.; Harvey, J.N. QM/MM studies of the electronic structure of the compound I intermediate in cytochrome c peroxidase and ascorbate peroxidase *J. Chem. Soc. Dalton Trans.* **2005**, 3470–3476.

90. Derat, E.; Cohen, S.; Shaik, S.; Altun, A.; Thiel, W. Principal active species of horseradish peroxidase compound I: A hybrid quantum mechanical/molecular mechanical study. *J. Am. Chem. Soc.* **2005**, *127*, 13611–13621.

91. Jensen, K.P.; Ryde, U. Importance of proximal hydrogen bonds in haem proteins. *Mol. Phys.* **2003**, *101*, 2003–2018.

92. Guallar, V.; Wallrapp, F.H. QM/MM methods: Looking inside heme proteins biochemisty. *Biophys. Chem.* **2010**, *149*, 1–11.

93. Vlasitsa, J.; Jakopitscha, C.; Bernroitnera, M.; Zamockya, M.; Furtmüllera, P.G.; Obingera, C. Mechanisms of catalase activity of heme peroxidases. *Arch. Biochem. Biophys.* **2010**, *500*, 74–81.

94. Harris, D.L.; Loew, G.H. Proximal ligand effects on electronic structure and spectra of compound I of peroxidases. *J. Porphyr. Phthalocyanins* **2001**, *5*, 334–344.

95. Nelson, D.R.; Goldstone, J.V.; Stegeman, J.J. The cytochrome P450 genesis locus: The origin and evolution of animal cytochrome P450s. *Phil. Trans. R. Soc. B* **2013**, *368*, 20120474.

96. Guengerich, F.P. Chapter 10 (6.45). In *Cytochrome P450: Structure, Mechanism, and Biochemistry*, 2nd ed.; Ortiz de Montellano, P.R., Ed.; Plenum Press: New York, NY, USA, 1995; pp. 450–452.

97. Shaik, S.; Kumar, D.; de Visser, S.P.; Altun, A.; Thiel, W. Theoretical perspective on the structure and mechanism of cytochrome P450 enzymes. *Chem. Rev.* **2005**, *105*, 2279–2328.

98. Rittle, J.; Green, M.T. Cytochrome P450 Compound I: Capture, characterization, and C-H Bond activation kinetics. *Science* **2010**, *330*, 933–937.

99. De Visser, S.P.; Ogliaro, F.; Sharma, P.K.; Shaik, S. Hydrogen bonding modulates the selectivity of enzymatic oxidation by P450: A chameleon oxidant behavior by compound I. *Angew. Chem. Int. Ed.* **2002**, *41*, 1947–1951.

100. De Visser, S.P.; Ogliaro, F.; Sharma, P.K.; Shaik, S. What factors affect the regioselectivity of oxidation by cytochrome p450? A DFT study of allylic hydroxylation and double bond epoxidation in a model reaction. *J. Am. Chem. Soc.* **2002**, *124*, 11809–11826.

101. Ogliaro, F.; Cohen, S.; de Visser, S.P.; Shaik, S. Medium polarization and hydrogen bonding effects on compound I of cytochrome P450: What kind of a radical it really is? *J. Am. Chem. Soc.* **2000**, *122*, 12892–12893.

102. Lonsdale, R.; Oláh, J.; Mulholland, A.J.; Harvey, J.N. Does compound I vary significantly between isoforms of cytochrome P450? *J. Am. Chem. Soc.* **2011**, *133*, 15464–15474.

103. Schmider, J.; Greenblatt, D.J.; Fogelman, S.M.; von Moltke, L.L.; Shader, R.I. Metabolism of dextromethorphan *in vitro*: Involvement of cytochromes P450 2D6 and 3A3/4, with a possible role of 2E1. *Biopharm. Drug. Dispos.* **1997**, *18*, 227–240.

104. Daly, J. Metabolism of acetanilides and anisoles with rat liver microsomes. *Biochem. Pharmacol.* **1970**, *19*, 2979–2993.

105. Bray, H.G.; James, S.P.; Thorpe, W.V.; Wasdell, M.R. The metabolism of ethers in the rabbit. 1. anisole and diphenyl ether. *Biochem. J.* **1953**, *54*, 547–551.

106. Olsen, L.; Rydberg, P.; Rod, T.H.; Ryde, U. Prediction of activation energies for hydrogen abstraction by cytochrome P450. *J. Med. Chem.* **2006**, *49*, 6489–6499.

107. Oláh, J.; Mulholland, A.J.; Harvey, J.N. Determinants of selectivity in drug metabolism by cytochrome P450: QM/MM modeling of dextromethorphan oxidation by CYP2D6. *Proc. Natl. Acad. Sci. USA* **2011**, *108*, 6050–6055.

108. Ingelman-Sundberg, M. Genetic polymorphisms of cytochrome P450 2D6 (CYP2D6): Clinical consequences, evolutionary aspects and functional diversity. *Pharmacogenomics J.* **2005**, *5*, 6–13.

109. Rowland, P.; Blaney, F.E.; Smyth, M.G.; Jones, J.J.; Leydon, V.R.; Oxbrow, A.K.; Lewis, C.J.; Tennant, M.G.; Modi, S.; Eggleston, D.S.; *et al*. Crystal structure of human cytochrome P450 2D6. *J. Biol. Chem.* **2006**, *281*, 7614–7622.

110. McLaughlin, L.A.; Paine, M.J.I.; Kemp, C.A.; Maréchal, J.D.; Flanagan, J.U.; Ward, R.; Sutcliffe, M.J.; Roberts, G.C.K.; Wolf, C.R. Why is quinidine an inhibitor of cytochrome P450 2D6? The role of key active-site residues in quinidine binding. *J. Biol. Chem.* **2005**, *280*, 38617–38624.

111. Flanagan, J.U.; Maréchal, J.D.; Ward, R.; Kemp, C.A.; McLaughlin, L.A.; Sutcliffe, M.J.; Roberts, G.C.K.; Paine, M.J.I.; Wolf, C.R. Phe120 contributes to the regiospecificity of cytochrome P450 2D6: Mutation leads to the formation of a novel dextromethorphan. *Biochem. J.* **2004**, *380*, 353–360.

112. Lonsdale, R.; Houghton, K.T.; Żurek, J.; Bathelt, C.M.; Foloppe, N.; de Groot, M.J.; Harvey, J.N.; Mulholland, A.J. Quantum mechanics/molecular mechanics modeling of regioselectivity of drug metabolism in cytochrome P450 2C9. *J. Am. Chem. Soc.* **2013**, *135*, 8001–8015.

113. Zhang, L.; Kudo, T.; Takaya, N.; Shoun, H. The B′ helix determines cytochrome P450nor specificity for the electron donors NADH and NADPH. *J. Biol. Chem.* **2002**, *277*, 33842–33847.

114. De Vries, S.; Schröder, I. Comparison between the nitric oxide reductase family and its aerobic relatives, the cytochrome oxidases. *Biochem. Soc. Trans.* **2002**, *30*, 662–667.

115. Richardson, D.; Felgate, H.; Watmough, N.; Thomson, A.; Baggs, E. Mitigating release of the potent greenhouse gas N(2)O from the nitrogen cycle—Could enzymic regulation hold the key? *Trends Biotechnol.* **2009**, *27*, 388–397.

116. Wink, D.A.; Hines, H.B.; Cheng, R.Y.S.; Switzer, C.H.; Flores-Santana, W.; Vitek, M.P.; Ridnour, L.A.; Colton, C.A.J. Nitric oxide and redox mechanisms in the immune response. *Leukocyte Biol.* **2011**, *89*, 873–891.

117. Chao, L.Y.; Rine, J.; Marletta, M.A. Spectroscopic and kinetic studies of nor1, a cytochrome p450 nitric oxide reductase from the fungal pathogen *Histoplasma capsulatum*. *Arch. Biochem. Biophys.* **2008**, *480*, 132–137.

118. Shiro, Y.; Fujii, M.; Iizuka, T.; Adachi, S.; Tsukamoto, K.; Nakahara, K.; Shoun, H. Spectroscopic and kinetic studies on reaction of cytochrome P450nor with nitric oxide. Implication for its nitric oxide reduction mechanism. *J. Biol. Chem.* **1995**, *270*, 1617–1623.

119. Harris, D.L. Cytochrome P450nor: A nitric oxide reductase—Structure, spectra, and mechanism. *Int. J. Quantum Chem.* **2002**, *288*, 183–200.

120. Tsukamoto, K.; Nakamura, S.; Shimizu, K. SAM1 semiempirical calculations on the catalytic cycle of nitric oxide reductase from *Fusarium oxysporum*, *J. Mol. Struct. (THEOCHEM)* **2003**, *624*, 309–322.

121. Averill, B.A. Dissimilatory nitrite and nitric oxide reductases. *Chem. Rev.* **1996**, *96*, 2951–2964.

122. Daiber, A.; Nauser, T.; Takaya, N.; Kudo, T.; Weber, P.; Hultschig, C.; Shoun, H.; Ullrich, V. Isotope effects and intermediates in the reduction of NO by P450NOR. *J. Inorg. Biochem.* **2002**, *88*, 343–352.

123. Lehnert, N.; Praneeth, V.K.K.; Paulat, F. Electronic structure of Fe(II)-porphyrin nitroxyl complexes: Molecular mechanism of fungal nitric oxide reductase (P450nor). *J. Comput. Chem.* **2006**, *27*, 1338–1351.

124. Krámos, B.; Menyhárd, D.K.; Oláh, J. Direct hydride shift mechanism and stereoselectivity of P450nor confirmed by QM/MM calculations. *J. Phys. Chem. B* **2012**, *116*, 872–885.

125. Suzuki, N.; Higuchi, T.; Urano, Y.; Kikuchi, K.; Uchida, T.; Mukai, M.; Kitagawa, T.; Nagano, T. First synthetic no-heme-thiolate complex relevant to nitric oxide synthase and cytochrome P450nor. *J. Am. Chem. Soc.* **2000**, *122*, 12059–12060.

126. Shimizu, H.; Obayashi, E.; Gomi, Y.; Arakawa, H.; Park, S.Y.; Nakamura, H.; Adachi, S.; Shoun, H.; Shiro, Y. Proton delivery in no reduction by fungal nitric-oxide reductase. cryogenic crystallography, spectroscopy, and kinetics of ferric-no complexes of wild-type and mutant enzymes. *J. Biol. Chem.* **2000**, *275*, 4816–4826.

127. Menyhárd, D.K.; Keserű, G.M. Binding mode analysis of the NADH cofactor in nitric oxide reductase: A theoretical study. *J. Mol. Graphics Model.* **2006**, *25*, 363–372.

128. Oshima, R.; Fushinobu, S.; Su, F.; Zhang, L.; Takaya, N.; Shoun, H. Structural evidence for direct hydride transfer from NADH to cytochrome P450nor. *J. Mol. Biol.* **2004**, *342*, 207–217.

129. Riplinger, C.; Neese, F. The reaction mechanism of cytochrome P450 NO reductase: A detailed quantum mechanics/molecular mechanics study. *ChemPhysChem* **2011**, *12*, 3192–3203.

130. Callens, M.; Tomme, P.; Kerstens-Hilderson, H.; Cornelis, W.; Vangrysperre, W.; de Bruyne, C.K. Metal ion binding to d-xylose isomerase from streptomyces violaceoruber. *Biochem. J.* **1988**, *250*, 285–291.

131. Farber, G.K.; Machin, P.; Almo, S.C.; Petsko, G.A.; Hajdu, J. X-ray laue diffraction from crystals of xylose isomerase. *Proc. Natl. Acad. Sci. USA* **1988**, *85*, 112–118.

132. Collyer, C.A.; Henrick, K.; Blow, D.M. Mechanism for aldose-ketose interconversion by D-Xylose isomerase involving ring opening followed by a 1,2-hydride shift. *J. Mol. Biol.* **1990**, *212*, 211–235.

133. Jenkins, J.; Janin, J.; Rey, F.; Chidmi, M.; Tilbeurgh, H.; Lasters, I.; Maeyer, M.; Belle, D.; Wodak, S.; Lauwereys, M.; *et al.* Protein engineering of xylose (Glucose) isomerase from actinoplanes missouriensis. 1. Crystallography and site-directed mutagenesis of metal binding sites. *Biochemistry* **1992**, *31*, 5449–5458.

134. Hu, H.; Liu, H.; Shi, Y. The reaction pathway of the isomerization of *d*-xylose catalyzed by the enzyme d-xylose isomerase: A theoretical study. *Proteins Struct. Funct. Genet.* **1997**, *27*, 545–555.

135. Fuxreiter, M.; Farkas, Ö.; Náray-Szabó, G. Molecular modeling of xylose isomerase catalysis: The role of electrostatics and charge transfer to metals. *Protein Eng.* **1995**, *8*, 925–933.

136. Fábián, P.; Asbóth, B.; Náray-Szabó, G. The role of electrostatics in the ring-opening step of xylose isomerase catalysis. *J. Mol. Struct. Theochem.* **1994**, *307*, 171–178.

137. Lambeir, A.M.; Lauwereys, M.; Stanssens, P.; Mrabet, N.T.; Snauwaert, J.; van Tilbeurgh, H.; Matthyssens, G.; Lasters, I.; de Maeyer, M.; Wodak, S.J.; *et al.* Protein engineering of xylose (glucose) isomerase from actinoplanes missouriensis. 3. Changing metal specificity and the PH profile by site-directed mutagenesis. *Biochemistry* **1992**, *31*, 5459–5466.

138. Garcia-Viloca, M.; Alhambra, C.; Truhlar, D.G.; Gao, J. Quantum dynamics of hydride transfer catalyzed by bimetallic electrophilic catalysis: Synchronous motion of Mg2+ and H- in xylose isomerase. *J. Am. Chem. Soc.* **2002**, *124*, 7268–7269.

139. Garcia-Viloca, M.; Alhambra, C.; Truhlar, D.G.; Gao, J. Hydride transfer catalyzed by xylose isomerase: Mechanism and quantum effects. *J. Comput. Chem.* **2003**, *24*, 177–190.

140. Masgrau, L.; Roujeinikova, A.; Johannissen, L.O.; Hothi, P.; Basran, J.; Ranaghan, K.E.; Mulholland, A.J.; Sutcliffe, M.J.; Scrutton, N.S.; Leys, D. Atomic description of an enzyme reaction dominated by proton tunneling. *Science* **2006**, *312*, 237–241.

141. Iyengar, S.S.; Sumner, I.; Jakowski, J. Hydrogen tunneling in an enzyme active site: A quantum wavepacket dynamical perspective. *J. Phys. Chem. B* **2008**, *112*, 7601–7613.

Biocatalytic Synthesis of Chiral Alcohols and Amino Acids for Development of Pharmaceuticals

Ramesh N. Patel

Abstract: Chirality is a key factor in the safety and efficacy of many drug products and thus the production of single enantiomers of drug intermediates and drugs has become increasingly important in the pharmaceutical industry. There has been an increasing awareness of the enormous potential of microorganisms and enzymes derived there from for the transformation of synthetic chemicals with high chemo-, regio- and enatioselectivities. In this article, biocatalytic processes are described for the synthesis of chiral alcohols and unntural aminoacids for pharmaceuticals.

Reprinted from *Biomolecules*. Cite as: Patel, R.N. Biocatalytic Synthesis of Chiral Alcohols and Amino Acids for Development of Pharmaceuticals. *Biomolecules* **2013**, *3*, 741-777.

1. Introduction

For preparation of drugs and their intermediates, the synthesis of single enantiomers has become increasingly important in the pharmaceutical industry [1]. Single enantiomers can be produced by either by chemical or biocatalytic routes. The advantages of biocatalysis over chemical synthesis are that enzyme-catalyzed reactions are often highly enantioselective and regioselective. They can be carried out under mild conditions at ambient temperature and atmospheric pressure, thus avoiding the use of more extreme reaction conditions which could cause problems with isomerization, racemization, epimerization, and rearrangement of compound. Microbial cells and wide variety and class of enzymes derived there from can be used for chiral synthesis. Enzymes can be immobilized and reused for many cycles. In addition, enzymes can be over expressed to make biocatalytic processes economically efficient, and enzymes with modified activity can be tailor-made. Directed evolution of biocatalysts can lead to increased enzyme activity, selectivity and stability [2–15]. A number of review articles [16–31] have been published on the use of enzymes in organic synthesis. This chapter provides some examples of the use of enzymes for the synthesis chiral alcohols, unnatural amino acids, and amines for synthesis of phamaceuticals.

2. Enzymatic Preparation of Chiral Alcohols

2.1. Hydroxy Buspirone (Antianxiety Drug): Enzymatic Preparation of 6-Hydroxybuspirone

Buspirone (Buspar®, **1**, Figure 1) is a drug used for treatment of anxiety and depression that is thought to produce its effects by binding to the serotonin 5HT1A receptor [32–34]. Mainly as a result of hydroxylation reactions, it is extensively converted to various metabolites and blood concentrations return to low levels a few hours after dosing [35]. A major metabolite, 6-hydroxybuspirone **2**, produced by the action of liver cytochrome P450 CYP3A4, is present at much higher concentrations in human blood than buspirone itself. For development of 6-hydroxybuspirone as a potential antianxiety drug, preparation and testing of the two enantiomers as well as the racemate was of interest. An enantioselective microbial reduction process was developed for reduction of 6-oxobuspirone **3**, to either (*R*)- and (*S*)-6-hydroxybuspirone **2**. About 150 microbial cultures were screened for the enantioselective reduction of **3**. *Rhizopus stolonifer* SC 13898, *Neurospora crassa* SC 13816, *Mucor racemosus* SC 16198, and *Pseudomonas putida* SC 13817 gave >50% reaction yields and >95% e.e.s of (*S*)-6-hydroxybuspirone. The yeast strains *Hansenula polymorpha* SC 13845 and *Candida maltosa* SC 16112 gave (*R*)-6-hydroxybuspirone **2** in >60% reaction yield and >97% e.e. [36]. The NADP-dependent (*R*)-reductase (RHBR) from *Hansenula polymorpha* SC 13845 was purified to homogeneity, its *N*-terminal and internal sequences were determined and cloned and expressed in *Escherichia coli*. To regenerate the cofactor NADPH required for reduction we have also cloned and expressed the glucose-6-phosphate dehydrogenase gene from *Saccharomyces cerevisiae* in *Escherichia coli*. Recombinant cultures expressing (*R*)-reductase (RHBR) catalyzed the reduction of 6-ketobuspirone to (*R*)-6-hydroxybuspirone in 99% yield and 99.9% e.e. at 50 g/L substrate input [37].

Figure 1. Hydroxy buspirone (antianxiety drug): Enzymatic preparation of 6-hydroxybuspirone.

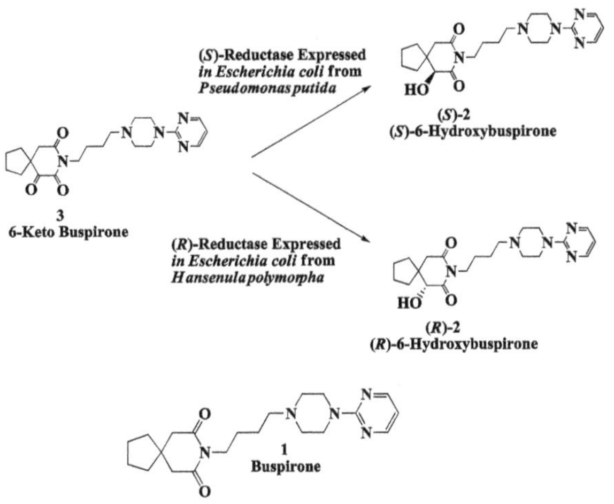

The NAD-dependent (*S*)-reductase (SHBR) from *Pseudomonas putida* SC 16269 was also purified to homogeneity, its *N*-terminal and internal sequences were determined and cloned and expressed in *Escherichia coli*. To regenerate the cofactor NADH required for reduction we have also cloned and expressed the NAD⁺ dependent formate dehydrogenase gene from *Pichia pastoris* in *Escherichia coli*. Recombinant *Escherichia coli* expressing (*S*)-reductase was used to catalyze the reduction of 6-ketobuspirone to (*S*)-6-hydroxybuspirone, in >98% yield and >99.8% e.e. at 50 g/L substrate input [37].

2.2. Cholesterol Lowering Agents: Enzymatic Preparation of (3S,5R)-Dihydroxy-6-(Benzyloxy) Hexanoic Acid, Ethyl Ester 4

Compound **4** (Figure 2) is a key chiral intermediate required for the chemical synthesis of compound **5**, Arotvastatin **6**, and Rosuvastatin all are anticholesterol drugs which acts by inhibition of HMG CoA reductase [38–42].

Figure 2. Cholesterol lowering agents: Enzymatic preparation of (3S,5R)-dihydroxy-6-(benzyloxy) hexanoic acid, ethyl ester.

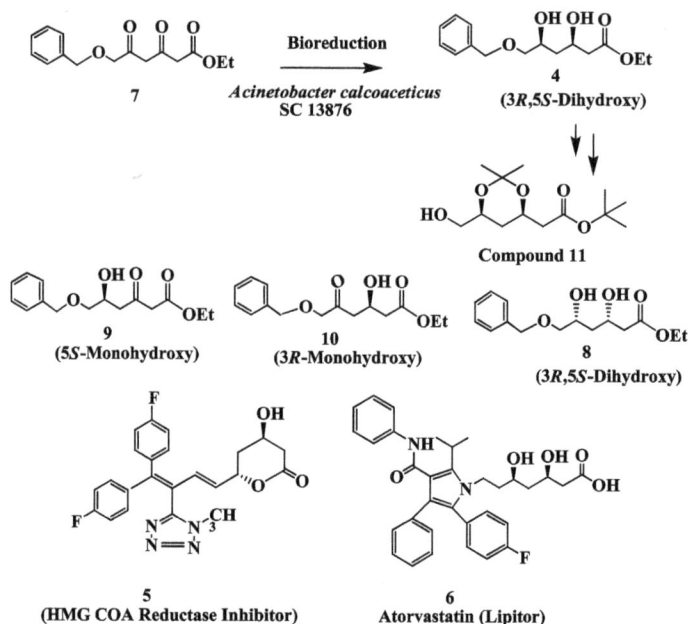

The enantioselective reduction of a diketone 3,5-dioxo-6-(benzyloxy) hexanoic acid, ethyl ester **7** to (3R,5S)-dihydroxy-6-(benzyloxy) hexanoic acid, ethyl ester **4** (Figure 2) was demonstrated by cell suspensions of *Acinetobacter calcoaceticus* SC 13876 [39,43]. On reduction of **7** by cell suspensions, the *syn*-**4** and *anti*-**8** dihydroxy esters were formed in the ratio of about 87:13, 83:17, 76:24 after 24 h at 2, 5 and 10 g/L of substrate input, respectively. There was no significant peak due to a monohydroxy ester. Chiral HPLC determined that the desired (3R,5S)-**4** was the major product with 99.4% e.e. Almost complete (>95%) conversion of the ethyl diketoester **7** to dihydroxy ester **4** in 24 h was seen up to a substrate concentration of 10 g/L and cell concentration of 200 g/L [39,43].

A mixture of ethyl 3-keto-5-hydroxy **9** (major) and 5-keto-3-hydroxy **10** (minor) was obtained from partial microbial reduction of ketoester **7**. These two mixtures were subjected to microbial reduction by *Acinetobacter* sp. SC13874 cells for 6 h (incomplete reduction). The reduction provided the dihydroxy esters with the isomeric composition. The results indicated that the second reduction of the monohydroxy compound by SC13874 cells was quite enantiospecific. Reduction of the

3-keto-5-hydroxy **9** provided predominantly the *(3R)*-hydroxy, while reduction of the 3-hydroxy-5-keto ester **10** provided predominantly the *(5S)*-hydroxy compound [43].

Cell extracts of A. *calcoaceticus* SC 13876 in the presence of NAD⁺, glucose, and glucose dehydrogenase reduced **7** to the corresponding monohydroxy compounds [3-hydroxy-5-oxo-6-(benzyloxy) hexanoic acid ethyl ester **9** and 5-hydroxy-3-oxo-6-(benzyloxy) hexanoic acid ethyl ester **10**]. Both **9** and **10** were further reduced to the *(3R,5S)*-dihydroxy compound **4** in 92% yield and 99% e.e. by cell extracts. *(3R,5S)*-**4** was converted to **11**, a key chiral intermediate for the synthesis of compound **5** and Atorvastatin **6**. Three different ketoreductases were purified to homogeneity from cell extracts of A. *calcoaceticus* SC 13876 and their biochemical properties were compared. Reductase I only catalyzes the reduction of ethyl diketoester **7** to its monohydroxy products whereas reductase II catalyzes the formation of dihydroxy products from monohydroxy substrates. A third reductase (III) was identified which catalyzes the reduction of diketoester **7** to *syn*-(3R,5S)-dihydroxy ester **4** [44], which now has been cloned and expressed in E. *coli* [44] and the reduction of diketoester **7** to *syn*-(3R,5S)-dihydroxy ester **4** was demonstrated by recombinant enzyme at 50 g/L substrate input with 10 g/L cell suspensions.

2.3. Atorvastatin: Enzymatic Preparation of (R)-4-Cyano-3-Hydroxybutyrate

An enzymatic process for the preparation of ethyl *(R)*-4-cyano-3-hydroxybutyric acid **12** (Figure 3), a key intermediate for the synthesis of Atorvastatin **6** was developed by Codexis [45]. In this process, first the enzymatic synthesis of ethyl *(S)*-4-chloro-3-hydroxybutyric acid derivatives **13** was carried out by ketoreductase-catalyzed conversion of 4-chloro-3-ketobutyric acid derivatives **14** [46]. The genes encoding halohydrin dehydrogenase from *Agrobacterium tumefaciens*, ketoreductase from *Candida magnoliae*, glucose dehydrogenase from *Bacillus subtilis* and formate dehydrogenase from *Candida boidinii* were separately cloned into *Escherichia coli* BL21. Each enzyme was then produced by fermentation, isolated and characterized. Then ethyl *(R)*-4-cyano-3-hydroxybutyrate **12** (Figure 3) was prepared from ethyl 4-chloroacetoacetate **14** by the following procedure: Ethyl 4-chloroacetoacetate 14 was incubated at pH 7.0 with ketoreductase, glucose dehydrogenase, and NADP⁺ for 40 h to produce ethyl *(S)*-4-chloro-3-hydroxybutyrate **13** which was extracted with ethyl acetate, dried, filtered and concentrated to yield ~97% pure ester. The dried ethyl *(S)*-4-chloro-3-hydroxybutyrate **13** was dissolved in phosphate buffer and mixed with halohydrin dehalogenase and sodium cyanide at pH 8.0. After 57 h, essentially pure ethyl *(R)*-4-cyano-3-hydroxybutyrate **12**, an intermediate used in HMG-CoA reductase inhibitors syntheses, was recovered [45].

Figure 3. Atorvastatin: Enzymatic preparation of *(R)*-4-cyano-3-hydroxybutyrate.

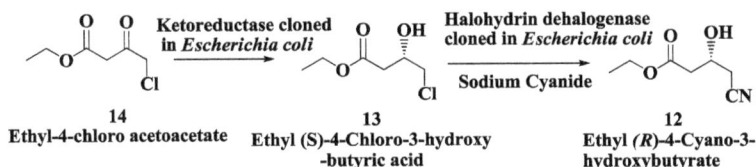

2.4. Preparation of (S)-4-Chloro-3-Hydroxybutanoic Acid Methyl Ester

(S)-4-chloro-3-hydroxybutanoic acid methyl ester **15** (Figure 4) is a key chiral intermediate in the total chemical synthesis of **16**, an inhibitor of HMG CoA reductase [46,47]. The reduction of 4-chloro-3-oxobutanoic acid methyl ester **17** to (S)-4-chloro-3-hydroxybutanoic acid methyl ester **15** (Figure 4) by cell suspensions of *Geotrichum candidum* SC 5469. In the biotransformation process, a reaction yield of 95% and e.e. of 96% were obtained for (S)-**15** by glucose-, acetate- or glycerol-grown cells (10% w/v) of *G. candidum* SC 5469 at 10 g/L substrate input. The e.e. of (S)-**15** was increased to 98% by heat-treatment of cell-suspensions (55 °C for 30 min) prior to conducting the bioreduction of **17** [48].

Figure 4. Chloesterol lowering agents: Preparation of (S)-4-chloro-3-hydroxybutanoic acid methyl ester.

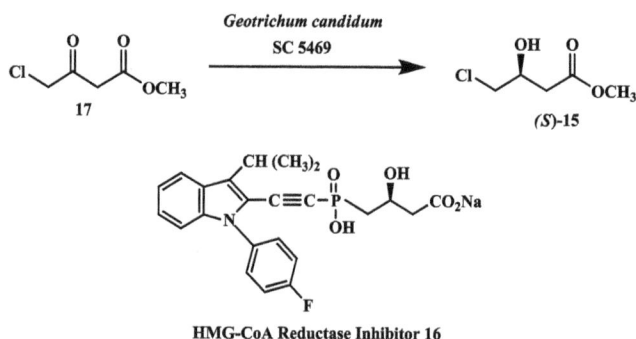

In an alternate approach, the asymmetric reduction of ethyl 4-chloroacetoacetate to (S)-4-chloro-3-hydroxybutonoate was demonstrated by a secondary alcohol dehydrogenase (PfODH) from *Pichia finlandica*. The gene encoding PfODH was cloned from *P. finlandica* and over expressed in *Escherichia coli*. Formate dehydrogenase was used to regenerate the cofactor NADH required for this reaction. Using recombinant *E. coli* coexpressing both PfODH and formate dehydrogenase from *Mycobacetrium* sp. produced to (S)-4-chloro-3-hydroxybutonoate in 98.5% yield and 99% e.e. at 32 g/L substrate input [49].

2.5. Rhinovirus Protease Inhibitor: Enzymatic Process for the Preparation of (R)-3-(4-Fluorophenyl)-2-Hydroxy Propionic Acid

(R)-3-(4-fluorophenyl)-2-hydroxy propionic acid **18** (Figure 5) is a building block for the synthesis of AG7088, a rhinovirus protease inhibitor **19** [50,51]. The preparation of **18** using a biocatalytic reduction of **20** in a membrane reactor [52]. A continuous enzymatic process for an efficient synthesis of (R)-3-(4-fluorophenyl)-2-hydroxy propionic acid at multikilogram scale with a high space-time yield (560 g/L/day) using a membrane reactor. The product was generated in excellent enantiomeric excess (e.e. >99.9%) and good overall yield (68%–72%).

Figure 5. Rhinovirus protease inhibitor: Enzymatic process for the preparation of (*R*)-3-(4-fluorophenyl)-2-hydroxy propionic acid.

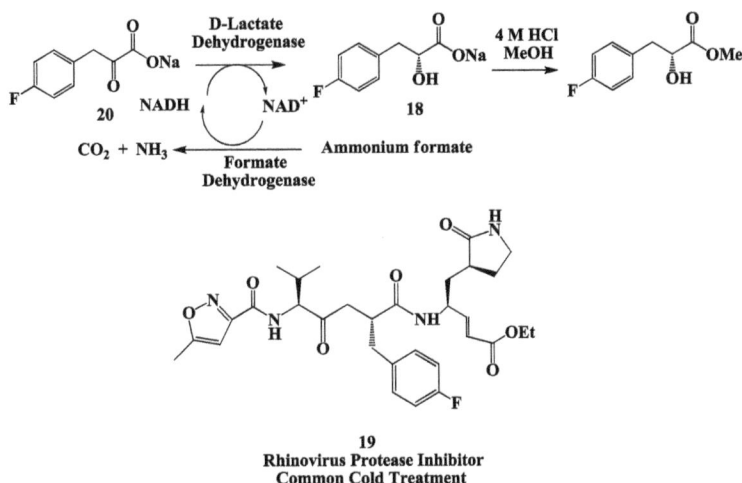

19
Rhinovirus Protease Inhibitor
Common Cold Treatment

Using this method, an overall quantity of 23 kg of **18** was prepared. The key step was an aqueous enzymatic reduction using D-lactate dehydrogenase (D-LDH) and formate dehydrogenase (FDH). Mechanistically, the keto acid salt **20** is stereoselectively reduced to the corresponding *R*-hydroxy acid **18** in the presence of D-lactate dehydrogenase by NADH. The cofactor itself is oxidized to NAD^+ in the process. Subsequently, in the presence of formate dehydrogenase, NAD^+ is reduced back to NADH by ammonium formate, which was oxidized to CO_2 and NH_3. In this fashion the expensive cofactor NAD^+ is regenerated by FDH, and only a catalytic amount of NAD^+ was required [52].

2.6. Enzymatic Preparation of Chiral Intermediates for Atazanavir

Atazanavir **21** (Figure 6) is an acyclic aza-peptidomimetic, a potent HIV protease inhibitor [53,54] approved by the Food and Drug Administration for treatment of Auto Immune Diseases (AIDS). An enzymatic process was developed for the preparation of (1*S*,2*R*)-[3-chloro-2-hydroxy-1-(phenylmethyl) propyl]carbamic acid, 1,1-dimethylethyl ester **22**, a key chiral intermediate required for the total synthesis of the HIV protease inhibitor atazanavir. The diastereoselective reduction of (1*S*)-[3-chloro-2-oxo-1-(phenylmethyl)propyl] carbamic acid, 1,1-dimethylethyl ester **23** was carried out using *Rhodococcus*, *Brevibacterium*, and *Hansenula* strains to provide **22**. Three strains of *Rhodococcus* gave >90% yield with a diastereomeric purity of >98% and an e.e. of 99.4% [55]. An efficient single-stage fermentation-biotransformation process was developed for the reduction of ketone **23** with cells of *Rhodococcus erythropolis* SC 13845 to yield **22** in 95% with a diasteromeric purity of 98.2% and an e.e. of 99.4% at substrate input of 10 g/L. The reduction process was further improved by generating mutants and selection of desired mutant for conversion of **23** to (1*S*,2*R*)-**22** at substrate input of 60 g/L [56]. (1*S*,2*R*)-**22** was converted to epoxide **24** and used in the synthesis of atazanavir. Chemical reduction of chloroketone **23** using NaBH₄ produces the undesired chlorohydrin diastereomer [57].

Figure 6. Atazanavir (antiviral agent): Enzymatic reparation of (1*S*,2*R*)-[3-chloro-2-hydroxy-1-(phenylmethyl) propyl]-carbamic acid,1,1-dimethyl-ethyl ester.

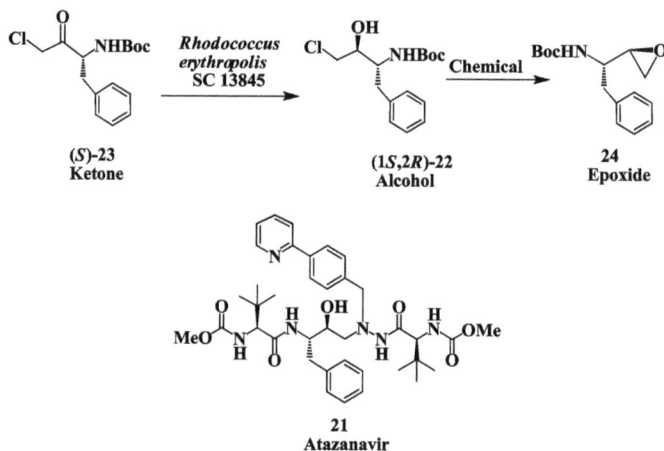

(S)-23
Ketone

(1S,2R)-22
Alcohol

24
Epoxide

21
Atazanavir

2.7. Enzymatic Reduction Process for Synthesis of Montelukast Intermediate

The discovery of the biological activity of the slow reacting substance of anaphylaxis (SRS-A) and its relation to the leukotrienes (LTC4, LTD4, and LTE4) and asthma, the search for leukotriene antagonists has been intensive. As part of an ongoing program for the development of specific LTD4 antagonists for the treatment of asthma and other associated diseases at Merck have identified Montelukast **25** (Figure 7) as LTD4 antagonist [58–60].

Merck has described the synthetic route for the production of montelukast, using a stereoselective reduction of a ketone **26** to the (*S*)-alcohol **27** as the key step. The alcohol subsequently undergoes a Sn2 displacement with a thiol to give the *R*-configured final product [59,60]. The reduction of the ketone **26** to produce the chiral alcohol **27** requires stoichiometric amounts of the chiral reducing agent (−)-flchlorodiisopino campheylborane [(−)-DIP-chloride]. (−)-DIP-chloride is selective and avoids the side reactions but it is corrosive and moisture-sensitive, causing burns if it is allowed to contact the skin. The reaction must be carried out at −20 to −25 °C to achieve the best stereoselectivity. The quench and extractive work-up generate large volumes of waste solvent, due to the product's low solubility. The potential advantages of biocatalytic transformation of ketone to alcohol were recognized early on by researchers at Merck. However, only two microorganisms were identified as having activity on the bulky and hydrophobic substrate [61]. Due to several reasons, an enzyme-catalyzed process for reduction of the ketone **26** was developed by Codexis. A ketoreductase was developed by directed evolution by high throughput screens using a slurry of the ketone substrate and high isopropanol concentration. Beneficial mutations among the various improved mutants were recombined in each round, and new mutations were made guided by ProSAR. The productivity of the final enzyme was improved 2,000-fold and stability was also substantially increased [62].

Figure 7. Enzymatic reduction process for synthesis (*S*)-alcohol **27** for Montelukast intermediate.

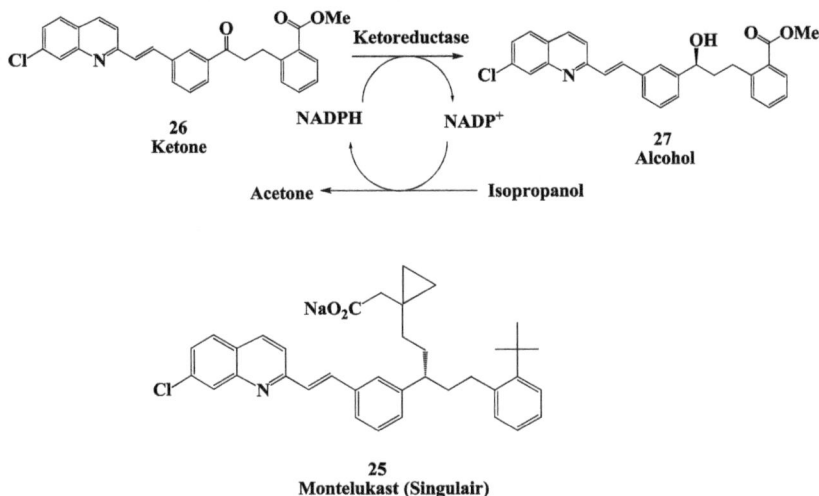

The final process was carried out as a slurry-to-slurry reaction at 45 °C, with the sparingly soluble ketone **26** being converted to an almost equally insoluble alcohol **27** at a concentration of 100 g/L substrate in aqueous isopropanol and toluene. A reaction yield of 99.3% and enantiomeric excess of 99.9% was obtained for alcohol 27 [62].

2.8. Anticancer Drug: Enzymatic Preparation of C-13 Paclitaxel Side-Chain Synthon

Among the antimitotic agents, paclitaxel (taxol®) **28** (Figure 8), a complex, polycyclic diterpene, exhibits a unique mode of action on microtubule proteins responsible for the formation of the spindle during cell division. Various types of cancers have been treated with paclitaxel and it was approved for use by the FDA for treatment of ovarian cancer and metastatic breast cancer [63–65]. A key precursor for the paclitaxel semi-synthetic process is the chiral C-13 paclitaxel side-chain **29**. An enzymatic enantioselective microbial reduction of 2-keto-3-(N-benzoylamino)-3-phenyl propionic acid ethyl ester **30** to yield (2*R*,3*S*)-*N*-benzoyl-3-phenyl isoserine ethyl ester **29** was demonstrated using two strains of *Hansenula* [66]. Preparative-scale bioreduction of ketone **30** was demonstrated using cell suspensions of *Hansenula polymorpha* SC 13865 and *Hansenula fabianii* SC 13894 in independent experiments. In both batches, a reaction yield of >80% and e.e.s of >94% were obtained for (2*R*,3*S*)-**29**. In a single-stage process, cells of *H. fabianii* were grown in a 15-L fermentor for 48 h, then the bioreduction process was initiated by addition of 30 g of substrate and 250 g of glucose and continued for 72 h. A reaction yield of 88% with an e.e. of 95% was obtained for (2*R*,3*S*)-**29**.

2.9. Antipsychotic Drug: Enzymatic Reduction of
1-(4-Fluorophenyl)4-[4-(5-Fluoro-2-Pyrimidinyl)1-Piperazinyl]-1-Butanone

The sigma receptor system in the brain and endocrine tissue has been target for development of new class of antipsychotic drugs [67,68]. Compound (R)-31 (Figure 9) is a sigma ligand and has a high affinity for sigma binding site and antipsychotic efficacy. The enantioselective microbial reduction process was developed for the conversion of ketone 32 to both enantiomers of alcohol 31 [69]. Various microorganisms screened for the enatioselective reduction of 1-(4-fluorophenyl)4-[4-(5-fluoro-2-pyrimidinyl)1-piperazinyl]-1butanone 32. From this screen, *Mortierella ramanniana* ATCC 38191 was identified to predominantly reduced compound 32 to (R)-31, while *Pullularia pullulans* ATCC 16623 was identified to predominantly reduced compound 32 to (S)-31. A single stage fermentation/biotransformation process was developed. Cells of *M. ramanniana* were grown in a 20-L fermentor and after 40 h growth period, the biotransformation process was initiated by addition of 40 g ketone 32 and 400 g glucose. The biotransformation process was completed in 24 h with a reaction yield of 100% and an e.e. of 98.9% for (R)-31. At the end of the biotransformation process, cells were removed by filtration and product was recovered from the filtrate in overall 80% yield [69].

Figure 8. Anticancer drug: Enzymatic preparation of C-13 paclitaxel side-chain synthon.

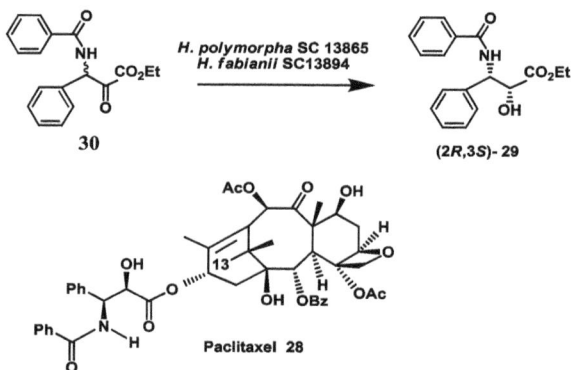

2.10. Retinoic Acid Receptpor Agonist: Enzymatic Preparation of
2-(R)-Hydroxy-2-(1',2',3',4'-Tetrahydro-1',1',4',4'-Tetramethyl-6'-Naphthalenyl)Acetate

Retinoic acid and its natural and synthetic analogs (retinoids) exert a wide variety of biological effects by binding to or activating a specific receptor or sets of receptors [70]. They have been shown to effect cellular growth and differentiation and are promising drugs for the treatment of cancers [71]. A few retinoids are already in clinical use for the treatment of dermatological diseases such as acne and psoriasis. (R)-3-Fluoro-4-[[hydroxy-(5,6,7,8-tetrahydro-5,5,8,8-tetramethyl -2-naphthalenyl)-acetyl]amino]benzoic acid 33 (Figure 10) is a retinoic acid receptor gamma-specific agonist potentially useful as a dermatological and anticancer drug [72].

Figure 9. Antipsychotic drug: Enzymatic reduction of 1-(4-fluorophenyl)4
-[4-(5-fluoro-2-pyrimidinyl)1-piperazinyl]-1-butanone.

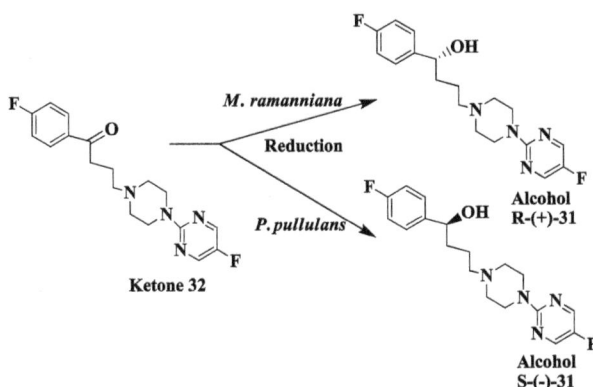

Figure 10. Retinoic acid receptor agonist: Enzymatic preparation of
2-(*R*)-hydroxy-2-(1′,2′,3′,4′-tetrahydro-1′,1′,4′,4′-tetramethyl-6′-naphthalenyl)acetate.

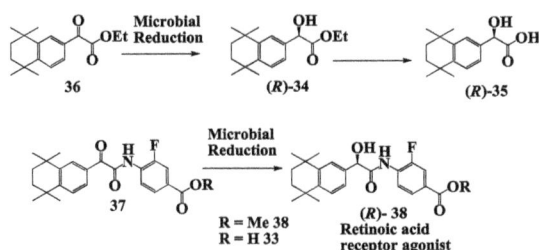

Ethyl 2-(*R*)-hydroxy-2-(1′,2′,3′,4′-tetrahydro-1′,1′,4′,4′-tetramethyl-6′-naphthalenyl)acetate **34** and the corresponding acid **35** were prepared as intermediates in the synthesis of the retinoic acid receptor gamma-specific agonist [73]. Enantioselective microbial reduction of ethyl 2-oxo-2-(1′,2′,3′,4′-tetrahydro-1′,1′,4′,4′-tetramethyl-6-naphthalenyl) acetate **36** to alcohol **34** was carried out using *Aureobasidium pullulans* SC 13849 in 98% yield and with an e.e. of 96%. At the end of the reaction, hydroxyester **34** was adsorbed onto XAD-16 resin and, after filtration, recovered in 94% yield from the resin with acetonitrile extraction. The recovered (*R*)-hydroxyester **34** was treated with Chirazyme L-2 or pig liver esterase to convert it to the corresponding (*R*)-hydroxyacid **35** in quantitative yield. The enantioselective microbial reduction of ketoamide **37** to the corresponding (*R*)-hydroxyamide **38** by *A. pullulans* SC 13849 has also been demonstrated [73].

2.11. Anti-Alzheimer's Drugs: Enzymatic Reduction of 5-Oxohexanoate and 5-Oxohexanenitrile

Ethyl-(*S*)-5-hydroxyhexanoate **39** and (*S*)-5-hydroxyhexanenitrile **40** (Figure 11) are key chiral intermediates in the synthesis of anti-Alzheimer's drugs [74]. Both chiral compounds have been prepared by enantioselective reduction of ethyl-5-oxohexanoate **41** and 5-oxohexanenitrile 42 by *Pichia methanolica* SC 16116 [75]. Reaction yields of 80%–90% and >95% e.e.s were obtained for each compound. In an alternate approach, the enzymatic resolution of racemic 5-hydroxyhexane nitrile **43** by enzymatic succinylation was demonstrated using immobilized lipase PS-30 to obtain (S)-5-hydroxyhexanenitrile **40** in 35% yield (maximum yield is 50%). (S)-5-Acetoxy-hexanenitrile **44** was prepared by enantioselective enzymatic hydrolysis of racemic 5-acetoxyhexanenitrile **45** by *Candida antarctica* lipase. A reaction yield of 42% and an e.e. of >99% were obtained [75].

Figure 11. Anti-Alzheimer's drugs: Enzymatic reduction of 5-oxohexanoate and 5-oxohexanenitrile.

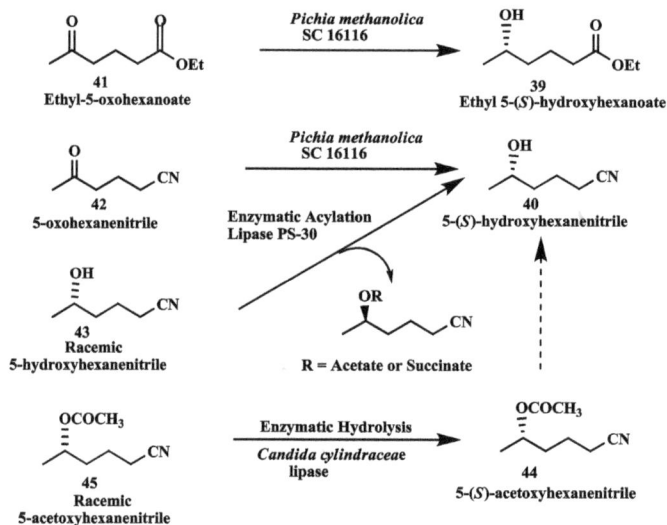

2.12. Enantioselective Microbial Reduction of Substituted Acetophenone

The chiral intermediates (S)-1-(2'-bromo-4'-fluorophenyl)ethanol **46** and (S)-methyl 4-(2'-acetyl-5'-fluorophenyl)-butanol **47** are potential intermediates for the synthesis of several potential anti-Alzheimer's drugs [76]. The chiral intermediate (S)-1-(2'-bromo-4'-fluoro phenyl)ethanol **46** (Figure 12A) was prepared by the enantioselective microbial reduction of 2-bromo-4-fluoro acetophenone **48** [77]. Organisms from genus *Candida, Hansenula, Pichia, Rhodotorula, Saccharomyces, Sphingomonas* and Baker's yeast reduced **48** to **46** in >90% yield and 99% enantiomeric excess (e.e.).

In an alternate approach, the enantioselective microbial reduction of methyl-4-(2'-acetyl-5'-fluorophenyl) butanoates **49** (Figure 12B) was demonstrated using strains of *Candida* and *Pichia*. Reaction yields of 40%–53% and e.e.s of 90%–99% were obtained for the corresponding (S)-hydroxy esters **47**. The reductase which catalyzed the enantioselective reduction of ketoesters was purified to homogeneity from cell extracts of *Pichia methanolica* SC 13825. It was cloned and expressed in *Escherichia coli* and recombinant cultures were used for the enantioselective reduction of the keto-methyl ester **49** to the corresponding (S)-hydroxy methyl ester **47**. On preparative scale, a reaction yield of 98% with an enantiomeric excess of 99% for **47** was obtained [77].

Figure 12. (**A**) Anti-Alzheimer's drugs: Enantioselective microbial reduction of substituted acetophenone; (**B**) Enantioselective microbial reduction of methyl-4-(2'-acetyl-5'-fluorophenyl) butanoates.

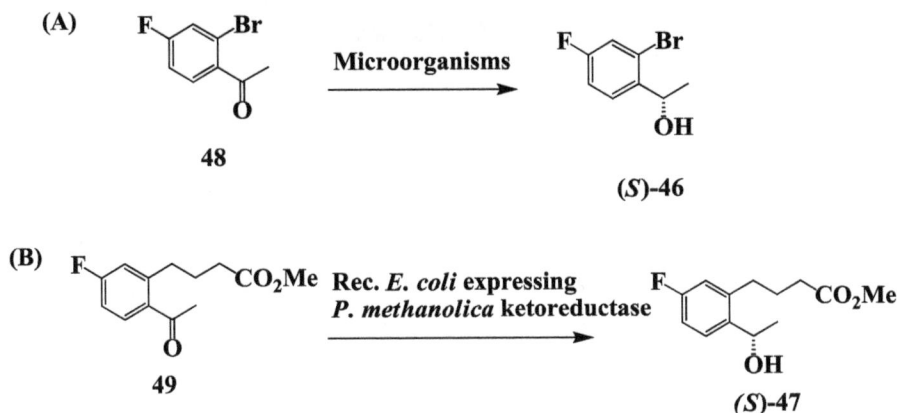

(**A**)

48

Microorganisms

(S)-46

(**B**)

49

Rec. *E. coli* expressing
P. methanolica ketoreductase

(S)-47

2.13. Anticancer Drug: Enzymatic Preparation of (S)-2-Chloro-1-(3-Chlorophenyl)Ethanol

The synthesis of the leading candidate compound **50** [78] in an anticancer program (IGF-1 receptor inhibitors) [79,80] required (S)-2-chloro-1-(3-chlorophenyl)ethanol **51** (Figure 13) as an intermediate. Other possible candidate compounds used are analogs of (S)-alcohol **51**. From microbial screen of the reduction of ketone **52** to (S)-alcohol **51**, two cultures namely *Hansenula polymorpha* SC13824 (73.8% enantiomeric excess) and *Rhodococcus globerulus* SC SC16305 (71.8% enantiomeric excess) were identified that had the highest enantioselectivity. A ketoreductase from *Hansenula polymorpha*, after purification to homogeneity, gave (S)-alcohol **51** with 100% ee [81]. The ketoreductase was cloned and expressed in *E. coli* together with a glucose-6-phosphate dehydrogenase from *Saccharomyces cerevisiae* to allow regeneration of the NADPH required for the reduction process. An extract of *E. coli* containing the two recombinant enzymes was used to reduce 2-chloro-1-(3-chloro-4fluorophenyl)ethanone **52**. Intact *E. coli* cells provided with glucose were used to prepare (S)-2-chloro-1-(3-chloro-4-fluorophenyl)ethanol **51** in 89% yield with 100% e.e. [81].

2.14. Thrombin Inhibitor: Enzymatic Preparation of (R)-2-Hydroxy-3,3-Dimethylbutanoic Acid

Thrombin is a trypsin-like protease enzyme that plays a critical role in intrinsic and extrinsic blood coagulation. As a result of the enzymatic activation of numerous coagulation factors, thrombin is activated to cleave fibrinogen, producing fibrin, which is directly responsible for blood clotting. An imbalance between these factors and their endogenous activators and inhibitors can give rise to a number of disease states such as myocardial infarction, unstable angina, stroke, ischemia, restenosis following angioplasty, pulmonary embolism, deep vein thrombosis, and arterial thrombosis [82,83]. Consequently, the aggressive search for a potent, selective, and bioavailable thrombin inhibitor is widespread [84]. An intensive effort by Merck has led to the identification of thrombin inhibitor **53** [85]. The synthesis of **53** required a key chiral intermediate (R)-hydroxy ester **54**. An enzymatic process

272

was developed for the asymmetric reduction of ketoester **55** to (*R*)-**54** using commercially available ketoreductase KRED1001 (Figure 14). The cofactor NADPH required for this reaction was regenerated using glucose dehydrogenase. The hydroxy ester (*R*)-**54** was isolated as an oil and then saponified to the corresponding enantiomerically pure hydroxy acid (*R*)-**56** without epimerization [86]. The enantiomerically pure (*R*)-**56** was obtained in 82% isolated yield (>99.5% e.e.).

Figure 13. Anticancer drug: Enzymatic preparation of (*S*)-2-chloro-1-(3-chlorophenyl)ethanol.

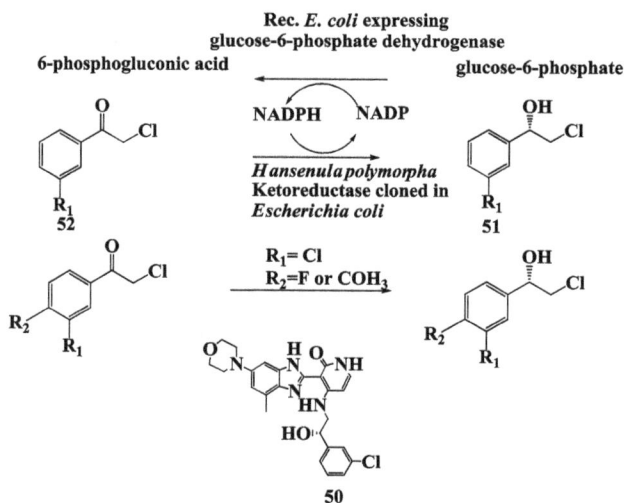

Figure 14. Thrombin inhibitor: Enzymatic preparation of (*R*)-2-Hydroxy-3,3-dimethylbutanoic acid.

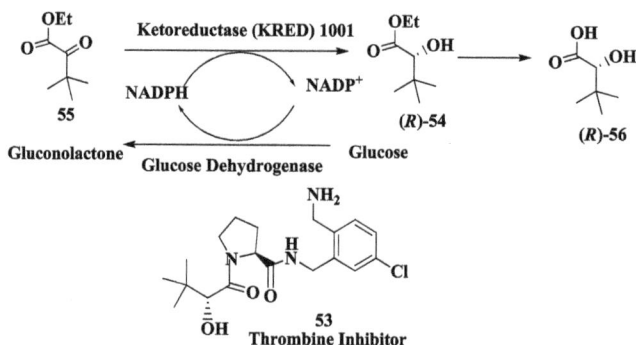

2.15. Endothelin Receptor Antagonist: Enantioselective Microbial Reduction of Keto Ester and Chloroketone

Endothelin is present in elevated levels in the blood of patients with hypertension, acute myocardial infarction and pulmonary hypertension. Two endothelin receptor sub-types have been identified which bind endothelin, thus causing vasoconstriction [87,88]. Endothelin receptor antagonists such as compound **57** (Figure 15) have potential therapeutic value. Synthesis of compound **57** required two key chiral intermediates (*S*)-alcohols **58** and **59**. Enantioselective microbial reduction of a ketoester **60** and a chlorinated ketone **61** to their corresponding (*S*)-alcohols **58** and **59** was demonstrated using *Pichia delftensis* MY 1569 and *Rhodotorula piliminae* ATCC 32762 to afford desired products in >98% e.e. and >99% e.e, respectively [89]. Reductions were scaled up to 23 L to produce the desired (*S*)-alcohols in 88% and 97% yields, respectively.

Figure 15. Endothelin receptor antagonist: Enantioselective microbial reduction of keto ester and chloroketone.

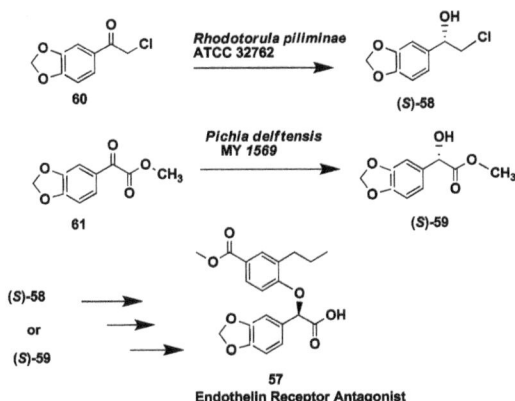

2.16. Calcium Channel Blocker: Preparation of
[(3R-cis)-1,3,4,5-Tetrahydro-3-Hydroxy-4-(4-Methoxyphenyl)-6-(Trifluromethyl)
-2H-1-Benzazepin-2-One]

Diltiazem **62** (Figure 16) a benzothiazepinone calcium channel blocking agent that inhibits influx of extracellular calcium through L-type voltage-operated calcium channels, has been widely used clinically in the treatment of hypertension and angina [90]. Since diltiazem has a relatively short duration of action [91], an 8-chloro derivative recently has been introduced into the clinic as a more potent analogue [92]. Lack of extended duration of action and little information on structure-activity relationships in this class of compounds led Floyd *et al.* [93] to prepare isosteric 1-benzazepin-2-ones; this led to identification of (*cis*)-3-(acetoxy)-1-[2-(dimethylamino)ethyl] -1,3,4,5-tetrahydro-4-(4-methoxyphenyl)-6-trifluoromethyl)-2H-1-benzazepin-2-one **63** as a longer lasting and more potent antihypertensive agent. A key intermediate in the synthesis of this compound was (3R-cis)-1,3,4,5-tetrahydro-3-hydroxy-4-(4-methoxyphenyl)-6-(trifluromethyl) -2H-1-benzazepin-2-one **64**. An enantioselective process was developed for the reduction of 4,5-dihydro-4-(4-methoxyphenyl)-6-(trifluoromethyl)-1H-1-benzazepin-2,3-dione **65** to **64** using *Nocardia salmonicolor* SC 6310, in 96% reaction yield with 99.8% e.e. [94].

Figure 16. Calcium channel blocker: Preparation of [(3*R-cis*)-1,3,4, 5-tetrahydro-3-hydroxy-4-(4-methoxyphenyl)-6-(trifluromethyl)-2*H*-1-benzazepin-2-one].

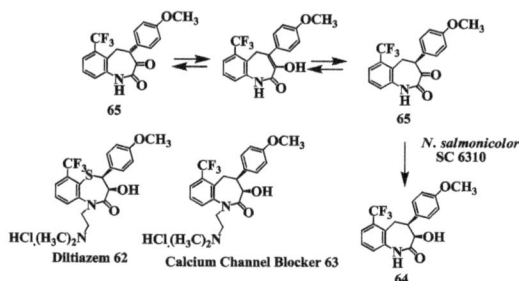

2.17. β3-Receptor Agonist: Reduction of 4-Benzyloxy-3-Methanesulfonylamino-2'-Bromo-Acetophenone

β3-Adrenergic receptors are found on the cell surfaces of both white and brown adipocytes and are responsible for lipolysis, thermogenesis, and relaxation of intestinal smooth muscle [95]. Consequently, several research groups are engaged in developing selective β3 agonists for the treatment of gastrointestinal disorders, type II diabetes, and obesity [96,97]. Biocatalytic syntheses of chiral intermediates required for the total synthesis of β3 receptor agonists **66** (Figure 17) has been demonstrated [98].

Figure 17. β3-Receptor agonist: Reduction of 4-benzyloxy-3-methanesulfonylamino-2-bromo-acetophenone.

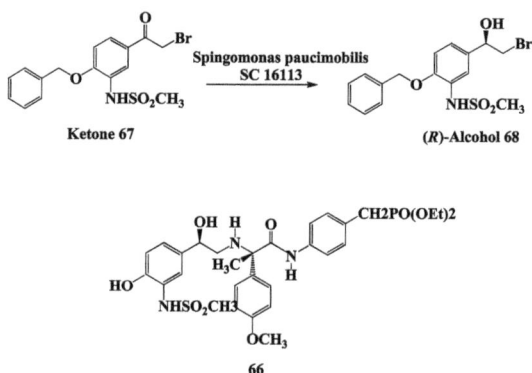

The microbial reduction of 4-benzyloxy-3-methanesulfonylamino-2'-bromo-acetophenone **67** to the corresponding (*R*)-alcohol **68** has been demonstrated [98] using *Sphingomonas. paucimobilis* SC 16113. The growth of *S. paucimobilis* SC 16113 was carried out in a 750-L fermentor and harvested cells (60 kg) were used to conduct the biotransformation in 10-L and 200-L preparative batches using 20% (wt/vol, wet cells). In some batches, the fermentation broth was concentrated 3-fold by microfiltration and subsequently washed with buffer by diafilteration and used directly in the bioreduction process. In all the batches, reaction yields of >85% and e.e.s. of >98% were obtained.

The isolation of alcohol **68** from the 200-L batch gave 320 g (80% yield) of product with an e.e. of 99.5%.

In an alternate process, frozen cells of *S. paucimobilis* SC 16113 were used with XAD-16 hydrophobic resin (50 g/L) adsorbed substrate at 10 g/L concentration. In this process, an average reaction yield of 85% and an e.e. of >99% were obtained for alcohol **68**. At the end of the biotransformation, the reaction mixture was filtered on a 100 mesh (150 μm) stainless steel screen, and the resin retained by the screen was washed with water. The product was then desorbed from the resin with acetonitrile and crystallized in 75% overall yield with a 99.8% e.e.[98].

2.18. Penem and Carbapenem: Enzymatic Preparation of (R)-1,3-Butanediol and (R)-4-Chloro-3-Hydroxybutonoate

(*R*)-1,3-Butanediol **69** (Figure 18) is a key starting material of azetidinone derivatives **70**, which are key chiral intermediates for the synthesis of penem **71** and carbapenem antibiotics [99]. From a microbial screen, the *Candida parapsilosis* strain IFO 1396 was identified which produced (*R*)-1,3-butanediol from the racemate. The (*S*)-1,3-butanediol oxidizing enzyme (CpSADH) which produced (*R*)-1,3-butanediol from the racemate was cloned in *Escherichia coli*. The recombinant culture catalyzed the enantioselective oxidation of secondary alcohols and also catalyzed the asymmetric reduction of aromatic and aliphatic ketones to their corresponding (*S*)-secondary alcohols. Using the recombinant enzyme, (*R*)-1,3-butanediol was produced in 97% yield and 95% e.e. using 150 g/L input of the racemate. Recombinant enzyme (CpSADH) was also used for reduction of ethyl 4-chloroacetoacetate **72** to produce ethyl-(*R*)-4-chloro-3-hydroxybutonoate **73** in 95% yield and 99% e.e. using 36 g/L substrate input. Isopropanol was used to regenerate the NADH required for this reduction. Ethyl-(*R*)-4-chloro-3-hydroxybutonoate is useful for the synthesis of L-carnitine **74** and (*R*)-4-hydroxyl pyrrolidone **75** [100,101]).

Figure 18. Penem and carbapenem: Enzymatic preparation of (*R*)-1,3-butanediol and (*R*)-4-chloro-3-hydroxybutonoate.

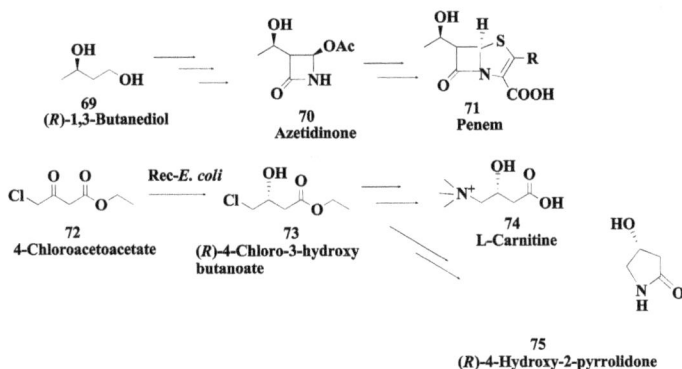

2.19. Integrin Receptor Agonist: Enzymatic Preparation of (R)-Allylic Alcohol

(R)-allylic alcohol **76** (Figure 19) was required as an intermediate for the synthesis of a desired monanoic derivate useful as an integrin receptor antagonist for the inhibition of bone desorption and treatment of osteoporosis [102]. A pilot scale whole cell process was developed for the enantioselective 1,2-reduction of prochiral alpha,beta-unsaturated ketone **77** to (R) allylic alcohol, (R)-**76** using *Candida chilensis* [103]. Initial development showed high enantiomeric excess (>95%) but low product yield (10%). Further process development, using a combination of statistically designed screening and optimization experiments, improved the desired alcohol yield to 90%. The fermentation growth stage, particularly medium composition and growth pH, had a significant impact on the bioconversion while process characterization identified diverse challenges including the presence of multiple enzymes, substrate/product toxicity, and biphasic cellular morphology. Manipulating the fermentation media allowed control of the whole cell morphology to a predominantly unicellular broth, away from the viscous pseudohyphae, which were detrimental to the bioconversion. The activity of a competing enzyme, which produced the undesired saturated ketone **78** and (R)-saturated alcohol **79**, was minimized to < or =5% by controlling the reaction pH, temperature, substrate concentration, and biomass level. Despite the toxicity effects limiting the volumetric productivity, a reproducible and saleable process was demonstrated at pilot scale with high enantioselectivity (e.e. > 95%) and overall yield greater than 80% [104]. The whole cell approach proved to be a valuable alternative to chemical reduction routes.

Figure 19. Integrin receptor agonist: Enzymatic preparation of (R)-allylic alcohol.

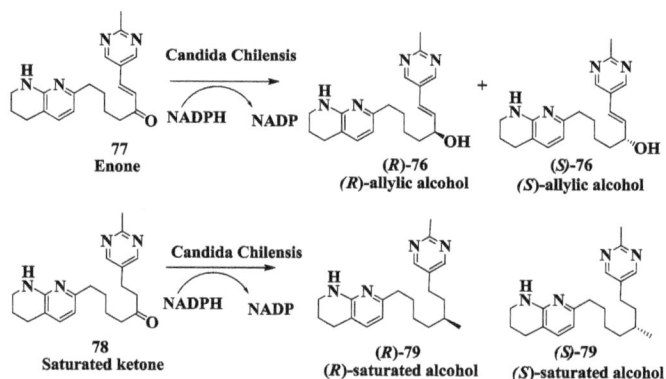

2.20. NK1 Receptor Antagonists: Enzymatic Synthesis of (S)-3,5-Bistrifluoromethylphenyl Ethanol

The synthesis of (S)-3,5-bistrifluoromethylphenyl ethanol, (S)-**80**, (Figure 20), an intermediate for the synthesis of NK-1 receptor antagonists **81** [104] was demonstrated from a ketone **82** via asymmetric enzymatic reduction process [105]. The isolated enzyme alcohol dehydrogenase from *Rhodococcus erythropolis* reduced the poorly water soluble substrate with an excellent enantiomeric excess (>99.9%) and good conversion (>98%). The optimized process was demonstrated up to pilot scale using concentration (390 mM) using a easy isolation process achieving overall isolation yields

(>90%). Process improvements at preparative scale, demonstrated increase in the substrate input to 580 mM achieving a space time yield of 260 g/L/day [105].

Figure 20. NK1 receptor antagonists: Enzymatic synthesis of (S)-3,5-bistrifluoromethylphenyl ethanol.

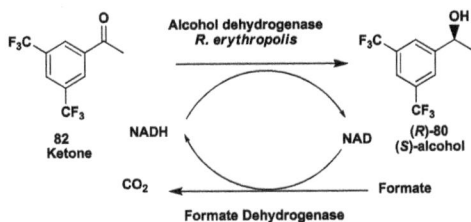

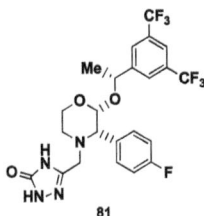

3. Enzymatic Preparation of Chiral Amino Acids

The reductive amination of α-keto acids using amino acid dehydrogenases to be one of the most useful methods because the enzymes have good stability, broad substrate specificity and very high enantioselectivity and can be used at high substrate concentrations as keto acids are soluble in aqueous system. The reductive aminations process coupled to an enzymatic cofactor regeneration system are most prominent method for preparation of chiral amino acids. For most enzymes, the required cofactor is NADH but NADPH is required in some cases. Yeast formate dehydrogenase is commonly used for NADH regeneration and glucose dehydrogenase usually from *Bacillus* species may be used for either NADH or NADPH regeneration. There are excellent reviews on the amino acid dehydrogenases and examples of their synthetic utilities [106–109].

3.1. Tigemonam: Enzymatic Synthesis of (S)-β-Hydroxyvaline

(S)-β-hydroxyvaline **83** (Figure 21), is a key chiral intermediate required for the total synthesis of orally active monobactam [110], Tigemonam **84**. Chiral amino acids have been made from corresponding keto acids by reductive amination process [111]. The synthesis of (S)-β-hydroxyvaline **83** from α-keto-β-hydroxyisovalerate **85** by reductive amination using leucine dehydrogenase from *Bacillus sphaericus* ATCC 4525 has been demonstrated [112]. The NADH required for this reaction was regenerated by either formate dehydrogenase from *Candida boidinii* or glucose dehydrogenase from *Bacillus megaterium*. The required substrate **85** was generated either from α-keto-β-bromoisovalerate or its ethyl esters by hydrolysis with sodium hydroxide *in situ*. In this process, an overall reaction yield of 98% and an enantiomeric excess of 99.8% were obtained for the L-β-hydroxyvaline **83**.

Figure 21. Tigemonam: Enzymatic synthesis of (S)-β-hydroxyvaline.

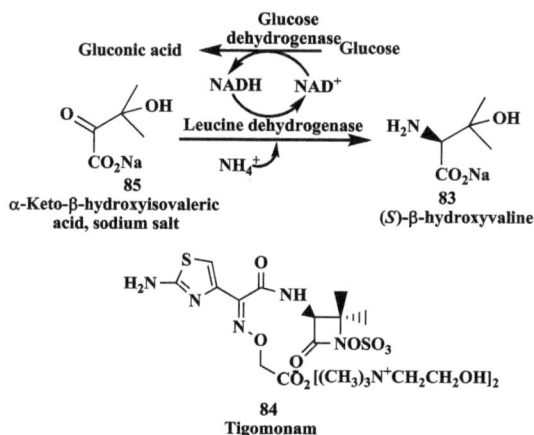

85
α-Keto-β-hydroxyisovaleric
acid, sodium salt

83
(S)-β-hydroxyvaline

84
Tigomonam

3.2. Atazanavir: Enzymatic Synthesis of (S)-Tertiary-Leucine

Atazanavir **86** is an acyclic aza-peptidomimetic, a potent HIV protease inhibitor [53,54]. Synthesis of atazanavir required (S)-tertiary leucine **87** (Figure 22). An enzymatic reductive amination of ketoacid **88** to amino acid **87** by recombinant *Escherichia coli* expressing leucine dehydrogenase from *Thermoactinimyces intermedius* has been demonstrated. The reaction required ammonia and NADH as a cofactor. NAD produced during the reaction was converted back to NADH using recombinant *Escherichia coli* expressing formate dehydrogenase from *Pichia pastoris*. A reaction yield of >95% with an e.e. of >99.5% was obtained for **87** at 100 g/L substrate [113]. Leucine dehydrogenase from *Bacillus* strain has also been cloned and expressed and used in reductive amination process [114,115].

3.3. Vanlev: Enzymatic Synthesis of (S)-6-Hydroxynorleucine

Vanlev **89** (Figure 23) is an antihypertensive drug which acts by inhibiting angiotensin-converting enzyme (ACE) and neutral endopeptidase (NEP) [116]. (S)-6-Hydroxynorleucine **90** is a key intermediate in the synthesis of Vanlev. The synthesis and complete conversion of 2-keto-6-hydroxyhexanoic acid **91** to (S)-6-hydroxynorleucine **90** was demonstrated by reductive amination using beef liver glutamate dehydrogenase [117]. As depicted, compound **91**, in equilibrium with 2-hydroxytetrahydropyran-2-carboxylic acid sodium salt **92**, was converted to **90**. The reaction requires ammonia and NADH. NAD produced during the reaction was recycled to NADH by the oxidation of glucose to gluconic acid using glucose dehydrogenase from *Bacillus megaterium*. The reaction was complete in about 3 h at 100 g/L substrate input with a reaction yields of 92% and e.e. of 99.8% for (S)-6-hydroxynorleucine. The synthesis and isolation of keto acid **91** required several steps. In a second, more convenient process the ketoacid was prepared by treatment of racemic 6-hydroxy norleucine **90** [produced by hydrolysis of 5-(4-hydroxybutyl) hydantoin **93**] with (*R*)-amino acid oxidase (Figure 24) After the e.e. of the unreacted (*S*)-6-hydroxynorleucine had risen to 99.8%, the reductive amination procedure was used to convert the mixture containing the 2-keto-6-hydroxyhexanoic acid entirely to (*S*)-6-hydroxynorleucine in 97% yield with 99.8% e.e. from racemic 6-hydroxynorleucine at 100 g/L substrate input [117]. The (*S*)-6-hydroxynorleucine prepared by the enzymatic process was converted chemically to Valev **89** [118].

Figure 22. Atazanavir (anti-viral agent): Enzymatic synthesis of (*S*)-tertiary-leucine.

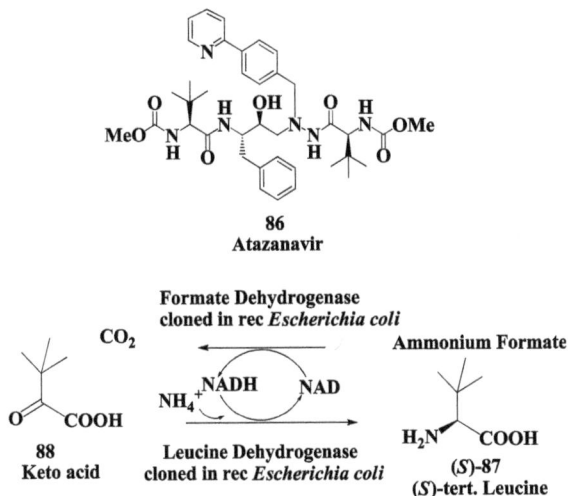

Figure 23. Vanlev: Enzymatic synthesis of (*S*)-6-hydroxynorleucine by reductive amination.

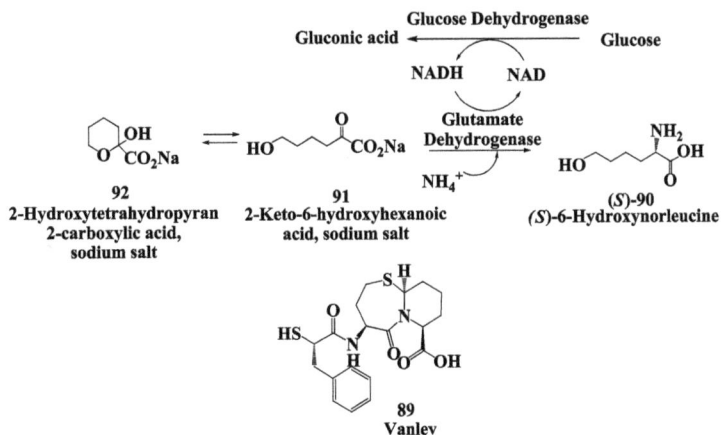

280

Figure 24. Vanlev: Enzymatic conversion of racemic 6-hydroxy norleucine to (S)-6-hydroxymorleucine.

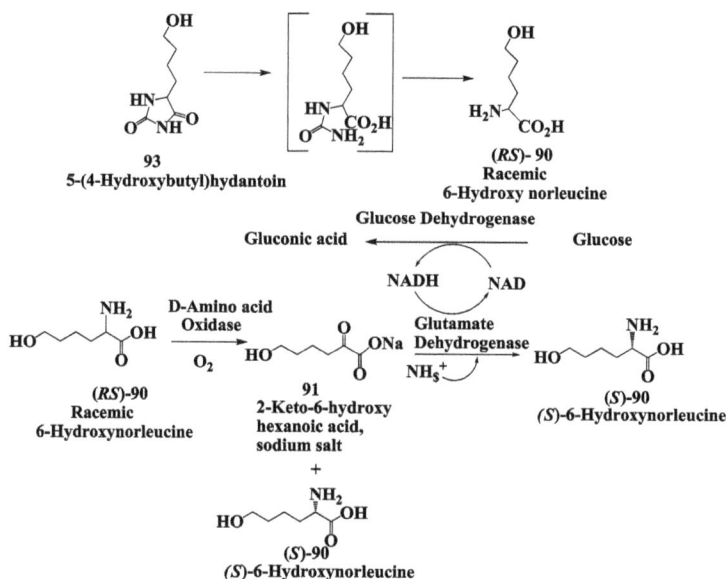

3.4. Vanlev: Enzymatic Synthesis of Allysine Ethylene Acetal

(S)-2-Amino-5-(1,3-dioxolan-2-yl)-pentanoic acid [(S)-allysine ethylene acetal] **94** (Figure 25) is one of three building blocks used in an alternative synthesis of Vanlev **89**. Synthesis of **94** was demonstrated by reductive amination of ketoacid acetal **95** using phenylalanine dehydrogenase [PDH] from *Thermoactinomyces intermedius* [119]. The reaction required ammonia and NADH; NAD produced during the reaction was recyled to NADH by the oxidation of formate to CO_2 using formate dehydrogenase [FDH]. *T. intermedius* PDH was cloned and expressed in *Escherichia coli* and recombinant culture was used as a source of PDH. Expression of *T. intermedius* PDH in *P. pastoris*, inducible by methanol, allowed generation of both enzymes in a single fermentation as methanol grown cells of *P. pastoris* also contained formate dehydrogease. A total of 197 kg of **94** was produced in three 1600-L batches using a 5% concentration of substrate **95** with an average yield of 91 M % and e.e. >98% [119]. (S)-allysine ethylene acetal was converted to Vanlev **89** [118].

3.5. Saxagliptin: Enzymatic Reductive Amination of 2-(3-Hydroxy-1-Adamantyl)-2-Oxoethanoic Acid

Dipeptidyl peptidase 4 (DPP-4) is a ubiquitous proline-specific serine protease responsible for the rapid inactivation of incretins, including glucagon-like peptide 1 (GLP-1) and glucose-dependent insulinotropic peptide. To alleviate the inactivation of GLP-1, inhibitors of DPP-IV are being evaluated for their ability to provide improved control of blood glucose for diabetics [120–123]. Januvia developed by Merck is a marketed DPP4 Inhibitor [122].

Figure 25. Vanlev: Enzymatic synthesis of allysine ethylene acetal.

89
Vanlev

95
Ketoacid Acetal

Formate dehydrogenase
CO$_2$ ← Ammonium formate

NADH
NH$_4^+$ → NAD

Phenylalanine dehydrogenase

(S)-94
(S)-Allysine Ethylene Acetal

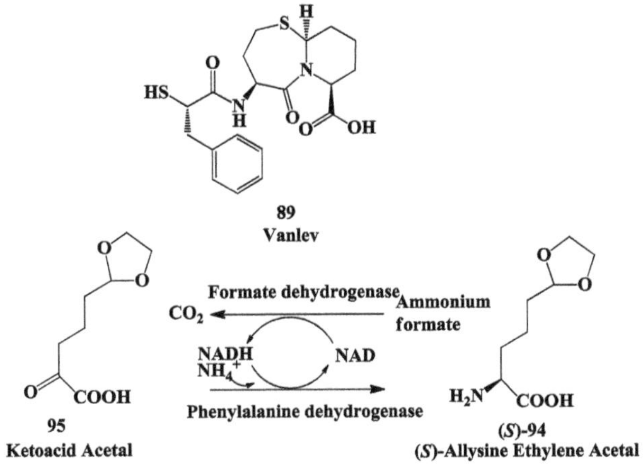

Saxagliptin **96** [121,122] (Figure 26), a DPP-IV inhibitor developed by Bristol-Myers Squibb and now approved for type 2 diabetic treatment by Food and Drug administration, requires (S)-N-boc-3-hydroxyadamantylglycine **97** as an intermediate. A process for conversion of the keto acids **98** to the corresponding amino acid **99** using (S)-amino acid dehydrogenases was developed. A modified form of a recombinant phenylalanine dehydrogenase cloned from *Thermoactinomyces intermedius* and expressed in *Pichia pastoris* or *Escherichia coli* was used for this process. NAD produced during the reaction was recycled to NADH using formate dehydrogenase. The modified phenylalanine dehydrogenase contains two amino acid changes at the C-terminus and a 12 amino acid extension of the C-terminus [124].

Figure 26. Saxagliptin: Enzymatic reductive amination of 2-(3-hydroxy-1-adamantyl)-2-oxoethanoic acid.

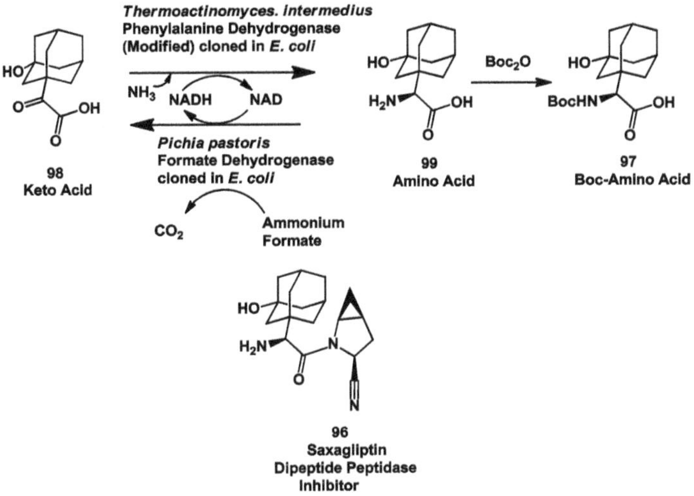

98
Keto Acid

Thermoactinomyces. intermedius
Phenylalanine Dehydrogenase
(Modified) cloned in *E. coli*

NH$_3$ NADH → NAD

Pichia pastoris
Formate Dehydrogenase
cloned in *E. coli*

CO$_2$ Ammonium Formate

99
Amino Acid

Boc$_2$O

97
Boc-Amino Acid

96
Saxagliptin
Dipeptide Peptidase
Inhibitor

Production of multi-kg batches was originally carried out with extracts of *Pichia pastoris* expressing the modified phenylalanine dehydrogenase from *Thermoactinomyces intermedius* and endogenous formate dehydrogenase. The reductive amination process was further scaled up using a preparation of the two enzymes expressed in single recombinant *E. coli*. The amino acid **99** was directly protected as its boc derivative without isolation to afford intermediate. Yields before isolation were close to 98% with 100% e.e. [124].

Reductive amination was also conducted using cell extracts from *E. coli* strain SC16496 expressing PDHmod and cloned FDH from *Pichia pastoris*. Cell extracts after polyethyleneamine treatment, clarification and concentration were used to complete the reaction in 30 h with >96% yield and >99.9% e.e. of product **99**. This process has now been used to prepare several hundred kg of boc-protected amino acid **97** to support the development of Saxagliptin [124].

3.6. Enzymatic Synthesis of (S)-Neopentylglycine

The enantioselective synthesis of (S)-neopentylglycine **100** (Figure 27) has been developed by Groeger *et al.* [125]. Recombinant whole cell containing leucine dehydrogenase and formate dehydrogenase was used in the reductive amination of the corresponding α-keto acid **101**. The desired (S)-neopentylglycine was obtained with >95% conversion and a high enantioselectivity of >99% e.e. at substrate concentrations of up to 88 g/L. Spiroheterocyclic compounds [morpholine-4-carboxylic acid amides of heterocyclic cyclohexylalanine and neopentylglycine derivatives and their analogs] are useful as reversible inhibitors of cysteine proteases such as cathepsin S useful in the treatment of variety of autoimmune diseases [126].

Figure 27. Enzymatic synthesis of (S)-neopentylglycine.

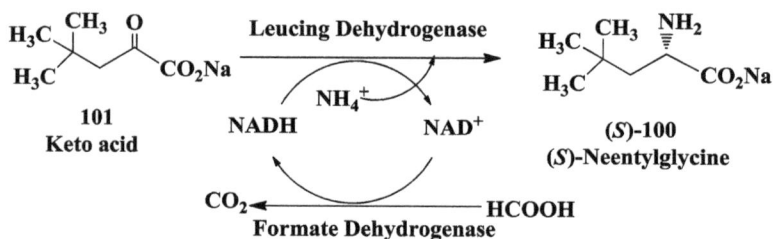

3.7. Glucogen like Peptide: Enzymatic Deracemization Racemic Amino Acid to (S)-Amino Acid

The (S)-amino-3-[3-{6-(2-methylphenyl)}pyridyl]-propionic acid 102 (Figure 28) is a key intermediate required for synthesis of GLP-1 mimics or GLP-1 receptor modulators. Such receptor modulators are potentially useful for the treatment of type II diabetes treatment [127,128].

Figure 28. Glucogen like peptide: The (S)-amino-3-[3-{6-(2-methylphenyl)}pyridyl]-propionic acid.

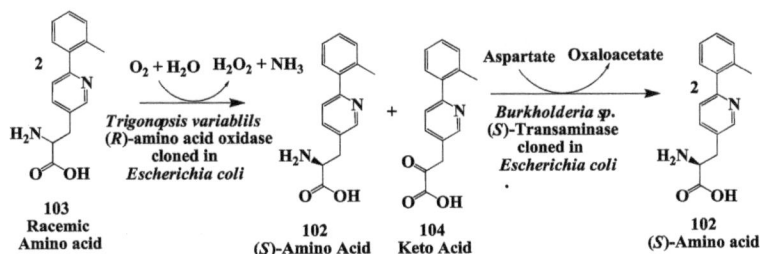

(S)-Amino-3-[3-{6-(2-methylphenyl)}pyridyl]-propionic acid was prepared by enzymatic deracemization process [129] in 72% isolated yield with >99.4% e.e. from racemic amino acid **103** using combination of two enzymes (R)-amino acid oxidase from *Trigonopsis variabilis* expressed in *Escherichia coli* and (S)-aminotransferase from *Sporosarcina ureae* cloned and expressed in *Escherichia coli*. (S)-aspartate was used as amino donor. A (S)-aminotransferase was also purified from a soil organism identified as *Burkholderia* sp. and cloned and expressed in *Escherichia coli* and used in this process [131]. In enzymatic process racemic amino acid was first treated with (R)-amino acid oxidase for 4 h to convert racemic amino acid to mixture of (S)-amino acid and keto acid **104**. Subsequently in the same reaction mixture (S)-aminotransferase was charged to convert keto acid **104** to (S)-amino acid **102** to get 85% yield at the end of the biotransformation process. This process was scaled up to 100 L scale at a substrate input of 1.5 kg.

In an alternate process, the enzymatic dynamic resolution of racemic amino acid **103** was also demonstrated. (R)-selective oxidation with celite-immobilized (R)-amino acid oxidase from *Trigonopsis variabilis* expressed in *Escherichia coli* in combination with chemical imine reduction with borane-ammonia gave a 75% in process yield and 100 e.e. of (S)-amino acid **102** [129].

3.8. Preparation of (R)-Amino Acid

(R)-Amino acids are increasingly becoming important building blocks in the production of pharmaceuticals and fine chemicals, and as chiral directing auxiliaries and chiral synthons in organic synthesis [130,131]. Using both rational and random mutagenesis, Rozzell and Novick [132] have created the broad substrate range, nicotinamide cofactor dependent, and highly stereoselective (R)-amino acid dehydrogenase. This new enzyme is capable of producing (R)-amino acids via the reductive amination of the corresponding 2-keto acid with ammonia. This biocatalyst was the result of three rounds of mutagenesis and screening performed on the enzyme *meso*-diaminopimelate (R)-dehydrogenase from *Corynebacterium glutamicum*. The first round targeted the active site of the wild-type enzyme and produced mutants that were no longer strictly dependent on the native substrate. The second and third rounds produced mutants that had an increased substrate range including straight- and branched-aliphatic amino acids and aromatic amino acids. The very high selectivity toward the (R)-enantiomer (95% to >99% e.e.) was shown to be preserved three rounds of mutagenesis and screening [132]. This new enzyme was active against variety of amino acids could complement and improve upon current methods for (R)-amino acid synthesis. The synthesis of (R)-cyclohexylalanine 105 (Figure 29) was developed by reductive amination of cyclohexylpyruvate 106 to yield (R)-105 in 98% yield and >99% e.e. (R)-105 is a potential chiral intermediate for the synthesis of thrombin inhibitor Inogatran 107 [133].

Figure 29. Thrombin inhibitor inogatran: Enzymatic synthesis of (R)-cyclohexylalanine.

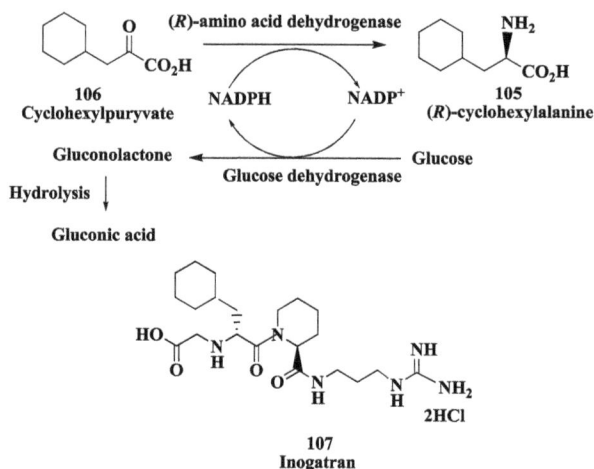

The deracemisation of DL-amino acids using L-amino acid oxidase from *Proteus myxofaciens* and amine-boranes as chemical reducing agents has been investigated. Amine-boranes were found to be of particular interest in terms of reactivity and chemoselectivity compared to sodium borohydride and cyanoborohydride. Starting from the racemic amino acids, a range of D-amino acids were prepared in yields of up to 90% and e.e. >99% [134].

3.9. Calcitonin Gene-Related Peptide Receptors (Antimigraine Drugs): Enzymatic Deracemization Process

The (R)-amino acid (R)-2-amino-3-(7-methyl-1 H-indazol-5-yl)propanoic acid (R)-**108**, (Figure 30) is a key intermediate needed for synthesis of antagonists of calcitonin gene-related peptide receptors **109** [135] Such antagonists are potentially useful for the treatment of migraine and other maladies [135,136].

(R)-Amino acid 108 was prepared in 68% isolated yield with >99% e.e. from racemic amino acid **110** using (S)-amino acid oxidase from *Proteus mirabilis* expressed in *Escherichia coli* in combination with a commercially available (R)-transaminase using (R)-alanine as amino donor [137]. The (R)-enantiomer was also prepared in 79% isolated yield with >99% e.e. from the corresponding keto acid **111** using the (R)-transaminase with racemic alanine as the amino donor. The rate and yield of this reaction could be accelerated by addition of lactate dehydrogenase (with NAD^+, formate and formate dehydrogenase to regenerate NADH) to remove the inhibitory pyruvate produced during the reaction. A (R)-transaminase was identified and purified from a soil organism identified as *Bacillus thuringiensis* and cloned and expressed in *Escherichia coli*. The recombinant (R)-transaminase was very effective for the preparation of (R)-**108** and gave a nearly complete conversion of **111** to (R)-**108** without the need for additional enzymes for pyruvate removal [137].

Figure 30. Calcitonin gene-related peptide receptors (antimigraine drugs): Enzymatic preparation of (R)-2-amino-3-(7-methyl-1H-indazol-5-yl)propanoic acid.

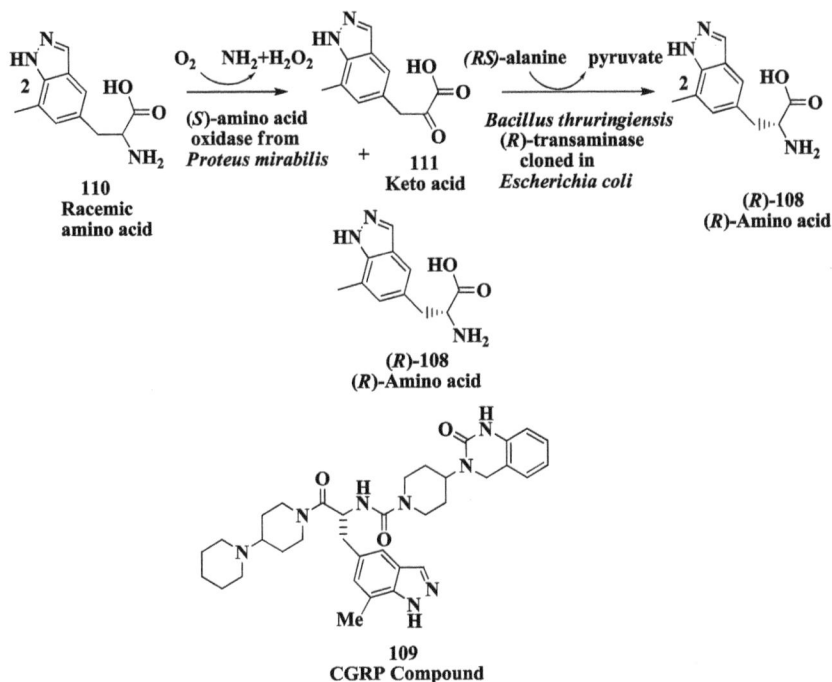

110
Racemic
amino acid

O$_2$ NH$_2$+H$_2$O$_2$

(S)-amino acid
oxidase from
Proteus mirabilis

+

111
Keto acid

(RS)-alanine   pyruvate

Bacillus thruringiensis
(R)-transaminase
cloned in
Escherichia coli

(R)-**108**
(R)-Amino acid

(R)-**108**
(R)-Amino acid

109
CGRP Compound

3.10. Corticotropin Releasing Factor (CRF)-1 Receptor Antagonist: Enzymatic Resolution by Transaminase

(R)-amines synthesis for Anxiety and depression are psychiatric disorders that constitute a major health concern worldwide. While numerous marketed treatments exits for both disorders, there continue to be need agents which may have increased efficacy and/or reduced side-effect profiles [138–140]. CRF-1 receptor antagonists have been proposed as novel pharmacological treatments for depression, anxiety and stress disorders [138–141]. (R)-sec-butylamine **112** and (R)-1-cyclopropylethylamine **113** (Figure 31) are key chiral intermediates for the synthesis of CRF-1 receptor antagonists such as **114** [141,142].

Figure 31. Corticotropin releasing factor (CRF)-1 receptor antagonist: Enzymatic synthesis of (*R*)-1-cyclopropylethylamine and (*R*)-*sec*-butylamine.

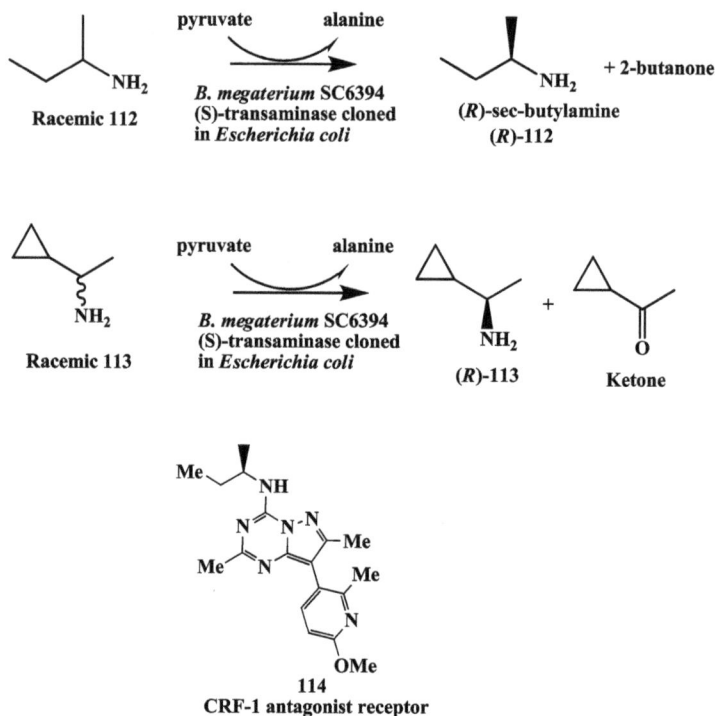

We have developed enzymatic resolution process for the preparation of (*R*)-sec-butylamine and (*R*)-1-cyclopropylethylamine [143]. Screening was carried out to identify strains useful for the preparation of (*R*)-1-cyclopropylethylamine and (*R*)-*sec*-butylamine from the racemic amines with an (*S*)-specific transaminase. Several *Bacillus megaterium* strains as well as several soil isolates were found to have the desired activity for the resolution of the racemic amines to give the (*R*)-enantiomers. Using an extract of the best strain, *Bacillus megaterium* SC6394, the reaction was shown to be a transamination requiring pyruvate as amino acceptor and pyridoxal phosphate as a cofactor. Initial batches of both amines were produced using whole cells of *Bacillus megaterium* SC6394. The transaminase was purified to homogeneity to obtain N-terminal as well as internal amino acid sequences. The sequences were used to design polymerase chain reaction (PCR) primers to enable cloning and expression of the transaminase in *Escherichia coli* SC16578. In contrast to using *Bacillus megaterium* process, pH control and aeration were not required for the resolution of sec-butylamine and an excess of pyruvate was not consumed by the recombinant cells. The resolution of sec-butylamine (0.68 M) using whole cells of *Escherichia coli* SC16578 was scaled up to give (*R*)-sec-butylamine ·1/2 H_2SO_4 in 46.6% isolated yield with 99.2% e.e. An alternative isolation procedure was also used to isolate (*R*)-sec-butylamine as the free base. Using the same recombinant (*S*)-tansaminase, (*R*)-1-cyclopropylethylamine was obtained in 42% isolated yield (theoretical max. 50%) and 99% e.e. [143].

4. Conclusions

The production of single enantiomers of drug intermediates is increasingly important in the pharmaceutical industry. Biocatalysis provides organic chemists an alternate opportunity to prepare pharmaceutically important chiral compounds. The examples presented in this review are only from a few selected articles for synthresis of chiral alcohols and unnatural amino acids. Different types of biocatalytic reactions are capable of generating a wide variety of chiral compounds useful in the development of drugs. The use of hydrolytic enzymes such as lipases, esterases, proteases, dehalogenases, acylases, amidases, nitrilases, epoxide hydrolases, and decarboxylases for the resolution of variety of racemic compounds and in the asymmetric synthesis of enantiomerically enriched chiral compounds. Dehydrogenases and aminotransferases has been successfully used along with cofactors and cofactor regenerating enzymes for the synthesis of chiral alcohols, aminoalcohols, amino acids and amines. Aldolases and decarboxylases have been effectively used in asymmetric synthesis by aldol condensation and acyloin condensation reactions. Monoxygenases have been used in enantioselective and regioselective hydroxylation, epoxidation, sulfoxidation and Baeyer-Villiger reactions. Dioxygenases have been used in the chemo-enzymatic synthesis of chiral diols. Enzymatic deracemization, dynamic resolution and stereoinversion, to achieve >50% yield and high e.e. by combination of chemo- and/or biocatalysts in sequential reactions or by a single biocatalyst. In the course of the last decade, progress in biochemistry, protein chemistry, molecular cloning, random and site-directed mutagenesis, directed evolution of biocatalysts under desired process conditions has opened up unlimited access to a variety of enzymes and microbial cultures as tools in organic synthesis. Future of bicatalysis for synthesis of chiral compounds looks very promising.

Acknowledgments

The author would like to acknowledge Ronald Hanson, Animesh Goswami, Amit Banerjee, Venkata Nanduri, Jeffrey Howell, Steven Goldeberg, Robert Johnston, Mary-Jo Donovan, Dana Cazzulino, Thomas Tully, Thomas LaPorte, Lawrence Parker, John Wasylyk, Michael Montana, Ronald Eiring, Rapheal Ko, Linda Chu, Clyde McNamee, Michael Montana for research collaboration.

Conflict of Interest

The authors declare no conflict of interest.

References

1. Food and Drug Administration. FDA's statement for the development of new stereoisomeric drugs. *Chirality* **1992**, *4*, 338–340.
2. Oliver, M.; Voigt, C.A.; Arnold, F.H. Enzyme engineering by directed evolution. In *Enzyme Catalysis in Organic Synthesis*, 2nd ed.; VCH, New York, USA, 2002; Volume 1, pp. 95–138.
3. Kazlauskas, R.J. Enhancing catalytic promiscuity for biocatalysis. *Curr. Opin. Chem. Biol.* **2005**, *9*, 195–201.

288

4. Schmidt, M.; Bauman, M.; Henke, E.; Konarzycka-Bessler, M.; Bornscheuer, U.T. Directed evolution of lipases and esterases. *Meth. Enzymol.* **2004**, *388*, 199–207.

5. Reetz, M.T.; Torre, C.; Eipper, A.; Lohmer, R.; Hermes, M.; Brunner, B.; Maichele, A.; Bocola, M.; Arand, M.; Cronin, A.; *et al.* Enhancing the enantioselectivity of an epoxide hydrolase by directed evolution. *Org. Lett.* **2004**, *6*, 177–180.

6. Rubin-Pitel, S.B.; Zhao, H. Recent advances in biocatalysis by directed enzyme evolution. *Comb. Chem. High T. Scr.* **2006**, *9*, 247–257.

7. Pollard, D.J.; Woodley, J.M. Biocatalysis for pharmaceutical intermediates: The future is now. *Trends Biotechnol.* **2007**, *25*, 66–73.

8. Otey, C.R.; Bandara, G.; Lalonde, J.; Takahashi, K.; Arnold, F.H. Preparation of human metabolites of propranolol using laboratory-evolved bacterial cytochromes P450. *Biotechnol. Bioeng.* **2006**, *93*, 494–499.

9. Huisman, G.W.; Lalonde, J.J. Enzyme evolution for chemical process applications. In *Biocatalysis in the Pharmaceutical and Biotechnology Industries*; Patel, R.N., Ed.; CRC Press: Boca Raton, FL, USA, 2007; pp. 717–742.

10. Arnold, F.; Volkov, A. Directed evolution of biocatalysts. *Curr. Opin. Chem. Biol.* **1999**, *3*, 54–59.

11. Patten, P.A.; Howard, R.J.; Stemmer, W.P. Applications of DNA shuffling to pharmaceuticals and vaccines. *Curr. Opin. Biotechnol.* **1997**, *8*, 724–733.

12. Hibbert, E.G.; Baganz, F.; Hailes, H.C.; Ward, J.M.; Lye, G.J.; Woodley, J.M.; Dalby, P.A. Directed evolution of biocatalytic processes. *Biomol. Eng.* **2005**, *22*, 11–19.

13. Sylvestre, J.; Chautard, H.; Cedrone, F.M. Directed evolution of biocatalysts. *Org. Process Res. Dev.* **2006**, *10*, 562–571

14. Turner, N.J. Directed evolution drives the next generation of biocatalysts. *Nat. Chem. Biol.* **2009**, *5*, 567–573.

15. Bornscheuer, U.T.; Huisman, G.W.; Kazlauskas, R.J.; Lutz, S.; Moore, J.C.; Robins, K. Engineering the third wave of biocatalysis. *Nature* **2012**, *485*, 185–194.

16. Wells, A.S.; Finch, G.L.; Michels, P.C.; Wong, J.W. Use of enzymes in the manufacture of active pharmaceutical ingredients—A science and safety-based approach to ensure patient safety and drug quality. *Org. Process Res. Dev.* **2012**, *16*, 1986–1993.

17. Reetz, M.T. Biocatalysis in organic chemistry and biotechnology: Past, present, and future. *J. Am. Chem. Soc.* **2013**, *135*, 12480–12496.

18. Huisman, G.W.; Collier, S.J. On the development of new biocatalytic processes for practical pharmaceutical synthesis. *Curr. Opin. Chem. Biol.* **2013**, *17*, 284–292.

19. Bryan, M.C.; Dillon, B.; Hamann, L.G.; Hughes, G.J.; Kopach, M.E.; Peterson, E.A.; Pourashraf, M.; Raheem, I.; Richardson, P.; Richter, D.; *et al.* Sustainable practices in medicinal chemistry: Current state and future directions. *J. Med. Chem.* **2013**, *56*, 6007–6021.

20. DiCosimo, R. Nitrilases and nitrile hydratases. In *Biocatalysis in the Pharmaceutical and Biotechnology Industries*; Patel, R.N., Ed.; CRC Press: Boca Raton, FL, USA, 2007; pp. 1–26.

21. Patel, R.N. Biocatalysis: Synthesis of chiral intermediates for pharmaceuticals. *Curr. Org. Chem.* **2006**, *10*, 1289–1321.

22. Simeo, Y.; Kroutil, W.; Faber, K. Biocatalytic deracemization: Dynamic resolution, stereoinversion, enantioconvergent processes, and cyclic deracemization. In *Biocatalysis in the Pharmaceutical and Biotechnology Industries*; Patel, R.N., Ed.; CRC Press: Boca Raton, FL, USA, 2007; pp. 27–51.

23. Patel, R.N. Biocatalysis: Synthesis of key intermediates for development of pharmaceuticals. *ACS Catal.* **2011**, *1*, 1056–1074.

24. Turner, N.J. Enzyme catalyzed deracemization and dynamic kinetic resolution reactions. *Curr. Opin. Chem. Biol.* **2004**, *8*, 114–119.

25. Ishige, T.; Honda, K.; Shimizu, S. Whole organism biocatalysis. *Curr. Opin. Chem. Biol.* **2005**, *9*, 174–180.

26. Zhao, H.; Chockalingom, K.; Chen, Z. Directed evolution of enzymes and pathways for industrial biocatalysis. *Curr. Opin. Biotechnol.* **2002**, *13*, 104–110.

27. Schulze, B.; Wubbolts, M. Biocatalysis for industrial production of fine chemicals. *Curr. Opin. Biotechnol.* **1999**, *10*, 609–611.

28. Steinreiber, A.; Faber, K. Microbial epoxide hydrolases for preparative biotransformations. *Curr. Opin. Biotechnol.* **2001**, *12*, 552–558.

29. Tao, J.; Xu, J.-H. Biocatalysis in development of green pharmaceutical processes. *Curr. Opin. Chem. Biol.* **2009**, *13*, 43–50.

30. Patel, R.N. Biocatalytic hydrolysis (esters, amides, epoxides, nitriles) and biocatalytic dynamic kinetic resolution. In *Comprehensive Chirality* **2012** *10*, 288-317.

31. Patel, R.N. Biocatalytic routes to chiral intermediates for development of drugs. In *Biocatalysis for Green Chemistry and Chemical Process Development*; Tao, J., Kazlauskas, R., Eds.; John Wiley & Sons, Inc.: Hoboken, NJ, USA, 2010.

32. Jajoo, H.; Mayol, R.; LaBudde, J.; Blair, I. Metabolism of the antianxiety drug buspirone in human subjects. *Drug Metab. Dispos.* **1989**, *17*, 634–640.

33. Mayol, R. Buspirone Metabolite for the Alleviation of Anxiety. US6150365A, June 6, 2000.

34. Yevich, J.; New, J.; Lobeck, W.; Dextraze, P.; Bernstein, E.; Taylor, D.; Yocca, F.; Eison, M.; Temple, D., Jr. Synthesis and biological characterization of α-(4-fluorophenyl)-4-(5-fluoro-2-pyrimidinyl)-1-piperazinebutanol and analogs as potential atypical antipsychotic agents. *J. Med. Chem.* **1992**, *35*, 4516–4525.

35. Yevich, J.; Mayol, R.; Li, J.; Yocca, F. (*S*)-6-Hydroxy-Buspirone for Treatment of Anxiety, Depression and Related Disorders. US2003022899, January 30, 2003.

36. Patel, R.; Chu, L.; Nanduri, V.; Jianqing, L.; Kotnis, A.; Parker, W.; Liu, M.; Mueller, R. Enantioselective microbial reduction of 6-oxo-8-[4-[4-(2-pyrimidinyl)-1-piperazinyl]butyl]-8-azaspiro[4.5]decane-7,9-dione. *Tetrahedron Asymmetry* **2005**, *16*, 2778–2783.

37. Goldberg, S.; Nanduri, V.; Chu, L.; Johnston, R.; Patel, R. Enantioselective microbial reduction of 6-oxo-8-[4-[4-(2-pyrimidinyl)-1-piperazinyl]butyl]-8-azaspiro[4.5]decane-7,9-dione: Cloning and expression of reductases. *Enzyme Microb. Technol.* **2006**, *39*, 1441–1450.

38. Patel, R.N.; Banerjee, A.; McNamee, C.; Brzozowski, D.; Hanson, R.; Szarka, L. Enantioselective microbial reduction of 3,5-dioxo-6-(benzyloxy) hexanoic acid, ethyl ester. *Enzyme Microb. Technol.* **1993**, *15*, 1014-1021.

39. Sit, S.; Parker, R.; Motoe, I.; Balsubramanian, H.; Cott, C.; Brown, P.; Harte, W.; Thompson, M.; Wright, J. Synthesis, biological profile, and quantitative structure activity relationship of a series of novel 3-hydroxy-3-methylglutaryl coenzyme A reductase inhibitors. *J. Med. Chem.* **1990**, *33*, 2982–2999.

40. Roth, B.D. The discovery and development of atorvastatin, a potent novel hypolipidemic agent. *Prog. Med. Chem.* **2002**, *40*, 1–22.

41. Law, M.; Rudinka, A.R. Statin safety: A systematic review. *Am. J. Cardiol.* **2006**, *97(8A)*, 52C–60C.

42. McTaggart, F.; Buckett, L.; Davidson, R.; Holdgate, G.; McCormick, A.; Schneck, D.; Smith, G.; Warwick, M. Preclinical and clinical pharmacology of Rosuvastatin, a new 3-hydroxy-3-methylglutaryl coenzyme A reductase inhibitor. *Am. J. Cardiol.* **2001**, *87*, 28B–32B.

43. Guo, Z.; Chen, Y.; Goswami, A.; Hanson, R.L.; Patel, R.N. Synthesis of ethyl and t-butyl (3*R*,5*S*)-dihydroxy-6-benzyloxyhexanoates via diastereo- and enantioselective microbial reduction. *Tetrahedron Asymmetry* **2006**, *17*, 1589–1602.

44. Goldberg, S.; Guo, Z.; Chen, S.; Goswami, A.; Patel, R.N. Synthesis of ethyl-(3*R*,5*S*)-dihydroxy-6-benzyloxyhexanoates via diastereo- and enantioselective microbial reduction: Cloning and expression of ketoreductase III from *Acinetobacter* sp. SC 13874. *Enzyme Microb. Technol.* **2008**, *43*, 544–549.

45. Davis, S.; Christopher, G.; John, H.; Gray, D.; Gruber, J.; Huisman, G.; Ma, S.; Newman, L.; Sheldon, R. Enzymatic Processes for the Production of 4-Substituted 3-Hydroxybutyric Acid Derivatives. US 7807423B2, 5NOctober 2010.

46. Jagoda, E.; Stouffer, B.; Ogan, M.; Tsay, H.M.; Turabi, N.; Mantha, S.; Yost, F.; Tu, J.I. Radioimmunoassay for hydroxyphosphinyl-3-hydroxybutanoic acid (SQ 33,600), a hypocholesterolemia agent. *Ther. Drug Monit.* **1993**, *15*, 213–219.

47. Wang, D.I.; Arnold, M.E.; Jemal, M.; Cohen. A.I. Determination of SQ 33,600, a phosphinic acid containing HMG CoA reductase inhibitor, in human serum by high-performance liquid chromatography combined with ionspray mass spectrometry. *Biol. Mass Spectrom.* **1992**, *21*, 189–194.

48. Patel, R.; McNamee, C.; Banerjee, A.; Howell, J.; Robison, R.; Szarka, L. Stereoselective reduction of β-keto ester by *Geotrich candidum*. *Enzyme Microb. Technol.* **1992**, *14*, 731–738.

49. Matsuyama, A.; Yamamoto, H.; Kobayashi, Y. Practical application of recombinant whole-cell biocatalysts for the manufacturing of pharmaceutical intermediates such as chiral alcohols. *Org. Process Res. Dev.* **2002**, *6*, 558–561.

50. Zalman, L.S.; Brothers, M.A.; Dragovich, P.S.; Zhou, R.; Prins, T.J.; Worland, S.T.; Patick, A.K. Inhibition of human rhinovirus-induced cytokine production by AG7088, a human rhinovirus 3C protease inhibitor. *Antimicrob. Agents Chemother.* **2000**, *44*, 1236–1241.

51. Dragovich, P.S.; Prins, T.J.; Zhou, R.; Webber, S.E.; Marakovits, J.T.; Fuhrman, S.A.; Patick, A.K.; Matthews, D.A.; Lee, C.A.; Ford, C.E.; *et al*. Structure-based design, synthesis, and biological evaluation of irreversible human rhinovirus 3C protease inhibitors. 4. incorporation of P_1 lactam moieties as l-glutamine replacements. *J. Med. Chem.* **1999**, *42*, 1213–1224.

52. Tao, J.; McGee, K. Development of a continuous enzymatic process for the preparation of (*R*)-3-(4-fluorophenyl)-2-hydroxy propionic acid. *Org. Process Res. Dev.* **2002**, *6*, 520–524.

53. Bold, G.; Faessler, A.; Capraro, H.-G.; Cozens, R.; Klimkait, T.; Lazdins, J.; JMestan, J.; Poncioni, B.; Roesel, J.; Stover, D.; *et al*. New aza-dipeptide analogs as potent and orally absorbed HIV-1 protease inhibitors: Candidates for clinical development. *J. Med. Chem.* **1998**, *41*, 3387–3401.

54. Robinson, B.S.; Riccardi, K.A.; Gong, Y.F.; Guo, Q.; Stock, D.A.; Blair, W.S.; Terry, B.J.; Deminie, C.A.; Djang, F.; Colonno, R.J.; *et al*. BMS-232632, a highly potent human immunodeficiency virus protease inhibitor that can be used in combination with other available antiretroviral agents. *Antimicrob. Agents Chemother.* **2000**, *44*, 2093–2099.

55. Patel, R.N.; Chu, L.; Mueller, R.H. Diastereoselective microbial reduction of (*S*)-[3-chloro-2-oxo-1-(phenylmethyl)propyl]carbamic acid, 1,1-dimethylethyl ester. *Tetrahedron Asymmetry* **2003**, *14*, 3105–3109.

56. Bowers, N.I.; Skonezny, P.M.; Stein, G.L.; Franceschini, T.; Chiang, S.-J.; Anderson, W.L.; You, L.; Xing, Z. Pocess for preparing (2*R*,3*S*)-1,2-epoxy-3-(protected)amino-4-substituted butane and intermediates thereof. WO 2006127180 A1, November 30, 2006

57. Xu, Z.; Singh, J.; Schwinden, M.D.; Zheng, B.; Kissick, T.P.; Patel, B.; Humora, M.J.; Quiroz, F.; Dong, L.; Hsieh, D.-M.; *et al*. Process research and development for an efficient synthesis of the HIV protease inhibitor BMS-232632. *Org. Process Res. Dev.* **2002**, *6*, 323–328.

58. King, A.O.; Corley, E.G.; Anderson, R.K.; Larsen, R.D.; Verhoeven, T.R.; Reider, P.J.; Xiang, Y.B.; Belley, M.; Leblanc, Y.; Labelle, M.; *et al*. An efficient synthesis of LTD4 antagonist L-699,392. *J. Org. Chem.* **1993**, *58*, 3731–3735.

59. Shinkai, I.; King, A.O.; Larsen, R.D. Practical asymmetric synthesis of LTD4 antagonist. *Pure Appl. Chem.* **1994**, *66*, 1551–1556.

60. Zhao, M.; King, A.O.; Larsen, R.D.; Verhoeven, T.R.; Reider, P.J. A convenient and economical method for the preparation of DIP-Chloride™ and its application in the asymmetric reduction of aralkyl ketones. *Tetrahedron Lett.* **1997**, *36*, 2641–2644.

61. Shafiee, A.; Motamedi, H.; King, A. Purification, characterization and immobilization of an NADPH-dependent enzyme involved in the chiral specific reduction of the keto ester M, an intermediate in the synthesis of an anti-asthma drug, Montelukast, from *Microbacterium campoquemadoensis* (MB5614). *Appl. Microbiol. Biotechnol.* **1998**, *49*, 709–717.

62. Liang, J., Lalonde, J., Borup, B., Mitchell, V., Mundorff, E., Trinh, N., Kochrekar, D.A., Cherat, R.N., Pai, G.G. Development of a biocatalytic process as an alternative to the (−)-DIP-Cl-mediated asymmetric reduction of a key intermediate of Montelukast. *Org. Proc. Res. Dev.* **2010**, *14*, 193-198.

63. Holton, R.; Biediger, R.; Joatman, P. Semisynthesis of taxol and taxotere. In *Taxol: Science and Application*; Suffness, M., Ed.; CRC Press: NewYork, NY, USA, 1995; pp. 97–123.

64. Kingston, D. Natural taxoids: Structure and chemistry. In *Taxol: Science and Application*; Suffness, M., Ed.; CRC press: New York, NY, USA, 1995; pp. 287–317.

65. Patel, R. Tour de paclitaxel: Biocatalysis for semisynthesis. *Annu. Rev. Microbiol.* **1995**, *98*, 361–395.

66. Patel, R.; Banerjee, A.; Howell, J.; McNamee, C.; Brozozowski, D.; Mirfakhrae, D.; Nanduri, V.; Thottathil, J.; Szarka, L. Microbial synthesis of (2R,3S)-N-benzoyl-3-phenyl isoserine ethyl ester-a taxol side-chain synthon. *Tetrahedron Asymmetry* **1993**, *4*, 2069–2084.

67. Junie, J.L.; Leonard, B.E. Drugs acting on sigma and phencyclidine receptors: A review of their nature, function, and possible therapeutic importance. *Clin. Neuropharmacol.* **1989**, *12*, 353–374.

68. Ferris, C.D.; Hirsch, D.J.; Brooks, B.P.; Snyder, S.H. σ Receptors: From molecule to man. *J. Neurochem.* **1991**, *57*, 729–737.

69. Patel, R.N.; Banerjee, A.; Liu, M.; Hanson, R.; Ko, R.; Howell, J.; Szarka, L. Microbial reduction of 1-(4-fluorophenyl)-4-[4-(5-fluoro-2-pyrimidinyl)-1-piperazinyl]butan-1-one. *Biotechnol. Appl. Biochem.* **1993**, *17*, 139–153.

70. Kagechika, H.; Kawachi, E.; Hashimoto, Y.; Shudo, K.; Himi, T. Retinobenzoic acids. 1. Structure-activity relationships of aromatic amides with retinoidal activity. *J. Med. Chem.* **1989**, *32*, 2583–2588.

71. Kagechika, H.; Shudo, K. Retinoids. Vitamin A for clinical applications. *Farumashia* **1990**, *26*, 35–40.

72. Moon, R.C.; Mehta, R.G. Anticarcinogenic effects of retinoids in animals. *Adv. Exp. Med. Biol.* **1986**, *206*, 399–411.

73. Patel, R.N.; Chu, L.; Chidambaram, R.; Zhu, J.; Kant, J. Enantioselective microbial reduction of 2-oxo-2-(1′,2′,3′,4′-tetrahydro-1′,1′,4′,4′-tetramethyl-6′-naphthalenyl)acetic acid and its ethyl ester. *Tetrahedron Asymmetry* **2002**, *13*, 349–355.

74. Prasad, C.V.C.; Wallace, O.B.; Noonan, J.W.; Sloan, C.P.; Lau, W.; Vig, S.; Parker, M.F.; Smith, D.W.; Hansel, S.B.; Polson, C.T.; *et al.* Hydroxytriamides as potent γ-secretase inhibitors. *Bioorg. Med. Chem. Lett.* **2004**, *14*, 3361–3371.

75. Nanduri, V.B.; Hanson, R.L.; Goswami, A.; Wasylyk, J.M.; LaPorte, T.L.; Katipally, K.; Chung, H.-J.; Patel, R.N. Biochemical approaches to the synthesis of ethyl 5-(S)-hydroxyhexanoate and 5-(S)-hydroxyhexanenitrile. *Enzyme Microb. Technol.* **2001**, *28*, 632–636.

76. Schenk, D.G.; Seubert, P. Potential treatment opportunities for Alzheimer's disease through inhibition of secretases and Aβ immunization. *J. Mol. Neurosci.* **2001**, *17*, 259–267.

77. Patel, R.N.; Goswami, A.; Chu, L.; Donovan, M.J.; Nanduri, V.; Goldberg, S.; Johnston, R.; Siva, P.J.; Nielsen, B.; Fan, J.; *et al.* Enantioselective microbial reduction of substituted acetophenones. *Tetrahedron Asymmetry* **2004**, *15*, 1247–1258.

78. Wittman, M.; Carboni, J.M.; Attar, R.; Balasubramanian, B.; Balimane, P.; Brassil, P.; Beaulieu, F.; Chang, C.; Clarke, W.; Dell, J.; *et al.* Discovery of a 1*H*-Benzoimidazol-2-yl)-1*H*-pyridin-2-one (BMS-536924) inhibitor of insulin-like growth factor I receptor kinase with *in vivo* antitumor activity. *J. Med. Chem.* **2005**, *48*, 5639–5643.

79. Carboni, J.M.; Hurlburt, W.W.; Gottardis, M.M. Synergistic methods and compositions for treating cancer. WO 2004030625 A2, April 15 2004.

80. Beaulieu, F.; Ouellet, C.; Zimmermann, K.; Velaparthi, U.; Wittman, M.D. Novel tyrosine kinase inhibitors WO 2004063151 A3, 9 December 2004

81. Hanson, R.L.; Goldberg, S.; Goswami, A.; Tully, T.P.; Patel, R.N. Purification and cloning of a ketoreductase used for the preparation of chiral alcohols. *Adv. Synth. Catal.* **2005**, *347*, 1073–1080.

82. Vacca, J.P. New advances in the discovery of thrombin and factor Xa inhibitors. *Curr. Opin. Chem. Biol.* **2000**, *4*, 394–400.

83. Gladwell, T.D. Bivalirudin: A direct thrombin inhibitor. *Clin. Ther.* **2002**, *24*, 38–58.

84. Fevig, J.M.; Wexler, R.R. Anticoagulants: Thrombin and factor Xa inhibitors. *Annu. Rep. Med. Chem.* **1999**, *34*, 81–100.

85. Williams, P.D.; Coburn, C.; Burgey, C.; Morrissette, M.M. Preparation of Triazolopyrimidines as Thrombin Inhibitors. WO 2002064211 A1, August 22, 2002.

86. Nelson, T.D.; LeBlond, C.R.; Frantz, D.E.; Matty, L.; Mitten, J.V.; Weaver, D.G.; Moore, J.C; Kim, J.M.; Boyd, R.; Kim, P.-Y.; *et al.* Stereoselective synthesis of a potent thrombin inhibitor by a novel P2-P3 lactone ring opening. *J. Org. Chem.* **2004**, *69*, 3620–3627.

87. Fukuroda, T.; Nishikibe, M. Enhancement of pulmonary artery contraction induced by endothelin-β receptor antagonism. *J. Cardiovasc. Pharmacol.* **1998**, *31*, S169–S171.

88. Sumner, M.J.; Cannon, T.R.; Mundin, J.W.; White, D.G.; Watts, I.S. Endothelin ETA and ETB receptors mediate vascular smooth muscle contraction. *Br. J. Pharmacol.* **1992**, *107*, 858–860.

89. Krulewicz, B.; Tschaen, D.; Devine, P.; Lee, S.S.; Roberge, C.; Greasham, R.; Chartrain, M. Asymmetric biosynthesis of key aromatic intermediates in the synthesis of an endothelin receptor antagonist. *Biocatal. Biotransformation* **2001**, *19*, 267–279.

90. Chaffman, M.; Brogden, R.N. Diltiazem. A review of its pharmacological properties and therapeutic efficacy. *Drugs* **1985**, *29*, 387–390.

91. Kawai, C.; Konishi, T.; Matsuyama, E.; Okazaki, H. Comparative effects of three calcium antagonists, diatiazem, verapamil and nifedipine, on the sinoatrial and atrioventricular nodes. Experimental and clinical studies. *Circulation* **1981**, *63*, 1035–1038.

92. Isshiki, T.; Pegram, B.; Frohlich, E. Immediate and prolonged hemodynamic effects of TA-3090 on spontaneously hypertensive (SHR) and normal Wistar-Kyoto (WKY) rats. *Cardiovasc. Drug Ther.* **1988**, *2*, 539–544.

93. Das, J.; Floyd, D.M.; Kimball, D.; Duff, K.J.; Lago, M.W.; Moquin, R.V.; Gougoutas, J.Z. Benzazepinone calcium channel blockers. 3. Synthesis and structure-activity studies of 3-alkylbenzazepinones. *J. Med. Chem.* **1992**, *35*, 773–780.

94. Patel, R.N.; Robison, R.S.; Szarka, L.J.; Kloss, J.; Thottathil, J.K.; Mueller, R.H. Stereospecific microbial reduction of 4,5-dihydro-4-(4-methoxyphenyl)-6-(trifluoromethyl-1*H*-1) -benzazepin-2-one. *Enzyme Microb. Technol.* **1991**, *13*, 906–912.

95. Arch, J.R.S. β3-adrenoceptors and other putative atypical β-adrenoceptors. *Pharmacol. Rev. Commun.* **1997**, *9*, 141–148.

96. Bloom, J.D.; Datta, M.D.; Johnson, B.D.; Wissner, A.; Bruns, M.G.; Largis, E.E.; Dolan, J.A.; Claus, T.H. Disodium (R,R)5-[2-(3-chlorophenyl)-2-hydroxyethyl]amino]propyl]-1, 3-benzodioxole-2,2-dicarboxylate. A potent β-adrenergic agonist virtually specific for β3 receptors. *J. Med. Chem.* **1989**, *35*, 3081–3084.

97. Fisher, L.G.; Sher, P.M.; Skwish, S.; Michael, I.M.; Seiler, S.; Dickinson, K.E.J. BMS-187257, a potent, selective, and novel heterocyclic β-3 adrenergic receptor agonist. *Bioorg. Med. Chem. Lett.* **1994**, *6*, 2253–2258.

98. Patel, R.N.; Banerjee, A.; Chu, L.; Brzozowski, D.; Nanduri, V.; Szarka, L.J. Microbial synthesis of chiral intermediates for β-3-receptor agonists. *J. Am. Oil Chem. Soc.* **1998**, *75*, 1473–1482.

99. Iwata, H.; Tanaka, R.; Ishiguro, M. Structures of the alkaline hydrolysis products of penem antibiotic, SUN5555. *J. Antibiot.* **1990**, *43*, 901–903.

100. Jean-Paul Vandecasteele, J.-P. Enzymatic synthesis of L-carnitine by reduction of an achiral precursor: The problem of reduced nicotinamide adenine dinucleotide recycling. *Appl. Environ. Microbiol.* **1980**, *39*, 327–334.

101. Yamamoto, H; Matsuyama, A.; Kobayashi, Y. Synthesis of (*R*)-1,3-butanediol by enantioselective oxidation using whole recombinant *Escherichia coli* cells expressing (*S*)-specific secondary alcohol dehydrogenase. *Biosci Biotechnol Biochem.* **2002**, *66*, 925–927.

102. Coleman, P.J.; Brashear, K.M.; Askew, B.C. Nonpeptide α vβ 3 antagonists. Part 11: Discovery and preclinical evaluation of potent α vβ3 antagonists for the prevention and treatment of osteoporosis. *J. Med. Chem.* **2004**, *47*, 4829–4837.

103. Pollard, D.J.; Telari, K.; Lane, J.; Humphrey, G.; McWilliams, C.; Nidositko, S.; Salmon, P.; Moore, J. Asymmetric reduction of alpha, beta-unsaturated ketone to (*R*) allylic alcohol by *Candida chilensis*. *Biotechnol. Bioeng.* **2006**, *93*, 674-684.

104. Brands, K.M.J.; Payack, J.F.; Rosen, J.D.; Nelson, T.D.; Candelario, A.; Huffman, M.A.; Zhao, M.M.; Bridgette, J.L.; Zhiguo, C.J.; Song, D.M.; *et al.* Efficient synthesis of NK1 receptor antagonist aprepitant using a crystallization-induced diastereoselective transformation. *J. Am. Chem. Soc.* **2003**, *125*, 2129–2135.

105. Pollard, D.; Truppo, M.; Pollard, J.; Chen, C.-Y.; Moore, J. Effective synthesis of (*S*)-3,5-bistrifluoro methylphenyl ethanol by asymmetric enzymatic reduction. *Tetrahedron Asymmetry* **2006**, *17*, 554–559.

106. Patel, R.N. Chemo-enzymatic synthesis of pharmaceutical intermediates. *Expert Opin. Drug Dis. Dev.* **2008**, *3*, 187–245.

107. Ohshima, T.; Soda, K. *Stereoselective Biocatalysis: Amino Acid Dehydrogenases and Their Applications in Stereoselective Biocatalysis*; Patel, R.N., Ed.; Marcel and Dekker Pub.: New York, New York, USA 2000, pp. 877–903.

108. Wandrey, C.; Wichman, R.; Leuchtenberger, W. Continuous Enzymic Transformation of Water-Soluble α-Keto Carboxylic Acids into the Corresponding Amino Acids. EP 0023346 B1 13 July 1983.

109. Brunhuber, N.M.; Blanchard, J.S. The biochemistry and enzymology of amino acid dehydrogenases. *Crit. Rev. Biochem. Mol. Biol.* **1994**, *29*, 415–467.

110. Gordon, E.M.; Ondetti, M.A.; Pluscec, J.; Cimarusti, C.M.; Bonner, D.P.; Sykes, R.B. *O*-Sulfated β-lactam hydroxamic acids (monosulfactams). Novel monocyclic β-lactam antibiotics of synthetic origin. *J. Am. Chem. Soc.* **1982**, *104*, 6053–6060.

111. Godfrey, J.D.; Mueller, R.H.; van Langen, D.J. β-Lactam synthesis: Cyclization *versus* 1,2-acyl migration-cyclization. The mechanism of the 1,2-acyl migration-cyclization. *Tetrahedron Lett.* **1986**, *27*, 2793–2796.

112. Hanson, R.L.; Singh, J.; Kissick, T.P.; Patel, R.N.; Szarka, L.; Mueller, R. Synthesis of L-β-hydroxyvaline from α-keto-β-hydroxyisovalerate using leucine dehydrogenase from *Bacillus* species. *Bioorg. Chem.* **1990**, *18*, 116–130.

113. Hanson, R., Goldberg, S., Patel, R. (unpublished results).

114. Stoyan, T.; Recktenwald, A.; Kula, M.R. Cloning, sequencing and overexpression of the leucine dehydrogenase gene from *Bacillus cereus*. *J. Biotechnol.* **1997**, *54*, 77–80.

115. Menzel, A.; Werner, H.; Altenbuchner, J.; Groger, H. From enzymes to "designer bugs" in reductive amination: A new process for the synthesis of L-tert-leucine using a whole cell. *Eng. Life Sci.* **2004**, *4*, 573–576.

116. Robl, J.; Sun, C.; Stevenson, J.; Ryono, D.; Simpkins, L.; Cimarusti, M.; Dejneka, T.; Slusarchyk, W.; Chao, S.; Stratton, L.; *et al.* Dual metalloprotease inhibitors: Mercaptoacetyl-based fused heterocyclic dipeptide mimetics as inhibitors of angiotensin-converting enzyme and neutral endopeptidase. *J. Med. Chem.* **1997**, *40*, 1570–1577.

117. Hanson, R.L.; Schwinden, M.D.; Banerjee, A.; Brzozowski, D.B.; Chen, B.-C.; Patel, B.P.; McNamee, C.G.; Kodersha, G.A.; Kronenthal, D.R.; Patel, R.N.; *et al.* Enzymatic synthesis of L-6-hydroxynorleucine. *Bioorg. Med. Chem.* **1999**, *7*, 2247–2252.

118. Patel, R. Enzymatic synthesis of chiral intermediates for Omapatrilat, an antihypertensive drug. *Biomol. Eng.* **2001**, *17*, 167–182.

119. Hanson, R.L.; Howell, J.; LaPorte, T.; Donovan, M.; Cazzulino, D.; Zannella, V.; Montana, M.; Nanduri, V.; Schwarz, S.; Eiring, R.; *et al.* Synthesis of allylsine ethylene acetal using phenylalanine dehydrogenase from *Thermoactinomyces intermedius. Enzyme Microb. Technol.* **2000**, *26*, 348–358.

120. Gallwitz, B. Glucagon-like peptide-1-based therapies for the treatment of type 2 diabetes mellitus. *Treat. Endocrinol.* **2005**, *4*, 361–370.

121. Sinclair, E.M.; Drucker, D.J. Glucagon-like peptide 1 receptor agonists and dipeptidyl peptidase IV inhibitors: New therapeutic agents for the treatment of type 2 diabetes. *Curr. Opin. Endocrinol. Diabet.* **2005**, *12*, 146–151.

122. Augeri, D.J.; Robl, J.A.; Betebenner, D.A.; Magnin, D.R.; Khanna, A.; Robertson, J.G.; Wang, A.; Simpkins, L.M.; Taunk, P.; Huang, Q.; *et al.* A highly potent, long-acting, orally active dipeptidyl peptidase IV inhibitor for the treatment of type 2 diabetes. *J. Med. Chem.* **2005**, *48*, 5025–5037.

123. David J Augeri, David A Betebenner, Lawrence G Hamann, David R Magnin, Jeffrey A Robl, Richard B Sulsky, Cyclopropyl-fused pyrrolidine-based inhibitors of dipeptidyl iv, processes for their preparation and their use. WO 2001068603 A2, 20 September 2001.

124. Hanson, R.L.; Goldberg, S.L.; Brzozowski, D.B.; Tully, T.P.; Cazzulino, D.; Parker, W.L.; Lyngberg, O.K.; Vu, T.C.; Wong, M.K.; Patel, R.N. Preparation of an amino acid intermediate for the dipeptidyl peptidase IV inhibitor, saxagliptin, using a modified phenylalanine dehydro genase. *Adv. Synth. Catal.* **2007**, *349*, 1369–1378.

125. Groeger, H.; May, O.; Werner, H.; Menzel, A.; Altenbuchner, J. A "second-generation process" for the synthesis of L-neopentylglycine: Asymmetric reductive amination using a recombinant whole cell catalyst. *Org. Process Res. Dev.* **2006**, *10*, 666–669.

126. Emmanuel, M.J.; Frye, L.L.; Hickey, E.R.; Liu, W.; Morwick, T.M.; Spero, D.M.; Sun, S.; Thomson, D.S.; Ward, Y.D.; Young, E.R.R. Novel Spiroheterocyclic Compounds [Morpholine-4-Carboxylic Acid Amides of Heterocyclic Cyclohexylalanine and Neopentylglycine Derivatives and Their Analogs], Useful as Reversible Inhibitors of Cysteine Proteases such as Cathepsin S. WO 2001019816 A1, 22 May 2001.

127. Haque, T.S.; Ewing, W.R.; Mapelli, C.; Lee, V.G.; Sulsky, R.B.; Riexinger, D.J.; Martinez, R.L.; Zhu. Y.Z. Human Glucagon-like-Peptide-1 Modulators and Their Use in the Treatment of Diabetes and Related Conditions. WO2007082264, A2, 11 January 2007.

128. Qian, F.; Ewing, W.R.; Mapelli, C.; Riexinger, D.J.; Lee, V.G.; Sulsky, R.B.; Zhu, Y.; Haque, T.S.; Martinez, R.L.; Naringrekar, V.; *et al.* Sustained release GLP-1 receptor modulators. US 20070099835 A1, 3 May 2007.

129. Chen, Y.; Goldberg, S.L.; Hanson, R.L.; Parker, W.L.; Gill, I.; Tully, T.P.; Montana, M.; Goswami, A.; Patel, R.N. Enzymatic preparation of an (*S*)-amino acid from a racemic amino acid. *Org. Process Res. Dev.* **2011**, *15*, 241–248.

130. Straathof, A.J.J.; Panke, S.A. The production of fine chemicals by biotransformations. *Curr. Opin. Biotechnol.* **2002**, *13*, 548–556.

131. Bommarius, A.S.; Schwarm, M.; Drauz, K. Biocatalysis to amino acid-based chiral pharmaceuticals-examples and perspectives. *J. Mol. Catal. B Enzym.* **1998**, *5*, 1–11.

132. Vedha-Peters, K.; Gunawardana, M.; Rozzell, J.D.; Novick, S.J. Creation of a broad-range and highly stereoselective D-amino acid dehydrogenase for the one-step synthesis of D-amino acids. *J. Am. Chem. Soc.* **2006**, *128*, 10923–10929.

133. Gustafsson, D.; Elg, M.; Lenfors, S.; Boerjesson, I.; Teger-Nilsso, A.-C. Effects of inogatran, a new low-molecular-weight thrombin inhibitor, in rat models of venous and arterial thrombosis, thrombolysis and bleeding time. *Blood Coagul. Fibrinolysis* **1996**, *7*, 69–79.

134. Alexandre, F.-R.; Pantaleone, D.P.; Taylor, P.P.; Fotheringham, I.G.; Ager, D.J.; Turner, N.J. Amine-boranes: Effective reducing agents for the deracemisation of DL-amino acids using L-amino acid oxidase from *Proteus myxofaciens. Tetrahedron Lett.* **2002**, *43*, 707–710.

135. Chaturvedula, P.V.; Chen, L.; Civiello, R.; Degnan, A.P.; Dubowchik, G.M.; Han, X.; Jiang, J.J.; Macor, J.E.; Poindexter, G.S.; Tora, G.O.; *et al.* Anti-Migraine Spirocycles. US 7842808 B2, 5 January 2007.

136. Han, X.; Civiello, R.L.; Conway, C.M.; Cook, D.A.; Davis, C.D.; Macci. R.; Pin, S.S.; Ren, S.X.; Schartman, R.; Signor, L.J.; *et al.* The synthesis and SAR of calcitonin gene-related peptide (CGRP) receptor antagonists derived from tyrosine surrogates. Part 1. *Bioorg Med Chem Lett.* **2012**, *22*, 4723-4727.

137. Hanson, R.L.; Davis, B.L.; Goldberg, S.L.; Johnston, R.M.; Parker, W.L.; Tully, T.P.; Montana, M.A.; Patel, R.N. Enzymatic preparation of a D-amino acid from a racemic amino acid or keto acid. *Org. Process Res. Dev.* **2008**, *12*, 1119–1129.

138. Ising, M.; Zimmermann, U.S.; Künzel, H.E.; Uhr, M.; Foster, A.C.; Learned-Coughlin, S.M.; Holsboer, F.; Grigoriadis, D.E. High-affinity CRF1 receptor antagonist NBI-34041: Preclinical and clinical data suggest safety and efficacy in attenuating elevated stress response. *Neuropsychopharmacology* **2007**, *32*, 1941–1949.

139. Overstreet, D.H.; Griebel, G. Antidepressant-like effects of CRF1 receptor antagonist SSR125543 in an animal model of depression. *Eur. J. Pharmacol.* **2004**, *497*, 49–53.

140. Tache, Y.; Martinez, V.; Wang, L.; Million, M. CRF1 receptor signaling pathways are involved in stress-related alterations of colonic function and viscerosensitivity: Implications for irritable bowel syndrome. *Br. J. Phamacol.* **2004**, *141*, 1321–1330.

141. Yu, W.-L.; Lawrence, F.; Wong, H.; Lelas, S.; Zhang, G.; Lindner, M.D.; Wallace, T.; McElroy, J.; Lodge, N.J.; Gilligan, P.; *et al.* The pharmacology of DMP696 and DMP904, non-peptidergic CRF1 receptor antagonists. *CNS Drug Rev.* **2006**, *11*, 21–52.

142. Gilligan, P.J.; Clarke, T.; He, L.; Lelas, S.; Li, Y.-W.; Heman, K.; Fitzgerald, L.; Miller, K.; Zhang, G.; Marshall, A.; *et al.* 8-(4-Methoxyphenyl)pyrazolo[1,5-*a*]-1,3,5-triazines: Selective and centrally active corticotropin-releasing factor receptor-1 (CRF1) antagonists. *J. Med. Chem.* **2009**, *52*, 3084–3092.

143. Hanson, R.L.; Davis, B.L.; Chen, Y.; Goldberg, S.L.; Parker, W.L.; Tully, T.P.; Montana, M.A.; Patel, R.N. Preparation of (*R*)-amines from racemic amines with an (*S*)-amine transaminase from *Bacillus megaterium*. *Adv. Synth. Catal.* **2008**, *350*, 1367–1375.

Improvement of Biocatalysts for Industrial and Environmental Purposes by Saturation Mutagenesis

Francesca Valetti and Gianfranco Gilardi

Abstract: Laboratory evolution techniques are becoming increasingly widespread among protein engineers for the development of novel and designed biocatalysts. The palette of different approaches ranges from complete randomized strategies to rational and structure-guided mutagenesis, with a wide variety of costs, impacts, drawbacks and relevance to biotechnology. A technique that convincingly compromises the extremes of fully randomized *vs.* rational mutagenesis, with a high benefit/cost ratio, is saturation mutagenesis. Here we will present and discuss this approach in its many facets, also tackling the issue of randomization, statistical evaluation of library completeness and throughput efficiency of screening methods. Successful recent applications covering different classes of enzymes will be presented referring to the literature and to research lines pursued in our group. The focus is put on saturation mutagenesis as a tool for designing novel biocatalysts specifically relevant to production of fine chemicals for improving bulk enzymes for industry and engineering technical enzymes involved in treatment of waste, detoxification and production of clean energy from renewable sources.

Reprinted from *Biomolecules*. Cite as: Valetti, F.; Gilardi, G. Improvement of Biocatalysts for Industrial and Environmental Purposes by Saturation Mutagenesis. *Biomolecules* **2013**, *3*, 778-811.

1. Introduction

Protein engineering allows exploration of mutational space under artificial evolutionary pressure and selection that could not be sampled by the natural environment of proteins. Advances in this field demonstrate how natural catalysts can be finely tuned to perform reactions that are new in terms of specificity [1–3], efficiency [4–6], stability of the enzyme, conditions [7,8] and chemistry of the reaction catalyzed [9–11]. Many of the biotechnological benefits of this "laboratory-driven evolution" have already been translated into practical applications, and many others can be foreseen to have a high impact in sustainable and innovative processes [12], environmental bioremediation, detoxification, and clean energy production [13–15].

New tools and strategies aiming at simplifying the experimental work required for a successful result in obtaining engineered enzymes are continuously being developed. The methods follow two main directions: the rational site-specific mutagenesis and the evolution-like random approach. Both are powerful but each suffer from different limitations in the performance of the outcome and in time necessary to achieve the results. The rational site-specific mutagenesis focuses on the mutation of one or more specific amino acids that are replaced with another residue. It needs to be supported by structural and functional data of the enzyme and it is frequently biased by the assumptions made by the researchers on the basis of previous knowledge. In this respect it might be less innovative and aim at less ambitious goals, although it remains a very precious strategy for testing hypothesis on the fine details and structural determinants of reaction mechanisms. Compared to the random evolution-like approach, it is less time consuming in the production of the mutants, but in the perspective of producing significantly improved biocatalysts for industrial applications, it often results in limited improvement of the desired property. Results are achieved through series of trial-and-error experiments that surely provide interesting data for theoretical speculation but that may require large amounts of time and resources.

On the other hand, laboratory evolution is based on the selection of random mutants with the desired features. It is not limited by the availability of the 3D structure of the enzyme and it mimics in the lab the evolution process that in nature has led to the selection of the best natural catalysts available: the enzymes. This approach establishes methods to introduce random genetic diversity in libraries of mutants (variants) that include various implementations of mutagenic PCR, oligonucleotide-assisted mutagenesis and *in vitro* recombination under mutagenic conditions, including DNA shuffling [16] and several specific techniques such as ITCHY [17], RACHITT [18] SHIPREC [19] and many others that have been extensively reviewed [20–25]. The time consuming process of obtaining the randomly mutated library and the requirement for a high-throughput screening procedure for selection of the desired properties among thousands of clones, is the severe drawback of a very powerful technique that otherwise has the advantage of providing entirely novel landscapes of mutants [26,27].

A specific type of laboratory-evolution method is the "targeted random mutagenesis" method, also called "saturation mutagenesis" that focuses on specific "hot spots" for mutational variability or on critical residues identified by structural comparison and modeling methods. It applies site-saturation mutagenesis (SSM), *i.e.*, the systematic replacement of one amino acid at a chosen site with all alternative encoded amino acids, to explore the performance of each possible variant in terms of structural or functional features of the resulting mutated enzyme. SSM may be applied at random positions but more often it is based on the assumption that most mutations are deleterious or neutral, and therefore the construction of mutant libraries by random methods is inefficient. Since the enzyme properties that are pursued are mainly codified in a small part of the enzyme corresponding to the active site or structural portions known to modulate protein stability, a rational choice of the sites to be targeted is usually preferred. This approach allows fine-tuning of the catalytic properties, particularly when performed as a refinement step after directed evolution. In fact, in fully random techniques a trade-off between the selected property and the overall enzyme performance might put an apparent threshold to the optimization of the target property [28]. Therefore, saturation mutagenesis is a precious tool for exploring and widening the landscape of the enzyme properties and applications. The advantages lie in a compromise solution combining the positive features of the rational mutagenesis and the random approach followed by laboratory selection, with minimum or negligible additive effect on the drawbacks. This is becoming clear in the last few years due to the increasing number of successful results obtained. A particular relevance is given in literature to positive results of this approach applied to enzymes used in fine chemical synthesis, industrial processing and bioremediation.

In order to improve the outputs and to obtain libraries with high abundance methods such as iterative Combinatorial Active Site Test (CAST) [29] and Iterative Saturation Mutagenesis (ISM) [30], all based on the same principle of SSM, were more recently implemented.

The methodology for Site Saturation Mutagenesis, Iterative Saturation Mutagenesis and other innovative methods will be presented highlighting advantages *vs.* site specific and random mutagenesis. Technical details and implications will be discussed, also tackling the issues of randomization and statistical evaluation of the library completeness and throughput efficiency of screening methods. Examples of successful applications covering different enzyme classes will be presented, focusing on cases that are relevant for the production of fine chemicals as well as bulk enzymes for industry, treatment of wastes, detoxification of pollutants and xenobiotics, and production of clean energy from renewable sources.

2. Experimental

Different methodologies pertaining saturation mutagenesis, leading to libraries of mutants relevant in terms of their size with minimal screening efforts, will be illustrated in the following paragraphs. The choice of alternative approaches bears crucial implications and must be carefully considered. Following the pattern of single site saturation mutagenesis and extending the strategies to various multiple combinations, a range of protocols have been proposed and tested. These are described and discussed here, together with the statistical analysis of library coverage and screening methods specifically for the saturation mutagenesis approaches.

2.1. Strategies for the Generation of Libraries of Mutants

2.1.1. Site Saturation Mutagenesis (SSM)

The SSM libraries are usually generated with protocols that follow the commercially available QuikChange™ kit commercialized by Stratagene [31] or using equivalent in house procedures [30]. Mutagenic and complementary primers that carry the desired mutation (Figure 1) are used in a PCR reaction to amplify the plasmid with high fidelity and thus inserting the desired mutations. The position chosen for mutagenesis can be randomized with the codon NNN (where N is any nucleotide), or with a codon NNK (where K is either a T or a G) that can produce codons for all the 20 amino acids and a stop codon. Compared to NNN degeneration, NNK has the advantage that it will produce 32 variants instead of 64, reducing screening effort and inserting one stop codon instead of three. The mutagenic primers are designed with the targeted position in the middle and at least 15 non-mutated bases before and after the point of mutation. The PCR product is digested with DpnI, a restriction enzyme that recognizes and cleaves the methylated template DNA, while the non-methylated newly synthesized and mutated DNA strands are not recognized nor digested. The mutated nicked plasmid is transformed in highly competent *E. coli* strain DH5α or XL1-Blue.

2.1.2. Iterative Saturation Mutagenesis (ISM)

The Iterative Saturation Mutagenesis (ISM) was proposed by Reetz and coworkers [30] and it combines, in an iterative manner, the SSM described above. While other strategies simply add mutations at rationally-chosen single sites by producing double or triple mutants that simply contain the positive mutation 1, 2, 3 *etc.*, in the ISM approach, a few sites in the protein sequence are identified as crucial by means of structural data or modeling, requiring a partially rational approach as in SSM, but saturation mutagenesis is then applied at the chosen sites in a combinatorial pattern. The site can be represented by a single amino acid or by a few neighboring amino acids, ideally not more than three, keeping in mind that an increase in the number of variants will then require screening of a large number of clones. These sites are then mutated according to the saturation mutagenesis approach. The novelty of this approach resides in the iterative feature given by selecting the best hit of the library obtained at each target site. For example, assume sites X, Y, Z have been selected for mutagenesis. These sites will lead to three libraries X, Y, Z, each giving as best variant X1, Y1, and Z1. Saturation mutagenesis is applied at the respective other sites: X1 will be subjected to SSM at site Y, providing library X1Y, and at site Z, providing library X1Z, as shown in the scheme of Figure 2.

Figure 1. Scheme of site saturation mutagenesis approach following the QuikChange™ kit.

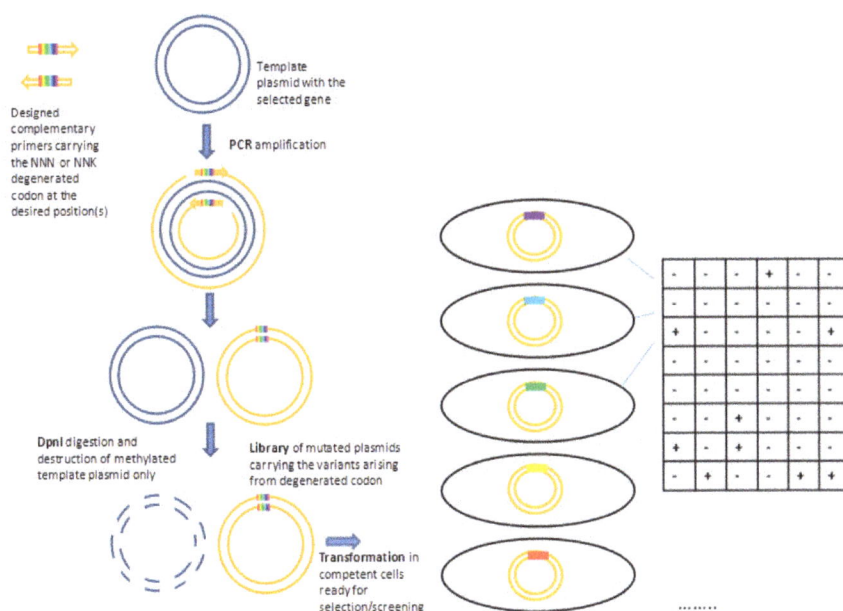

This branching process, iterated by applying SSM to a single site one or more times, can theoretically extend very quickly. For example, iterating each SSM at three sites results in 12 libraries as shown in Figure 2. In practice, non-productive branches will stop the process, as the example highlighted in red in Figure 2, while a pathway leading to synergistically improved mutants (*i.e.*, not resulting from the simple sum of single mutations) can be efficiently defined, reducing the library size. The productive pathway is highlighted in green, while yellow is shown as another branch producing variants with limited improvement. Each new cycle of ISM maximizes the probability of obtaining additive and/or cooperative effects of newly introduced mutations, which optimize the fitness landscape in a defined region of protein sequence space. This is not the case when the best-hit mutant of each library is simply added to a double or multiple mutant, where the effect can be non additive or even detrimental to the desired protein property. ISM has been demonstrated to achieve impressive results especially in enhancing enantio-selectivity [32] and thermostability of enzymes. Notably, the ISM strategy was also tested on libraries that initially did not contain improved variants, by applying the iterative cycle even to inferior mutants as templates. This was done within the systematical testing of features of 24 alternative pathways to improved variants of a biocatalyst (epoxide hydrolase from *Aspergillus niger*) and the performance evaluation of the ISM when reaching a local minimum [33]. The results showed that applying ISM resulted in successfully escaping from the local minimum.

Figure 2. Scheme of iterative saturation mutagenesis showing the branching process and highlighting the productive pathway (in green), non-productive mutants that stop the process simplifying the screening procedure (in red). Highlighted in yellow are mutants produced with moderate to low improvement that can be discarded or reconsidered for further processing in a second phase.

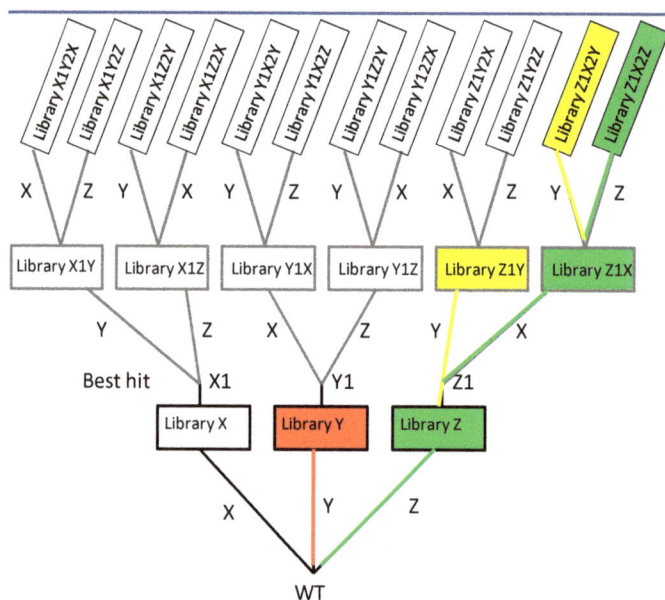

2.1.3. Combinatorial Active-Site Saturation Test (CAST)

Strategies for evolving properties such as substrate recognition and catalysis specificity, including stereochemistry of reaction and selection of improved enzyme for resolution of racemic mixtures and precise enantio-selectivity, have been proposed over the last 5 years by selecting one or more amino acids in the active site pocket or in its close proximity. The best example of a systematic approach to this end is represented by the Combinatorial Active-site Saturation Test (CAST). In this approach, pairs of amino acid residues pointing towards the active site of an enzyme are chosen for complete randomization. The selection of residues is made on the basis of geometric assumptions that suggest choosing amino acid pairs along the sequence of loops, helices or β-sheets. For example, two residues pointing both to the catalytic pocket will for instance be n and n + 2 along the sequence in a β-sheet and n and n + 4 in a α-helix. The randomization of each pair generates a CAST library with

20^2, *i.e.*, 400 possible variants. The limited size of each CAST library allows an oversampling of 3000 clones for statistically significant screening coverage, thus drastically reducing time and cost efforts. The results from each CAST library can then be combined pairwise by multiple mutations or by iterative strategies and re-randomized as explained above. The impressive results obtained with enzyme specificity and enantio-selectivity [32,34] highlight the suitability of the method to evolve new functions for biocatalysts. Lipases are a good example of the powerful application of CAST. The results achieved on lipases support the suitability of SSM-based methods for biocatalysts improvement, as lipases certainly constitute the core business in key industrial processes such as detergent additives, food processing and biomass pretreatment, bearing a significant impact on the global biocatalysts market that is expected to reach \$7.6 billion by 2015 [35]. The availability of the CASTER software provides a very powerful tool for assigning the residue pairs for randomization on the basis of a crystal structure or a homology model. This makes the approach easy to test with several different enzymes in reproducible conditions. The main group working with this approach is that of Reetz [29], but recent applications from other research groups highlighted equally important results [36]. The limitation of the method, that requires as ideal starting point a substrate-bound crystal structure of the biocatalyst to be targeted, can be overcome in most cases by homology modeling, docking tools and in general by available bio-computing techniques.

2.1.4. B-Factor Iterative Test (B-FIT)

The focus of the B-factor iterative test (B-FIT) is the protein scaffold stability, more so than the detail of the catalytic pocket, and therefore it can guide the improvement of parameters such as thermostability that is known to not necessarily relate to the active site residues. The B-factor, or "temperature-factor", can be calculated from crystallographic data and indicates the static or dynamic mobility of an atom or groups of atoms. The B-FIT approach therefore relies on the principle of ISM combined with criteria for selecting the crucial sites that are based on the availability of B-factor values, *i.e.*, on information about the protein scaffold mobility. The hot spots are identified using software called the B-FITTER. This averages the B-factors available from X-ray crystallographic structures and it relies on the principle that high B-factors are signature of very flexible regions of the protein scaffold. Iterative mutagenesis at these flexible sites of the enzyme aims at increasing their rigidity and therefore improving the thermal stability of the enzymes to be used in industrial processes or bulk applications. The test cases that show the most impressive results to date are once more regarding the lipases, enzymes that need to be thermostable as they are typically added to detergents for mid to high temperature biological activity. The availability of the crystal structure is much more of a prerequisite here and therefore the bottleneck. Another limiting point could be the matching of an increased rigidity for thermostability [37,38] and also for stability against denaturing agents such as organic solvents [39], together with an adequate dynamic range necessary for the structural rearrangements that occur in many enzymes during catalysis. The interesting further proof that the approach is based on a measurable parameter directly correlated with flexibility and thermolability is the re-engineering of the thermostable lipase from *Pseudomonas aeruginosa*. This enzyme maintains catalytic features while dramatically decreasing its thermal stability, with Tm halved from 72 °C to 36 °C. This was achieved by reversing the approach illustrated above, by selecting and randomizing few chosen positions with a lower *B*-value according to the B-FITTER software to achieve destabilization of the original enzyme [40].

Another recent strategy able to select regions of potential protein flexibility and therefore hot spots to be subjected to saturation mutagenesis for tuning thermostability was named Coevolving-Site Saturation Mutagenesis (CSSM) [41]. The method relies on computational algorithm [42] and sequence alignment to select coevolving residues and/or pairs of co-evolutionary interactions that are then targeted with saturation mutagenesis to generate variants selected for improved thermostability.

2.1.5. Cassette Mutagenesis and Other Approaches for Multisite Saturation Mutagenesis

Cassette mutagenesis is one of the classical approaches for systematic mutagenesis at fixed positions [43] that can be chosen for multisite saturation mutagenesis. It is usually applied when a relatively short DNA sequence is to be mutated by synthetic oligonucleotide primers designed to introduce multiple mutations at targeted amino acids in the same stretch of primary sequence. The excision and re-introduction of the mutated cassette by molecular biology techniques, such as introduction of restriction sites and ligation in the original vector, makes it a time consuming procedure. Likewise, methods that follow the classical Kunkel mutagenesis approach using ssDNA also suffer from the same drawbacks. However, a recent novel approach named PFunkel [44] has been proposed that re-interprets the Kunkel methodology and that can be performed in one day in a single test tube (Figure 3). This was applied to create a library with site-saturation at four distal sites and it was tested on TEM-1 β-lactamase gene to produce a library of 18,081 designed variants: library sequencing attested that a 97% coverage of the expected variants were present in the library, and this was then screened for variants resistant to the ß-lactamase inhibitor tazobactam.

Figure 3. Schematic of PFunkel mutagenesis strategy (adapted from Firnberg *et al.* [44]).

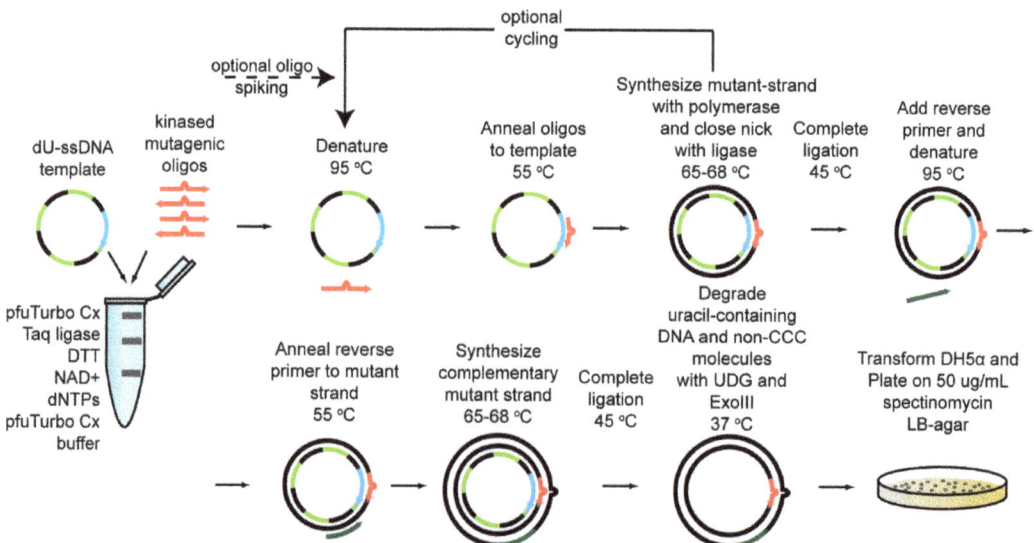

Another recent strategy to simultaneously introduce saturation mutagenesis at multiple sites (up to five codons) was proposed by Schwaneberg and co-workers [45]. The scheme of this approach, named OmniChange is reported below (Figure 4).

Figure 4. The 4-step strategy for the simultaneous saturation of 5 independent codons by OmniChange (adapted from Dennig *et al.* [45]).

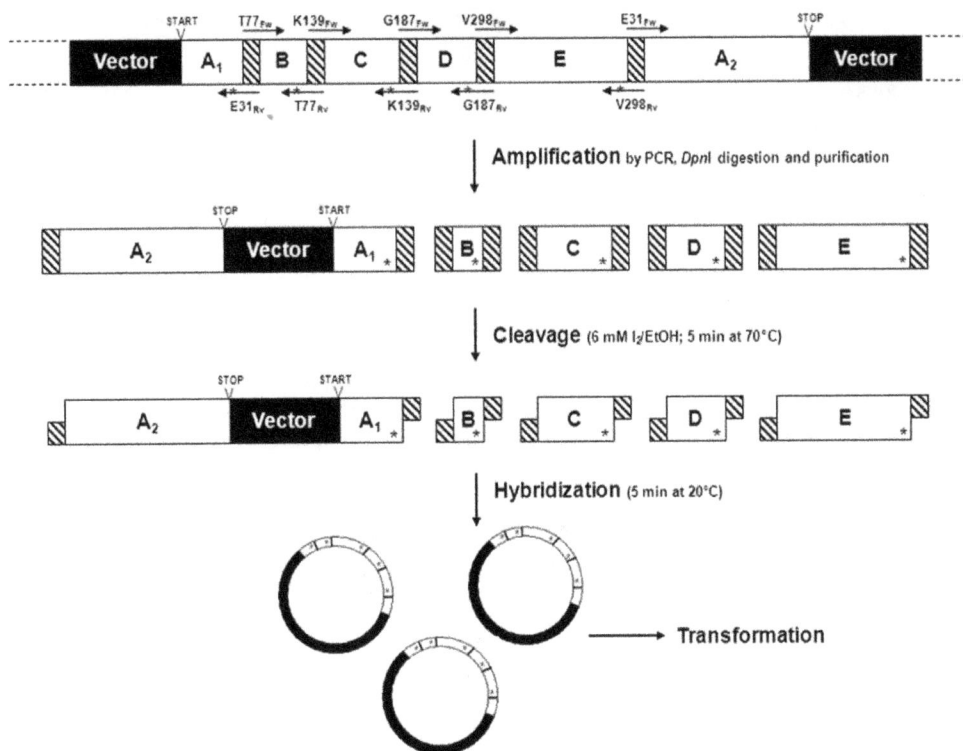

2.1.6. Reducing Amino Acid Alphabet

The query for strategies that can reduce library size without limiting functional variants has led to several attempts to restrict the amino acid alphabet. All "reducing amino acid alphabet" approaches aim at defining a small set of a few representative amino acids that can efficiently function as building blocks for all proteins. Saturation mutagenesis performed with a restricted alphabet at multiple sites has the advantage of generating smaller and potentially smarter libraries. The risk is to over-simplify the subset and exclude subtle and specific properties of some amino acids. The design of the subset chosen is therefore a very delicate step. The main efforts in this direction came from Hilvert [46] and Reetz [47] and co-workers who respectively proposed a reduced alphabet of 9 and 12 representative amino acids applied to the design of an enzyme able to function as chorismate mutase [46] and to the engineering of the active site of an epoxide hydrolase [47]. Although the function of these enzymes can efficiently be complied by this simplified catalyst, the stability of the protein was not entirely satisfactory, as an undesired enhanced flexibility was observed in the enzyme designed with the 9 amino acid reduced alphabet [46]. In other cases the reduced amino acid alphabet was specifically designed on the basis of sequence alignment and consensus variants and the strategy applied to the focused mutagenesis of a phenyl acetone monooxygenase [48]. The main advantage of this method is well highlighted by the rigorous comparison of library coverage when randomizing multiple positions with the alternative codon NNK for the 20 amino acids and with the codon NDT (D: adenine/guanine/thymine) encoding for the reduced 12 amino acid alphabet. The number of variants to be screened in the NDT library for 95% coverage is less than 500 for a two position randomized mutant and 5000 for a three position mutant. In the case of NNK library for a two positions mutant a screening of 3000 is required, while for a three positions mutant the screening of 10,000 variants only covers 25% [49]. For the purpose of reducing library redundancy, and consequently screening efforts, a more convincing strategy has recently been proposed by designing appropriate mutagenic primers that can cover the 20 amino acids with only 22 codons [50].

2.2. Statistical Robustness of the Method and Requirements for Library Screenings

A key point of all laboratory evolution techniques is library screening and variant selection, which is tightly intertwined with the statistical analysis of library coverage. Although SSM is a focused strategy among the wider landscape of directed evolution approaches, the importance of these two aspects is crucial and bears implications for judging SSM and evaluating its potential application. Therefore a brief coverage of the topic will be presented below with a focus on relevance to SSM strategy.

The saturation mutagenesis methods usually aim at the production of relatively small and high quality libraries, whose screening could cover all different variants with an established degree of confidence. It is therefore crucial to acknowledge the importance of statistics [51–54] for estimating the number of analyses to be performed and determining the sample size to be screened. In most methods, with the exception of recently proposed alphabet reducing [47] and redundancy reducing approaches [50], the distribution of encoded amino acids is impaired in frequency due to the genetic code redundancy. Thus a library constructed with NNN configuration will have leucine represented six times for every tryptophan. As a result, the sample size should always be calculated on the basis of nucleotide rather than amino acid diversity. The statistics of the process is described by the following equation [54].

$$L \approx -V \ln\left(-\frac{\ln P_c}{V}\right)$$ (1)

where V is the number of possible variants (64 for NNN degeneracy, 32 for NNK degeneracy of a single codon), L is the number of clones in the library, Pc is the probability of completeness of the library. Thus, the equation correlates the number of clones in the library with the probability that each clone is actually present in the library at least once. The same holds for the screening. As an example, the screening of 360 clones obtained by a NNK degenerated library at a single site, providing 32 different codon variants, ensures a probability of 99.96% that each variant has been tested at least once, while lowering the screened clones to 247 lowers the probability to 98.59%. The assumption is of course that the NNK or NNN degeneracy and the SSM protocol applied is not affected by biases and that the incorporation of each codon is equally possible. This is not always the case and controls of library completeness can be performed by sequencing the entire library mixture (Figure 5) and/or randomly selecting a few clones (either positive or negative) to demonstrate that a good variability of codons for different amino acids are actually present [55].

Figure 5. DNA sequencing of the three libraries produced for evaluation of the randomization efficiency on selected position in hydrogenase gene: the targeted position is properly randomized for NNK in library A and C (K either a T or a G), while only partial degeneration is present in library B.

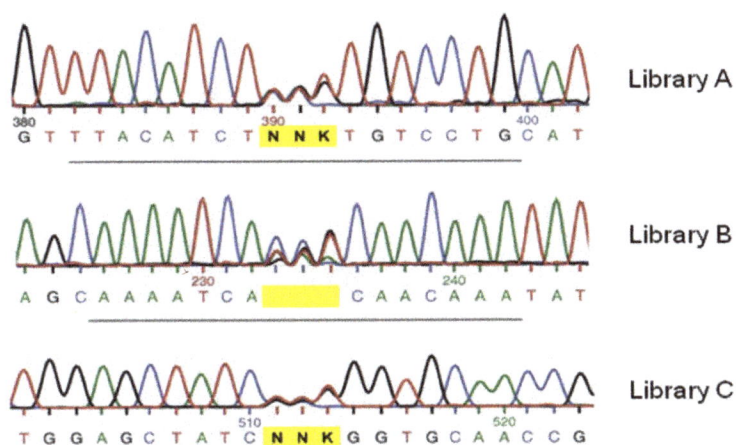

The higher the degeneracy of the library, the higher the number of clones to be screened in order to have a significant probability of coverage of all mutants. For example, to achieve 95% (the threshold for significance is usually set to this value) probability to cover all mutants in a 1024-fold degenerated library, it has been estimated that about 3,000 clones should be screened. Most SSM experiments reported in the literature cover the mutated library between two to four times on a basis of nucleotide diversity (e.g., 64–128 clones are usually screened for a 32-fold degenerated library). Often incomplete screenings of large libraries can allow identification of variants with desirable features [56]. This strategy is, however, prone to the statistical uncertainty of missing clones with remarkable properties. To reduce the library size and overcome genetic code redundancy, mixtures of highly specific primers can be used instead of a degenerated primer. Therefore, 19 primers (one for each specific amino acid alternative to the WT amino acid) can be used to randomize each codon. This can also be applied when a bias in codon incorporation is present (Figure 3 library B) and a properly randomized library cannot be synthesized.

Recent novel techniques and designed primers were proposed to further reduce codon redundancy and to ensure equal probability of coding each amino acid, by limiting the code to 22 triplets covering the 20 standard amino acids [50].

The researcher in the laboratory designs the selection of desired variants by the application of an appropriate screening method. The general rule that "you get what you screen for" indicates that this step is a particularly crucial one and often represents the bottleneck for the success of directed evolution in developing improved or new biocatalysts. The selection method must be rapid, sensitive and allow for the clear identification of the desired properties, implying that the screening must not be marred by undesired selection criteria.

The fully randomized methods of shuffling or error prone PCR implies the production of very large libraries and therefore the requirement for equally powerful high-throughput screening techniques, such as phage display or other more recent molecular display methods [57,58]. These methods enable the screening of up to 10^{12} protein variants, but usually rely on costly equipment and are only suitable for very focused applications. On the contrary, *in vivo* selection of suitable enzymes by setting experimental parameters so that conditional cell survival is linked to the desired biocatalyst function usually is low cost and allows high-throughput performance. Unfortunately, instances have been reported in literature in which surviving cells bypassed the desired enzyme expression. Also by setting a high threshold there is the probability that low activity variants with potential interest are excluded.

The application of spectrophotometric [59] or fluorimetric [60] platform that can screen for the desired product formation or at least for substrates and co-substrates consumption by the biocatalyst of interest is a more versatile option that can be extended to very specific catalysis, such as stereo-specific production of chiral compounds [61], biodegradation of recalcitrant poly-aromatic hydrocarbons [62], for the synthesis of drug metabolites [63,64] and the turnover of novel chemical entities for drug synthesis, such as 1,2,5-Oxadiazole derivatives [65], for hydrogen evolution and uptake [55,66]. The superior specificity and versatility of such assays is reached at the cost of lowering the through-put efficiency, even for quick assays that can be performed on multi-well plates, directly on cell lysates or colonies (Figure 6) [55]. Compared to fully randomized methods, saturation mutagenesis, which provides small but high quality libraries, allows the application of such focused and function-specific screenings whilst maintaining statistically sound library coverage.

Figure 6. (**a**) Scheme of the principle of on-colonies activity test for a [FeFe] hydrogenase [55]; (**b**) Example of the screening results.

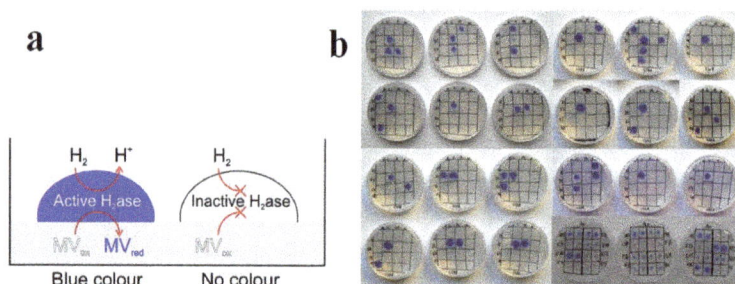

3. Recent Successful Applications

An increasing number of recent papers proposes the application of saturation mutagenesis to biocatalysts of applicative interest, for "greener" industrial processes [67,68] improved bulk enzymes [41,69,70], biotechnology [71,72] bioremediation [73], fine chemical synthesis [74–80], biofuels production [55,81,82] and biomass exploitation [82–85].

A selection of relevant successful examples published in the past 5 years is presented below. The report is divided in two sections: (1) enzyme classes with high impact on industrial processes and fine chemistry (*3.1*) and (2) enzyme classes with applications in environmental care and production of clean energy (*3.2*). Some classes, for example oxygenases, are relevant to both and therefore are listed twice.

3.1. Enzymes Relevant for Industry

3.1.1. Lipases

Lipases are considered as benchmark enzymes for biocatalysis: Lipolase®Ultra and LipoPrime® are the first examples of engineered lipases for commercial distribution in detergent industry. They are also exploited in other industrial large-scale processes and as dedicated catalysts for highly stereo-specific catalysis in fine chemistry. Saturation mutagenesis has played a key role in engineering several lipases both for thermal stability and enantio-selectivity, with at least 20 research papers published in the last 5 years. Among groups involved in lipases engineering, Reetz and co-workers achieved relevant results [29,32,34] by applying SSM, ISM and CAST for enhancing enantio-selectivity and B-FIT for tuning thermal stability properties. The SSM approach was applied to *Pseudomonas aeruginosa* lipase, a well-known catalyst applied to hydrolysis of carboxylic acid esters and transesterification of primary and secondary alcohols, with the aim of redesigning the substrate recognition pocket to enable catalysis on more bulky substrates, such as benzoic acid esters. Ser 82, the key residue for the stabilization of the oxyanion intermediate, was not addressed by the mutagenesis since it structurally belongs to a more distant portion of the enzyme, while the CAST strategy guided the selection of five pairs of residues pointing towards the active site and defining the recognition determinants of the hydrophobic portion of the ester. Five libraries were produced by simultaneous saturation mutagenesis at the two defined positions, that is library A to E: Met16/Leu17, Leu118/Ile 121, Leu131/Val 135, Leu159/Leu162, and Leu231/Val 232 (Figure 7).

The five libraries of 3000 variants each were then screened with a spectrophotometric method by testing 11 different substrates. The total reactions performed (165,000) allowed to select eight hits from libraries A and D, consistent with the focus on hot spots even within the restricted region analyzed. Although the success rate in this case was lower than for other SSM reported approaches, the few selected variants showed an impressive gain in function, for instance by binding adamantyl carboxylic acid esters that are not recognized by the WT, as well as showing a 100 fold increase in the rate of hydrolytic activity on substrates that are poorly recognized by the WT [29]. Further works on the same enzyme by ISM highlighted the enormous potentiality of iterative saturation versus other methods such as error prone PCR, shuffling and even the previous SSM, in particular for enhancing the stereospecificity of reactions. In fact, a more recent paper reports, on the same enzyme, the gain of function for the bulky 2-phenylalkanoic acid esters that are not recognized by the WT and the selection of variants with enantio-selectivity of E = 436, achieved with only small mutant libraries and thus a minimum of screening effort [34].

310

Figure 7. Scheme of the structure of *P. aeruginosa* lipase active site pocket (PDB: 1EX9) with the targeted sites (library A: Met16/Leu17 in red; library B: Leu118/Ile 121 in orange; library C: Leu131/Val 135 in yellow; library D: Leu159/Leu162 in green; and library E: Leu231/Val 232 in cyan). Ser82, Asp229, and His251 (in violet) represent the catalytic triad. A substrate analogue (RC-(RP,SP)-1,2-dioctylcarbamoyl-glycero-3-*O*-octylphosphonate) covalently bound to Ser 82 is shown in blue.

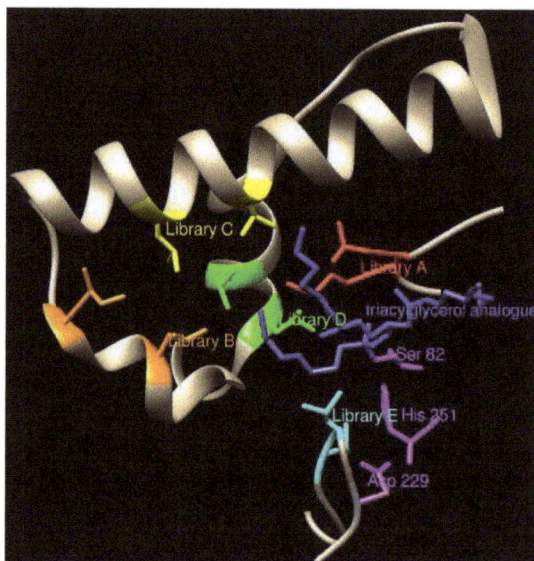

Also, the selection of a *Pseudomonas aeruginosa* lipase engineered variant with an enatioselectivity of E = 594 for the kinetic resolution of a chiral ester from an ISM library upon screening only 10,000 transformants is an unprecedented result [32], given that by directed evolution based on DNA shuffling, only a best variant value of E = 51 (ee > 95% at 24% conversion) could be obtained by screening about 50,000 transformants [86]. In the specific case of variant 1B2, characterized by a high E value of 594, this was produced by ISM starting from three libraries with simultaneous randomization at two near sites each, namely library A (Met16/Leu17), B (Leu159/Leu162), and C (Leu231/Val232). The selection of a best hit from library B with E = 8 (Leu162Asn) was followed by a second round of randomization on library A with DNT codon that simplifies amino acid alphabet by excluding Leu and therefore back-mutating to the original amino acid Leu17. This led to the highly optimized 1B2 variant (Met16Ala/Leu17Phe/Leu162Asn).

A very recent paper [70] reports the application of ISM and CAST to the engineering of *Candida antarctica* lipase B (CALB; Novozyme 435), a top industrial biocatalyst applied in kinetic resolution of racemic alcohols and amines, desymmetrization of diols and in other stereoselective synthesis of chiral intermediates for pharmaceuticals, polymer chemistry, and protection/deprotection technology. CAST guided selection of active site residues and ISM cycles with restricted alphabet using NDT degeneracy allowed for the isolation of two best mutants that were tested on several substrates for enhancement of activity and S- or R-stereospecificity. These two best hits, named RG401 and SG303 were tested on four representative chiral α-substituted carboxylic acid esters. Specificity constants k_{cat}/K_M from 13 to 270 fold higher than WT were achieved for SG303 with E (S) up to 64. The other mutant, RG401, acquired an enantio-specificity with E (R) up to 68 although the specificity constants were only slightly higher or of the same order of magnitude of WT. On *Candida antarctica* lipase A (CALA), Bäckvall and co-workers [36] applied the CAST strategy to enhance the performance of the catalyst by building two reduced libraries based on the NDT degeneracy: library FI (Phe149 and Ile150) with side chains directed toward the R-methyl group of the substrate and library FG (Phe233 and Gly237) with side chains defining the acyl-recognizing pocket of the active site. The reduced library size allowed a high coverage (>95%) by screening only 600 variants per library and allowed to select variants with E values of 45–276 (WT E value is only up to 20) and up to 30 fold increased activity for seven different esters used for the preparation of enantiomerically pure 2-arylpropionic acids, important building blocks for the synthesis of non-steroidal anti-inflammatory drugs such as Naproxen, Ibuprofen, and Flurbiprofen. The same group recently reported a further enhancement where CALA variants with high activity and E value of 100 towards an ester of ibuprofen were obtained. This substrate had failed to be recognized efficiently and with high stereospecificity by variants selected previously [80].

The robustness of the saturation mutagenesis methods, in particular with the B-FIT strategy, for thermal stabilization and destabilization of lipases for catalysis at desired optimal temperature, has already been discussed (Section 2.1.4) [37,41] and the same approach has proven to be suitable for stabilization towards other denaturing agents such as organic solvents [39].

3.1.2. Esterases and Other Hydrolases

Esterases are also extensively used in biocatalysis: saturation mutagenesis strategies have been applied to some enzymes of this class, in particular for the esterase from *Pseudomonas fluorescens*. Enhancement of enantio-selectivity [87] of this enzyme was pursued by the use of simultaneous saturation mutagenesis at four hot spots, with restricted alphabets chosen on the basis of more frequently represented amino acids in structurally equivalent positions on the basis of 1750 known sequences. This approach granted variants with improved rates (up to 240-fold) and enantioselectivities (up to E(true) = 80) towards 3-phenylbutyric acid esters with the advantage of a relatively limited effort for screening these "small but smart" libraries. As for thermal stabilization, the same enzyme was targeted at three sites, selected by B-FIT strategies, granting an enhanced stability of almost 10 °C higher than the starting catalyst [88].

Other class 3 hydrolytic enzymes that were targeted by saturation mutagenesis for improved catalysts development include epoxide hydrolases, already mentioned as test cases for the development of focused restricted alphabet libraries [46]. A limonene epoxide hydrolase from *Rhodococcus erythropolis*, performing a rare one-step mechanism, was also targeted by ISM to select variants with high stereoselectivity on substrates different from the natural limonene epoxide. Active site binding pocket residues were selected and the codons randomized with a reduced amino acid alphabet strategy. Variants obtained from 5000 screened hits can catalyze the desymmetrization of cyclopentene-oxide with stereoselective production of (*R*,*R*)- or (*S*,*S*)-enantiomers, the desymmetrization of other meso-epoxides and kinetic resolution of racemic substrates [89].

Because of its potential usefulness in β-lactam antibiotics synthesis, α-amino acid ester hydrolases were also chosen for improvement by saturation mutagenesis. A study was performed on 13 residues not directly involved in substrate recognition (based on the crystal structure of a protein-cefprozil complex) that were individually randomized in the enzyme from *Xanthomonas rubrillineans*. Mutants were selected with improved synthetic activity of *p*-hydroxylcephalosporins with a 23%, 17% and 64% increase in product yield for cefadroxil, cefprozil and cefatrizine, respectively [90].

Another biocatalyst relevant for bulk applications and belonging to the hydrolase class is represented by phytase, commercialized as an additive to poultry and swine feeding preparation in order to enhance digestibility of phytate and increase phosphorus assimilation. The challenge for enzyme engineering here is to enhance the stability of the catalyst not only to temperature but also to gastric degradation and to very low pH environment of the digestive tract so that the enzyme can still be active during the feeding process. Industry interest in this biocatalyst and in mutagenesis approaches aiming at improving its performance is testified by a paper dating back to 2004 [91] published on a research carried out by the company Diversa Corporation, San Diego, CA, USA. The dhlA phytase encoding gene from *Rhodococcus* was chosen to apply saturation mutagenesis with NNK codon systematically to all 431 positions of the protein sequence and screening was performed on at least 150 clones for each individually produced library. By isolating the best single mutants for enhanced low pH stability after heat treatment of the variants, therefore combining a selection for two desired properties, the authors selected 14 single mutants with improved properties and performed a combinatorial strategy and a second screening to isolate synergic and additive effects of multiple mutations. Variant Phy9X, with eight combined mutations, led to a novel biocatalyst with the ability to reversibly renature upon heat treatment and also function at process temperatures of 65 °C, with specific activity at the same level of WT but extending to below pH 2.5 and a 3.5 fold enhanced stability to gastric degradation.

3.1.3. Oxygenases and Other Redox Enzymes

Among redox enzymes, oxygenases have been key examples of the possible improvements brought by protein engineering to the efficiency of enzymes, and particularly of biocatalysts: the focus on cytochromes P450 and Baeyer-Villiger monooxygenases has always been maintained when proposing rational, semi-rational and randomized techniques of laboratory evolution with the seeding work of the groups of Arnold and Reetz, respectively and of many other groups that proposed directed evolution of these versatile biocatalysts. More recently, in particular for P450s, an increasing number of papers proposed saturation mutagenesis alone, or in combination with random techniques, to refine particular applications supported by this class of enzymes in fine chemical synthesis. This also extends to other non-heme iron oxygenases used for enantioselective synthesis of pharmaceutical compounds and chiral sulfoxides [74].

Starting from P450s, saturation mutagenesis seems to be the preferred method to enable enhancement of both regio- and stereo-selectivity for the C-H hydroxylation reactions that are of interest in fine chemistry. Steroid hydroxylation by cytochromes P450 in controlled positions leading to enantiomerically pure products is one of the most targeted goals of industry. The results achieved with saturation mutagenesis in the last few years benefit from the knowledge in terms of key spots relevant to improving enzyme performance acquired through directed evolution. Further specific improvements have been made possible by saturation mutagenesis. A very recent work by Glieder and co-workers [75] addressed the two active site residues 216 and 483 by saturation mutagenesis to generate all 400 possible combinations of amino acids. A double mutant of WT CYP2D6 resulted in a high regio-selectivity for hydroxylation at the 2β-position, instead of the 6β-position, suggesting that the mutation F483G could be preferential to the reported F483I for regio-selectivity in the well-known protein hot spot F483. Moreover, a previously obtained mutant F87A of P450 BM3, was further targeted by ISM for selective hydroxylation of testosterone in either of the two possible products 2β- and 15β-alcohols [92]. The CAST approach was applied to choose appropriate sites surrounding the binding pocket. The 20 residues selected as possible candidates for ISM were grouped into nine sites of neighboring amino acids, as this is known to maximize the cooperativity more than the additive effects and it is obviously useful to reduce the library size. Site A (Arg47, Thr49, Tyr51), and site B (Val78, Ala82) were targeted (Figure 8) first with NDC codon degeneracy at the three spots of site A with the need to screen only 430 transformants for a 95% coverage.

The two-residues at site B were randomized using NNK codon degeneracy. From this first screening, highly 2β-selective mutants (97%) were obtained from library A while 15β-selective variants, also reaching 91% regio-selectivity on testosterone, were found mainly in library B. The best variant from library B was then subjected to randomization at site A with some variants reaching 96% regio-selectivity on testosterone (R47Y/T49F/V78L/A82M/F87A) while a variant from library B only selected on testosterone (V78V/A82N/F87A) was able to reach a 100% regio-selectivity on other steroidal substrates such as progesterone. Moreover, some mutated variants displayed increased coupling of product formation with NADPH consumption. This ISM approach was also characterized by a limited amount of screening, the step that is normally considered the bottleneck of directed evolution.

A refinement of previously evolved mutants of P450 BM3 was also proposed in 2008 for production of indigo and indirubin by indole hydroxylation [93]. Starting from a variant A74G/F87V/L188Q obtained by random methods and directed evolution, and by applying saturation mutagenesis as a refinement of catalyst properties, granted two variants with increased catalytic efficiency up to six times that of the starting variant, with improved regio-selectivity for 3-hydroxyindole, leading to 93% indigo production *vs.* the initial 72%. One of the variants also showed increased coupling efficiency with NADH. The overall result nicely supports the importance of synergy of random and saturation mutagenesis approaches for optimized catalysts production.

Recently, another study has been published [94] on P450sca-2 from *Streptomyces carbophilus* to be employed in the synthesis of the cholesterol-lowering drug pravastatin. Here the saturation mutagenesis was applied to enhance electron transfer efficiency in a hybrid P450sca-2/Pdx/Pdr functional system by targeting residues at the interface between the electron transfer moiety putidaredoxin (Pdx) and the catalytic P450sca-2. Three rounds of ISM granted a variant with a 10 fold improved catalytic performance.

Figure 8. Structure of P450 BM3 heme domain (PDB: 2HPD) showing the target sites A (Arg47, Thr49, Tyr51) in green and B (Val78, Ala82) in blue. Heme is shown in red, the Fe coordinating Cys 400 is in magenta.

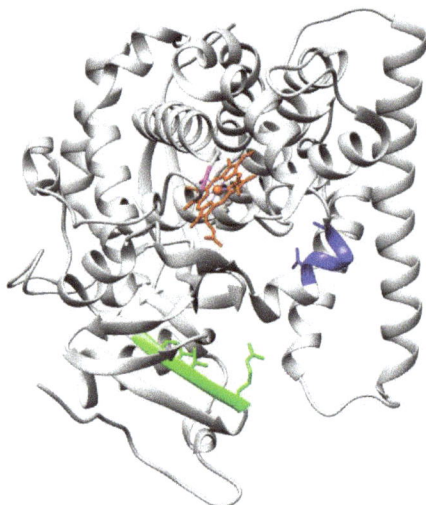

The other important enzymes belonging to the oxygenase class and successfully targeted for improvement by saturation mutagenesis [95,96] are represented by the Baeyer-Villiger monoxygenases (BVMO), able to perform specific reactions on racemic mixture of various ketones to obtain enantiopure lactones, conversion of prochiral ketones in chiral lactones and oxidation of organic sulfides. Although novel Baeyer-Villiger monoxygenases with tuned substrate specificity can be found in diverse microbial populations [97–99], there is the need to evolve BVMOs with specific performance in biosynthesis. This can be done with random or SSM laboratory techniques.

A thermostable phenylacetone monoxygenase (PAMO) belonging to the BVMO group was successfully engineered by saturation mutagenesis to perform catalysis on 2-aryl, 2-alkylcyclohexanones and a bicyclic ketone that are not recognized as substrates by the WT enzyme [96]. Given that a CAST approach previously applied to positions 441–444 belonging to a loop next to the binding pocket, were only partially successful [48], only positions 440 and 437 were targeted instead, where the first amino acid is located in the second sphere, and therefore not in direct contact with the substrate (Figure 9). Pro440 was identified to play a key role, since several mutants generated at this position granted an enhanced percentage of conversions and improved enantio-selectivity for substrates not recognized by the WT. Since in this case the library was apparently not covering the entire range of variants at position 440, the missing variants Pro440Tyr and Pro440Trp were produced by site-specific mutagenesis, with the aim of exploring the entire range of amino acid properties at this position for the enhancement of the biocatalyst performance. Further work on the same enzyme [95] targeted positions 93 and 94, located in site distal from the binding pocket chosen on the basis of the crystal structure, with a simultaneous saturation mutagenesis using a NDT codon to reduce degeneracy. A double mutant Gln93Asn/Pro94Asp was selected for its acquired activity on an otherwise inert 2-substituted cyclohexanone derivatives and it was found to be able to catalyze the conversion to the corresponding lactones with high enantio-selectivity. These results have been rationalized by a rearrangement of the H-bonds and salt-bridge networks in the protein, much alike an induced allosteric effect.

Figure 9. Scheme of the active site of PAMO (PDB: 1W4X) with targeted residues Pro440, Pro437, Gln93 and Pro94 (in black). FAD is shown in orange; Arg 337, involved in catalysis, is shown in blue.

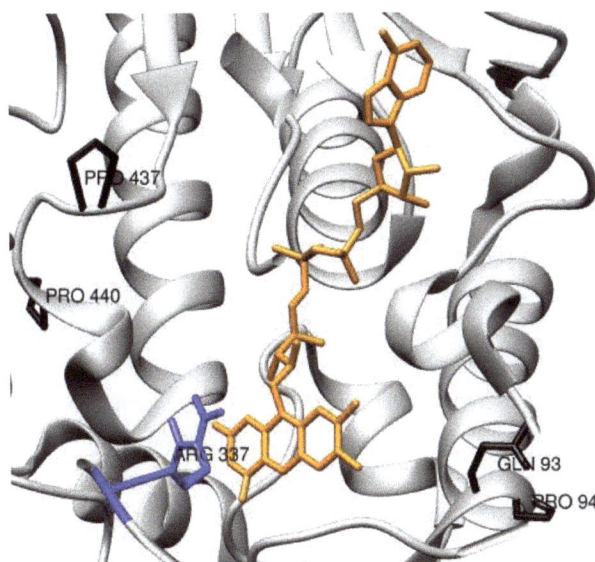

In order to enhance the performance of biocatalysts for fine chemistry, for example, for the synthesis of chiral sulfoxides and asymmetric ketone reduction, other redox enzymes such as nitrobenzene dioxygenase [77], alcohol dehydrogenase [78] and carbonyl reductase [79] were also recently optimized by saturation mutagenesis.

An interesting example of active site saturation mutagenesis recently published, targeted an unusual non-heme iron dioxygenase, belonging to the class of α-ketoglutarate dependent dioxygenase [74]. This enzyme is involved in the biosynthesis of carbapenem-3-carboxylic acid, the core building block of the all carbapenems, including Meropenem and Imipenem. This is a relatively new class of β-lactam antibiotics of great importance as therapeutic agents given the increasing bacterial resistance to an older class of antibiotics. In order to dissect and better understand the molecular determinants of the biocatalyst that promote the epimerization and desaturation crucial for the biosynthesis of the core of cabapenem, SSM was applied to six active sites and four second sphere residues of the dioxygenase, generating point as well as double mutant libraries. The importance of Tyr 67 for catalyst engineering was highlighted together with the advantage of promoting a two step reaction mechanism, including epimerization and desaturation, with release and rebound of the intermediate to ensure complete desaturation and avoid the frequent aborted cycles that are observed in the native enzyme due to a difficult rotation of the intermediate required in the catalytic pocket in the full reaction.

Other redox enzymes optimized by SSM include dehydrogenases as the previously cited alcohol dehydrogenase from *Thermoethanolicus brockii* [78] and the meso-diaminopimelate dehydrogenase from *Symbiobacterium thermophilum* [100] successfully exploited for the synthesis of D-phenylalanine, thanks to a 35-fold increase in specific activity of the variant compared to the WT.

3.2. Enzymes Relevant to Environmental and Clean Energy Approaches

The use of enzymes in environmental applications include biocatalysts able to detoxify pesticides such as atrazine, chlorinated polyaromatic hydrocarbons, DDT, toxic compounds in industrial wastes such as phenols, organic solvents, aniline, drugs, explosives and chemicals resulting from military operations, among which trinitrotoluene (TNT) and G-series organophosphorus toxins contained in nerve agents like Sarin and Cyclosarin. These are usually xenobiotics particularly recalcitrant to degradation by bacteria and fungi, given that their natural enzymes, though powerful catalysts for bioremediation [101], have not evolved under the selective pressure of such compounds, as these organisms were not massively exposed to these compounds until very recently. In this respect, protein engineering by laboratory-driven evolution is of unique importance for what it can deliver. Several important results have been achieved in this respect by random directed evolution approaches both on P450 enzymes acting on pollutants [1,4,62] and on hydrolytic enzymes, for example on paraoxonases (PON) for detoxification of organophosphorus toxins [102], but an increasing number of works have recently tackled the same problem by applying SSM methods.

SSM relevance for improvement of lipase applications as an industrial catalyst has already been discussed in Section 3.1. Lipases are also relevant for clean energy issues in the transesterification of triacylglyerol with methanol for biodiesel production [81,103]. These have many advantages over traditional base or acid catalyzed approaches, but natural lipases often lack the required stability and efficiency in the high methanol concentrations used for biodiesel synthesis, limiting their practical use. Directed evolution techniques were very recently applied to the lipase from *Proteus mirabilis* to enhance methanol tolerance and allow its industrial application as a biocatalyst. The dieselzyme variant 4, evolved by randomized methods (error prone PCR) and site-directed mutagenesis to combine beneficial mutations, shows a 30-fold increase in the half-inactivation time to temperature (50 °C) and a 50-fold longer half-inactivation time in 50% aqueous methanol [81]. Although saturation mutagenesis was not the chosen technique for this approach, the authors foresee the application of CAST and structure guided ISM for further refinement of the obtained catalyst.

Enhancement of performance of enzymes such as cellulases and ligninases, present in nature in a restricted number of organisms, is of high relevance to the production of clean and sustainable energy from renewable sources. These enzymes offer precious tools for waste and poor-value biomass recycling, acting both on recovery of resources for energy production and on management of wastes [104].

The frontier of environmental care and clean energy production is the setup of hybrid systems based on biocatalysts, often interfaced with semiconductor materials [105,106] with the ability to mimic nature in efficient solar energy harvesting and energy storage in transportable fuels of low impact to the delicate equilibrium of our planet. In this respect, photosystems, light activated proteins, CO_2 fixing enzymes and biocatalysts able to produce fuels such as biohydrogen, bioethanol and biodiesel, are the ideal target of engineering approaches. Many clean-energy production related enzymes (in particular photosystems and hydrogenases) are generally difficult to purify, manipulate and engineer, and therefore the laboratory evolution approaches are still at their first steps of development, but it is foreseen that increasing interest will be devoted to engineering, particularly with SSM methods applied to hydrogenases, nitrogenases, formate-dehydrogenase.

Here a choice of examples, grouped as in Section 3.1 by enzyme classes or subclasses, focus on the three aspects: detoxification, biomass degradation and clean energy production.

3.2.1. Oxygenases and Other Oxidoreductases for Bioremediation

Oxygenases and more in general redox enzymes represent a class of biocatalysts spanning from P450s to non-heme iron mono- and di-oxygenases and flavoenzymes widely used for the oxidation of toxic compounds. The addition of one or two hydroxyls to a poorly reactive C-H bond, for example in aromatic and aliphatic hydrocarbons, is usually crucial for the initiation of the detoxification and clearance process. The increasing amount of pollutants with halogenated substitutions in aromatic rings, for example in pesticides, and the presence of compounds recalcitrant to biodegradation, poses difficult challenges to protein engineers. SSM techniques are often the selected method to test and modify redox enzymes to recognize a broader substrate range and to attack xenobiotics with a sustainable approach, recovering carbon sources for safe microorganism growth. The catabolic pathways that enable many microorganisms to degrade large classes of aromatic pollutants, often relay on non-heme iron dioxygenases and monoxygenases. These include di-iron oxo-bridged monoxygenases such as methane-monoxygenase, phenol hydroxylase, toluene 4-monoxygenase and toluene-o-xylene monoxygenase. The last two enzymes have been target of early applications of SSM [107,108], as well as refinement of previous successful directed evolution approaches [109]. Further work, more focused on developing enzyme catalysts for bioremediation, has been developed on dioxygenases containing a single iron atom such as ring-cleaving dioxygenases acting on polychlorinated biphenyls [110], aniline [111,112], dinitrotoluene [113] and chlorinated catechols [114]. The engineering of the extradiol dioxygenase (DoxG) that displays a low activity in 3,4-dihydroxybiphenyls ring cleavage was achieved by a combination of error-prone PCR, SSM at hot spots and DNA shuffling applied in sequence. Four residues located within 14 Å of the enzyme active site iron, highlighted by error prone PCR to be relevant for enzyme activity on the screening substrate, were targeted by saturation mutagenesis applied in pairs, grouping Ile-154 and Leu242, Leu-190 and Ser-191. The two resulting libraries were screened with coverage of 99.9% of the possible diversity resulting in variants with 2–10-fold increases in 3,4-dihydroxybiphenyl cleavage rates. After DNA shuffling, a further improvement generated a variant with a k_{cat}/K_M towards 3,4-dihydroxybiphenyl increased by 770 fold when compared to WT, confirming the feasibility and advantage of a coupled random and saturation mutagenesis approach in biocatalysts activity enhancement. SSM was also applied to an aniline dioxygenase isolated from *Acinetobacter* sp. strain YAA [112]. Substrate-binding pocket residues were selected and the V205A mutation that is possibly responsible for enlarging the binding pocket, was highlighted to lead the oxidation of 2-isopropylaniline, a substrate not recognized by the WT enzyme. The same mutants also shift the substrate specificity from 2,4-dimethylaniline, a good substrate for WT, to 2-isopropylaniline. Another variant, I248L, improved activity towards aniline and

2,4-dimethylaniline by approximately 2 fold. Both residues I248 and V205 were not previously reported to influence substrate recognition, therefore the finding also granted basic information on the enzyme active site determinants for substrate specificity. A further refinement by random mutagenesis on mutant V205A generated variant 3-R21, with improvement in activity towards the carcinogenic 2,4-dimethylaniline of 3.5 fold and retaining WT activity levels towards the natural substrate aniline. Therefore it can be concluded that the laboratory evolution of this biocatalyst generated a powerful tool to detoxify highly hazardous compounds. Another pollutant that has received attention in view of bioremediation strategies is 2,4,6-Trinitrotoluene (TNT), the most common explosive found in past and present war sites, and the intermediates of its synthesis 2,6-dinitrotoluene (2,6-DNT) and 2,4-dinitrotoluene (2,4-DNT) found as soil and water contaminants at TNT production facilities. 2,4-DNT dioxygenase of *Burkholderia* sp. strain DNT can catalyze the oxidation of 2,4-DNT to form 4-methyl-5-nitrocatechol and nitrite, but it has poor activity on other DNTs and nitrotoluens. By applying saturation mutagenesis at position I204 of the catalytic subunit and selecting for nitro-catechol producing mutants (signature of activity on the screened substrate), variants I204L and I204Y were identified [113]. These showed unprecedented activity on 2,3-DNT and 2,5-DNT and 2 to 8 fold improved activity towards 2,4-DNT, 2,6-DNT, 2NT and 4NT. The activity reported on 2,5-DNT, never observed for an enzyme, confirms that new biocatalysts unexplored by natural evolution can be generated by laboratory-driven evolution.

A gain of function on unnatural substrates and an inversion of specificity were also achieved by site directed and site-saturation mutagenesis on a catechol 1,2 dioxygenase from *Acinetobacter radioresistens* S13 [114]. Catechols are the converging metabolites of several aromatic degrading pathways, although natural enzymes usually cannot efficiently oxidize highly chlorinated or variously substituted catechols originated from chloroaromatic, biphenil and nitroaromatic compounds. The advantage of catechol dioxygenases is that these enzymes do not require any supply of reducing equivalent to perform the dihydroxylation and ring-cleavage of substrates, and therefore have a simpler architecture, higher stability and no need for expensive cofactors such as NAD(P)H to perform catalysis. Encapsulated and immobilized forms are also available [115], making them ideal biocatalysts. Mutagenesis on the active site was performed on residues L69 and A72 with a combined site-specific and SSM approach. This led to a series of variants with improved activity on the rarely recognized substrate 4,5-dichlorocatechol (by 2 fold in variant A72S), inversion of specificity for 4-chlorocatechol instead of catechol (variants L69A and L69A-A72G) and gain-of-function for recognition and catalysis on 4-*tert*-butyl catechol, a contaminant of cosmetics and foodstuff banned by EU since it can give sensitizations in patch testing at low concentrations (1%). The effect of active site re-shaping of the chosen mutational sites is shown in Figure 10, together with an example of the SSM obtained variants. An influence on the oxygen binding properties of mutants *vs.* WT was recently highlighted [116] and further work is ongoing in our labs for SSM at other catalytic pocket sites and for production of multiple site variants.

Figure 10. (a) Structure of active site of catechol 1,2 dioxygenase highlighting the residue that define the active site pocket (PDB file from crystallographic structure in [117]); (b) The effect of reshaping by mutagenesis and SSM on model of substrate/pocket interaction; (c) The list of identified and characterized mutants for SSM on position 72 are reported in the table (related to studies published in [114]).

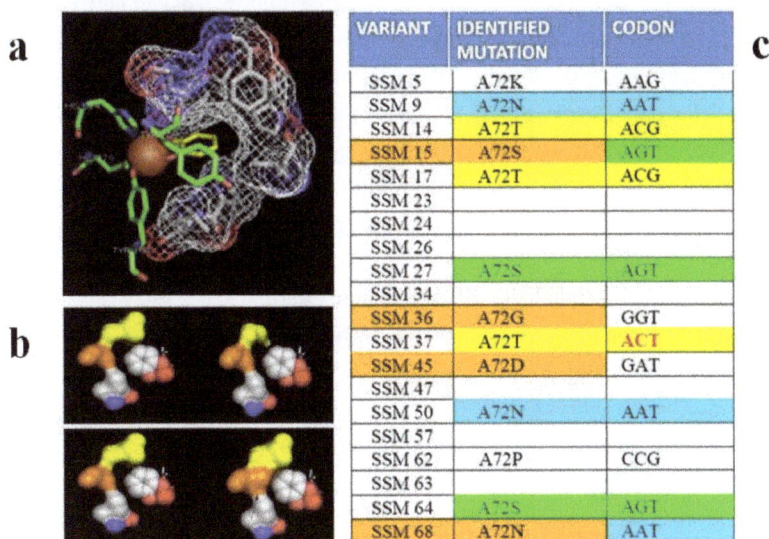

VARIANT	IDENTIFIED MUTATION	CODON
SSM 5	A72K	AAG
SSM 9	A72N	AAT
SSM 14	A72T	ACG
SSM 15	A72S	AGT
SSM 17	A72T	ACG
SSM 23		
SSM 24		
SSM 26		
SSM 27	A72S	AGT
SSM 34		
SSM 36	A72G	GGT
SSM 37	A72T	ACT
SSM 45	A72D	GAT
SSM 47		
SSM 50	A72N	AAT
SSM 57		
SSM 62	A72P	CCG
SSM 63		
SSM 64	A72S	AGT
SSM 68	A72N	AAT

Cytochrome P450 enzymes were also targeted by directed evolution for enhancing the degradation of recalcitrant aromatic and aliphatic pollutants. A recent work by Arnold and co-workers [118] compares combinatorial SSM strategies to the results obtained by random directed evolution. Although in this case it seems that the notable achievements obtained by error prone PCR and several round of random mutagenesis cannot be fully matched by SSM, the paper reports an improved activity on propane and ethane hydroxylation. In this case, nonetheless, a simpler approach by two rounds of error-prone PCR and back-crossing with parental DNA devised in our group on the same P450 BM3, led to variants that are active on highly recalcitrant polyaromatic hydrocarbon (PAH) pollutants, more relevant for environmental concerns, such as chrysene and pyrene [62].

A detoxification activity specifically improved by SSM on lactaldehyde oxidoreductase [72] is of relevance for detoxification of furfural, a toxic compound that originates from pre-treatment of cellulosic material. In this perspective the optimized catalyst obtained by SSM, a L7F mutant with a 10-fold higher activity than WT, is crucial both for lowering a toxic compound in an environment and for direct application in cell factory systems to enable cells to improve growth on treated lignocellulosic material. In the cited paper the variant obtained by SSM was also tested for performance in *E. coli* cells and showed a 2-fold higher rate of furfural metabolism during fermentation.

3.2.2. Cellulases, Haloalkane Dehalogenase and Other Hydrolases for Waste Degradation

Hydrolytic enzymes such as cellulases, endoglucanases, xylosidases and β-glycosidases, are increasingly being applied in lignocellulosic waste pre-treatment in combination or in alternative to steam-explosion and chemical treatments for enhanced saccharification of the biomass and lowered environmental impact. The SSM approach to enhance applicability of this class of biocatalysts has been focusing on improvement of thermal stability by the same research group both for an endoglucanase [84] and more recently on a β-glycosidase [85]. In the first case the endoglucanase CelA from *Clostridium thermocellum* was chosen for SSM at protein surface position Ser329. All the variants with improved thermal stability (approximately 5-fold increase in half-life of inactivation) and maintaining hydrolytic activity at WT levels, showed the presence of the S329G mutation. This finding suggested a systematic analysis of other possible substitutions to Gly of surface Ser residues, in line with reported works that Ser to Gly mutations on protein surface may improve thermostability. Thr and His surface residues were also selected on the basis that His and Thr, along with Ser, are generally substituted by Gly on the surface of proteins with enhanced thermal stability compared to their thermo-sensitive homologous. Few residues were also tested for substitution to Pro. A final variant S329G/S269P/H194G, generated by a combination of SSM and site-directed mutagenesis resulted in a 10-fold increase in half-life of inactivation at 86 °C.

A more recent paper from the same group [85] reports a consensus-based semi rational approach that benefits from the results of the previous work to enhance thermal stability of a β-glycosidase BglY from *Thermus thermophilus*.

An SSM approach applied to β-D-Xylosidase/α-L-arabinofuranosidase from *Selenomonas ruminantium* to residue W145 was instead focused on modulating the inhibitory effect of glucose and xylose on this enzyme for application to the saccharification of lignocellulosic waste biomass for biofuels production and as microbial substrate for other biotechnological processes [119]. While the β-D-Xylosidase/α-L-arabinofuranosidase can promote the hydrolytic cleavage of 1,4-β-D-xylooligosaccharides to D-xylose, the high affinity for the product D-xylose as well as for D-glucose hinders its excellent performance as a catalyst. Three variants isolated by screening the SSM library, W145F, W145L, and W145Y, showed decreased inhibition by the monosaccharides and increased catalytic activities up to 70% greater than that of the WT enzyme.

Another hydrolase applied to a different perspective of waste recycling is represented by a haloalkane dehalogenase DhaA from *Rhodococcus rhodochrous*. This enzyme is able to convert 1,2,3-trichloropropane (TCP) into (*R*)- or (*S*)-2,3-dichloropropan-1-ol, which can be converted into optically active epichlorohydrins, industrially important building blocks for the synthesis of fine chemicals. Enatioselectivity of the WT DhaA was further improved [120] by a pair-wise SSM approach applied to 16 active-site residues not directly involved in the catalytic reaction. A further refinement was then applied to the best R- and S-enantioselective variants by site directed mutagenesis including residues that are not part of the active site. A multi-site mutagenesis protocol with restricted codon usage allowed to finalize two variants, r5-90R and r5-97S with 13 and 17 mutations, that generate (*R*)-epichlorohydrin with 90% ee and (*S*)-epichlorohydrin with 97% ee, respectively.

3.2.3. Hydrogenases and Other Enzymes Relevant to Clean Energy Production

The energy issue has driven a great interest towards hydrogenases as powerful and efficient catalysts for hydrogen production in cell factory systems and in biohybrid fuel cells or solar harvesting devices as catalysts instead of platinum or other expensive rare-metal based materials [105]. Among the three classes of reported hydrogenases, [FeFe] hydrogenases are in this respect the most efficient catalysts due to their high turnover numbers, reaching turnover frequencies up to 10^4 s^{-1} [121] with a bias toward hydrogen production, but with relatively low overpotential needed as a driving force for catalysis in either direction. Interestingly, perspectives are also discussed in literature on [NiFe] hydrogenases for application in molecular hydrogen conversion for biofuel cells and in $NAD(P)^+$ cofactor regeneration.

Some limiting features, such as oxygen sensitivity, and the interest to further investigate the complex mechanism of the catalytic center, are increasingly pointing towards the application of saturation mutagenesis techniques to refine hydrogenases for desired applications. Although until now not many papers have been published on this topic [55,122] and in general on mutagenesis and laboratory evolution of all classes of hydrogenases [66,123–128], a very recent review from a leading group in the field of [FeFe] hydrogenase foresees imminent development in this direction [129]. In our group we applied saturation mutagenesis to a key residue in the active site of [FeFe] hydrogenase from *C. acetobutylicum* (CaHydA) recombinantly expressed in *E. coli*. This residue, namely cysteine 298, is involved in proton delivery to the active site; therefore it is crucial for substrate supply and product release, since the protons are converted reversibly to molecular hydrogen. In this case, accounting for proton pathways and local delivery engineering, means not only a matter of pH stability and fine regulation, but also of controlling the substrate concentration. We are also pursuing the same SSM strategy on other active site positions. The results of the focused approach on the conserved residue Cys 298, the final amino acid of a proton transfer chain to the active H-cluster [124] and believed to relay proton to the dithiolate bridging group that funnel them to the distal Fe, are reported in a recent publication [55]. Upon saturation mutagenesis with the NNK codon, a colorimetric screening performed on colonies allowed to reach 99.8% coverage of the library. Clones containing an active enzyme (with a detection threshold of 14% of original WT activity) were identified resulting in selection of only WT revertants or Cys-to-Asp mutants. The C298D variant shows a retained activity of 50%, which is interesting since the Cys residue is fully conserved in evolution, and therefore novel mutational spaces were explored, attesting that Asp can functionally replace Cys in proton relay and is structurally compatible (Figure 11).

Figure 11. Model of CaHydA structure illustrating C298 (**left**) and replacement at 298 position with aspartic acid (**right**) (adapted from Morra *et al.* [55]).

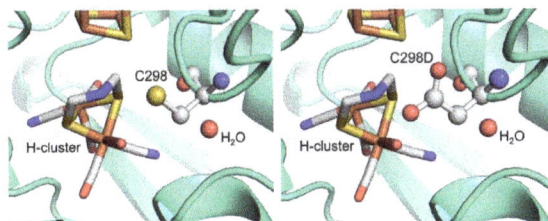

The frequency of WT revertants and Asp mutants matched the expected value on the basis of encoding codon frequency. To confirm the library completeness, selected clones were sequenced, showing a good and balanced codon randomization [55].

The SSM approach reported on [NiFe]-hydrogenase [122], performed in combination with directed evolution techniques such as error-prone PCR and shuffling is, as a matter of fact, the first random protein engineering of a hydrogenase. This work targeted the large subunit (HycE) of *Escherichia coli* hydrogenase 3. Hydrogenase 3 is responsible for synthesizing hydrogen from $2H^+$ and $2e^-$ within the supramolecular complex of formate hydrogen lyase (FHL), that also contains a formate dehydrogenase-H for forming $2H^+$, $2e^-$, and CO_2 from HCOOH: the overall FHL catalyses therefore hydrogen production from formate. A C-terminal truncated variant of HycE, generated by this combined random and SSM approach, showed increased hydrogen production by 30-fold.

Formate processing enzymes other than the cited subunit of *E. coli* hydrogenase are also relevant for the energy and sustainable process issues in their reversible activity of CO_2 conversion. The possibility of CO_2 sequestering and conversion of formate to methanol and methane is an intriguing perspective for research and applications [130]. Also the formate/CO_2 conversion is coupled to reduction of NAD^+ to NADH. Formate dehydrogenase from the yeast *Candida boidinii* catalyses the reaction with a selectivity for NAD^+ only, while $NADP^+$ is not recognized as a productive cofactor for the redox reaction and only gives minimal activity. SSM applied to two specific residues, Asp195 and Tyr196, of the dinucleotide-binding region, allowed an improvement in catalytic efficiency with $NADP^+$ of the order of 10^7 [131]. The selected variant Asp195Gln/Tyr196His is relevant for cofactor recycling systems with specificity for NADPH, preferred in enzymes such as cytochrome P450 monooxygenases that are largely applied in industry. The recovery of reduced cofactor is basically the natural strategy for storing solar energy in photosynthetic and chemical energy in chemosynthetic organisms, and therefore the control of biocatalysts performance in this reaction is a step forward in the direction of exploiting and mimicking nature in a sustainable manner.

4. Conclusions

The huge number of successful applications of SSM methods to enzymes reported in the last years underlines the feasibility of a semi-random approach to enzyme engineering. The results in activity, specificity and stability enhancement obtained are in several respects more cost-effective and less time-consuming than their counterparts, purely based on random approach and directed evolution. A factor of about ten, comparing enhancement of 20–50 fold by directed evolution and up to 700 for SSM, put SSM far ahead of fully randomized methods achievement-wise. In addition, the number of screened variants required for sound library coverage is generally 2–3 orders of magnitude smaller, allowing for application of more specific screening methods, able to precisely select the desired feature. Generating small and smart libraries is certainly a common and important goal also for the random directed evolution approach. The positive and negative results of both strategies in this direction can give important inputs and shared benefits. The drawback of SSM, *i.e.*, the required knowledge of structural data, is becoming less relevant given the increasingly available 3D models that can be calculated by homology with existing structural data and/or *ab-initio* modeling methods. These indirect structural data might not provide details of mechanisms and functions, but they are very indicative for intelligent planning of experimental approaches in SSM. Therefore, at least for technical enzymes, the SSM methods can be foreseen playing a major role in enzyme evolution. In combination with site-directed and random approaches, the methods have the potential to make a difference in exploring novel landscapes for biocatalysts most ambitious refinement, enhancement and application. The challenges remain in the development of biocatalysts performing entirely novel activities. In this respect, the importance of information in the details of mechanism of natural and successfully engineered enzymes is crucial. The role played by rational site-directed mutagenesis in elucidating mechanism and substrate specificity has been of paramount importance. A very recent review focused on an important class of enzymes foresees a similarly important role for SSM [132].

The next generation of engineered biocatalysts can certainly reach unprecedented performances [133] and this can be achieved due to the choices available to scientists to select among different strategies, whose advantages and limitations have to be carefully balanced. The versatility of SSM and the various modifications of this general approach, together with the chance to combine with other strategies, equip protein engineers with an already powerful toolbox. How to apply the tools is not simple to rationalize or give rules for, but this is certainly the undefined area that must remain open, in which scientists can propose original experimental design and improved methods.

Conflicts of Interest

The authors declare no conflict of interest.

References

1. Peters, M.W.; Meinhold, P.; Glieder, A.; Arnold, F.H. Regio- and enantioselective alkane hydroxylation with engineered cytochromes P450 BM-3. *J. Am. Chem. Soc.* **2003**, *125*, 13442–13450.
2. Bocola, M.; Otte, N.; Jaeger, K.E.; Reetz, M.T.; Thiel, W. Learning from directed evolution: Theoretical investigations into cooperative mutations in lipase enantioselectivity. *Chembiochem* **2004**, *5*, 214–223.
3. Bartsch, S.; Kourist, R.; Bornscheuer, U.T. Complete inversion of enantioselectivity towards acetylated tertiary alcohols by a double mutant of a *Bacillus subtilis* esterase. *Angew. Chem. Int. Ed.* **2008**, *47*, 1508–1511.
4. Glieder, A.; Farinas, E.T.; Arnold, F.H. Laboratory evolution of a soluble, self-sufficient, highly active alkane hydroxylase. *Nat. Biotechnol.* **2002**, *20*, 1135–1139.
5. Schmidt, D.M.Z.; Mundorff, E.C.; Dojka, M.; Bermudez, E.; Ness, J.E.; Govindarajan, S.; Babbitt, P.C.; Minshull, J.; Gerlt, J.A. Evolutionary potential of (β/α)(8)-barrels: Functional promiscuity produced by single substitutions in the enolase superfamily. *Biochemistry* **2003**, *42*, 8387–8393.
6. Bosma, T.; Danborsky, J.; Stucki, G.; Janssen, D.B. Biodegradation of 1,2,3-trichloropropane through directed evolution and heterologous expression of a haloalkane dehalogenase gene. *Appl. Environ. Microbiol.* **2002**, *68*, 3582–3587.
7. Reetz, M.T.; Soni, P.; Acevedo, J.P.; Sanchis, J. Creation of an amino acid network of structurally coupled residues in the directed evolution of a thermostable enzyme. *Angew. Chem. Int. Ed. Engl.* **2009**, *48*, 8268–8272.

8. Zumarraga, M.; Bulter, T.; Shleev, S.; Polaina, J.; Martinez-Arias, A.; Plou, F.J.; Ballesteros, A.; Alcalde, M. *In vitro* evolution of a fungal laccase in high concentrations of organic cosolvents. *Chem. Biol.* **2007**, *14*, 1052–1064.

9. Siegel, J.B.; Zanghellini, A.; Lovick, H.M.; Kiss, G.; Lambert, A.R.; St. Clair, J.L.; Gallaher, J.L.; Hilvert, D.; Gelb, M.H.; Stoddard, B.L.; *et al.* Computational design of an enzyme catalyst for a stereoselective bimolecular Diels-Alder reaction. *Science* **2010**, *329*, 309–313.

10. Khersonsky, O.; Kiss, G.; Röthlisberger, D.; Dym, O.; Albeck, S.; Houk, K.N.; Baker, D.; Tawfik, D.S. Bridging the gaps in design methodologies by evolutionary optimization of the stability and proficiency of designed Kemp eliminase KE59. *Proc. Natl. Acad. Sci. USA* **2012**, *109*, 10358–10363.

11. Merski, M.; Shoichet, B.K. Engineering a model protein cavity to catalyze the Kemp elimination. *Proc. Natl. Acad. Sci. USA* **2012**, *109*, 16179–16183.

12. Savile, C.K.; Janey, J.M.; Mundorff, E.C.; Moore, J.C.; Tam, S.; Jarvis, W.R.; Colbeck, J.C.; Krebber, A.; Fleitz, F.J.; Brands, J.; *et al.* Biocatalytic asymmetric synthesis of chiral amines from ketones applied to sitagliptin manufacture. *Science* **2010**, *329*, 305–309.

13. Janssen, D.B. Evolving haloalkane dehalogenases. *Curr. Opin. Chem. Biol.* **2004**, *8*, 150–159.

14. Pavlova, M.; Klvana, M.; Prokop, Z.; Chaloupkova, R.; Banas, P.; Otyepka, M.; Wade, R.C.; Tsuda, M.; Nagata, Y.; Damborsky, J. Redesigning dehalogenase access tunnels as a strategy for degrading an anthropogenic substrate. *Nat. Chem. Biol.* **2009**, *5*, 727–733.

15. Fasan, R.; Meharenna, Y.T.; Snow, C.D.; Poulos, T.L.; Arnold, F.H. Evolutionary history of a specialized p450 propane monooxygenase. *J. Mol. Biol.* **2008**, *383*, 1069–1080.

16. Stemmer, W.P. Rapid evolution of a protein *in vitro* by DNA shuffling. *Nature* **1994**, *370*, 389–391.

17. Ostermeier, M.; Shim, J.H.; Benkovic, S.J. A combinatorial approach to hybrid enzymes independent of DNA homology. *Nat. Biotechnol.* **1999**, *17*, 1205–1209.

18. Pelletier, J.N. A RACHITT for our toolbox. *Nat. Biotechnol.* **2001**, *19*, 314–315.

19. Sieber, V.; Martinez, C.A.; Arnold, F.H. Libraries of hybrid proteins from distantly related sequences. *Nat. Biotechnol.* **2001**, *19*, 456–460.

20. Wang, M.; Si, T.; Zhao, H. Biocatalyst development by directed evolution. *Bioresour. Technol.* **2012**, *115*, 117–125.

21. Bornscheuer, U.T.; Huisman, G.W.; Kazlauskas, R.J.; Lutz, S.; Moore, J.C.; Robins, K. Engineering the third wave of biocatalysis. *Nature* **2012**, *485*, 185–194.

22. Yuan, L.; Kurek, I.; English, J.; Keenan, R. Laboratory-directed protein evolution. *Microbiol. Mol. Biol. Rev.* **2005**, *69*, 373–392.

23. Bloom, J.D.; Meyer, M.M.; Meinhold, P.; Otey, C.R.; MacMillan, D.; Arnold, F.H. Evolving strategies for enzyme engineering. *Curr. Opin. Struct. Biol.* **2005**, *15*, 447–452.

24. Valetti, F.; Gilardi G. Directed evolution of enzymes for product chemistry. *Nat. Prod. Rep.* **2004**, *21*, 490–511.

25. Farinas, E.T.; Bulter, T.; Arnold, F.H. Directed enzyme evolution. *Curr. Opin. Biotechnol.* **2001**, *12*, 545–551.

26. Romero, P.A.; Arnold, F.H. Exploring protein fitness landscapes by directed evolution. *Nat. Rev. Mol. Cell. Biol.* **2009**, *10*, 866–876.

27. Turner, N.J. Directed evolution drives the next generation of biocatalysts. *Nat. Chem. Biol.* **2009**, *5*, 567–573.

28. Guo, F.; Xu, H.; Xu, H.; Yu, H. Compensation of the enantioselectivity-activity trade-off in the directed evolution of an esterase from *Rhodobacter sphaeroides* by site-directed saturation mutagenesis. *Appl. Microbiol. Biotechnol.* **2013**, *97*, 3355–3362.

29. Reetz, M.T.; Bocola, M.; Carballeira, J.D.; Zha, D.; Vogel, A. Expanding the range of substrate acceptance of enzymes: Combinatorial active-site saturation test. *Angew. Chem. Int. Ed. Engl.* **2005**, *44*, 4192–4196.

30. Reetz, M.T.; Carballeira, J.D. Iterative saturation mutagenesis (ISM) for rapid directed evolution of functional enzymes. *Nat. Protoc.* **2007**, *2*, 891–903.

31. Loke, P.; Sim, T.S. A comparison of three site-directed mutagenesis kits. *Z. Naturforsch. C* **2001**, *56*, 810–813.

32. Reetz, M.T.; Prasad, S.; Carballeira, J.D.; Gumulya, Y.; Bocola, M. Iterative saturation mutagenesis accelerates laboratory evolution of enzyme stereoselectivity: Rigorous comparison with traditional methods. *J. Am. Chem. Soc.* **2010**, *132*, 9144–9152.

33. Gumulya, Y.; Sanchis, J.; Reetz, M.T. Many pathways in laboratory evolution can lead to improved enzymes: How to escape from local minima. *Chembiochem* **2012**, *13*, 1060–1066.

34. Prasad, S.; Bocola, M.; Reetz, M.T. Revisiting the lipase from *Pseudomonas aeruginosa*: Directed evolution of substrate acceptance and enantioselectivity using iterative saturation mutagenesis. *Chemphyschem* **2011**, *12*, 1550–1557.

35. http://www.reportlinker.com/p0747897-summary/World-Enzymes-Industry.html

36. Engström, K.; Nyhlén, J.; Sandström, A.G.; Bäckvall, J.E. Directed evolution of an enantioselective lipase with broad substrate scope for hydrolysis of alpha-substituted esters. *J. Am. Chem. Soc.* **2010**, *132*, 7038–7042.

37. Wen, S.; Tan, T.; Zhao, H. Improving the thermostability of lipase Lip2 from *Yarrowia lipolytica*. *J. Biotechnol.* **2012**, *164*, 248–253.

38. Gumulya, Y.; Reetz, M.T. Enhancing the thermal robustness of an enzyme by directed evolution: Least favorable starting points and inferior mutants can map superior evolutionary pathways. *Chembiochem* **2011**, *12*, 2502–2510.

39. Reetz, M.T.; Soni, P.; Fernández, L.; Gumulya, Y.; Carballeira, J.D. Increasing the stability of an enzyme toward hostile organic solvents by directed evolution based on iterative saturation mutagenesis using the B-FIT method. *Chem. Commun. (Camb.)* **2010**, *46*, 8657–8658.

40. Reetz, M.T.; Soni, P.; Fernández, L. Knowledge-guided laboratory evolution of protein thermolability. *Biotechnol. Bioeng.* **2009**, *102*, 1712–1717.

41. Wang, C.; Huang, R.; He, B.; Du, Q. Improving the thermostability of alpha-amylase by combinatorial coevolving-site saturation mutagenesis. *BMC Bioinformatics* **2012**, *13*, e263.

42. Gouveia-Oliveira, R.; Pedersen, A.G. Finding coevolving amino acid residues using row and column weighting of mutual information and multi-dimensional amino acid representation. *Algorithms Mol. Biol.* **2007**, *2*, 12.

43. Derbyshire, K.M.; Salvo, J.J.; Grindley, N.D. A simple and efficient procedure for saturation mutagenesis using mixed oligodeoxynucleotides. *Gene* **1986**, *46*, 145–152.

44. Firnberg, E.; Ostermeier, M. PFunkel: Efficient, expansive, user-defined mutagenesis. *PLoS One* **2012**, *7*, e52031.

45. Dennig, A.; Shivange, A.V.; Marienhagen, J.; Schwaneberg, U. OmniChange: The sequence independent method for simultaneous site-saturation of five codons. *PLoS One* **2011**, *6*, e26222.

46. Walter, K.U.; Vamvaca, K.; Hilvert, D. An active enzyme constructed from a 9-amino acid alphabet. *J. Biol. Chem.* **2005**, *280*, 37742–37746.

47. Reetz, M.T.; Kahakeaw, D.; Sanchis, J. Shedding light on the efficacy of laboratory evolution based on iterative saturation mutagenesis. *Mol. Biosyst.* **2009**, *5*, 115–122.

48. Reetz, M.T.; Kahakeaw, D.; Lohmer, R. Addressing the numbers problem in directed evolution. *Chembiochem* **2008**, *9*, 1797–1804.

49. Reetz, M.T.; Wu, S. Greatly reduced amino acid alphabets in directed evolution: Making the right choice for saturation mutagenesis at homologous enzyme positions. *Chem. Commun. (Camb.)* **2008**, 5499–5501, doi:10.1039/B813388C.

50. Kille, S.; Acevedo-Rocha, C.G.; Parra, L.P.; Zhang, Z.G.; Opperman, D.J.; Reetz, M.T.; Acevedo, J.P. Reducing codon redundancy and screening effort of combinatorial protein libraries created by saturation mutagenesis. *ACS Synth. Biol.* **2013**, *2*, 83–92.

51. Bosley, A.D.; Ostermeier, M. Mathematical expressions useful in the construction, description and evaluation of protein libraries. *Biomol. Eng.* **2005**, *22*, 57–61.

52. Mena, M.A.; Daugherty, P.S. Automated design of degenerate codon libraries. *Protein Eng. Des. Sel.* **2005**, *18*, 559–561.

53. Firth, A.E.; Patrick, W.M. Statistics of protein library construction. *Bioinformatics* **2005**, *21*, 3314–3315.

54. Patrick, W.M.; Firth, A.E.; Blackburn, J.M. User-friendly algorithms for estimating completeness and diversity in randomized protein-encoding libraries. *Protein Eng.* **2003**, *16*, 451–457.

55. Morra, S.; Giraudo, A.; di Nardo, G.; King, P.W.; Gilardi, G.; Valetti, F. Site saturation mutagenesis demonstrates a central role for cysteine 298 as proton donor to the catalytic site in CaHydA [FeFe]-hydrogenase. *PLoS One* **2012**, *7*, e48400.

56. Koga, Y.; Kato, K.; Nakano, H.; Yamane, T. Inverting enantioselectivity of *Burkholderia cepacia* KWI-56 lipase by combinatorial mutation and high-throughput screening using single-molecule PCR and *in vitro* expression. *J. Mol. Biol.* **2003**, *331*, 585–592.

57. Levin, A.M.; Weiss, G.A. Optimizing the affinity and specificity of proteins with molecular display. *Mol. Biosyst.* **2006**, *2*, 49–57.

58. Granieri, L.; Baret, J.C.; Griffiths, A.D.; Merten, C.A. High-throughput screening of enzymes by retroviral display using droplet-based microfluidics. *Chem. Biol.* **2010**, *17*, 229–235.

59. Tsotsou, G.E.; Cass, A.E.G.; Gilardi, G. High throughput assay for cytochrome P450 BM3 for screening libraries of substrates and combinatorial mutants. *Biosens. Bioelectron.* **2002**, *17*, 119–131.

60. Despotovic, D.; Vojcic, L.; Prodanovic, R.; Martinez, R.; Maurer, K.H.; Schwaneberg, U. Fluorescent assay for directed evolution of perhydrolases. *J. Biomol. Screen.* **2012**, *17*, 796–805.

61. Sass, S.; Kadow, M.; Geitner, K.; Thompson, M.L.; Talmann, L.; Bottcher, D.; Schmidt, M.; Bornscheuer, U.T. A high-throughput assay method to quantify Baeyer-Villiger monooxygenase activity. *Tetrahedron* **2012**, *68*, 7575–7580.

62. Sideri, A.; Goyal, A.; di Nardo, G.; Tsotsou, G.E.; Gilardi, G. Hydroxylation of non-substituted polycyclic aromatic hydrocarbons by cytochrome P450 BM3 engineered by directed evolution. *J. Inorg. Biochem.* **2013**, *120*, 1–7.

63. Tsotsou, G.E.; Sideri, A.; Goyal, A.; di Nardo, G.; Gilardi, G. Identification of mutant Asp251Gly/Gln307His of cytochrome P450 BM3 for the generation of metabolites of diclofenac, ibuprofen and tolbutamide. *Chemistry* **2012**, *18*, 3582–3588.

64. Di Nardo, G.; Gilardi, G. Optimization of the Bacterial Cytochrome P450 BM3 System for the production of human drug metabolites. *Int. J. Mol. Sci.* **2012**, *13*, 15901–15924.

65. Tsotsou, G.E.; di Nardo, G.; Sadeghi, S.J.; Fruttero, R.; Lazzarato, L.; Bertinaria, M.; Gilardi, G. A rapid screening for cytochrome P450 catalysis on new chemical entities: Cytochrome P450 BM3 and 1,2,5-oxadiazole derivatives. *J. Biomol. Screen.* **2013**, *18*, 211–218.

66. Stapleton, J.A.; Swartz, J.R. A cell-free microtiter plate screen for improved [FeFe] hydrogenases. *PLoS One* **2010**, *5*, e10554.

67. Chuah, J.A.; Tomizawa, S.; Yamada, M.; Tsuge, T.; Doi, Y.; Sudesh, K.; Numata, K. Characterization of site-specific mutations in a short-chain-length/medium-chain-length polyhydroxyalkanoate synthase: *In vivo* and *in vitro* studies of enzymatic activity and substrate specificity. *Appl. Environ. Microbiol.* **2013**, *79*, 3813–3821.

68. Jakoblinnert, A.; van den Wittenboer, A.; Shivange, A.V.; Bocola, M.; Heffele, L.; Ansorge-Schumacher, M.; Schwaneberg, U. Design of an activity and stability improved carbonyl reductase from *Candida parapsilosis*. *J. Biotechnol.* **2013**, *165*, 52–62.

69. Vojcic, L.; Despotovic, D.; Maurer, K.H.; Zacharias, M.; Bocola, M.; Martinez, R.; Schwaneberg, U. Reengineering of subtilisin Carlsberg for oxidative resistance. *Biol. Chem.* **2013**, *394*, 79–87.

70. Wu, Q.; Soni, P.; Reetz, M.T. Laboratory evolution of enantiocomplementary *Candida antarctica* lipase B mutants with broad substrate scope. *J. Am. Chem. Soc.* **2013**, *135*, 1872–1881.

71. Nallaseth, F.S.; Anderson, S. A screen for over-secretion of proteins by yeast based on a dual component cellular phosphatase and immuno-chromogenic stain for exported bacterial alkaline phosphatase reporter. *Microb. Cell Fact.* **2013**, *12*, e36.

72. Zheng, H.; Wang, X.; Yomano, L.P.; Geddes, R.D.; Shanmugam, K.T.; Ingram, L.O. Improving *Escherichia coli* FucO for furfural tolerance by saturation mutagenesis of individual amino acid positions. *Appl. Environ. Microbiol.* **2013**, *79*, 3202–3208.

73. Zhou, H.; Qu, Y.; Kong, C.; Shen, E.; Wang, J.; Zhang, X.; Ma, Q.; Zhou, J. The key role of a non-active-site residue Met148 on the catalytic efficiency of meta-cleavage product hydrolase BphD. *Appl. Microbiol. Biotechnol.* **2013**, doi:10.1007/s00253-013-4814-0.

74. Phelan, R.M.; Townsend, C.A. Mechanistic insights into the bifunctional non-heme iron oxygenase carbapenem synthase by active site saturation mutagenesis. *J. Am. Chem. Soc.* **2013**, *135*, 7496–7502.

75. Geier, M.; Braun, A.; Fladischer, P.; Stepniak, P.; Rudroff, F.; Hametner, C.; Mihovilovic, M.D.; Glieder, A. Double site saturation mutagenesis of the human cytochrome P450 2D6 results in regioselective steroid hydroxylation. *FEBS J.* **2013**, *280*, 3094–3108.

76. Molloy, E.M.; Field, D.; O'Connor, P.M.; Cotter, P.D.; Hill, C.; Ross, R.P. Saturation mutagenesis of lysine 12 leads to the identification of derivatives of nisin A with enhanced antimicrobial activity. *PLoS One* **2013**, *8*, e58530.

77. Shainsky, J.; Bernath-Levin, K.; Isaschar-Ovdat, S.; Glaser, F.; Fishman, A. Protein engineering of nitrobenzene dioxygenase for enantioselective synthesis of chiral sulfoxides. *Protein Eng. Des. Sel.* **2013**, *26*, 335–345.

78. Agudo, R.; Roiban, G.D.; Reetz, M.T. Induced axial chirality in biocatalytic asymmetric ketone reduction. *J. Am. Chem. Soc.* **2013**, *135*, 1665–1668.

79. Jakoblinnert, A.; Wachtmeister, J.; Schukur, L.; Shivange, A.V.; Bocola, M.; Ansorge-Schumacher, M.B.; Schwaneberg, U. Reengineered carbonyl reductase for reducing methyl-substituted cyclohexanones. *Protein Eng. Des. Sel.* **2013**, *26*, 291–298.

80. Sandström, A.G.; Wikmark, Y.; Engström, K.; Nyhlén, J.; Bäckvall, J.E. Combinatorial reshaping of the *Candida antarctica* lipase A substrate pocket for enantioselectivity using an extremely condensed library. *Proc. Natl. Acad. Sci. USA* **2012**, *109*, 78–83.

81. Korman, T.P.; Sahachartsiri, B.; Charbonneau, D.M.; Huang, G.L.; Beauregard, M.; Bowie J.U. Dieselzymes: Development of a stable and methanol tolerant lipase for biodiesel production by directed evolution. *Biotechnol. Biofuels* **2013**, *6*, e70.

82. Anbar, M.; Bayer, E.A. Approaches for improving thermostability characteristics in cellulases. *Methods Enzymol.* **2012**, *510*, 261–271.

83. Sygmund, C.; Santner, P.; Krondorfer, I.; Peterbauer, C.K.; Alcalde, M.; Nyanhongo, G.S.; Guebitz, G.M.; Ludwig, R. Semi-rational engineering of cellobiose dehydrogenase for improved hydrogen peroxide production. *Microb. Cell Fact.* **2013**, *12*, e38.

84. Yi, Z.L.; Pei, X.Q.; Wu, Z.L. Introduction of glycine and proline residues onto protein surface increases the thermostability of endoglucanase CelA from *Clostridium thermocellum*. *Bioresour. Technol.* **2011**, *102*, 3636–3638.

85. Yi, Z.L.; Zhang, S.B.; Pei, X.Q.; Wu, Z.L. Design of mutants for enhanced thermostability of β-glycosidase BglY from *Thermus thermophilus*. *Bioresour. Technol.* **2013**, *129*, 629–633.

86. Reetz, M.T.; Wilensek, S.; Zha, D.; Jaeger, K.E. Directed evolution of an enantioselective enzyme through combinatorial multiple-cassette mutagenesis. *Angew. Chem. Int. Ed. Engl.* **2001**, *40*, 3589–3591.

87. Jochens, H.; Bornscheuer, U.T. Natural diversity to guide focused directed evolution. *Chembiochem* **2010**, *11*, 1861–1866.

88. Jochens, H.; Aerts, D.; Bornscheuer, U.T. Thermostabilization of an esterase by alignment-guided focussed directed evolution. *Protein Eng. Des. Sel.* **2010**, *23*, 903–909.

89. Zheng, H.; Reetz, M.T. Manipulating the stereoselectivity of limonene epoxide hydrolase by directed evolution based on iterative saturation mutagenesis. *J. Am. Chem. Soc.* **2010**, *132*, 15744–15751.

90. Ye, L.J.; Wang, L.; Pan, Y.; Cao, Y. Changing the specificity of α-amino acid ester hydrolase toward para-hydroxyl cephalosporins synthesis by site-directed saturation mutagenesis. *Biotechnol. Lett.* **2012**, *34*, 1719–1724.

91. Garrett, J.B.; Kretz, K.A.; O'Donoghue, E.; Kerovuo, J.; Kim, W.; Barton, N.R.; Hazlewood, G.P.; Short, J.M.; Robertson, D.E.; Gray, K.A. Enhancing the thermal tolerance and gastric performance of a microbial phytase for use as a phosphate-mobilizing monogastric-feed supplement. *Appl. Environ. Microbiol.* **2004**, *70*, 3041–3046.

92. Kille, S.; Zilly, F.E.; Acevedo, J.P.; Reetz, M.T. Regio- and stereoselectivity of P450-catalysed hydroxylation of steroids controlled by laboratory evolution. *Nat. Chem.* **2011**, *3*, 738–743.

93. Li, H.M.; Mei, L.H.; Urlacher, V.B.; Schmid, R.D. Cytochrome P450 BM-3 evolved by random and saturation mutagenesis as an effective indole-hydroxylating catalyst. *Appl. Biochem. Biotechnol.* **2008**, *144*, 27–36.

94. Ba, L.; Li, P.; Zhang, H.; Duan, Y.; Lin, Z. Semi-rational engineering of cytochrome P450sca-2 in a hybrid system for enhanced catalytic activity: Insights into the important role of electron transfer. *Biotechnol. Bioeng.* **2013**, doi:10.1002/bit.24960.

95. Wu, S.; Acevedo, J.P.; Reetz, M.T. Induced allostery in the directed evolution of an enantioselective Baeyer-Villiger monooxygenase. *Proc. Natl. Acad. Sci. USA* **2010** 107, 2775–2780.

96. Reetz, M.T.; Wu, S. Laboratory evolution of robust and enantioselective Baeyer-Villiger monooxygenases for asymmetric catalysis. *J. Am. Chem. Soc.* **2009**, *131*, 15424–15432.

97. Willetts, A.; Joint, I.; Gilbert, J.A.; Trimble, W.; Mühling, M. Isolation and initial characterization of a novel type of Baeyer-Villiger monooxygenase activity from a marine microorganism. *Microb. Biotechnol.* **2012**, *5*, 549–559.

98. Minerdi, D.; Zgrablic, I.; Sadeghi, S.J.; Gilardi, G. Identification of a novel Baeyer-Villiger monooxygenase from *Acinetobacter radioresistens*: Close relationship to the *Mycobacterium tuberculosis* prodrug activator EtaA. *Microb. Biotechnol.* **2012**, *5*, 700–716.

99. Mascotti, M.L.; Juri Ayub, M.; Dudek, H.; Sanz, M.K.; Fraaije, M.W. Cloning, overexpression and biocatalytic exploration of a novel Baeyer-Villiger monooxygenase from *Aspergillus fumigatus* Af293. *AMB Express* **2013**, *3*, e33.

100. Gao, X.; Huang, F.; Feng, J.; Chen, X.; Zhang, H.; Wang, Z.; Wu, Q.; Zhu, D. Engineering the meso-diaminopimelate dehydrogenase from *Symbiobacterium thermophilum* by site-saturation mutagenesis for D-phenylalanine synthesis. *Appl. Environ. Microbiol.* **2013**, *79*, 5078–5081.

101. Paul, D.; Pandey, G.; Pandey, J.; Jain, R.K. Accessing microbial diversity for bioremediation and environmental restoration. *Trends Biotechnol.* **2005**, *23*, 135–142.

102. Goldsmith, M.; Ashani, Y.; Simo, Y.; Ben-David, M.; Leader, H.; Silman, I.; Sussman, J.L.; Tawfik, D.S. Evolved stereoselective hydrolases for broad-spectrum G-type nerve agent detoxification. *Chem. Biol.* **2012**, *19*, 456–466.

103. Du, W.; Li, W.; Sun, T.; Chen, X.; Liu, D. Perspectives for biotechnological production of biodiesel and impacts. *Appl. Microbiol. Biotechnol.* **2008**, *79*, 331–337.

104. Parawira, W. Enzyme research and applications in biotechnological intensification of biogas production. *Crit. Rev. Biotechnol.* **2012**, *32*, 172–186.

105. King, P.W. Designing interfaces of hydrogenase-nanomaterial hybrids for efficient solar conversion. *Biochim. Biophys. Acta* **2013**, *1827*, 949–957.

106. Morra, S.; Valetti, F.; Sadeghi, S.J.; King, P.W.; Meyer, T.; Gilardi, G. Direct electrochemistry of an [FeFe]-hydrogenase on a TiO_2 electrode. *Chem. Commun. (Camb.)* **2011**, *47*, 10566–10568.

107. Vardar, G.; Wood, T.K. Protein engineering of toluene-o-xylene monooxygenase from *Pseudomonas stutzeri* OX1 for synthesizing 4-methylresorcinol, methylhydroquinone, and pyrogallol. *Appl. Environ. Microbiol.* **2004**, *70*, 3253–3562.

108. Tao, Y.; Fishman, A.; Bentley, W.E.; Wood, T.K. Altering toluene 4-monooxygenase by active-site engineering for the synthesis of 3-methoxycatechol, methoxyhydroquinone, and methylhydroquinone. *J. Bacteriol.* **2004**, *186*, 4705–4713.

109. Canada, K.A.; Iwashita, S.; Shim, H.; Wood, T.K. Directed evolution of toluene ortho-monooxygenase for enhanced 1-naphthol synthesis and chlorinated ethene degradation. *J. Bacteriol.* **2002**, *184*, 344–349.

110. Fortin, P.D.; MacPherson, I.; Neau, D.B.; Bolin, J.T.; Eltis, L.D. Directed evolution of a ring-cleaving dioxygenase for polychlorinated biphenyl degradation. *J. Biol. Chem.* **2005**, *280*, 42307–42314.

111. Ang, E.L.; Obbard, J.P.; Zhao, H. Directed evolution of aniline dioxygenase for enhanced bioremediation of aromatic amines. *Appl. Microbiol. Biotechnol.* **2009**, *81*, 1063–1070.

112. Ang, E.L.; Obbard, J.P.; Zhao, H. Probing the molecular determinants of aniline dioxygenase substrate specificity by saturation mutagenesis. *FEBS J.* **2007**, *274*, 928–939.

113. Leungsakul, T.; Keenan, B.G.; Yin, H.; Smets, B.F.; Wood, T.K. Saturation mutagenesis of 2,4-DNT dioxygenase of *Burkholderia* sp. strain DNT for enhanced dinitrotoluene degradation. *Biotechnol. Bioeng.* **2005**, *92*, 416–426.

114. Caglio, R.; Valetti, F.; Caposio, P.; Gribaudo, G.; Pessione, E.; Giunta, C. Fine-tuning of catalytic properties of catechol 1,2-dioxygenase by active site tailoring. *Chembiochem* **2009**, *10*, 1015–1024.

115. Di Nardo, G.; Roggero, C.; Campolongo, S.; Valetti, F.; Trotta, F.; Gilardi, G. Catalytic properties of catechol 1,2-dioxygenase from Acinetobacter radioresistens S13 immobilized on nanosponges. *Dalton Trans.* **2009**, *7*, 6507–6512.

116. Caglio, R.; Pessione, E.; Valetti, F.; Giunta, C.; Ghibaudi, E. An EPR, thermostability and pH-dependence study of wild-type and mutant forms of catechol 1,2-dioxygenase from *Acinetobacter radioresistens* S13. *Biometals* **2013**, *26*, 75–84.

117. Micalella, C.; Martignon, S.; Bruno, S.; Pioselli, B.; Caglio, R.; Valetti, F.; Pessione, E.; Giunta, C.; Rizzi, M. X-ray crystallography, mass spectrometry and single crystal microspectrophotometry: A multidisciplinary characterization of catechol 1,2 dioxygenase. *Biochim. Biophys. Acta* **2011**, *1814*, 817–823.

118. Chen, M.M.; Snow, C.D.; Vizcarra, C.L.; Mayo, S.L.; Arnold, F.H. Comparison of random mutagenesis and semi-rational designed libraries for improved cytochrome P450 BM3-catalyzed hydroxylation of small alkanes. *Protein Eng. Des. Sel.* **2012**, *25*, 171–178.

119. Jordan, D.B.; Wagschal, K.; Fan, Z.; Yuan, L.; Braker, J.D.; Heng, C. Engineering lower inhibitor affinities in β-D-xylosidase of *Selenomonas ruminantium* by site-directed mutagenesis of Trp145. *J. Ind. Microbiol. Biotechnol.* **2011**, *38*, 1821–1835.

120. Van Leeuwen, J.G.; Wijma, H.J.; Floor, R.J.; van der Laan, J.M.; Janssen, D.B. Directed evolution strategies for enantiocomplementary haloalkane dehalogenases: From chemical waste to enantiopure building blocks. *Chembiochem* **2012**, *13*, 137–148.

121. Frey, M. Hydrogenases: Hydrogen-activating enzymes. *Chembiochem* **2002**, *3*, 153–160.

122. Maeda, T.; Sanchez-Torres, V.; Wood, T.K. Protein engineering of hydrogenase 3 to enhance hydrogen production. *Appl. Microbiol. Biotechnol.* **2008**, *79*, 77–86.

123. Buhrke, T.; Lenz, O.; Krauss, N.; Friedrich, B.J. Oxygen tolerance of the H_2-sensing [NiFe] hydrogenase from *Ralstonia eutropha* H16 is based on limited access of oxygen to the active site. *Biol. Chem.* **2005**, *280*, 23791–23796.

124. Cornish, A.J.; Gartner, K.; Yang, H.; Peters, J.W.; Hegg, E.L. Mechanism of proton transfer in [FeFe]-hydrogenase from *Clostridium pasteurianum*. *J. Biol. Chem.* **2011**, *286*, 38341–38347.

125. Knorzer, P.; Silakov, A.; Foster, C.E.; Armstrong, F.A.; Lubitz, W.; Happe, T. Importance of the protein framework for catalytic activity of [FeFe]-hydrogenases. *J. Biol. Chem.* **2012**, *286*, 38341–38347.

126. Lautier, T.; Ezanno, P.; Baffert, C.; Fourmond, V.; Cournac, L.; Fontecilla-Camps, J.C.; Soucaille, P.; Bertrand, P.; Meynial-Salles, I.; Léger, C. The quest for a functional substrate access tunnel in FeFe hydrogenase. *Faraday Discuss* **2011**, *148*, 385–407.

127. Stapleton, J.A.; Swartz, J.R. Development of an *in vitro* compartmentalization screen for high-throughput directed evolution of [FeFe] hydrogenases. *PLoS One* **2010**, *5*, e15275.

128. Bingham, A.S.; Smith, P.R.; Swartz, J.R. Evolution of an [FeFe] hydrogenase with decreased oxygen sensitivity. *Int. J. Hydrogen Energy* **2012**, *37*, 2965–2976.

129. Winkler, M.; Esselborn, J.; Happe, T. Molecular basis of [FeFe]-hydrogenase function: An insight into the complex interplay between protein and catalytic cofactor. *Biochim. Biophys. Acta* **2013**, *1827*, 974–985.

130. Reda, T.; Plugge, C.M.; Abram, N.J.; Hirst, J. Reversible interconversion of carbon dioxide and formate by an electroactive enzyme. *Proc. Natl. Acad. Sci. USA* **2008**, *105*, 10654–10658.

131. Andreadeli, A.; Platis, D.; Tishkov, V.; Popov, V.; Labrou, N.E. Structure-guided alteration of coenzyme specificity of formate dehydrogenase by saturation mutagenesis to enable efficient utilization of $NADP^+$. *FEBS J.* **2008**, *275*, 3859–3869.

132. Andrews, F.H.; McLeish, M.J. Using site-saturation mutagenesis to explore mechanism and substrate specificity in thiamin diphosphate-dependent enzymes. *FEBS J.* **2013**, doi:10.1111/febs.12459.

133. Goldsmith, M.; Tawfik, D.S. Directed enzyme evolution: Beyond the low-hanging fruit. *Curr. Opin. Struct. Biol.* **2012**, *22*, 406–412.

Biocatalysis for Biobased Chemicals

Rubén de Regil and Georgina Sandoval

Abstract: The design and development of greener processes that are safe and friendly is an irreversible trend that is driven by sustainable and economic issues. The use of Biocatalysis as part of a manufacturing process fits well in this trend as enzymes are themselves biodegradable, require mild conditions to work and are highly specific and well suited to carry out complex reactions in a simple way. The growth of computational capabilities in the last decades has allowed Biocatalysis to develop sophisticated tools to understand better enzymatic phenomena and to have the power to control not only process conditions but also the enzyme's own nature. Nowadays, Biocatalysis is behind some important products in the pharmaceutical, cosmetic, food and bulk chemicals industry. In this review we want to present some of the most representative examples of industrial chemicals produced *in vitro* through enzymatic catalysis.

Reprinted from *Biomolecules*. Cite as: de Regil, R.; Sandoval, G. Biocatalysis for Biobased Chemicals. *Biomolecules* **2013**, *3*, 812-847.

1. Introduction

It is becoming evident that in order to sustain the standard way of life of the developed and in-development world, it will be necessary to make some adjustments either to our consumption habits or to our sources of supplies of energy and materials. In the latter case, Biotechnology, as a diversified discipline in which chemistry, physics, biology, optics, electro-magnetism and thermodynamics converge, possess the knowledge tools to play a relevant and vital role to address the challenges of growth, ageing, employment, limited sources of raw materials, energy and water supply and living standard. Industrial biobased processes will increasingly become the *de facto* alternative to build a sustainable economy. It is estimated that, by 2030, the products of white biotechnology and bioenergy will account for 30% of industrial production worth €300 bn [1].

Conversion of biomass by Biocatalysis is likely to become standard technology which will contribute significantly to open up access to large feedstock supplies for bioprocesses and the production of transport fuels. On the health and ageing field, personalized nutrition, tailor-made medicine will become a reality in the coming years thanks to novel, specific biotech drugs and regenerative medicine obtained by more efficient and greener processes.

Biocatalysis refers to the transformation of substances of chemical or biological origin through the use of the enzymes produced by diverse living organisms. Enzymes may carry out reactions in a free, or immobilized form, or within the living cell in which they naturally live.

Isolated enzymes obtained as purified and concentrated extracts, whether used immobilized onto a support or in free form, may produce neater products than when the whole microorganism cell is used for the biotransformation. This is because of the absence of other kinds of enzymes from the internal cell machinery, which may subsequently modify the product, and the absence of internal cellular components during the lysis-extraction step. This advantage of isolated enzymes has a positive impact on yield and purification costs. However, isolated enzymes are known to be less stable in a purified form than within the cell. The lower stability of free enzymes has been improved to some extent by immobilization and crosslinking techniques, the results of which vary depending on the type of enzyme, pH memory, extent of crosslinking, immobilization support and the procedure itself.

Whole microorganism cells, obtained in sufficient amount by fermentation, are used instead of isolated enzymes when their enzymes become highly unstable or non-functional outside the inner environment of the cell, so catalysis is confined within the cell and products are later extracted from it.

Chemical synthesis in the food, feed, industrial and pharma sectors is the field to which Biocatalysis has contributed the most, but it has also contributed to the bioremediation sector, another field in which enzymes are having a significant role.

The relative success of Biocatalysis applied to Synthetic Chemistry has been due mainly to the high enantio- and regioselectivities that enzymes exhibit towards their substrates, because enzymes speed up chemical processes that would otherwise run very slowly or without selectivity, and because enzymes function under mild reaction conditions. These advantages have allowed chemists to avoid the burden of group-protecting procedures, saving time, materials (including the harsh, dangerous or toxic ones) and energy costs. Other advantages of enzymes are that they are easy to control and biodegradable. Thus, Biocatalysis has proved in many cases to be a superior pathway than conventional chemical synthesis pathways, not only in the simplicity of accomplishing the reactions, but also from an economical and environmental point of view.

An important landmark in Biocatalysis was the use of organic solvents as reaction media, as it was thought that enzymes may only work in aqueous medium, naturally. Organic solvents became an important aid in dissolving organic, hydrophobic molecules, which account for much of the library of organic chemicals used in Synthetic Chemistry. The possibility to carry out reactions in organic media favored the reactions rate precisely because of the better solubility of reactants. Purification steps became shorter and easier because the avoidance of surfactants needed in aqueous media and the use of low boiling point solvents easy to evaporate. Moreover, hydrolytic, secondary, water-dependent reactions responsible for lower product yields, and growth of microbes in containers and pipes, is avoided because of the absence of water and the harsh effects of solvents to living cells.

However, Biocatalysis still needs to overcome some limitations such as the enzyme costs of production and the relative narrow stability window of many enzymes under diverse reaction conditions, which restricts their applications onto broader industrial processes. Chemicals used in industrial settings are mostly derived from fossil oil, whereas active ingredients in pharmaceutical processes may be new and/or structurally complex. In general, a vast number of chemicals used in industry are artificial, new man-made chemicals for which enzymes did not evolve to work with and thus are not suitable for the synthetic needs in industry. So there are high discrepancies between the enzyme's function in nature and the functions needed in the transformation industry. High throughput enzyme screening and protein engineering techniques, particularly Directed Evolution, are some of the tools being employed to advance faster in this aim to find enzymes for artificial substrates, and to create enzymes with new capabilities.

In this review we want to present some of the most representative examples of industrial chemicals produced *in vitro* through enzymatic catalysis, and hence, *in vivo* fermentation products are not included.

2. Enzymes in Food Industry

Applications of enzymes in the food industry are found in almost every sector of this industry: confectionary and sweeteners, fruit and vegetables, dairy, brewery and beverages, meat, dietary and the nutraceuticals niche [2]. However, most of these applications are of hydrolytic nature focused in debranching, improving solubility, clarification, and hydrolysis aimed at diverse goals depending on the food being treated.

2.1. Prebiotics and Sweeteners

There are some examples of food chemicals being synthesized by enzymes. One of them is Disaccharide Difructose Anhydride III (DFA III), which is a non-reducing, non-cariogenic sweetener with probiotic properties [3]. DFA III can be synthesized by enzyme inulase II (EC 2.4.1.93), (Figure 1), which was first identified in *Arthrobacter ureafaciens* [4] and later in other bacteria [5–7]. However, native enzymes are not thermotolerant enough to resist high temperatures required for a large scale process. Thus, the *ift*-gene encoding for the inulase II from Buo141, a thermotolerant strain, was cloned and expressed into *E. coli* XL1-blue and further modified and immobilized to obtain the biocatalyst which was reported to have 1.7×10^6 U/L [3].

Prebiotics is another field in which enzymes are being used. Oligosaccharides are non-digestible saccharide polymers containing 3–10 monomeric sugar units that are found in low amounts in human milk [8,9], onion, garlic, banana, soybean and chicory [10]. They are classified as prebiotics because they selectively promote the growth of bifidobacteria and lactobacilli in the intestine, which are regarded to have a beneficial effect to human health [10–14].

Figure 1. Enzymatic synthesis of Difructose Anhydride III (DFA III) from Inulin using enzyme inulase II, an inulin fructo-transferase.

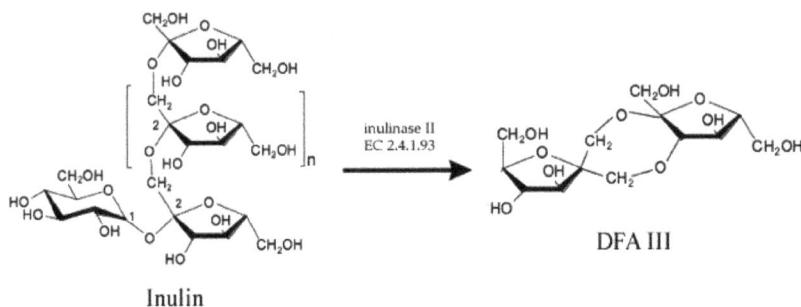

Oligosaccharides composed either of fructose or galactose units are named fructo-oligosaccharides (FOS) and galacto-oligosaccharides (GOS) respectively.

Galacto-oligosaccharides (GOS) can be synthesized from lactose when this sugar acts as the acceptor and transgalactosylation is catalyzed by β-galactosidase (Figure 2). In addition to the prebiotic activity, GOS have also been reported to contribute to (i) reduction of serum cholesterol and lipid level; (ii) synthesis of B-complex vitamins; (iii) enhance absorption of dietary calcium [14–16]; (iv) protection from infection and decrease of pathogenic bacteria; (v) stimulate absorption of some minerals [17]. However, these health promoting properties vary depending on the chemical composition, structure and degree of polymerization and these features depend, in turn, on the origin of the β-galactosidase [18].

Figure 2. Simplified enzymatic reaction to produce Galacto-oligosaccharides (GOS) from lactose using β-galactosidase. Subscript n may range from 0–6 though most native enzymes produce GOS with n between 1–2.

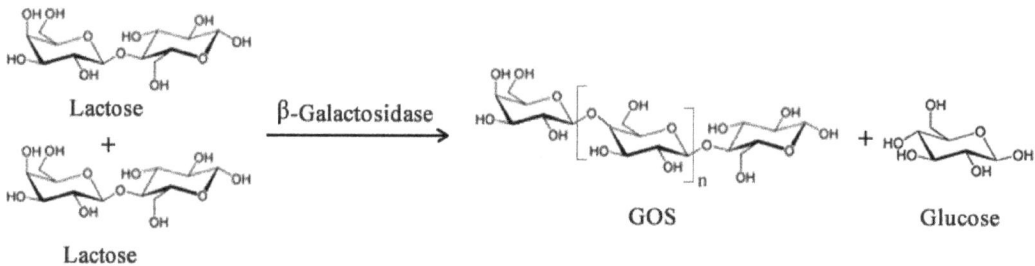

Lactose + Lactose → β-Galactosidase → GOS + Glucose

The most recurring means of the synthesis of GOS is by enzymatic catalysis from lactose using glycosyltransferases (EC 2.4) or glycoside hydrolases (EC 3.2.1) [19]. Glycosyltransferases are not used in the synthesis of GOS due to their low availability, the need for nucleotide sugar substrates and prohibitive prices. Instead, glycoside hydrolases are used, despite the fact that they are less stereoselective than the former [20]. Glycoside hydrolases from archeas (*Sulfolobus solfactaricum* and *Pyrococcus furiosus*), bacteria (*Saccharopolyspora* sp., *Bifidobacterium* sp., *Thermotoga* sp., *Thermus* sp., *Bacillus* sp., *Geobacillus* sp., *Caldicellulosiruptor sp.*, *Lactobacillus* sp., *Streptococcus* sp., *Enterobacter* sp., *Escherichia* sp.) and yeasts (*Aspergillus* sp., *Penicillinum* sp., *Talaromyces* sp., *Trichoderma* sp., *Kluyveromyces* sp., *Sirobasidium* sp., *Sterigmatomyces* sp., *Rhodotorula* sp., *Sporobolomyces* sp., *Rhizopus* sp.) have been tested for the synthesis of GOS [19,21].

Milk whey is a lactose-rich source which has been regarded in the past as a waste by-product from cheese production highly contaminant. So β-galactosidases have become a valued natural tool to produce a beneficial product out from a contaminant waste in a single step.

As a general finding, reports show that GOS yields average 30%–35% of total sugars [22,23] and are directly proportional to the initial lactose concentration. The major product is the trisaccharide accounting for as much as 80% of total GOS synthesized [12,24]. It was estimated that at least 3500 tons of GOS are enzymatically synthesized from whey lactose, out of 30,000 tons of total world annual production [25]. They are commercialized to enrich mainly infant formulas.

Just like GOS, Fructo-oligosaccharides (FOS) have low caloric value and have much the same prebiotic properties due to their indigestibility in the upper gastrointestinal tract: they are non-cariogenic and have ability to promote the activity of beneficial colonic lactic acid bacteria and to modulate the intestinal immune response [26–28]. However, unlike GOS, FOS are naturally occurring sugars biosynthesized by numerous plants such as asparagus, sugar beet, onion, artichoke, *etc.* [29,30]. Two main types of FOS can be found in nature, the inulin type, which are fructose polymers with linkages β(2–1) biosynthesized by inulosucrases (E.C. 2.4.1.9), and the levan type, which are fructose polymers with linkages β(2–6) biosynthesized by levansucrases (E.C. 2.4.1.10) [31–33].

Two different classes of FOS mixtures are produced commercially, one is based on inulin by controlled enzymatic hydrolysis, and the other is based on sucrose by a transfructosylation processes with fructosyltransferases, as shown in Figure 3 (β-fructofuranosidase, E.C. 3.2.1.26 or β-d-fructosyltransferase, EC 2.4.1.9) [34,35]. FOS from inulin hydrolysis contain longer fructose chains (Degree of Polymerization, DP 2–9) and may have either a fructose or glucose unit at the end of the chain. On the other hand, FOS from sucrose transfructosylation contain shorter polymer chains (DP 2–4) and always end with a glucose unit [35].

Figure 3. Simplified enzymatic reactions used commercially to obtain Fructo-oligosaccharides (FOS).

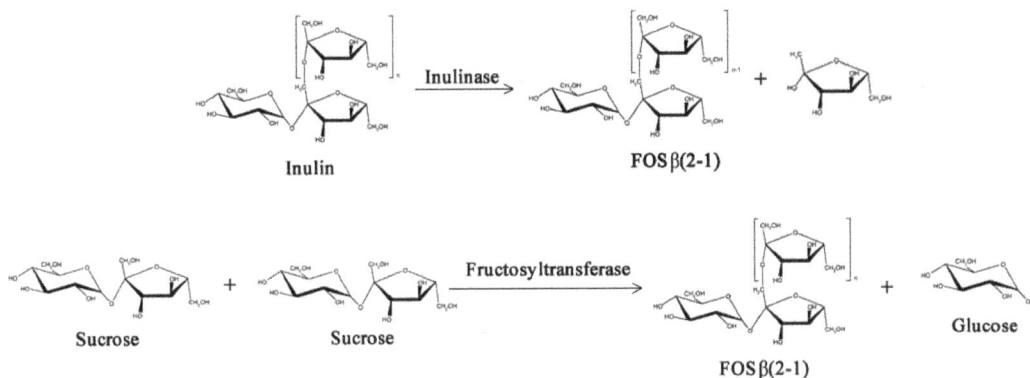

A commercial enzyme Pectinex Ultra SP-L was used immobilized onto Eupergit C to synthesize FOS from a 600 g/L of sucrose solution. Reactions were carried out at 65 °C in pH 6.5 during 24 h with a yield of 57% FOS of total sugars [36].

Despite the big production numbers that prebiotics have, the overall European market for prebiotics is still at the beginning stage, with the $87-million fructan (inulin and fructo-oligosaccharide) segment as the most developed part. In US the prebiotics market is estimated to reach US$198.3 million in 2014 [37].

2.2. Structured Lipids

Specialty fats and oils are lipids with special functional or nutritional effects in the human body. Among these, structured lipids (SLs) have a predominant importance within this field [38,39]. SLs are tailor-made fats and oils which incorporate specific new fatty acids to triacylglycerols, or have different composition and positional distribution of existing fatty acids, within its glycerol backbone. Among the various types of SLs, the MLM (medium, long, medium fatty acid chain length esterified at the *sn*-1, *sn*-2 and *sn*-3 positions of the glycerol backbone respectively) have been a subject of great interest because of their ability to provide quick energy through the pancreatic lipase hydrolytic release of the medium chain fatty acids which become rapidly oxidized by the liver [40]. The remaining long chain *sn*-2-monoacylglyceride is left to be absorbed through the lymphatic system [41]. This long chain monoacylglyceride can be an omega-6 fatty acid or any other poly unsaturated fatty acid (PUFA) which will provide the already known health benefits to the body [42].

SLs are claimed to have a modulation effect on the immune system, to improve the lipid clearance in the blood [43], and as a fat for special nutritional feeding [44]. Fatty acids at the *sn*-2 position are more readily absorbed *in vivo* than those at the *sn*-1 or 3 positions, thus, SLs of the type MLM that include an essential fatty acid in the *sn*-2 position are desirable nutrition sources for people who suffer from malabsorption or a pancreatic condition [44,45].

SLs can be obtained either chemically or enzymatically using lipases [42]. The high regioselectivity of lipases makes Biocatalysis particularly well suited for the synthesis of SLs, avoiding the synthesis of unwanted by-products, which lower the yields [46]. However, enzymatic synthesis of SLs has yet to be optimized in order to avoid the high costs of large-scale purification of unreacted substrates (Free fatty acids, Triacyglicerides, Diacylgricerides, Esters) which must be removed upon completion of reaction [47].

Two basic approaches have been followed to carry out the enzymatic synthesis of MLM SLs: (1) Transesterification and (2) Acidolysis [48]. Lipase transesterifications for the synthesis of MLM SLs have been performed using different vegetal and fish oils as source of essential long PUFAs, and coconut and palm kernel oil as a source of medium chain fatty acids (C6:0–C12:0) to be incorporated in the *sn*-1 and *sn*-3 positions [42,49]. Thus, to synthesize MLM SLs, *sn*-1 and *sn*-3, regiospecific lipases are favored. In Figure 4 these two approaches are depicted using a *sn*-1,3-specific lipase.

Casas-Godoy *et al*. [50] incorporated caprilyc and capric acid into olive oil using *Yarrowia lipolytica* immobilized on Accurel. Their optimized reaction allowed them to obtain an incorporation rate of 25% and 21% for capylic and capric acid respectively within 2 days at 40 °C and 5% (w/w) enzyme load.

Figure 4. The main two approaches to synthesize MLM Structured Lipids enzymatically: **(A)** Transesterification and **(B)** Acidolysis. Subproducts like LML Structured lipids may also be obtained, but only the product of interest is shown. L = Long Chain; M = Medium Chain; MCFA = Medium Chain Fatty Acid; MCFAEt = Medium Chain Fatty Acid Ester (see also [48]).

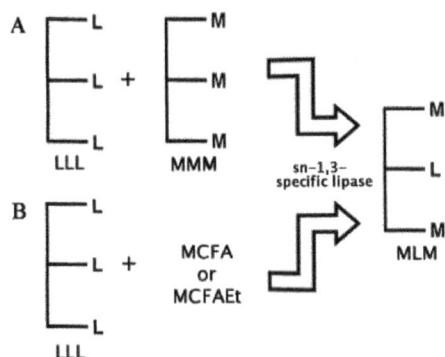

In another work, castor oil was dehydrated, isomerized and then transesterified with methyl laurate using *Thermomyces lanuginosa* and *Carica papaya*. The incorporation and transesterification yields were 59% and 88% for *T. lanuginosa* and 44% and 67% for *C. papaya*, respectively. This was achieved in 72 h at 60 °C with a 10% (w/w) enzyme load. Transesterification in the *sn*-2 position was observed and accounted for less than 8% [51].

Palm oil trolein has been subject to enrichment in its *sn*-2 position with DHA and ARA through acidolysis using Novozym 435. The research Group achieved an incorporation of 11% of DHA at *sn*-2 position (17% total) and 5.5% of ARA at *sn*-2 position (7% total) in 24 h at 60 °C and 10% enzyme load [52]. In a similar work, Khodadadi *et al.* [49] transesterified palm oil with tricaprylin in order to modify the former. Their results showed that Linolenic acid chains in palm oil are more easily transesterified than Linoleic or Oleic. Their best results were around 20% incorporation of caprylic chains into *sn*-1, *sn*-2 and *sn*-3 positions of which around a half corresponded to *sn*-2 position. The experiments were carried out with Novozym 435, Lipozyme TL-IM, Lipozyme RM-IM and Amano DF, though the best results were with Novozym 435, 24 h of reaction time, 50 °C and 1% enzyme load. Tecelão *et al.* [53] recently achieved 21% and 8% of incorporation of oleic acid and DHA respectively, to tripalmitin using *Carica papaya* latex at 60 °C, in a solvent-free system during 24 h.

Nagao *et al.* [54] achieved almost 100% of fatty acid incorporation with a DHA-rich by-product waste from a tuna oil industrial, hydrolysis process employed to extract DHA. Their reaction conditions were 30 °C, 120 h, vacuum at 2 kPa and 10% of Novozym 435 load. The degree of esterification with DHA was 51% and 17% at *sn*-1,3 and *sn*-2 position respectively.

3. Enzymes in the Bulk Chemistry Industry

Although industrial biotransformations are mainly used for the production of fine chemicals, there are a few examples where Biocatalysis is also used to produce commodity chemicals such as

340

acrylamide, and biodiesel. The use of biocatalysts employed to assist in synthetic routes to complex molecules of industrial interest is growing steadily [55–57].

3.1. Biodiesel

The lipase-catalyzed synthesis of biodiesel offers advantages over conventional methods for its production: lipases are able to work in gentle conditions and with a variety of triglyceride substrates, including waste oils and fats, corrosion problems present in chemical synthesis are avoided in the lipase-catalyzed synthesis, easy recovery of biocatalyst and glycerol, high levels of Free Fatty Acids (FFA) may also be esterified by lipases, and low environmental impact [58,59]. Furthermore, the separation and purification step of biodiesel is easier [60,61], resulting in a more attractive technical and environmental process. Numerous lipases have been studied for biodiesel production, with diverse triglyceride substrates and acyl acceptors. The use of edible oils is today not an option due to the food *vs.* fuel issue, which also makes them a more expensive raw material. Research studies so far have converted a series of non-edible fats and oils replacing the traditional alkaline transesterification. Process flow, reactor design and cost performance have been some of the main elements studied. It has been shown that high productivity, enzyme reuse and low reaction times can be achieved [62–64]. Nevertheless, enzymatic biodiesel still faces technical and economic challenges and has room for improvement to make enzymatic biodiesel a more attractive option for industrial production.

The most used method to produce enzymatic biodiesel is by transesterification of oil with an alcohol as acyl acceptor (Figure 5). Acyl acceptors, pose a challenge because the most available and cheap ones for industrial production and those who meet international specifications for biodiesel, are methanol and ethanol, which exert a strong denaturating action towards lipases [65]. Nevertheless, relatively successful efforts to overcome this inconvenience have emerged, like a pioneering work on stepwise alcohol addition [66], acyl acceptor alterations [67,68] and solvent engineering [69,70] which have sorted out this problem with relatively efficacy. Isopropanol [71], Isobutanol [72], 1-butanol [71], 2-butanol [72], 2-ethyl-1-hexanol [73], methyl acetate [74] and ethyl acetate [68] have been reported to be used as acyl acceptors. It was later documented that glycerol, a by-product of biodiesel synthesis, exerted lipase inhibition as well, which is more likely due to mass transfer limitation in the immobilized lipase [75].

Free and immobilized lipases of fungal and yeast origin such as *Mucor* sp., *Rhizopus* sp., *Candida* sp., *Aspergillus* sp., *Thermomyces* sp., *Penicillinum* sp. *and Pseudomonas* sp. have shown to be good biocatalysts for biodiesel synthesis as yields for most of them are reported to be 80%–95% [58]. Enzyme immobilization is a cost which greatly influences the economic viability when scaling-up industrial biodiesel projects; thus, alternative methods of preparing the enzyme is a current active topic in the field [76].

Figure 5. Enzymatic reaction of transesterification of oils with alcohol to produce fatty acid esters (biodiesel).

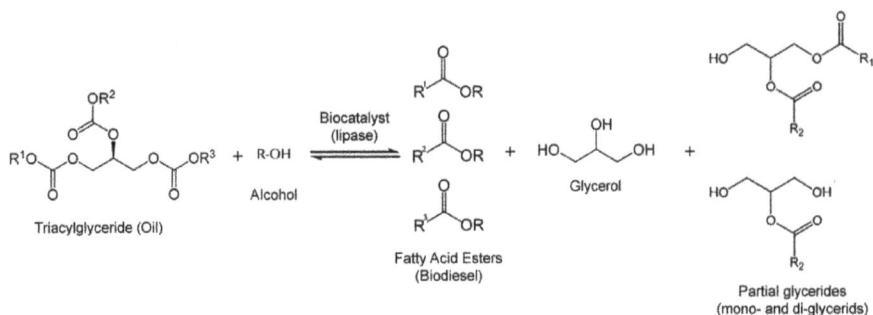

Organic solvents have been used to solve problems like substrate solubility and mass transfer [63]. Hydrophobic organic solvents have been used because they improve trygliceride and fatty substrates solubility [77], but leave viscous glycerol insoluble, which poses mass transfer limitations as stated above. Despite the denaturing effects of hydrophilic organic solvents over enzymes [78,79], some solvents like 1,4-dioxane and *tert*-butanol have been proven to generate high transesterification yields [69,70,80]. Incubation of lipases in alcohols with carbon number ≥ 3 has been documented to improve enzymatic activity in the synthesis of methyl esters [81]. Acetone has also been tested; however, the maximum yields of biodiesel have reached 40% [82].

The use of waste animal fat from slaughterhouses as raw material for the production of biodiesel by transesterification with ethanol was recently evaluated by Rivera *et al.* [69]. Enzymes N435 and Lipozyme RM IM at 45 °C at a 2% (w/w) enzyme load, in an organic (*tert*-butanol) and solvent-free systems were used. The biodiesel yields were 80% for the solvent-free system after 2 days of reaction, and 65% for the organic system after 1 day of reaction.

Recently, solvents like supercritical carbon dioxide have been used and biodiesel yields accounted for as much as 81% at 60 °C with a 15% (w/w) enzyme load during 4 h [83]. Ionic liquids have also been used for biodiesel synthesis [84,85] and one of the best results was achieved after 12 h at 50 °C in 1-ethyl-3-methylimidazolium trifluoromethane-sulfonate ([C2mim][OTf]) with an 80 % yield [86].

Intracellular lipases in the form of whole-cell biocatalysts, present a feasible alternative for biodiesel production as well. Their main advantage is the lack of laborious and costly extraction and purification procedures needed when an isolated, free or immobilized, enzyme is used [87]. In order to use whole-cell Biocatalysis, immobilization is advocated. One of the most accepted whole-cell biocatalyst systems for industrial applications is the use of filamentous fungi immobilized onto biomass support particles (BSPs) [88–90]. A*spergillus* sp. and *Rhizopus* sp., have been identified as robust for whole-cell immobilization, and thus have become the most widely studied fungi for biodiesel production [58]. Oils from yeasts and fungi are an alternative source of oils for biodiesel, as they can accumulate long-chain triacylglycerols with 16 and 18 carbons. The oil contents obtained from several yeast strains such as *Cryptococcus, Lipomyces, and Rhodotorula* species have reached 60%–70% of their dry weight [91].

3.2. Industrial Polymers

Biocatalysis has opened new synthetic strategies for organic chemists because it has been applied to synthetic chemistry in order perform stereochemical complex reactions in a relatively simple, straightforward way, which otherwise would require laborious protection-deprotection steps, toxic reactants and/or high-temperature/pressure procedures [92,93]. Thus, these advantages of using enzymes have been adopted in the field of polymer synthesis, in which most polymers are difficult to produce or to control by conventional chemical methods. Polymers with specific structures can be prepared enzymatically. In contrast, attempts to attain similar levels of polymer structural control by conventional chemical methods may prove to be a true challenge. From an environmental stand point, polymers derived from enzyme-mediated catalysis, whether polyesters, polyphenols, polysaccharides, proteins, or other polymers, are in most cases biodegradable, a feature highly sought after these days.

The most common type of enzymes which are capable to catalyze polymerization reactions are: Transferases, Oxidoreductases and Hydrolases.

3.2.1. Transferases

Transferases transfer a glycosyl group from a sugar nucleotide donor to specific nucleophilic acceptors. Despite they impose a high degree of regio- and stereochemical control to the glycosidic bond they form, and thus having a great synthetic potential for interesting polymeric materials, their use for synthesis *in vitro* is limited and even prohibitive by both, the availability of enzymes due to expression and solubility, and by the high costs of expensive activated donor sugars such as uridine diphosphate. They are very sensitive biocatalysts so their isolation and use on a larger scale is not practical, and they are mostly reserved for specialty research endeavors [94].

3.2.2. Oxidoreductases

On the other hand, Oxidoreductases and particularly Hydrolases are more robust enzymes, less sensitive and easier to obtain and use *in vitro*. Polymers typically produced by these three types of enzymes are shown in Table 1.

Polyaromatics

Polyaromatics are widely found in nature such as lignin, and flavonoid compounds. Much of their role in nature is as structural component conferring structural strength to living systems, in the case of lignin, and as a bioactive molecule in the case of flavonoids. Phenol is the single aromatic most important compound for industrial applications. Current polymeric materials produced commercially from phenolic compounds as industrial plastics include Bakelite and poly-2,6-dimethyl-1,4-phenylene oxide) (PPO) which bear good toughness and temperature-resistant properties. However, the oxidative polymerization of phenol with a conventional catalyst usually gives insoluble products with uncontrolled structure [95]. Moreover, as Bakelite and PPO are phenol-formaldehyde resins, the toxicity of formaldehyde has brought limitations on their industrial production.

Table 1. Common enzymes and the typical polymers synthesized by them.

Enzymes	Polymers synthesized
Oxidoreductases	
Peroxidases	
Laccases	Polyphenols, polyanilines, vinyl polymers
Tyrosinases	
Glucose oxidases	
Transferases	
Glycosyl transferases	Polysaccharides, cyclic oligosaccharides, polyesters
Acyl transferases	
Hydrolases	
Glycosidases	
Lipases	Polysaccharides, polyesters, polycarbonates,
Peptidases	polyamides, polythioesters, polyphosphates
Proteases	

On the other hand, an enzyme-catalyzed polymerization, offers not only the typical benefits of Biocatalysis, but the possibility to have a better control over polymerization [96].

In a recent work, Salvachúa *et al.* [97] used Versatil peroxidase (VP) to crosslink several monomeric lignans and peptides. Results show lignan oligomers of a maximum DP of 9 with a Number Average Molecular Weight M_n = 3300. As per the reactions with peptides, peptide oligomers with a maximum DP of 11 and a M_n = 6500 were obtained. Hetero-oligomers between lignans and peptides were also synthesized by VP. Oligomers of a DP = 6 and a M_n = 2300 were obtained where the ratio peptide: lignan was 1:5. The reactions were done at room temperature with 1.5 U mL^{-1} of VP, 0.1 mM H_2O_2 and 0.1 mM Mn^{2+}, during 24 h.

A peroxidase-catalyzed polymerization was performed under mild reaction conditions, using an aqueous buffer alcohol resulting in a soluble polyphenol with M_n of 3000–6000 [98,99]. The catalysts included horseradish peroxidase (HRP) and soybean peroxidase (SBP). The polymer solubility increased with increasing the oxyphenylene unit content (32%–59%) which was controlled by varying the methanol amount [100], and the solution pH [101]. Monodisperse polymer particles (250 nm diameter) were synthesized from phenol and subsituted phenols like m-cresol, p-cresol and polyphenylphenol, with HRP in a dispersion system 1,4-dioxane/buffer [102,103]. The mechanism of a peroxidase-catalyzed polymerization of phenols comprises three stages: Radical formation, Radical transfer and Radical coupling, shown in Figure 6.

It was revealed that meta-substituted phenol polymerizations catalyzed by HRP and SBP give rise both to higher yields when small and large-bulky substituents are used, respectively [105]. Cardanol, a natural phenol derived from cashew nut shell liquid (CNSL) with a C15 unsaturated alkyl meta-substituent, has good perspectives for industrial utilization such as resins, friction lining materials, and surface coatings. Therefore, an enzymatic approach to develop derivatives from this compound is attractive. Kobayashi *et al.* [106] obtained an artificial polymer structurally similar to "urushi", a Japanese lacquer, through an SBP-polymerization of Cardanol. The polymer had a molecular weight between 2000–4000 Da., soluble in polar organic solvents and possessed a tough and hard property as a film with a glossy surface finish. Kim *et al.* [107] also synthesized polycardanol with SBP and found it had better anti-biofouling activity to *Pseudomonas fluorescens* compared to polypropylene.

Figure 6. Mechanism of phenol polymer formation (see also [104]).

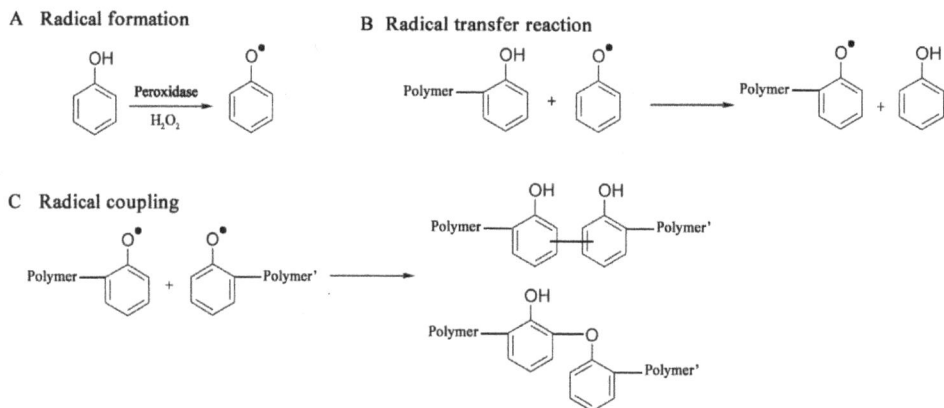

Various other m-substituted phenols have been polymerized by HRP and SBP, for example meta-alkylphenols, meta-halogenated phenols, and meta-phenylphenol [108]. These enzymatically synthesized m-substituted polymers were applied to positive-type photoresists for printed wire boards, because of their high solubility toward alkaline solution and high thermal stability [108,109].

Ortho-substituted phenols have been polymerized with SBP affording a variety of oligophenols (dimers to pentamers) and some of their oxidation products, including quinones and demethylated quinones. Some of these are considered to serve as biologically important compounds with therapeutic potentials [110]. In separate reaction systems, it was possible to synthesize poly(phenylene oxide) (PPO) from two different *o*-substituted phenols, 2,6-dimethylphenol and 3,5-dimethoxy-4-hydroxybenzoic acid (syringic acid), using HRP, SBP and a laccase [111–113]. The polymers were formed exclusively of 2,6-dimethyl- or 2,6-dimethoxy-1,4-oxyphenylene units respectively, which are similar in structure to a widely used high-performance engineering plastic PPO.

Para-alkylphenols were polymerized by HRP in an aqueous 1,4-dioxane solution to synthesize polymers with Mn of several thousands, whereby the polymer yield increased as the n-alkyl chain length increased from 1 to 5 [102,114]. Oxidative polymerization of natural *para*-substituted phenols like tyrosine ethyl ester or methyl ester or phenol derivative hydroquinone-β-D-glucopyranoside (arbutin) [115] were carried out using HRP catalyst in an aqueous buffer solution. A mixture of phenylene and oxyphenylene units was observed in the tyrosine polymer, whereas the arbutin polymer, after degycosilation, consisted of C-C *o*-position hydroquinone units. Resulting polymers had a molecular weight from 1500–4000. Reactions catalyzed by HRP proceeded, involving radical species, yet took place chemoselectively. *Para*-phenylphenol is one well-studied *para*-substituted phenols in peroxidase-catalyzed polymerizations. Polymers up to 26,000 Da have been synthesized with HRP [99]. However, the polymerization of *para*-phenylphenol lacks precise structure control due to the existence of both stabilized *ortho*- and *para*-single electron radical species, causing different kinds of linkages and leading to a complex structural polymer [116].

Other numerous reports manage different aspects of the enzymatic polymerization of phenols: use of mixtures of aqueous-organic solvents with 1,4-dioxane, methanol, DMF [117], or total organic systems (isooctane) [118], ionic liquids [119], using cyclodextrins as a phenol solubilizing agent [120], incorporating PEG as a template aid [121], or carrying out the reaction in micelles and reverse micelles [122] or in capsules [123].

An important group of natural phenols widely distributed throughout the plant kingdom are flavonoids. Flavonoids are benzo-γ-pyrone compounds consisting of phenolic and pyrane rings. Their biological and pharmacological effects as antioxidant, antimutagenic, anticarcinogenic, antiviral and antiinflammatory have been extensively reviewed [124–127].

Flavanols or commonly known as catechins are the major group of polyphenols present in green tea. The main catechins in green tea are (+)-catechin, (−)-epicatechin (EC), (−)-epigallocatechin (EGC), (−)-epicatechin gallate (ECG), and (−)-epigal-locatechin gallate (EGCG). Poly(cathechin) has been synthesized by HRP in aqueous-organic solvents having yields of DMF-soluble polymers around 30% and molecular weights of 3000 [128]. It has also been polymerized by a laccase derived from *Myceliophthore* (ML) in a mixture of acetone-buffer pH 5 rendering an 8000 Da polymer [129]. In this case, as in other phenol polymerizations [100], the organic solvent/buffer ratio greatly affected the solubility of the synthesized polymer. The antioxidant properties of catechins and ECGC, not only remained, but increased in a concentration dependent manner in poly(catechin) and poly(ECGC) synthesized by HRP and ML [129,130]. Superoxide anion scavenging activity of poly(ECGC) was much superior than monomeric ECGC and poly(catechin) [130]. Inhibitory activity of Xanthine oxidase, which was negligible in monomeric catechin or ECGC, was markedly observed in poly(catechin) and in poly(ECGC), inclusive was higher than allopurinol, a commercial inhibitor frequently used for gout treatment [129,131]. Recently, a laccase was used to polymerize catechin in order to attach it to biomedical catheters in order to reduce bacterial biofilm formation [132].

Rutin has also been polymerized in organic-aqueous systems by Laccase ML-mediated catalysis. Yields superior to 70% were mostly observed and molecular weights between 7–9 kDa were registered [133].

Flavonols (quercetin) and isoflavones were also subject to an enzymatic oxidative polymerization by HRP and SBP in aqueous-organic solvent systems. Weight Average Molecular Weight Mw and Number Average Molecular Weight Mn for poly(quercetin) was 10,000 and 2500 respectively, with a yield around 50%. Poly(rutin), poly(catechin), poly(daidzein), poly(formononetin) and others were also obtained in similar numbers [128].

Functionalization of polymers with flavonoids has also been investigated. Quercetin-functionalized chitosan has been the most studied system to yield antimicrobial products [134–137]. However, naringin-PVDF, morin-resin, catechin-inulin systems have also been reported [138–140].

3.2.3. Hydrolases

Hydrolases are the enzyme class with most widespread use and applications in the world. Around 75% of all commercialized industrial enzymes are hydrolytic in action. Despite proteases and carbohydrases are the most demanded subclass of enzymes accounting for around 40% of world's enzyme sales, lipases remain as the biocatalyst subclass most widely used in organic chemistry [141,142].

Lipases have been used to catalyze reactions in polycondensations of dicarboxylic acids with diols [143], ring-opening polymerization (ROP) of lactones [144], cyclic carbonates [145] and polycondensations of hydroxycarboxylic acids [146]. More examples are described in the following sections.

3.2.4. Polyesters

Polyesters occupy the 4th place among the most important biomacromolecules in living systems. They are macromolecules with good biodegradability, biocompatibility and permeability, and thus are highly suitable for biomedical applications, such as implant biosorbable materials, for tissue engineering and delivery vehicles for drug or genes [147]. Polyesters are very valuable industrial materials that are broadly used like poly(ethylene terephthalate) (PET), poly(butylene succinate) (PBS), poly(ε-caprolactone) (PCL), and poly(lactic acid) (PLA).

Two major approaches can be taken to perform enzymatic polyester synthesis: (1) polycondensation and (2) ring-opening polymerization (ROP). PET and PBS are produced in large-scale by polycondensation whereas PCL and PLA are produced via ROP. Classical cationic, anionic or metallic chemical synthesis of polyesters may render them unsuitable for biomedical applications due to the toxicity of these reagents. Enzyme catalyzed synthesis of esters has circumvented this and other problems since enzymatic reactions do not require high energy input (temperature or pressure), most enzymes can carry out regio-, chemo- and enantiospecific reactions with no need of protecting groups, exhibit high catalytic activity, they may be reused and as a consequence of all this, reactions are environmentally and health safer than the conventional chemical route [148].

3.2.5. Polycondensations

Lipase-Catalyzed Polycondensations

In lipase-catalyzed polycondensations dicarboxylic acids are esterified with diols to produce polyesters. Reactions have been realized mostly in organic solvents, in solvent-free media and in aqueous systems. However, there have been studies in ionic liquids [149] and supercritical fluids as well [150]. In the early years of exploration of these systems, Okumura et al. [151] set a series of reactions with dicarboxylic acids and diols in aqueous systems using a lipase from *Aspergillus niger* and he obtained oligomers of 3–7 units. Extracting water molecules from the system, either with molecular sieves or applying vacuum, seemed to improve the polymer size up to a DP of 20 in an adipic acid-1,4-butanediol reaction [152], and up to a Mn = 77 kDa in an adipic acid-1,6-hexanediol reaction [153]. Organic solvents with high boiling points were identified to favor the polyester synthesis. In an aim to study natural hydroxy-acids, Gómez-Patiño et al. [154] obtained oligomers from tomato cuticle monomer, 10,16-dihydroxyhexadecanoic acid and its methyl ester. *Candida antarctica* B was the best performer among the 5 lipases tested in organic media reactions obtaining the largest oligomer with a DP = 3 and Mw = 1206.

Reactions between dicarboxylic acids and diols conducted in water with *Candida antarctica* (N435), but with a continuous dehydrating process, are claimed to give rise to good yields [155].

Polycondensations with structurally different monomers have been realized, for example siloxane-containing diacids with diols (Mw = 20,000) [156], diacids with glycerol (Mw = 2000–6000) [157,158], thio-glycerol with diacids (Mw = 170,000) [159], diacids with a variety of sugars, sorbitol, erythritol, xylitol, ribitol, mannitol, glucitol, galactitol yielded polyesters with Mw = 10 kDa for galactitol and 75 kDa for Mannitol. The regioselecitivy of the sugar esterifications was mostly consistent in all the sugars to be on the primary hydroxyl groups [160].

Activation of dicarboxylic acids has been employed by means of esterification the carboxylic groups with methanol or ethanol [161], by esterification [162] or by vinyl activation [163]. Azim *et al.* [164], in an interesting strategy, firstly polymerized succinic acid with 1,4-butanediol to obtain a cyclic oligomer, which later was repolymerized by ring-opening to obtain a high molecular weight polymer (Mw = 130 kDa). Activation of dicarboxylic acids by means of esterification the carboxylic groups with halogenated alcohols like 2-chloroethanol, 2,2,2-trifluroethanol and 2,2,2-trichloroethanol lead to an increase of Mw by a factor of 5 [162]. However, the halogenated alcohols produced as a consequence of the reaction may damage the biocatalyst. Activation of carboxylic groups by vinyl esterification produced in most cases polyesters with Mw around 25 kDa [103,165,166].

Through reaction optimizations, Yao *et al.* [167] were able to achieve a polyester Mw = 16.6 kDa using 1,8-octanediol, adipic acid and L-malic acid as monomers. The incorporation of a sugar to be used as a third monomer is a likely means to modify the properties of conventional polymers, and an interesting strategy to prepare a variety of functional materials.

Recently it was reported the polymerization of β-alanine by a lipase catalyzed polycondensation reaction between β-alanine esters. Lipase B from *Candida antarctica* aggregated in CLEAs was the biocatalyst that converted β-alanine esters into polymers in high yield (up to 90%) and with high DP (up to 53 units). The best results were obtained by using methyl esters and methyl-tert-butyl ether (MTBE) as the solvent medium at 50 °C for 16 h [168].

Protease-Catalyzed Polycondensations

Proteases, like some other hydrolases, catalyze not only hydrolytic reactions (peptide hydrolysis in this case) but also peptide bond formation under appropriate conditions to give polypeptides. There exist several oligopeptides with varied biologically active properties that have been synthesized widely using proteases as catalysts via condensation reactions [169]. Some examples include, aspartame synthesized by thermolysin [170], oxytocin by papain, thermolysin, and chymotrypsin, and somatostatin by thermolysin, and chymotrypsin [171]. Various attempts to synthesize long-chain polyaminoamides were done by a protease-catalyzed polycondensation using chymotrypsin, trypsin, subtilisin and papain. However, only lower molecular weight polymers were obtained [172].

3.2.6. Polyamides

It was recently reported the synthesis of polyamides by lipase Novozym 435 in high yields (93%) and a short lapse of time (30 min). Authors attribute this high productivity to the use of "designed" monomers of the type: ω-amino-α-alkoxy acetic acid ethyl ester, which bears an ω-amino group and an oxygen atom in β position. The reactions were performed in bulk at 80 °C with an enzyme load of 45% (v/v) and the resultant polyamides had a DP = 15 (PDI = 1.6) and a Mw between 3000–4000 [173].

3.2.6. Vinyl Polymers

One field that has expanded tremendously in the past two decades is the enzyme-initiated radical polymerization of aromatic and vinyl monomers [149]. Vinyl monomers studied for enzymatic polymerization are basically classified into (meth)acrylic type and styryl type, which both involve the formation of a radical species. HRP and Laccase peroxidases have been reported to perform well in the meth(acrylic)-type polymerization of acrylamide. In a HRP-mediated free radical polymerization of vinyl monomers, the HRP-mediator system has three components: enzyme, oxidant (H_2O_2) and an initiatior, such as β-diketones which are commonly used. On the other hand, when several oxidoreductases, such as laccase, lipoxidase, and sarcosine oxidase, were used as catalysts, the acrylamide polymerization proceeded even without H_2O_2 or β-diketones. This was the case for laccase from *Pycnoporus coccineus* which induced the acrylamide polymerization in water at 50–80 °C under argon to produce poly(acrylamide) with Mn = 1×10^6, Mw/Mn ≈ 2 for 4–24 h and up to 81% yields [174]. Since the laccase-mediator system (LMS) may induce the radical polymerization of vinyl monomer with no H_2O_2 and is environmentally benign, different conditions for polymerization with commercial laccase *Myceliophthora thermophila* were further examined and optimal conditions were found as slightly acidic reaction media at around 50 °C using β-diketones and O_2 as the initiator and oxidant respectively. The molecular weight of poly(acrylamide) was Mn 6–28 × 10^4; Mw/Mn = 2.5–3.2 and could be controlled through the ratio of monomer to enzyme [175].

Poly(acrylamide) polymers of Mn of 1.5–4.6 × 10^5 with Mw/Mn 2.0–2.4, and acrylamide conversion between 70%–90% were synthesized by HRP in water at room temperature with 2,4-pentanedione as an initiator intermediate [176].

Enzyme-catalyzed vinyl polymerizations have been demonstrated in recent years with significant control of polymer molecular weight and yield depending on reaction conditions [149]. Resins of poly(sodium acrylate) are used as water-absorbent materials for cleaning surfaces, in water and oil conditioning, personal care products, and disposable materials for medical applications [177].

3.2.7. Nylons

Polyamides, also called nylons, display improved physical properties compared with polyolefins and polyesters due to the directionally specific inter-chain hydrogen bonds and significantly enhanced melting points [178]. Nylons can be synthesized either by polycondensation or by ROP. Ragupathy *et al.* [179] presented two and three step polycondensation and ROP methods to enzymatically produce nylon-8,10, nylon-8,13, nylon-6,13, and nylon-12,13. He used 1,8-diaminooctane (DAO) and diethyl sebacate (DES) for the polycondensations and DAO and lactone ethyleneridecanoate (ETD) for ROP. Novozym 435 in diphenyl ether at 150 °C carried out the polymerizations. Monomer conversion reached 97% and 90% and polyamides synthesized had an Mw of 5000 and 8000 for polycondensation and ROP reactions respectively.

3.2.8. Acrylate and Styrene Polymerization

Methyl-methacrylate (MMA) was polymerized by en enzyme-catalyzed reaction using the ternary system (enzyme, oxidant, and initiator) in water and water-miscible organic cosolvents such as DMF, acetone, dioxane, and THF. Soybean peroxidase in aqueous solution afforded a 48% yield of poly(methyl methacrylate) (PMMA) with $Mn = 9.3 \times 10^5$ and $Mw/Mn = 6.8$. When HRP II (type II) was used, a 45% yield of PMMA was obtained with $Mn = 6.3 \times 10^5$ and $Mw/Mn = 3.0$. It was found that yields of PMMA increased when cosolvents with low dielectric constant like dioxane and THF were used [180].

Respect to styrenic polymerizations, HRP in water was used to polymerize styrene and some derivatives. The polymerization was investigated using several β-diketones as initiators, and proceeded in a mixed solution of $H_2O/THF = 3$ (v/v). Polystyrene synthesized using 2,5-cyclopentanedione as initiator resulted in 60% yield with Mn and Mw/Mn of 6.7×10^4 and 1.9 respectively. Polymer yield, Mn and Mw/Mn of the resulting polystyrene depended on the type of initiator used. Synthesis of polymers from styrene derivatives, 4-methylstyrene and 2-vinylnaphthalene were also investigated and afforded polystyrenes in a >90% yield of polymer with a Mn of 1.15×10^5 and $Mw/Mn = 2.28$ [181].

3.2.9. Ring-Opening Polymerizations (ROP)

Among the two major synthetic polymerization approaches, ring-opening polymerization (ROP) has been most extensively studied to polyester synthesis.

Polymerization of lactones via ring-opening catalysis carried out by lipases has been studied since the early 1990s. This catalytic activity for ROP of lactone monomers has been the research field on diverse lipases such as *Pseudomonas fluorescens*, *Pseudomonas cepacia*, *Candida rugosa*, *Candida cylindracea*, *Candida antarctica*, *Aspergillus niger*, *Mucor miehei*, *Penicillium roqueforti*, *Rhizopus japanicus*. *Yarrowia lipolytica*, *Carica papaya* and porcine pancreas lipase [182–189]. Cutinase from *Humicola insolens* (HiC) has also been reported to carry out ROP [190].

Poly(1,4-dioxan-2-one) (polyDO) is a desirable biocompatible polymer with good flexibility and tensile strength which might be considered for biomedical applications. This polyester was synthesized by ROP of 1,4-dioxan-2-one by lipase B from *Candida antarctica* at 60 °C, resulting in a polymer of $Mw = 41,000$ [191]. In another study, Jiang *et al.* [192] claimed to synthesize by ring-opening copolymerization a polyester from 1,4-dioxan-2-one (DO) with pentadecalactone (PDL) to give a copolyester of poly(DO-co-PDL) with $Mw > 30,000$. They used *Candida antarctica* B lipase in toluene or diphenyl ether at 70 °C for 26 h.

Lipase 2 from *Yarrowia lipolytica* and *Carica papaya* latex were recently employed to polymerize ε-CL in bulk. Lipase 2 from *Y. lipolytica* was found to be very efficient as catalyst for several reactions [193] and latex from *C. papaya* is a low-cost auto-immobilized biocatalyst. The polymerization yields were 74% and 40% with an Mw of 1350 and 1100 respectively. Reactions were realized at 150 °C and 6 h for *Y. lipolytica* and 70 °C and 24 h for *C. papaya* [182].

As to macrolides, lipase *Pseudomonas fluorescens* was able to polymerize 11-undecanolide (12-membered, UDL), 12-dodecanolide (13-membered, DDL), 15-pentadecanolide (16-membered,

PDL), and 16-hexadecanolide (17-membered, HDL) [114,186–189,194–196]. Lipases from *Candida cylindracea* and *Pseudomonas fluorescens* catalyzed the ROP of UDL in bulk with quantitative yields affording polyesters of Mn of 23,000 and 25,000 [197,198]. In another study, ROP by lipases CA, lipase CC, lipase PC, lipase PF, or PPL in bulk at 45–75 °C for 5 days was done over HDL, the largest unsubstituted lactone monomer studied so far. The study showed the synthesis of polyHDL with Mn reaching to 5,800 in high yields [199]. It was discovered that a larger ring monomer, like PDL showed a greater reactivity towards polymerization than a smaller monomers like 1,4-polydioxan-2-one (DO) [192].

Ebata *et al.* obtained a poly(ε-CL) from a cyclic dimer of ε-CL (14-memberd) that was polymerized at 70 °C in toluene by lipase B from *Candida antarctica*, affording quantitatively a poly(ε-CL) with Mn of 18,000 [200]. This research Group, under the same strategy used to produce oligomers which are then subject to subsequent polymerization, claimed that a poly(butylene-succiante) (PBS) polyester of Mw 130,000 was obtained from cyclic dimers of butylene-succiante of Mn = 390. The reaction was carried out in toluene at 120 °C using 40% (w/w) of lipase *Candida antarctica* B for 24 h [201].

It was found that among ε-CL substituted monomers, ω-methyl ε-CL showed the least reactivity towards the lipase-catalytic ROP [202]. On the other hand, α-methyl or δ-methyl ε-CL afforded polymers of Mw = 8400–11,000 with yields of 74% and 93% respectively [203].

An equilibrium phenomenon was observed between the synthesis of cyclic and linear polymers in a lipase-catalyzed ROP reaction of lactones. Cyclic oligomers in addition to major linear polyesters coexist in equilibrium [204,205]. This cyclic-linear equilibrium is solvent-dependent, for example Novozym 435 was used to catalyze the ROP of ε-CL at 60 °C in bulk or in an organic solvent. In bulk, the polymer products coexisted as a cyclic dimer of ε-CL and linear poly(ε-CL) in 2% and in 98% abundance, respectively. When the reaction was carried out in in acetonitrile, THF or 1,4-dioxane the same proportion was observed, as for example the equilibrium yields in acetonitrile were 70% for the cyclic oligomers (17% of dilactone and 53% of cyclic oligomers) and 30% for linear poly(ε-CL). When the reaction was carried out in isooctane, the proportion inverted to 3% and 97%, respectively, as in the bulk reaction [204].

Another hydrolase enzyme, a depolymerase, was found to catalyze ROP reactions *in vitro*. This depolymerase is a poly(hydroxybutyrate) (PHB) (EC 3.1.1.75), and was extracted from *Pseudomonas stutzeri*, *Alcaligenes faecalis* and *Pseudomonas lemoignei*. *A. faecalis* PHB depolymerase was assayed with a series of small, medium and large lactones and the best polimerization activity (93% yield) was obtained with β-butyrolactone, resulting in the formation of polyesters with a Mw = 16,000. On the other hand, medium and large lactones (ε-caprolactone, 11-undecanolide, and 12-dodecanolide), which are readily polymerized by lipases, were scarcely polymerized by PHB depolymerase [206].

3.3. Commodity Chemicals

One of the most noteworthy cases of biocatalytic production of a commodity chemical is the bioconversion of acrylonitrile to acrylamide [207]. This reaction, schematically simplified in Figure 7, is carried out by a nitrile hydratase whose catalytic activity transforms a cyanide group into an amide.

Mitsubishi Rayon Co., Ltd. (Tokyo, Japan) currently produces over 20,000 tons annually of acrylamide using a third-generation biocatalyst, *Rhodococcus rhodochrous* J1, developed for commercial use by Nitto Chemical Industries. Acrylamide is produced from acrylonitrile in a continuous system of fixed-bed reactors at 10 °C with polyacrylamide-immobilized J1 cells. The process achieves conversion of acrylonitrile to acrylamide in ~99.9% yield, and the catalyst productivity is >7000 g of acrylamide per g dry cell weight [208].

Figure 7. Enzymatic conversion of acrylonitrile to acrylamide by means of a nitrile hydratase.

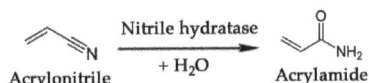

Lonza Guangzhou Fine Chemicals produces nicotinamide through a chemoenzymatic process shown in Figure 8 [209,210]. They start from 2-methyl-1,5-diaminopentane, a byproduct from production of nylon-6,6, which is converted to 3-methylpyridine, which in turn is ammoxidized. The resulting 3-cyanopyridine is hydrolyzed to nicotinamide using immobilized *Rhodococcus rhodochrous* J1 cells [211,212]. The Plant's capacity is 3400 tons per year of nicotinamide. The enzymatic process affords the desired amide at >99.3% selectivity at 100% conversion, whereas the chemical process requires caustic hydrolysis of 3-cyanopyridine but also produces 4% nicotinic acid as byproduct.

Figure 8. Chemoenzymatic route to obtain nicotinamide developed by Lonza [209,210].

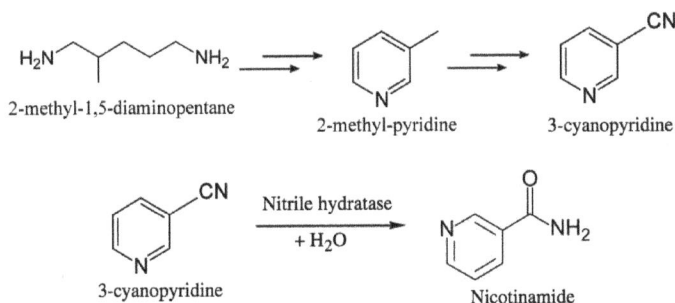

A commodity chemical which is aimed to substitute to some extent the universally oil-derived terephthalic acid is 2,5-furandicarboxylic acid (FDC) [213]. Terephthalic acid is one of the main raw materials to produce polyesters. FDC relies in the supply of 5-hydroxymethylfurfural (HMF), which is the product of the dehydration of hexoses. Oxidation of HMF yields FDC and may be realized by using heterogeneous or electrochemical catalysis [214,215]. However, two biocatalytic processes have been devised to help in having a reliable and sustainable supply for HMF: a whole-cell biocatalytic approach using a recombinant *Pseudomonas putida* hosting an oxidoreductase from *Cupriavidus basilensis*. This process is able to produce 30 g/L of 2,5-furandicarboxylic acid from HMF having a yield of 0.97 mol/mol [216]. The productivity of the whole process is 0.21 g/(L·h) under aerobic fed-batch conditions. The second approach consists of the use of a chloroperoxidase and *C. antarctica* lipase B [217,218].

4. Enzymes in the Fine Chemicals Industry

The role of Biocatalysis in the pharmaceutical and fine-chemical industries is clearly expanding. There are estimated to be around 150 implemented biocatalytic processes in industry, and the majority of these are in the pharmaceutical sector [219]. As stereoisomerism is quite relevant in pharmaceutics and fine chemistry, and a single swap in hydrogen position may mean a great difference in the bioactive function of a compound, Biocatalysis fits well to meet these challenges. Besides the enantio-, regio- and chemoselectivity that enzymes exhibit, their ability to perform complex catalysis procedures in a simple step, which otherwise, under a chemical approach, might require laborious treatments, toxic reagents or high energy input, has provided a strong basis for their usage in the fine chemicals industry. Some examples of the contribution of Biocatalysis to this field are described below.

A precursor of aspartame, *N*-(benzyloxycarbonyl)-L-aspartyl-L,-phenylalanine methyl ester (Z-APM) has been synthesized from *N*-(benzyloxycarbonyl)-L-aspartic acid (Z-L-ASP) and L-phenylalanine methyl ester (L-PM) with thermolysin [220]. By reverting the peptide-bond hydrolytic nature of thermolysin, this precursor is synthesized on a multi-thousand ton per year scale by a DSM/Tosoh joint venture (Holland Sweetener Company, Geleen, The Netherlands).

Pyrethroids now constitute the majority of commercial household insecticides. A novel industrial application of a lyase enzyme is to produce a pyrethroid intermedieate, (*S*)-*m*-phenoxy-benzaldehyde cyanohydrin (sPBC). Hydroxynitrile lyase, is an enzyme that catalyzes the addition of HCN to aldehydes and ketones [221]. Thus, the production of sPBC from *m*-phenoxybenzaldehyde by hydroxynitril lyase has been carried out on a multi-ton scale by DSM.

L-carnitine is a quaternary ammonium compound biosynthesized from the amino acids lysine and methionine [222]. Within mammal cells, L-carnitine is required for the transport of fatty acids from the cytosol into the mitochondria during the lipids oxidation [223]. Due to this role in lipid oxidation, L-carnitine is often advertised to improve fat metabolism, reduce fat mass, and increase muscle mass, which is widely available as an over-the-counter nutritional. L-carnitine is produced by Lonza (Basel, Switzerland) on an industrial scale using an enzyme from strain *Agrobacterium* HK1349 in a whole cell biotransformation process [224]. The process actually comprises a dehydrogenation of γ-butyrobetaine to 4-(trimethylamino)-butenoic acid followed by selective addition of a water molecule by L-carnitine lyase.

L-*tert*-leucine is an important chiral building block and intermediate of many ligands in chemo-catalysis in the pharmaceutical industry [225]. Menzel *et al.* [226] presented a process to produce L-*tert*-leucine in a whole-cell Biocatalysis system using a recombinant *E. coli* host expressing the two enzymes required by the process: a leucine hydrogenase and a formate dehydrogenase. The former catalyzes the main reaction, reductive amination of an α-keto acid, and the latter serves as a NADH regenerator. A yield of 84% in 24 h and an enantiomeric purity of ee > 99% was obtained. The process has been scaled up to tons level. Degussa-Hüls has used a similar whole-cell Biocatalysis system to produce L-*tert*-leucine, which has taken to a commercial scale [227].

Lonza produces 5-methylpyrazine-2-carboxylic acid on a commercial scale from the *p*-xylene analogue 2,5-dimethylpyrazine. This compound is used as a blood-lowering drug of the sulfenyl urea class commercialized as Glycotrol. The synthesis is carried out in *P. putida* ATCC33015 as a whole-cell biocatalyst, expressing a series of enzymes (a monooxygenase and two dehydrogenases) [224].

Japan Energy (Saitama, Japan) produces alkyloxiranes and phenyloxiranes on an industrial scale, especially the chiral building block 2-(trifluoromethyl)oxirane from 3,3,3- trifluoropropene through an oxidative reaction, using a whole-cell biocatalyst from *Nocardia corallina* [228].

Vanillin, the main component of vanillin extract, a natural flavoring, whose demand has long exceeded the supply, should be synthesized chemically from guaiacol, in order meet demand. Nevertheless, a whole-cell biocatalytic synthesis of vanillin from glucose has now been elaborated. Glucose is transformed into vanillic acid by a recombinant *E. coli* biocatalyst under fed-batch fermentor conditions. Then reduction of vanillic acid to vanillin is carried out by aryl aldehyde dehydrogenase isolated from *Neurospora crassa*. The biocatalytic route avoids the use of carcinogenic reagents and non-renewable petroleum derivatives (guaiacol) [229].

Aresta *et al.* used a carboxylase in the synthesis of 4-hydroxy benzoic acid, which is an intermediate for the synthesis of preservatives. The carboxylase enzyme is extracted from the bacteria *Thauera aromatica*, and it acts over the phenyl-phosphate moeity carboxylating it with 100% selectivity and 90% yield at 300 °K, P_{CO2} = 0.1 MPa [230].

Alfuzosin, a quinazoline derivative, against Benign prostatic hyperplasia (BPH), is synthesized through intermediate compund tetrahydro-*N*-[3-(methylamino)-propyl]-2-furan-carboxamide. This intermediate was traditionally produced in a three-steps chemical route from 2-tetrahydrofuroic acid involving a series of chemicals and distillation. The enzyme-catalyzed reaction with lipase B from *Candida antacrtica*, afforded the intermediate in two steps in which the same enzyme catalyzed the two reactions: esterification and amidation. This biocatalytic procedure simplyfied and made more environmentally friendly the previous chemical synthesis [231].

Another important intermediate in the synthesis of antiviral nucleosides such as 3'-deoxy-3'-azi-dothymidine (AZT), is thymidine. Production of thymidine is currently based in the hydrolysis of DNA from natural sources. A new biocatalytic approach for its production has been developed. It consists of transfering the 2'-deoxy-ribose moiety of 2'-deoxyinosine to thymine. The purine nucleoside phosphorylase of *Bacillus stearothermophilus* was used to carry out this reaction. A xantine oxidase is added in order to convert the concomitant hypoxanthine produced to uric acid, and thus draw the thermodynamic equilibrium towards the synthesis of thymidine (Figure 9). The yield of thymidine of this whole-cell biocatalytic route reached 68% under mild conditions [232].

Many catalytic functions that enzymes perform in the pharmaceutical industry is in resolution of racemic mixtures, in which one enantiomer is acylated or hydrolyzed selectively affording an easier separation of both enantiomers. One recent example of this is the resolution of pro-drug (R,S)-2-bromophenylacetic acid octyl ester. Rivera *et al.* [234] accomplished its resolution with high enantioselectivity using lipases embedded in crude latex from *Carica papaya*. An enantioselectivity *E*-value E > 200 was achieved using decane as solvent, 50 mM of substrate and 50 mg/mL enzyme/reaction medium. Furthermore, the E-value doubled after purifying latex and removing proteases.

Figure 9. Biocatalytic synthesis of thymidine using a Purine Nucleoside Phosphorilase (PNPase) and the biocatalytical removal of hypoxanthine with a Xanthine Oxidase (XAO) to obtain uric acid. Compounds: 1: 2'deoxyinosine; 2: Thymine; 3: Thymidine; 4: Hypoxanthine; 5: Uric acid (see also [233]).

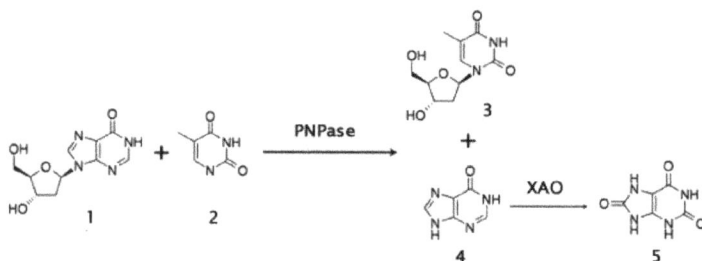

5. Conclusions

As outlined above, Biocatalysis is currently employed in a number of processes and products in diverse fields, and certainly new areas of application will be added. Advances in computational power have enabled the advent of bioinformatics, genomic sequencing and powerful analytic methods in physics, chemistry and molecular biology, which have allowed us to understand the dynamics, *in vivo* and *in vitro*, of biomacromolecules. The convergence of these tools has led to an improved access to more biocatalysts and to a deeper knowledge of them. In the case of enzymes, it has allowed us to explore their behavior, stability, specificity and even to begin to modify their very own nature through protein engineering. Larger availability of biocatalysts with superior qualities has been the main force behind the development of new industrial biocatalytic processes. The continued progress and interest in enzymes, serves as stimulus to make further efforts and ensure a steady success in meeting new synthetic challenges.

As per the environmental and economic benefits already reaped by the use of Biocatalysis in industry, it is possible to tell that the use of Biocatalysis is only expected to grow. This might be achieved with isolated enzymes but will probably be more successful using genetically engineered organisms where new pathways might be designed. The development of more robust, versatile, efficient enzymes via protein engineering, faster optimization of reaction conditions, microscale processing and better capabilities in design and machining new equipment will open new perspectives for the manufacture of many more products via Biocatalysis.

Future developments in Biocatalysis for industrial applications should be directed into the expansion of capabilities of current biocatalysts, to obtain new biocatalytic activities able to transform the vast amount of non-natural compounds found in industry and to achieve productivities comparable to current chemical processes. There is no doubt that modern biological tools, such as protein engineering and directed evolution will play an important role in meeting these challenges. As biodiversity remains largely unexplored, developing high-throughput screening methods to discover new efficient enzymes will also impact upon the development of biocatalyzed process for production of biobased chemicals.

Acknowledgments

We would like to thank to CONACYT for the scholarship provided to first author and for project CB 2008-01-104429.

Conflicts of Interest

The authors declare no conflict of interest.

References

1. Council of European Union. *En Route to the Knowledge-Based Bio-Economy*; German Presidency of the Council of European Union: Cologne, Germany, 2007.
2. Sandoval, G.; Plou, F.G. *Obtención enzimática de compuestos bioactivos a partir de recursos naturales iberoamericanos*; Consejo Superior de Instigaciones Cientificas (CSIC): Madrid, Spain, 2012; pp. 1–336.
3. Jahnz, U.; Schubert, M.; Baars, H.; Klaus, V. Process for producing the potential food ingredient DFA III from inulin-screening, genetic engineering, fermentation and immobilisation of inulase II. *Int. J. Pharm.* **2003**, *256*, 199–206.
4. Uchiyama, T.; Niwa, S.; Tanaka, K. Purification and properties of *Arthrobacter ureafaciens* inulase II. *Biochim. Biophys. Acta* **1973**, *315*, 412–420.
5. Kim, G.E.; Lee, S. Efficient production of DFA III (di-D-fructofuranose-dianhydride) from chicory root. In *Abstracts of the World Congress on Biotechnology*; DECHEMA: Berlin, Germany, 2000; Volume 272.
6. Yokota, A.; Hirayama, S.; Enomoto, K.; Miura, Y.; Takao, S.; Tomita, F. Production of inulin fructotransferase (depolymerizing) by *Arthrobacter* sp. H65–7 and preparation of DFA III from inulin by the enzyme. *J. Ferm. Bioeng.* **1991**, *72*, 258–261.
7. Kawamura, M.; Takahashi, S.; Uchiyama, T. Purification and some properties of inulin fructotransferase (depolymerizing) from Arthrobacter ilicis. *Agric. Biol. Chem.* **1988**, *52*, 3209–3210.
8. Gosling, A.; Stevens, G.W.; Barber, A.R.; Kentish, S.E.; Gras, S.L. Recent advances refining galactooligosaccharide production from lactose. *Food Chem.* **2010**, *121*, 307–318.
9. Rastall, R.A.; Gibson, G.R.; Gill, H.S.; Guarner, F.; Klaenhammer, T.R.; Pot, B.; Reid, G.; Rowland, I.R.; Sanders, M.E. Modulation of the microbial ecology of the human colon by probiotics, prebiotics and synbiotics to enhance human health: An overview of enabling science and potential applications. *FEMS Microbiol. Ecol.* **2005**, *52*, 145–152.
10. Sanz, J.I. Production of Glactooligo-Saccharidedes from Lactose by Immobilized β-Galactosidase and Posterioir Chromatographic Spearation. Ph.D. Thesis, Ohio State University, Columbus, OH, USA, 2009.
11. Gullón, B.; Gómez, B.; Martínez-Sabajanesb, M.; Yáñez, R.; Parajó, J.C.; Alonso, J.L. Pectic oligosaccharides: Manufacture and functional properties. *Trends Food Sci. Technol.* **2013**, *30*, 153–161.

12. Neri, D.F.M.; Balcão, V.M.; Costa, R.S.; Rocha, I.C.A.P.; Ferreira, E.M.F.C.; Torres, D.P.M.; Rodrigues, L.R.M.; Carvalho, L.B., Jr.; Teixeira, J.A. Galacto-oligosaccharides production during lactose hydrolysis by free *Aspergillus oryzae* β-galactosidase and immobilized on magnetic polysiloxane-polyvinyl alcohol. *Food Chem.* **2009**, *115*, 92–99.

13. Barreteau, H.; Delattre, C.; Michaud, P. Production of oligosaccharides as promising new food additive generation. *Food Technol. Biotechnol.* **2006**, *44*, 323–333.

14. Gaur, R.; Pant, H.; Jain, R.; Khare, S.K. Galacto-oligosaccharide synthesis by immobilized *Aspergillus oryzae* β-Galactosidase. *Food Chem.* **2006**, *97*, 426–430.

15. Whisner, C.M.; Weaver, C.M. Galacto-oligosaccharides: Prebiotic effects on calcium absorption and bone health. In *Nutritional Influences on Bone Health*; Burckhardt, P., Dawson-Hughes, B., Weaver, C.M., Eds.; Springer: London, UK, 2013; pp. 315–323.

16. Perugino, G.; Trincone, A.; Rossi, M.; Moracci, M. Oligosaccharide synthesis by glycosynthases. *Trends Biotech.* **2004**, *22*, 31–37.

17. Dias, L.G.; Veloso, A.C.A.; Correia, D.M.; Rocha, O.; Torres, D.; Rocha, I.; Rodrigues, L.R.; Peres, A.M. UV spectrophotometry method for the monitoring of galacto-oligosaccharides production. *Food Chem.* **2009**, *113*, 246–252.

18. Rodríguez, B.; Poveda, A.; Jiménez, J.; Ballesteros, A.O.; Plou, F.J. Galacto-oligosaccharide synthesis from lactose solution or skim milk using the β-galactosidase from *Bacillus circulans*. *J. Agric. Food Chem.* **2012**, *60*, 6391–6398.

19. Torres, D.; Gonçalves, M.D.P.F.; Teixeira, J.A.; Rodrigues, L. Galacto-oligosaccharides: Production, properties, applications, and significance as prebiotics. *Compr. Rev. Food Sci. F.* **2010**, *9*, 438–454.

20. Tzortzis, G.; Vulevic, J. Galacto-oligosaccharide prebiotics. In *Prebiotics and Probiotics Science and Technology*; Charalampopoulos, D., Rastall, R.A., Eds.; Springer: New York, NY, USA, 2009; pp. 207–244.

21. Park, H.Y.; Kim, H.J.; Lee, J.K.; Kim, D.; Oh, D.K. Galactooligosaccharide production by a thermostable β-galactosidase from *Sulfolobus solfataricus*. *World J. Microb. Biot.* **2008**, *24*, 1553–1558.

22. Rodriguez, B.; de Abreu, M.A.; Fernandez, L.; de Beer, R.; Poveda, A.; Jimenez, J.; Haltrich, D.; Ballesteros, A.O.; Fernandez, M.; Plou, F.J. Production of galacto-oligosaccharides by the β-galactosidase from *Kluyveromyces lactis*: Comparative analysis of permeabilized cells *versus* soluble enzyme. *J. Agric. Food Chem.* **2011**, *59*, 10477–10484.

23. Hsu, C.A.; Lee, S.L.; Chou, C.C. Enzymatic production of galactooligosaccharides by β-galactosidase from *Bifidobacterium longum* BCRC 15708. *J. Agric. Food Chem.* **2007**, *55*, 2225–2230.

24. Hansson, T.; Adlercreutz, P. Optimization of galactooligosaccharide production from lactose using β-glycosidases from hyperthermophiles. *Food Biotechnol.* **2001**, *15*, 79–97.

25. UBIC Europe Marketing Consulting. *The World GOS Market*; UBIC Europe Press: Sierre, Switzerland, 2010.

26. Padalino, M.; Perez-Conesa, D.; López-Nicolás, R.; Frontela-Saseta, C.; Berruezo, G. Effect of fructooligosaccharides and galactooligosaccharides on the folate production of some folate-producing bacteria in media cultures or milk. *Int. Dairy J.* **2012**, *27*, 27–33.

27. Fanaro, S.; Boehm, G.; Garssen, J.; Knol, J.; Mosca, F.; Stahl, B.; Vigi, V. Galacto-oligosaccharides and long-chain fructo-oligosaccharides as prebiotics in infant formulas: A review. *Acta Paediatr. Suppl.* **2005**, *94*, 22–26.

28. Watzl, B.; Girrbach, S.; Roller, M. Inulin, oligofructose and immunomodulation. *Br. J. Nutr.* **2005**, *93*, S49–S55.

29. Bornet, F.R.; Brouns, F.; Tashiro, Y.; Duvillier, V. Nutritional aspects of short-chain fructooligosaccharides: Natural occurrence, chemistry, physiology and health implications. *Dig. Liver Dis.* **2002**, *34*, S111–S120.

30. Yun, J.W. Fructooligosaccharides—Occurrence, preparation, and application. *Enzyme Microb. Tech.* **1996**, *19*, 107–117.

31. Arrizon, J.; Urias-Silvas, J.E.; Sandoval, G.; Mancilla-Margalli, N.A.; Gschaedler, A.C.; Morel, S.; Monsan, P. Production and bioactivity of fructan-type oligosaccharides. In *Food Oligosaccharides: Production, Analysis and Bioactivity*; Moreno, F.J., Sanz, M.L., Eds.; Wiley-Blackwell: Hoboken, NJ, USA, 2013; in press.

32. Beine, R.; Morarua, R.; Nimtz, M.; Na'amniehc, S.; Pawlowskic, A.; Buchholz, K.; Seibel, J. Synthesis of novel fructooligosaccharides by substrate and enzyme engineering. *J. Biotechnol.* **2008**, *138*, 33–41.

33. Castillo, E.; López-Munguía, A. Synthesis of levan in water-miscible organic solvents. *J. Biotechnol.* **2004**, *114*, 209–217.

34. Vega, R.J.; Zúniga, M.E. Potential application of commercial enzyme preparations for industrial production of short-chain fructooligosaccharides. *J. Mol. Catal. B Enzym.* **2012**, *76*, 44–51.

35. Singh, R.S.; Singh, R.P. Production of fructooligosaccharides from inulin by endoinulinases and their prebiotic potential. *Food Technol. Biotech.* **2010**, *48*, 435–450.

36. Tanriseven, A.; Aslan, Y. Immobilization of Pectinex Ultra SP-L to produce fructooligosaccharides. *Enzyme Microb. Technol.* **2005**, *36*, 550–554.

37. Guío, F.; Rodríguez, M.A.; Alméciga, C.J.; Sánchez, O.F. Recent trends in fructooligosaccharides production. *Recent Pat. Food Nutr. Agric.* **2009**, *1*, 221–230.

38. Jala, R.C.R.; Hu, P.; Yang, T.; Jiang, Y.; Zheng, Y; Xu, X. Lipases as biocatalysts for the synthesis of structured lipids. In *Lipases and Phospholipases. Methods in Molecular Biology*; Sandoval, G., Ed.; Springer-Humana Press: New York, NY, USA, 2012; Volume 861, Chapter 23.

39. Xu, X.; Akoh, C.C. Enzymatic production of Betapol and other specialty fats. In *Lipid Biotechnology*; Marcel Dekker: New York, NY, USA, 2002; pp. 461–478.

40. Odle, J. New insights into the utilization of medium-chain triglycerides by the neonate: Observations from a piglet model. *J. Nutr.* **1997**, *127*, 1061–1067.

41. Bugaut, M. Occurrence, absorption and metabolism of short chain fatty acids in the digestive tract of mammals. *Comp. Biochem. Physiol. B Biochem. Mol. Biol.* **1987**, *86*, 439–472.

42. Osborn, H.T.; Akoh, C. Structured lipids: Novel fats with medical, nutraceutical, and food applications. *Compr. Rev. Food Sci. F.* **2002**, *1*, 110–120.

43. Xu, X.; Hoy, C.E.; Balchen, S.; Adler-Nissen, J. Specific-Structured Lipid: Nutritional Perspectives and Production Potentials. In Proceedings of International Symposium on the Approach to Functional Cereals and Oils, CCOA, Beijing, China, 9–14 November 1997.

44. Trivedi, R.; Singh, R.P. Modification of oils and fats to produce structured lipids. *J. Oleo Sci.* **2005**, *54*, 423–430.

45. Hellner, G.; Tőke, E.R.; Nagy, V.; Szakács, G.; Poppe, L. Integrated enzymatic production of specific structured lipid and phytosterol ester compositions. *Process Biochem.* **2010**, *45*, 1245–1250.

46. Lee, K.T.; Akoh, C.C. Characterization of enzymatically synthesized structured lipids containing eicosapentaenoic, docosahexaenoic, and caprylic acids. *J. Am. Oil Chem. Soc.* **1998**, *75*, 495–499.

47. Akoh, C.C. Structured lipids. In *Food Lipids Chemistry, Nutrition, and Biotechnology*; Akoh, C.C., Min, D.B., Eds.; Marcel Dekker: New York, NY, USA, 1998; pp. 699–727.

48. Iwasaki, Y.; Yamane, T. Enzymatic synthesis of structured lipids. *J. Mol. Catal. B Enzym.* **2000**, *10*, 129–140.

49. Khodadadi, M.; Aziz, S.; St-Louis, R.; Kermash, S. Lipase-catalyzed synthesis and characterization of flaxseed oil-based structured lipids. *J. Funct. Foods* **2013**, *5*, 424–433.

50. Casas-Godoy, L.; Marty, A.; Sandoval, G.; Ferreira-Dias, S. Optimization of medium chain length fatty acid incorporation into olive oil catalyzed by immobilized Lip2 from *Yarrowia lipolytica*. *Biochem. Eng. J.* **2013**, *77*, 20–27.

51. Villeneuve, P.; Barouh, N.; Baréa, B.; Piombo, G.; Figueroa-Espinoza, M.C.; Turon, M.C.; Pina, M.; Lago, R. Chemoenzymatic synthesis of structured triacylglycerols with conjugated linoleic acids (CLA) in central position. *Food Chem.* **2007**, *100*, 1443–1452.

52. Nagachinta, S.; Akoh, C.C. Enrichment of palm olein with long chain polyunsaturated fatty acids by enzymatic acidolysis. *LWT Food Sci. Technol.* **2012**, *46*, 29–35.

53. Tecelão, C.; Rivera, I.; Sandoval, G.; Ferreira-Dias, S. *Carica papaya* latex: A low-cost biocatalyst for human milk fat substitutes production. *Eur. J. Lipid Sci. Technol.* **2012**, *114*, 266–276.

54. Nagao, T.; Watanabe, Y.; Maruyama, M.; Momokawa, Y.; Kishimoto, N.; Shimada, Y. One-pot enzymatic synthesis of docosahexaenoic acid-rich triacylglycerols at the sn-1(3) position using by-product from selective hydrolysis of tuna oil. *New Biotechnol.* **2011**, *28*, 7–13.

55. Buchholtz, K.; Volker, K.; Borscheuer, U.T. *Biocatalysts and Enzyme Technology*; Wiley-VCH: Berlin, Germany, 2005; pp. 1–465.

56. Bornscheuer, U.T.; Kazlauskas, R.J. *Hydrolases in Organic Synthesis—Regio- and Stereoselective Biotransformations*; Wiley-VCH: Berlin, Germany, 1999; pp. 1–355.

57. Cao, L. *Carrier-Bound Immobilized Enzymes*; Wiley-VCH: Berlin, Germany, 2005; pp. 1–578.

58. Gog, A.; Roman, M.; Toşa, M.; Paizs, C.; Irimie, F.D. Biodiesel production using enzymatic transesterification—Current state and perspectives. *Renew. Energ.* **2012**, *39*, 10–16.

59. Véras, I.C.; Silva, F.A.; Ferrão-Gonzales, A.D.; Moreau, V.H. One-step enzymatic production of fatty acid ethyl ester from high-acidity waste feedstocks in solvent-free media. *Bioresour. Technol*. **2011**, *102*, 9653–9658.

60. Fan, X.; Niehus, X.; Sandoval, G. Lipases as biocatalyst for biodiesel production. In *Lipases and Phospholipases. Methods in Molecular Biology*; Sandoval, G., Ed.; Springer-Humana Press: New York, NY, USA, 2012; Volume 861, Chapter 27.

61. Fukuda, H.; Kondo, A.; Noda, H. Biodiesel fuel production by transesterification of oils. *J. Biosci. Bioeng*. **2001**, *92*, 405–416.

62. Maleki, E.; Aroua, M.K.; Sulaiman, N.M.N. Improved yield of solvent free enzymatic methanolysis of palm and jatropha oils blended with castor oil. *Appl. Energ*. **2013**, *104*, 905–909.

63. Hama, S.; Kondo, A. Enzymatic biodiesel production: An overview of potential feedstocks and process development. *Bioresour. Technol.* **2013**, *135*, 386–395.

64. Al-Zuhair, S.; Hasan, M.; Ramachandran, K.B. Kinetics of the enzymatic hydrolysis of palm oil by lipase. *Process Biochem*. 2003, *38*, 1155–1163.

65. Salis, A.; Pinna, M.; Monduzzi, M.; Solinas, V. Biodiesel production from triolein and short chain alcohols through biocatalysis. *J. Biotechnol*. **2005**, *119*, 291–299.

66. Shimada, Y.; Watanabe, Y.; Samukawa, T.; Sugihara, A.; Noda, H.; Fukuda, H.; Tominaga, Y. Conversion of vegetable oil to biodiesel using immobilized *Candida antarctica* lipase. *J. Am. Oil Chem. Soc*. **1999**, *76*, 789–793.

67. Li, Q.; Xu, J.; Du, W.; Li, Y.; Liu, D. Ethanol as the acyl acceptor for biodiesel production. *Renew. Sust. Energ. Rev*. **2013**, *25*, 742–748.

68. Modi, M.K.; Reddy, J.R.; Rao, B.V.; Prasad, R.B. Lipase mediated conversion of vegetable oils into biodiesel using ethyl acetate as acyl acceptor. *Bioresour. Technol*. **2007**, *98*, 1260–1264.

69. Rivera, I.; Villanueva, G.; Sandoval, G. Biodiesel production from animal grease wastes by enzymatic catalysis. *Grasas Aceites* **2009**, *60*, 468–474.

70. Royon, D.; Daz, M.; Ellenrieder, G.; Locatelli, S. Enzymatic production of biodiesel from cotton seed oil using t-butanol as a solvent. *Bioresour. Technol*. **2007**, *98*, 648–653.

71. Abigor, R.D.; Uadia, P.O.; Foglia, T.A.; Haas, M.J.; Jones, K.C.; Okpefa, E.; Obibuzor, J.U.; Bafor, M.E. Lipase-catalysed production of biodiesel fuel from some Nigerian lauric oils. *Biochem. Soc. Trans*. **2000**, *28*, 979–981.

72. Nelson, L.; Foglia, T.; Marmer, W.N. Lipase-catalyzed production of biodiesel. *J. Am. Oil Chem. Soc*. **1996**, *73*, 1191–1195.

73. Linko, Y.Y.; Lamsä, M.; Huhtala, A.; Rantanen, O. Lipase biocatalysis in the production of esters. *J. Am. Oil Chem. Soc.* **1995**, *72*, 1293–1299.

74. Du, W.; Xu, Y.; Liu, D.; Zeng, J. Comparative study on lipase-catalyzed transformation of soybean oil for biodiesel production with different acyl acceptors. *J. Mol. Catal. B Enzym*. **2004**, *30*, 125–129.

360

75. Watanabe, Y.; Shimada, Y.; Sugihara, A.; Noda, H.; Fukuda, H.; Tominaga, Y. Continuous production of biodiesel fuel from vegetable oil using immobilized *Candida antarctica* lipase. *J. Am. Oil Chem. Soc.* **2000**, *77*, 355–360.

76. Zhang, B.; Weng, Y.; Xu, H.; Mao, Z. Enzyme immobilization for biodiesel production. *Appl. Microbiol. Biotechnol.* **2012**, *93*, 61–70.

77. Soumanou, M.M.; Bornscheuer, U.T. Lipase-catalyzed alcoholysis of vegetable oils. *Eur. J. Lipid Sci. Technol.* **2003**, *105*, 656–660.

78. Zhu, X.; Zhou, T.; Wu, X.; Cai, Y.; Yao, D.; Xie, C.; Liu, D. Covalent immobilization of enzymes within micro-aqueous organic media. *J. Mol. Catal. B Enzym.* **2011**, *3–4*, 145–149.

79. Zaks, A.; Klibanov, A.M. Enzyme-catalyzed processes in organic solvents. *Proc. Natl. Acad. Sci. USA* **1985**, *82*, 3192–3196.

80. Iso, M.; Chen, B.; Eguchi, M.; Kudo, T.; Shrestha, S. Production of biodiesel fuel from triglycerides and alcohol using immobilized lipase. *J. Mol. Catal. B Enzym.* **2001**, *16*, 53–58.

81. Chen, J.W.; Wu, W.T. Regeneration of immobilized *Candida antarctica* lipase for transesterification. *J. Biosci. Bioeng.* **2003**, *95*, 466–469.

82. Nie, K.; Xie, F.; Wang, F.; Tan, T. Lipase catalyzed methanolysis to produce biodiesel: optimization of the biodiesel production. *J. Mol. Catal. B Enzym.* **2006**, *43*, 142–147.

83. Ciftci, O.N.; Temelli, F. Enzymatic conversion of corn oil into biodiesel in a batch supercritical carbon dioxide reactor and kinetic modeling. *J. Supercrit. Fluids.* **2013**, *75*, 172–180.

84. Lin, Y.C.; Yang, P.M.; Chen, S.C.; Lin, J.F. Improving biodiesel yields from waste cooking oil using ionic liquids as catalysts with a microwave heating system. *Fuel Process. Technol.* **2013**, *115*, 57–62.

85. Earle, M.J.; Plechkova, N.V.; Seddon, K.R. Green synthesis of biodiesel using ionic liquids. *Pure Appl. Chem.* **2009**, *81*, 2045–2057.

86. Ha, S.H.; Lan, M.N.; Lee, S.H.; Hwang, S.M.; Koo, Y.M. Lipase-catalyzed biodiesel production from soybean oil in ionic liquids. *Enzyme Microb. Technol.* **2007**, *41*, 480–483.

87. Koda, R.; Numata, T.; Hama, S.; Tamalampudi, S.; Nakashima, K.; Tanaka, T; Ogino, C.; Fukuda, H.; Kondo, A. Ethanolysis of rapeseed oil to produce biodiesel fuel catalyzed by *Fusarium heterosporum* lipase-expressing fungus immobilized whole-cell biocatalysts. *J. Mol. Catal. B Enzym.* **2010**, *68*, 101–104.

88. Adachi, D.; Koha, F.; Hamab, S.; Ogino, C.; Kondo, A. A robust whole-cell biocatalyst that introduces a thermo- and solvent-tolerant lipase into *Aspergillus oryzae* cells: Characterization and application to enzymatic biodiesel production. *Enzyme Microb. Technol.* **2013**, *52*, 331–335.

89. Fukuda, H.; Hama, S.; Tamalampudi, S.; Noda, H. Whole-cell biocatalysts for biodiesel fuel production. *Trends Biotechnol.* **2008**, *26*, 668–673.

90. Atkinson, B.; Black, G.M.; Lewis, P.J.S.; Pinches, A. Biological particles of given size, shape, and density for use in biological reactors. *Biotechnol. Bioeng.* **1979**, *21*, 193–200.

91. Meng, X.; Yang, J.; Xu, X.; Zhang, L.; Nie, Q.; Xian, M. Biodiesel production from oleaginous microorganisms. *Renew. Energ.* **2009**, *34*, 1–5.

92. Turner, N.J.; Truppo, M.D. Biocatalysis enters a new era. *Curr. Opin. Chem. Biol.* **2013**, *17*, 212–214.

93. Woodley, J. New opportunities for biocatalysis: Making pharmaceutical processes greener. *Trends Biotechnol.* **2008**, *26*, 321–327.

94. Kittl, R.; Withers, S.G. New approaches to enzymatic glycoside synthesis through directed evolution. *Carbohyd. Res.* **2010**, *345*, 1272–1279.

95. Hay, A.S. Polymerization by oxidative coupling: Discovery and commercialization of PPO®. *J. Polym. Sci. Pol. Chem.* **1998**, *36*, 505–517.

96. He, F.; Li, S.; Garreau, H.; Vert, M.; Zhuo, R. Enzyme-catalyzed polymerization and degradation of copolyesters of ε-caprolactone and γ-butyrolactone. *Polymer* **2005**, *46*, 12682–12688.

97. Salvachúa, D.; Prieto, A.; Mattinen, M.L.; Tamminen, T.; Liitiä, T.; Lille, M.; Willför, S.; Martínez, A.T.; Martínez, M.J.; Faulds, C.B. Versatile peroxidase as a valuable tool for generating new biomolecules by homogeneous and heterogeneous cross-linking. *Enzyme Microb. Technol.* **2013**, *52*, 303–311.

98. Oguchi, T.; Tawaki, S.; Uyama, H.; Kobayashi, S. Enzymatic synthesis of soluble polyphenol. *Bull. Chem. Soc. Jpn.* **2000**, *73*, 1389–1396.

99. Dordick, J.S.; Marletta, M.A.; Klibanov, A.M. Polymerization of phenols catalyzed by peroxidase in nonaqueous media. *Biotech. Bioeng.* **1987**, *30*, 31–36.

100. Oguchi, T.; Tawaki, S.; Uyama, H.; Kobayashi, S. Soluble polyphenol. *Macromol. Rapid Commun.* **1999**, *20*, 401–403.

101. Mita, N.; Oguchi, T.; Tawaki, S.; Uyama, H.; Kobayashi, S. Control of structure and molecular weight of polyphenols in enzymatic oxidative polymerization. *Polymer Prepr.* **2000**, *41*, 223–224.

102. Kurioka, H.; Komatsu, I.; Uyama, H.; Kobayashi, S. Enzymatic oxidative polymerization of alkylphenols. *Macromol. Rapid Commun.* **1994**, *15*, 507–510.

103. Uyama, H.; Kurioka, H.; Kobayashi, S. Preparation of polyphenol particles by dispersion polymerization using enzyme as catalyst. *Chem. Lett.* **1995**, *24*, 795–796.

104. Uyama, H. Enzymatic polymerization. In *Future Directions in Biocatalysis*; Matsuda, T., Ed.; Elsevier Science: Cambridge, MA, USA, 2007; pp. 1–2.

105. Reihmann, M.; Ritter, H. Synthesis of phenol polymers using peroxidases. *Adv. Polym. Sci.* **2006**, *194*, 1–49.

106. Kobayashi, S.; Uyama, H.; Ikeda, R. Artificial Urushi. *Chem. Eur. J.* **2001**, *7*, 4755–4760.

107. Kim, Y.H.; An, E.S.; Song, B.K.; Kim, D.S.; Chelikani, R. Polymerization of cardanol using soybean peroxidase and its potential application as anti-biofilm coating material. *Biotechnol. Lett.* **2003**, *25*, 1521–1524.

108. Tonami, H.; Uyama, H.; Kobayashi, S.; Kubota, M. Peroxidase-catalyzed oxidative polymerization of m-substituted phenol derivatives. *Macromol. Chem. Phys.* **1999**, *200*, 2365–2371.

109. Kadota, J.; Fukuoka, T.; Uyama, H.; Hasegawa, K.; Kobayashi, S. New Positive-type photoresists based on enzymatically synthesized polyphenols. *Macromol. Rapid Commun.* **2004**, *25*, 441–444.

110. Antoniotti, S.; Santhanam, L.; Ahuja, D.; Hogg, M.G.; Dordick, J.S. Structural diversity of peroxidase-catalyzed oxidation products of o-methoxyphenols. *Org. Lett.* **2004**, *6*, 1975–1978.

111. Mita, N.; Tawaki, S.I.; Uyama, H.; Kobayashi, S. Laccase-catalyzed oxidative polymerization of phenols. *Macromol. Biosci.* **2003**, *3*, 253–257.

112. Ikeda, R.; Sugihara, J.; Uyama, H.; Kobayashi, S. Poly(2,6-dihydroxy-l,4-oxyphenylene synthesis of a new poly(phenylene oxide) derivative. *Polym. Bull.* **1997**, *38*, 273–277.

113. Ikeda, R.; Sugihara, J.; Uyama, H.; Kobayashi, S. Enzymatic oxidative polymerization of 2,6-dimethylphenol. *Macromolecules* **1996**, *29*, 8702–8705.

114. Uyama, H.; Kurioka, H.; Sugihara, J.; Komatsu, I.; Kobayashi, S. Oxidative polymerization of p-alkylphenols catalyzed by horseradish peroxidase. *J. Polym. Sci. Pol. Chem.* **1997**, *35*, 1453–1459.

115. Wang, P.; Martin, B.D.; Parida, S.; Rethwisch, D.G.; Dordick, J.S. Multienzymic synthesis of poly(hydroquinone) for use as a redox polymer. *J. Am. Chem. Soc.* **1995**, *117*, 12885–12886.

116. Akkara, J.A.; Senecal, K.J.; Kaplan, D.L. Synthesis and characterization of polymers produced by horseradish peroxidase in dioxane. *J. Polym. Sci. Pol. Chem.* **1991**, *29*, 1561–1574.

117. Akita, M.; Tsutsumi, D.; Kobayashi, M.; Kise, H. Structural change and catalytic activity of horseradish peroxidase in oxidative polymerization of phenol. *Biosci. Biotech. Bioch.* **2001**, *65*, 1581–1588.

118. Angerer, P.S.; Studer, A.; Witholt, B.; Li, Z. Oxidative polymerization of a substituted phenol with ion-paired horseradish peroxidase in an organic solvent. *Macromolecules* **2005**, *38*, 6248–6250.

119. Eker, B.; Zagorevski, D.; Zhu, G.; Linhardt, R.J.; Dordick, J.S. Enzymatic polymerization of phenols in room-temperature ionic liquids. *J. Mol. Catal. B Enzym.* **2009**, *59*, 177–184.

120. Mita, N.; Tawaki, S.; Uyama, H.; Kobayashi, S. Enzymatic oxidative polymerization of phenol in an aqueous solution in the presence of a catalytic amount of cyclodextrin. *Macromol. Biosci.* **2002**, *3*, 127–130.

121. Kim, Y.J.; Uyama, H.; Kobayashi, S. Regioselective synthesis of poly(phenylene) as a complex with poly(ethylene glycol) by template polymerization of phenol in water. *Macromolecules* **2003**, *36*, 5058–5060.

122. Kommareddi, N.S.; Tata, M.; Karayigitoglu, C.; John, V.T.; McPherson, G.L.; Herman, M.F.; Oconnor, C.J.; Lee, Y.S.; Akkara, J.A.; Kaplan, D.L. Enzymatic polymerizations using surfactant microstructures and the preparation of polymer-ferrite composites. *Appl. Biochem. Biotechnol.* **1995**, *51–52*, 241–252.

123. Ghan, R.; Shutava, T.; Patel, A.; John, V.T.; Lvov, Y. Enzyme-catalyzed polymerization of phenols within polyelectrolyte microcapsules. *Macromolecules* **2004**, *37*, 4519–4524.

124. Marín, F.R.; Frutos, M.J.; Pérez-Alvarez, J.A.; Martinez-Sánchez, F.; del Río, J.A. Flavonoids as nutraceuticals: Structural related antioxidant properties and their role on ascorbic acid preservation. *Stud. Nat. Prod. Chem.* **2002**, *26*, 741–778.

125. Di Carlo, G.; Mascolo, N.; Izzo, A.A.; Capasso, F. Flavonoids: Old and new aspects of a class of natural therapeutic drugs. *Life Sci.* **1999**, *65*, 337–353.

126. Rice-Evans, C.A.; Miller, N.J.; Paganga, G. Structure-antioxidant activity relationships of flavonoids and phenolic acids. *Free Radic. Biol. Med.* **1996**, *20*, 933–956.

127. *Flavonoids in Biology and Medicine III—Current Issues in Flavonoids Research*; Das, N.P., Cheeseman, K.H., Eds.; Informa Healthcare: London, UK, 1991; Volume 14, pp. 77–78.

128. Mejias, L.; Reihmann, M.H.; Sepulveda-Boza, S.; Ritter, H. New polymers from natural phenols using horseradish or soybean peroxidase. *Macromol. Biosci.* **2002**, *2*, 24–32.

129. Kurisawa, M.; Chung, J.E.; Uyama, H.; Kobayashi, S. Laccase-catalyzed synthesis and antioxidant property of poly(catechin). *Macromol. Biosci.* **2003**, *3*, 758–764.

130. Kurisawa, M.; Chung, J.E.; Uyama, H.; Kobayashi, S. Oxidative coupling of epigallocatechin gallate amplifies antioxidant activity and inhibits xanthine oxidase activity. *Chem. Commun.* **2004**, doi:10.1039/B312311A.

131. Kurisawa, M.; Chung, J.E.; Kim, Y.J.; Uyama, H.; Kobayashi, S. Amplification of antioxidant activity and xanthine oxidase inhibition of catechin by enzymatic polymerization. *Biomacromolecules* **2003**, *4*, 469–471.

132. Gonçalves, I.; Matamá, T.; Cavaco-Paulo, A.; Silva, C. Laccase coating of catheters with poly(catechin) for biofilm reduction. *Biocatal. Biotransform.* **2013**, in press.

133. Kurisawa, M.; Chung, J.E.; Uyama, H.; Kobayashi, S. Enzymatic synthesis and antioxidant properties of poly(rutin). *Biomacromolecules* **2003**, *4*, 1394–1399.

134. Božič, M.; Gorgieva, S.; Kokol, V. Laccase-mediated functionalization of chitosan by caffeic and gallic acids for modulating antioxidant and antimicrobial properties. *Carbohyd. Polym.* **2012**, *87*, 2388–2398.

135. Brzonova, I.; Steiner, W.; Zankel, A.; Nyanhongo, G.S. Enzymatic synthesis of catechol and hydroxyl-carboxic acid functionalized chitosan microspheres for iron overload therapy. *Eur. J. Pharm. Biopharm.* **2011**, *79*, 294–303.

136. Fras-Zemljič, L.; Kokol, V.; Čakara, D. Antimicrobial and antioxidant properties of chitosan-based viscose fibres enzymatically functionalized with flavonoids. *Text. Res. J.* **2011**, *81*, 1532–1540.

137. Sousa, F.; Guebitz, G.M.; Kokol, V. Antimicrobial and antioxidant properties of chitosan enzymatically functionalized with flavonoids. *Process Biochem.* **2009**, *44*, 749–756.

138. Pina-Luis, G.; Rosquete-Pina, G.; Valdés, A.C.; Ochoa, A.; Rivero, I.; Díaz-García, M.E. Morin functionalized Merrifield's resin: A new material for enrichment and sensing heavy metals. *React. Funct. Polym.* **2012**, *72*, 61–68.

139. Donato, L.; Chiappetta, G.; Drioli, E. Naringin-imprinted polymer layer using photo polymerization method. *Sep. Sci. Technol.* **2011**, *46*, 1555–1562.

364

140. Spizzirri, U.G.; Parisi, O.I.; Iemma, F.; Cirillo, G.; Puoci, F.; Curcio, M.; Picci, N. Antioxidant-polysaccharide conjugates for food application by eco-friendly grafting procedure. *Carbohyd. Polym.* **2010**, *79*, 333–340.

141. Jaeger, K.E.; Eggert, T. Lipases for biotechnology. *Curr. Opin. Biotechnol.* **2002**, *13*, 390–397.

142. Sharma, R.; Chisti, Y.; Banerjee, U.C. Production, purification, characterization and applications of lipases. *Biotechnol. Adv.* **2001**, *19*, 627–662.

143. Yu, Y.; Wu, D.; Liu, C.; Zhao, Z.; Yang, Y.; Li, Q. Lipase/esterase-catalyzed synthesis of aliphatic polyesters via polycondensation: A review. *Process Biochem.* **2012**, *47*, 1027–1036.

144. Yang, Y.; Yu, Y.; Zhang, Y.; Liu, C.; Shi, W.; Li, Q. Lipase/esterase-catalyzed ring-opening polymerization: A green polyester synthesis technique. *Process Biochem.* **2011**, *46*, 1900–1908.

145. He, F.; Wang, Y.P.; Liu, G.; Jia, H.L.; Feng, J.; Zhuo, R.X. Synthesis, characterization and ring-opening polymerization of a novel six-membered cyclic carbonate bearing pendent allyl ether group. *Polymer* **2008**, *49*, 1185–1190.

146. Runge, M.; O'Hagan, D.; Haufe, G. Lipase-catalyzed polymerization of fluorinated lactones and fluorinated hydroxycarboxylic acids. *J. Polym. Sci. Pol. Chem.* **2000**, *38*, 2004–2012.

147. Zinck, P. One-step synthesis of polyesters specialties for biomedical applications. *Rev. Environ. Sci. Biotechnol.* **2009**, *8*, 231–234.

148. Kobayashi, S.; Makino, A. Enzymatic polymer synthesis: An opportunity for green polymer chemistry. *Chem. Rev.* **2009**, *109*, 5288–5353.

149. Uyama, H.; Takamoto, T.; Kobayashi, S. Enzymatic synthesis of polyesters in ionic liquids. *Polym. J.* **2002**, *34*, 94–96.

150. Chaudhary, A.K.; Beckman, E.J.; Russell, A.J.; Rational control of polymer molecular weight and dispersity during enzyme-catalyzed polyester synthesis in supercritical fluids. *J. Am. Chem. Soc.* **1995**, *117*, 3728–3733.

151. Okumura, S.; Iwai, M.; Tominaga, T. Synthesis of ester oligomer by *Aspergillus niger* lipase. *Agr. Biol. Chem. (Tokyo)* **1984**, *48*, 2805–2813.

152. Binns, F.; Roberts, S.M.; Taylor, A.; Williams, C.F. Enzymic polymerization of unactivated diol/diacid system. *J. Chem. Soc. Perkin Trans.* **1993**, *1*, 899–904.

153. Linko, Y.Y.; Seppala, J. Producing high molecular weight biodegradable polyesters. *Chem. Tech.* **1996**, *26*, 25–31.

154. Gómez-Patiño, M.B.; Cassani, J.; Jaramillo-Flores, M.E.; Zepeda-Vallejo, L.G.; Sandoval, G.; Jimenez-Estrada, M.; Arrieta-Baez, D. Oligomerization of 10,16-dihydroxyhexadecanoic acid and methyl 10,16-dihydroxyhexadecanoate catalyzed by lipases. *Molecules* **2013**, *18*, 9317–9333.

155. Kobayashi, S.; Uyama, H.; Suda, S.; Namekawa, S. Dehydration polymerization in aqueous medium catalyzed by lipase. *Chem. Lett.* **1997**, *26*, 105–107.

156. Poojari, Y.; Palsule, A.S.; Cai, M.; Clarson, S.J.; Gross, R.A. Synthesis of organosiloxane copolymers using enzymatic polyesterification. *Eur. Polym. J.* **2008**, *44*, 4139–4145.

157. Yang, Y.; Lu, W.; Cai, J.; Hou, Y.; Ouyang, S.; Xie, W.; Gross, R.A. Poly(oleicdiacid-co-glycerol): Comparison of polymer structure resulting from chemical and lipase catalysis. *Macromolecules* **2011**, *44*, 1977–1985.

158. Korupp, C.; Weberskirch, R.; Muller, J.J.; Liese, A.; Hilterhaus, L. Scaleup of lipase-catalyzed polyester synthesis. *Org. Process. Res. Dev.* **2010**, *14*, 1118–1124.

159. Fehling, E.; Bergander, K.; Klein, E.; Weber, N.; Vosmann, K. Thiol-functionalized copolymeric polyesters by lipase-catalyzed esterification and transesterification of 1,12-dodecanedioic acid and its diethyl ester, respectively, with 1-thioglycerol. *Biotechnol. Lett.* **2010**, *32*, 1463–1471.

160. Hu, J.; Gao, W.; Kulshrestha, A.S.; Gross, R.A. Sweet polyesters: Lipase-catalyzed condensation polymerization of alditols. *Macromolecules* **2006**, *39*, 6789–6792.

161. Uyama, H.; Kobayashi, S. Enzymatic synthesis of polyesters via polycondensation. *Adv. Polym. Sci.* **2006**, *194*, 133–158.

162. Brazwell, E.M.; Filos, D.Y.; Morrow, C.J. Biocatalytic synthesis of polymers. III. Formation of a high molecular weight polyester through limitation of hydrolysis by enzyme-bound water and through equilibrium control. *J. Polym. Sci. Pol. Chem.* **1995**, *33*, 89–95.

163. Kobayashi, S. Recent developments in lipase-catalyzed synthesis of polyesters. *Macromol. Rapid Commun.* **2009**, *30*, 237–266.

164. Azim, H.; Dekhterman, A.; Jiang, Z.; Gross, R.A. *Candida antarctica* lipase B-catalyzed synthesis of poly(butylene succinate): Shorter chain building blocks also work. *Biomacromolecules* **2006**, *7*, 3093–3097.

165. Mesiano, A.J.; Beckman, E.J.; Russell, A.J. Biocatalytic synthesis of fluorinated polyesters. *Biotechnol. Prog.* **2000**, *16*, 64–68.

166. Uyama, H.; Yaguchi, S.; Kobayashi, S. Lipase-catalyzed polycondensation of dicarboxylic acid-divinyl esters and glycols to aliphatic polyesters. *J. Polym. Sci. Pol. Chem.* **1999**, *37*, 2737–2745.

167. Yao, D.; Li, G.; Kuila, T.; Li, P.; Kim, N.H.; Kim, S.I.; Lee, J.H. Lipase-catalyzed synthesis and characterization of biodegradable polyester containing l-malic acid unit in solvent system. *J. Appl. Polym. Sci.* **2011**, *120*, 1114–1120.

168. Steunenberg, P.; Uiterweerd, M.; Sijm, M.; Scott, E.L.; Zuilhof, H.; Sanders, J.P.M.; Franssen, M.C.R. Enzyme-catalyzed polymerization of β-alanine esters, a sustainable route towards the formation of poly-β-alanine. *Curr. Org. Chem.* **2013**, *17*, 682–690.

169. Kumar, D.; Bhalla, T.C. Microbial proteases in peptide synthesis: Approaches and applications. *Appl. Microbiol. Biotechnol.* **2005**, *68*, 726–736.

170. Kuhn, D.; Durrschmidt, P.; Mansfeld, J.; Ulbrich-Hofmann, R. Boilysin and thermolysin in dipeptide synthesis: A comparative study. *Biotechnol. Appl. Biochem.* **2002**, *36*, 71–76.

171. Bille, V.; Ripak, C.; Assche, I.; Forni, L.; Degelaen, J.; Searso, J. Semi-enzymic synthesis of somatostatin. In Proceedings of 21st European Peptide Symposium, Platja d'Aro, Spain, 2–8 September 1990.

172. Gu, Q.M.; Maslanka, W.W.; Cheng, H.N. Enzyme-catalyzed polyamides and their derivatives. In *Polymer Biocatalysis and Biomaterials II*; *ACS Symposium Series 999*; Cheng, H.N., Gross, R.A., Eds.; Oxford University Press: Washington, DC, USA, 2008; pp. 309–319.

173. Poulhès, F.; Mouysset, D.; Gil, G.; Bertrand, M.P.; Gastaldi, S. Speeding-up enzyme-catalyzed synthesis of polyamides using ω-amino-a-alkoxy-acetate as monomer. *Polymer* **2013**, *54*, 3467–3471.

174. Ikeda, R.; Tanaka, H.; Uyama, H.; Kobayashi, S. Laccase-catalyzed polymerization of acrylamide. *Macromol. Rapid Commun.* **1998**, *19*, 423–425.

175. Hollmann, F.; Gumulya, Y.; Tölle, C.; Liese, A.; Thum, O. Evaluation of the laccase from *Myceliophthora thermophila* as industrial biocatalyst for polymerization reactions. *Macromolecules* **2008**, *41*, 8520–8524.

176. Emery, O.; Lalot, T.; Brigodiot, M.; Maréchal, E. Free-radical polymerization of acrylamide by horseradish peroxidase-mediated initiation. *J. Polym. Sci. Pol. Chem.* **1997**, *35*, 3331–3333.

177. Mucientes, A.E.; Santiago, F.; Carrero, A.M.; Talavera, B. Superabsorbent hydrogels of poly(sodium acrylate) with crude and exfoliated vermiculites. *J. Polym. Eng.* **2013**, *33*, 61–69.

178. Jones, N.A.; Atkins, E.D.T.; Hill, M.J.; Cooper, S.J.; Franco, L. Chain-folded lamellar crystals of aliphatic polyamides. comparisons between nylons 44, 64, 84, 104, and 124. *Macromolecules* **1996**, *29*, 6011–6018.

179. Ragupathy, L.; Ziener, U.; Dyllick-Brenzinger, R.; von Vacano, B.; Landfester, K. Enzyme-catalyzed polymerizations at higher temperatures: Synthetic methods to produce polyamides and new poly(amide-co-ester)s. *J. Mol. Catal. B Enzym.* **2012**, *76*, 94–105.

180. Kalra, B.; Gross, R.A. Horseradish peroxidase mediated free radical polymerization of methyl methacrylate. *Biomacromolecules* **2000**, *1*, 501–505.

181. Singh, A.; Ma, D.C.; Kaplan, D.L. Enzyme-mediated free radical polymerization of styrene. *Biomacromolecules* **2000**, *1*, 592–596.

182. Sandoval, G.; Rivera, I.; Barrera-Rivera, K.A.; Martínez-Richa, A. Biopolymer synthesis catalyzed by tailored lipases. *Macromol. Symp.* **2010**, *289*, 135–139.

183. Varma, I.K.; Albertsson, A.C.; Rajkhowa, R.; Srivastava, R.K. Enzyme catalyzed synthesis of polyesters. *Prog. Polym. Sci.* **2005**, *30*, 949–981.

184. Kobayashi, S. Enzymatic polymerization: A new method of polymer synthesis. *J. Polym. Sci. Pol. Chem.* **1999**, *37*, 3041–3056.

185. Kobayashi, S.; Uyama, H.; Ohmae, M. Enzymatic polymerization for precision polymer synthesis. *Bull. Chem. Soc. Jpn.* **2001**, *74*, 613–635.

186. Uyama, H.; Kikuchi, H.; Takeya, K.; Kobayashi, S. Lipase-catalyzed ring-opening polymerization and copolymerization of 15-pentadecanolide. *Acta Polym.* **1996**, *47*, 357–360.

187. Uyama, H.; Takeya, K.; Kobayashi, S. Enzymatic ring-opening polymerization of lactones to polyesters by lipase catalyst: Unusually high reactivity of macrolides. *Bull. Chem. Soc. Jpn.* **1995**, *68*, 56–61.

188. Uyama, H.; Takeya, K.; Hoshi, N.; Kobayashi, S. Lipase-catalyzed ring-opening polymerization of 12-dodecanolide. *Macromolecules* **1995**, *28*, 7046–7050.

189. Bisht, K.S.; Henderson, L.A.; Gross, R.A. Enzyme-catalyzed ring-opening polymerization of ω-pentadecalactone. *Macromolecules* **1997**, *30*, 2705–2711.

190. Hunsen, M.; Azim, A.; Mang, H.; Wallner, S.R.; Ronkvist, A.; Xie, W.C.; Gross, R.A. A cutinase with polyester synthesis activity. *Macromolecules* **2007**, *40*, 148–150.

191. Nishida, H.; Yamashita, M.; Nagashima, M.; Endo, T.; Tokiwa, Y. Synthesis of metal-free poly(1,4-dioxan-2-one) by enzyme-catalyzed ring-opening polymerization. *J. Polym. Sci. Pol. Chem.* **2000**, *38*, 1560–1567.

192. Jiang, Z.; Azim, H.; Gross. R.A. Lipase-catalyzed copolymerization of ω-pentadecalactone with *p*-dioxanone and characterization of copolymer thermal and crystalline properties. *Biomacromolecules* **2007**, *8*, 2262–2269.

193. Fickers, P.; Marty, A.; Nicaud, J.M. The lipases from *Yarrowia lipolytica*: Genetics, production, regulation, biochemical characterization and biotechnological applications. *Biotechnol. Adv.* **2011**, *29*, 632–644.

194. Uyama, H.; Kikuchi, H.; Takeya, K.; Hoshi, N.; Kobayashi, S. Immobilized lipase showing high catalytic activity toward enzymatic ring-opening polymerization of macrolides. *Chem. Lett.* **1996**, *25*, 107–108.

195. Kobayashi, S.; Uyama, H. Precision enzymatic polymerization to polyesters with lipase catalysts. *Macromol. Symp.* **1999**, *144*, 237–246.

196. Kobayashi, S.; Uyama, H.; Namekawa, S. *In vitro* biosynthesis of polyesters with isolated enzymes in aqueous systems and organic solvents. *Polym. Degrad. Stabil.* **1998**, *59*, 195–201.

197. Kumar, A.; Kalra, B.; Dekhterman, A.; Gross, R.A. Efficient ring-opening polymerization and copolymerization of ε-caprolactone and ω-pentadecalactone catalyzed by *Candida antartica* lipase B. *Macromolecules* **2000**, *33*, 6303–6309.

198. Kobayashi, S.; Uyama, H.; Namekawa, S.; Hayakawa, H. Enzymatic ring-opening polymerization and copolymerization of 8-octanolide by lipase catalyst. *Macromolecules* **1998**, *31*, 5655–5659.

199. Namekawa, S.; Uyama, H.; Kobayashi, S. Lipase-catalyzed ring-opening polymerization of 16-hexadecanolide. *P. Jpn. Acad. B* **1998**, *74*, 65–68.

200. Ebata, H.; Toshima, K.; Matsumura, S. Lipase-catalyzed transformation of poly(ε-caprolactone) into cyclic dicaprolactone. *Biomacromolecules* **2000**, *1*, 511–514.

201. Sugihara, S.; Toshima, K.; Matsumura, S. New strategy for enzymatic synthesis of high-molecular-weight poly(butylene succinate) via cyclic oligomers. *Macromol. Rapid Commun.* **2006**, *27*, 203–207.

202. Kikuchi, H.; Uyama, H.; Kobayashi, S. Lipase-catalyzed ring-opening polymerization of substituted lactones. *Polym. J.* **2002**, *34*, 835–893.

203. Küllmer, K.; Kikuchi, H.; Uyama, H.; Kobayashi, S. Lipase-catalyzed ring-opening polymerization of α-methyl-δ-valerolactone and α-methyl-ε-caprolacton. *Macromol. Rapid. Commun.* **1998**, *19*, 127–130.

204. Cordova, A.; Iversen, T.; Martinelle, M. Lipase-catalysed formation of macrocycles by ring-opening polymerisation of ε-caprolactone. *Polymer* **1998**, *39*, 6519–6524.

205. Namekawa, S.; Uyama, H.; Kobayashi, S. Lipase-catalyzed ring-opening and copolymerization of β-propiolactione. *Polym. J.* **1996**, *28*, 730–731.

206. Suzuki, Y.; Taguchi, S.; Hisano, T.; Toshima, K.; Matsumura, S.; Doi, Y. Correlation between structure of the lactones and substrate specificity in enzyme-catalyzed polymerization for the synthesis of polyesters. *Biomacromolecules* **2003**, *4*, 537–543.

207. Nagasawa, T.; Shimizu, H.; Yamada, H. The superiority of the third-generation catalyst, *Rhodococcus rhodochrous* J1 nitrile hydratase, for industrial production of acrylamide. *Appl. Microbiol. Biotechnol.* **1993**, *40*, 189–195.

208. Thomas, S.M.; DiCosimo, R.; Nagarajan, V. Biocatalysis: Applications and potentials for the chemical industry. *Trends Biotechnol.* **2002**, *20*, 238–242.

209. Chassin, C. A biotechnological process for the production of nicotinamide. *Chim. Oggi.* **1996**, *14*, 9–12.

210. Nagasawa, T.; Matthew, C.D.; Mauger, J.; Yamada, H. Nitrile hydratase-catalyzed production of nicotinamide from 3-cyanopyridine in *Rhodococcus rhodochrous* J1. *Appl. Environ. Microbiol.* **1988**, *54*, 1766–1769.

211. Robins, K.T.; Nagasawa, T. Process for Preparing Amides. PCT Int. Appl. US 7,666,635 B2, 23 February 2010.

212. Heveling, J.; Armbruster, E.; Utiger, L.; Rhoner, M.; Dettwiler, H.R.; Chuck, R.J. Process for Preparing Nicotinamide. US Patent 5,719,045, 17 February 1998.

213. Straathof, A.J.J. Transformation of biomass into commodity chemicals using enzymes or cells. *Chem. Rev.* **2013**, doi:10.1021/cr400309c.

214. Vuyyuru, K.R.; Strasser, P. Oxidation of biomass derived 5-hydroxymethylfurfural using heterogeneous and electrochemical catalysis. *Catal. Today* **2012**, *195*, 144–154.

215. Casanova, O.; Iborra, S.; Corma, A. Biomass into chemicals: Aerobic oxidation of 5-hydroxymethyl-2-furfural into 2,5-furandicarboxylic acid with gold nanoparticle catalysts. *ChemSusChem* **2009**, *2*, 1138–1144.

216. Koopman, F.; Wierckx, N.; de Winde, J.H.; Ruijssenaars, H.J. Efficient whole-cell biotransformation of 5-(hydroxymethyl)furfural into FDCA, 2,5-furandicarboxylic acid *Bioresour. Technol.* **2010**, *101*, 6291–6296.

217. Krystof, M.; Pérez-Sánchez, M.; Domínguez de María, P. Lipase-mediated selective oxidation of furfural and 5-hydroxymethylfurfural. *ChemSusChem* **2013**, *6*, 826–830.

218. Van Deurzen, M.P.J.; van Rantwijk, F.; Sheldon, R.A. Chloroperoxidase-catalyzed oxidation of 5-hydroxymethylfurfural. *J. Carbohydr. Chem.* **1997**, *16*, 299–309.

219. Panke, S.; Wubbolts, M. Advances in biocatalytic synthesis of pharmaceutical intermediates. *Curr. Opin. Chem. Biol.* **2005**, *9*, 188–194.

220. Ooshima, H.; Mori, H.; Harano, Y. Synthesis of aspartame precursor by solid thermolysin in organic solvent. *Biotechnol. Lett.* **1985**, *7*, 789–792.

221. Griengl, H.; Klempier, N.; Pochlauer, P.; Schmidt, M.; Shi, N.Y.; Zabelinskaja-Mackova, A.A. Enzyme catalysed formation of (S)-cyanohydrins derived from aldehydes and ketones in a biphasic solvent system. *Tetrahedron* **1998**, *54*, 14477–14486.

222. Bieber, L.L. Carnitine. *Annu. Rev. Biochem.* **1988**, *57*, 261–283.

223. Fritz, I.B. Action of carnitine on long chain fatty acid oxidation by liver. *Am. J. Physiol.* **1959**, *197*, 297–304.

224. Meyer, H.P.; Kiener, A.; Imwinkelried, R.; Shaw, N. Biotransformations for fine chemicals production. *Chimia* **1997**, *51*, 287–289.

225. Bommarius, A.S.; Schwarm, M.; Stingl, K.; Kottenhahn, M.; Huthmacher, K.; Drauz, K. Synthesis and use of enantiomerically pure *tert*-leucine. *Tetrahedron Asymmetry* **1995**, *6*, 2851–2888.

226. Menzel, A.; Werner, H.; Altenbuchner, J.; Gröger, H. From enzymes to "designer bugs" in reductive amination: A new process for the synthesis of L-*tert*-leucine using a whole cell-catalyst. *Eng. Life Sci.* **2004**, *4*, 573–576.

227. Krix, G.; Bommarius, A.S.; Drauz, K.; Kottenhahn, M.; Schwarm, M.; Kula, M.R. Enzymatic reduction of α-keto acids leading to L-amino acids, D- or L-hydroxy acids. *J. Biotechnol.* **1997**, *53*, 29–39.

228. Furuhashi, K. Biological routes to optically active epoxides. In *Chirality in Industry*; Collins, A.N., Sheldrake, G.N., Crosby, J.C., Eds.; John Wiley & Sons: NJ, USA, 1992; pp. 167–186.

229. Li, K.; Frost, J. Synthesis of vanillin from glucose. *J. Am. Chem. Soc.* **1998**, *120*, 10545–10546.

230. Aresta, M.; Quaranta, E.; Liberio, R.; Dileo, C.; Tommasi, I. Enzymatic synthesis of 4-OH-benzoic acid from phenol and CO_2: The first example of a biotechnological application of a carboxylase enzyme. *Tetrahedron* **1998**, *54*, 8841–8846.

231. Baldessari, A. Lipases as catalysts in synthesis of fine chemicals. In *Lipases and Phospholipases. Methods in Molecular Biology*; Sandoval, G., Ed.; Springer-Humana Press: New York, NY, USA, 2012; Volume 861, pp. 445–448.

232. Pal, S.; Nair, V. Enzymatic synthesis of thymidine using bacterial whole cells and isolated purine nucleoside phosphorylase. *Biocatal. Biotransform.* **1997**, *15*, 147–158.

233. Liese, A.; Villela-Filho, M. Production of fine chemicals using biocatalysis. *Curr. Opin. Biotechnol.* 1999, *10*, 595–603.

234. Rivera, I.; Mateos, J.C.; Marty, A.; Sandoval, G.; Duquesne, S. Lipase from Carica papaya latex presents high enantioselectivity toward the resolution of prodrug (R,S)-2-bromophenylacetic acid octyl ester. *Tetrahedron Lett.* **2013**, *54*, 5523–5526.

Biotechnological Applications of Transglutaminases

Natalie M. Rachel and Joelle N. Pelletier

Abstract: In nature, transglutaminases catalyze the formation of amide bonds between proteins to form insoluble protein aggregates. This specific function has long been exploited in the food and textile industries as a protein cross-linking agent to alter the texture of meat, wool, and leather. In recent years, biotechnological applications of transglutaminases have come to light in areas ranging from material sciences to medicine. There has also been a substantial effort to further investigate the fundamentals of transglutaminases, as many of their characteristics that remain poorly understood. Those studies also work towards the goal of developing transglutaminases as more efficient catalysts. Progress in this area includes structural information and novel chemical and biological assays. Here, we review recent achievements in this area in order to illustrate the versatility of transglutaminases.

Reprinted from *Biomolecules*. Cite as: Rachel, N.M.; Pelletier, J.N. Biotechnological Applications of Transglutaminases. *Biomolecules* **2013**, *3*, 870-888.

1. Introduction

Harnessing the catalytic properties of enzymes is a field of research that continues to receive increasing attention. One of the most attractive characteristics of biocatalysts is that they are often highly chemo-, regio-, and stereo-selective. This provides potential for highly specific chemical transformations of complex, functionalized molecules. Additionally, biocatalysts are non-toxic, degradable, and functional in aqueous media at moderate temperatures and pressure, making them of high interest in the development of environmentally respectful synthetic methodologies. Due to these desirable properties, chemists are increasingly incorporating enzymes into their reaction schemes.

The synthesis of amide bonds has the potential to benefit greatly from biocatalysis. The high stability of the amide functionality makes it one of the most favorable and commonly used in organic synthesis [1]. Some examples of compounds containing biocatalyzed amide bonds are found in the large-scale production of Atorvastatin (commercialized as Lipitor™), Nylon, penicillin, and aspartame. The high activation barrier to amide-bond formation is synthetically challenging; further development of biocatalysts for formation of a broad range of compounds remains of interest. Transglutaminases (TGases) are a family of enzymes (EC 2.3.2.13) that catalyze an acyl-transfer reaction between the γ-carboxamide group of a protein- or peptide-bound glutamine and the ε-amino group of a lysine residue, resulting in the formation of a relatively protease-resistant isopeptide bond [2] (Figure 1). TGases, having evolved to catalyze the formation of amide bonds with little competition from the reverse hydrolytic reaction, are a promising biocatalytic alternative to classical organic chemistry for amide bond synthesis.

Figure 1. Amide bond formation catalyzed by TGase. Peptide- or protein-bound glutamines and lysines serve as substrates, releasing ammonia in the process.

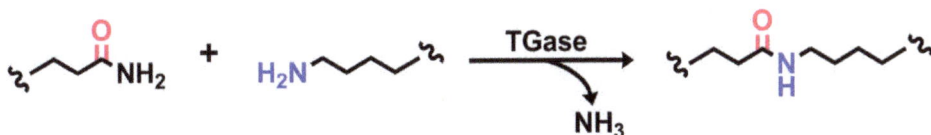

TGases have been identified in many different of taxonomic groups, including microorganisms, plants, invertebrates, and mammals [3]. With respect to application, the vast majority of research has been done on two forms of the enzyme: the first is a calcium-dependant TGase found in tissues of animals and humans, referred to as transglutaminase 2 (TG2). TG2 is implicated in a number of physiological roles including endocytosis, cell-matrix assembly, apoptosis, and cellular adhesive processes [4–6]. There is much interest in studying TG2 from a medical standpoint to better understand its role in disease, including cataract formation [7], celiac sprue [8], and psoriasis [9]. The second enzyme is a calcium-independent, microbial transglutaminase (MTG), which was first isolated from *Streptomyces mobaraense* [10] and has since been isolated from other microbial strains, including, but not limited to, *S. griseocarneum*, *S. hygroscopicus*, and *B. subtilis* [11,12]. Both types of TGases have been studied extensively in academia and industry. Mechanisms for the reaction catalyzed by both TGase types have been proposed. The catalytic triad characteristic to cysteine proteases is present in the human factor XIII TGase (Cys314, His373, and Asp396) [13]. These residues correspond to Cys276, His334, and Asp358 in the highly conserved active site of guinea pig TG2 [14]. In the proposed mechanism, the cysteine and the histidine residues are principally involved in the acyl transfer reaction, where the aspartic acid residue hydrogen bonds with the histidine, maintaining a catalytically-competent orientation. The crystal structure of MTG revealed that this triad is not conserved; rather, it was proposed that MTG uses a cysteine protease-like mechanism in which Asp255 plays the role of the histidine residue in factor XIII-like TGases [15].

Of the two, MTG is more robust, and is commonly employed as a tool in the food industry to catalyze the cross-linking of meat, soy, and wheat proteins to improve and modify their texture and tensile properties [11,16]. Despite the medical importance of TG2 and widespread industrial use of MTG, many properties such as ligand binding, catalytic mechanism, and function in health and disease remain poorly understood, ultimately hindering further successful integration of these enzymes into novel applications and processes. Nonetheless, researchers are continually looking for ways to exploit the cross-linking activity of TGases for novel applications outside of the fields of human physiology and the food industry. Examples include tissue engineering [17], as well as textile and leather processing [18]. These applications generally utilize TGase to serve the same purpose it does in the food industry: non-specific protein cross-linking to provide improved physical and textural properties. A recent example involved increasing the mechanical strength of amniotic membrane, for applications in regenerative medicine [19]. The advances made in these fields have been covered in recent reviews [20,21], and will not be discussed in detail here. This review focuses on recent advances made in studying TGases in the scope of biotechnology and characterization, including advances in assay development, site-specific modification of biomacromolecules, and protein labeling.

2. Production and Engineering of TGases

2.1. Transglutaminase Expression and Purification

Both TG2 and MTG are readily recombinantly expressed and purified in bacterial hosts [22,23]. Using these methods, the production of TG2 in a hexa-histidine labeled form has become routine [22,24,25], although other forms of TG2 can remain a challenge to obtain in good yield. A complementary technique for the purification of hTG2 was recently reported, in which hTG2 was expressed as a fusion with glutathione *S*-transferase (GST) and followed by a one-step affinity chromatography purification [26]. Unlike TG2, the purification of the most widely used MTG (from *S. mobaraensis* and homologs) is complicated by the fact that the native enzyme is expressed as a zymogen (pro-MTG); a 46-residue *N*-terminal pro-sequence must be proteolytically cleaved in order for MTG to be rendered functional. There are reports of other MTGs that can be directly expressed as recombinant, active enzymes [27,28], however these are not as well characterized. Three solutions to this problem have been reported: (1) expression of pro-MTG followed by *in vitro* activation using a protease[29,30]; (2) direct expression of insoluble MTG lacking its *N*-terminal pro-sequence (mature MTG) followed by refolding [23]; or (3) co-expression of pro-MTG with the activating protease in *Streptomyces* [31] or *E. coli* [32]. Each of these strategies has limitations: the first strategy can achieve high yields and activity, but involves lengthy activation methodologies (N.M. Rachel and J.N. Pelletier, unpublished observations). The second often leads to a low expression or insoluble protein, while the third strategy can result in protein degradation, affecting the yield [33].

Recently, MTG from *S. hygroscopicus* was successfully produced in its active form in *E. coli* by simultaneously expressing the pro-sequence and mature MTG as separate polypeptides under the control of a single T7 promoter [34]. Expression of the pro-sequence prior to the mature MTG polypeptide was found to be essential for activity, as well as an *N*-terminal pelB sequence for periplasmic localization. This supports the hypothesis that the pro-sequence is required for proper folding and soluble expression of MTG. Improved efficiency of MTG maturation in *Streptomyces* was also recently reported, by engineering more protease-labile linkers into the pro-propeptide [35]. The structural basis for this requirement can be understood upon observing the crystal structure of pro-MTG, which was determined at 1.9-Å resolution [36] (Figure 2). The pro-sequence folds into an α-helix, covering the putative active site cleft by adopting an L-shaped conformation. The active site cleft is predominantly composed of two flexible loop regions, explaining how the presence of this ordered helix stimulates proper folding, in a fashion similar to that of the pro-sequences for subtilisin BPN' and other proteases [37].

Two biophysical studies focusing on the detailed mechanism of unfolding and refolding of MTG were reported by Suzuki and colleagues [38,39]. In the first, a two-step refolding process of acid-denatured MTG was proposed after probing the effect of pH and salt concentration. The authors then applied this protocol to pro-MTG in the second report, such that by partially unfolding the enzyme, the internal residues would be exposed when in the presence of a deuterated solvent. This solvent exposure is often necessary so that hydrogen back-exchange occurs for all residues in the protein, allowing for accurate measurements using nuclear magnetic resonance (NMR) spectroscopy to be taken. Complete back-exchanges for internal residues of pro-MTG were observed by NMR spectroscopy, and the authors were able to recover the properly folded form of both pro-MTG and mature MTG, reporting refolding yields of 84% and 40%, respectively.

Figure 2. Crystal structure of MTG (PDB ID: 3IU0). The active site of the zymogen is covered (left) by an α-helix (gold), which is cleaved upon activation, exposing the active site cysteine residue (right, yellow spheres) that is critical for activity.

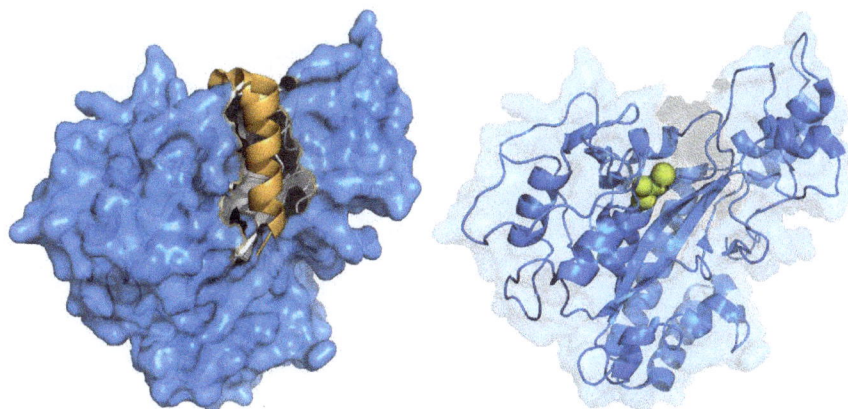

2.2. Engineering TGases for Altered Function and Properties

The design of enzymes with improved or non-native properties has become a common approach [40–42]. Engineering TGases may provide solutions to increase their applicability in biocatalytic contexts. TG2 has been engineered towards catalyzing amide bond formation between various synthetic substrates, by altering its substrate specificity [43]. A model peptide substrate, benzyloxycarbonyl-L-glutaminylglycine (Z-QG), was modified to yield a fluorescent umbelliferyl ester derivative (Z-GU) in order to screen for variants of TG2 with altered transpeptidase activity. Two separate point mutations were identified, which broaden the substrate scope of TG2, resulting in variants that can accept threonine methyl ester. To the best of our knowledge, this remains the only study focused on evolving TG2, and so the efforts in this field remain largely conservative.

With respect to MTG, logistical complications of expressing the mature enzyme and the lack of a simple, high-throughput screening assay remain major challenges for engineering. Nonetheless, enhancing the activity and thermostability of MTG has been probed by two different studies. Pietzsch and colleagues [44] performed random mutagenesis using a microtiter plate-based screening method adapted to the standard hydroxamate assay [45] to measure activity. A library of 5500 clones generated randomly by error-prone PCR was initially screened, 70 of which showed higher activity following incubation at 60 °C. Following another round of mutagenesis, the nine clones with the highest residual activity were further characterized. The single-residue variant Ser2Pro was found to have an optimal functioning temperature of 55 °C, an improvement of 5 °C compared to the native enzyme. More recent efforts using saturation mutagenesis and DNA-shuffling by the same group yielded a triply substituted variant of MTG exhibiting a 12-fold and 10-fold higher half-life at 60 °C and 50 °C, respectively [46], although the Ser2Pro variant remained the most active at 55 °C. Chen and colleagues also evolved thermostable variants of MTG by combining saturation mutagenesis and the deletion of various N-terminal residues [47]. The variant Del 1-4E5D, which lacks the first four N-terminal residues and substitutes the fifth residue, exhibits a modest 1.85-fold higher specific activity and a 2.7-fold higher half-life at 50 °C compared to the wild-type enzyme.

Determining what residues to be the focus of mutagenesis is key to the success of any protein engineering initiative. In order to probe which residues may be necessary for MTG activity, an alanine screen of 29 residues that are either located in proximity to, or constitute the putative active site, was performed [48]. Docking and molecular dynamics simulations were also performed in order to propose the manner in which the model peptide substrate Z-QG binds to the enzyme, and the mutagenesis results were interpreted in the context of the docking results. The results suggest that an extended surface along the active site cleft is involved in binding of a protein substrate. Furthermore, it appears that a number of hydrophobic and aromatic residues are important for interacting with Z-QG, which is summarized in Figure 3. Despite this data, further evolution of TGases has yet to be reported.

3. Substrate Specificity

While the acyl-transfer reaction catalyzed by TGase between the peptide- or protein-bound glutamine and lysine substrates is well characterized, the preference the enzymes display towards a specific peptide sequence is not obvious. Most glutamine and lysine residues will serve as a substrate, with varying degrees of reactivity, as long as they are accessible to TGase [49]. This limits the application scope of TGases where reactivity towards a specific substrate is required, such as protein labeling. Ten years ago, highly-reactive glutamine-containing substrates for TG2 were reported, which in some cases are related to physiologically-relevant targets [25], and in other cases were empirically designed and contain more than one glutamine for increased reactivity [50]. The secondary structure surrounding the glutamine appears to be important in defining reactivity [25]. With respect to MTG, the native substrates and physiological function of the enzyme are not known. This has led researchers to approach the question of TGase's poorly understood substrate preferences from two different perspectives. The first is to probe the specificity of the enzyme towards specific peptide or protein substrates of interest by analyzing which glutamine or lysine residues are reactive and to what degree. The second is to screen libraries of peptide sequences or other compounds with the goal of either identifying a preferred sequence pattern, or to identify highly reactive substrates. Recent advances with both of these approaches TGase substrate specificity offer further insight into the utility as well as the remaining limitations of these enzymes toward their biotechnological application.

Figure 3. Surface representation of MTG (PDB ID: 1UI4), illustrating active site residues investigated by mutagenesis (pink and orange regions) [48]. The active site cleft is indicated by an asterisk. Residues in orange, upon substitution to alanine, resulted in activity of 5% or less than the wild type, revealing their importance.

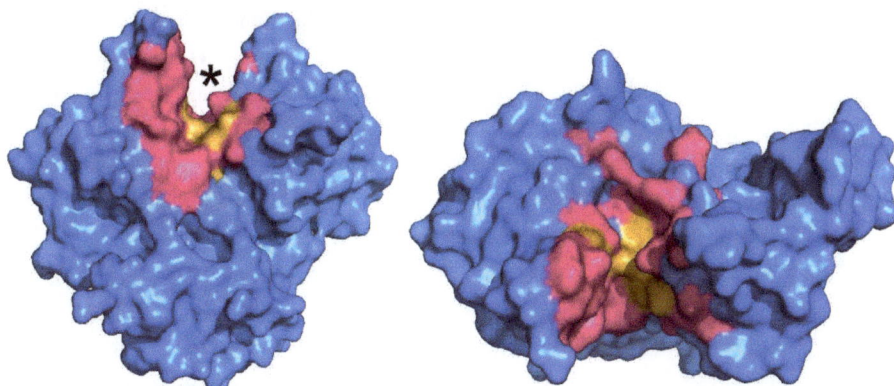

The reactivity of MTG towards glutamine residues on several different proteins has been recently investigated. Using the sensitivity of mass spectrometry (MS), the identification of the glutamine residues most reactive towards MTG-catalyzed PEGylation was described [51]. In that study, a monodisperse Boc-PEG-NH$_2$ was used as the amine substrate on three model proteins: granulocyte colony stimulating factor (GCSF), human growth hormone (hGH), and apomyoglobin (apoMb). The former two proteins were selected for their importance as therapeutic proteins, and apoMb for being a model protein regarding the investigation of protein structure, folding, and stability. Despite the fact that GCSF, hGH, and apoMb have 17, 13, and 6 glutamine residues, respectively, only one or two per protein were modified by MTG. All effectively PEGylated glutamines were within disordered regions, suggesting that a flexible polypeptide substrate facilitates binding of MTG to target glutamines. A similar study used type I collagen as a protein substrate [52]. The resulting intermolecular collagen cross-links were quantified by digesting the collagen sample and separating of the fragments by HPLC. No more than five cross-links were formed out of a maximum of 27 possible. At least half of the cross-links were located within the triple helical region of the collagen molecule; however, the specific residues that were modified by MTG were not identified. Importantly, the cross-links were introduced by MTG only after the collagen had been at least partially heat-denatured, supporting the correlation between structural disorder of the target and recognition by MTG. To further investigate the importance of secondary structure and MTG's apparent preference for flexible polypeptide regions, the reactivity of MTG towards apoMb, α-lactalbumin (α-LA) and fragment 205–316 of thermolysin was analyzed [53]. These extensively studied proteins are models of α-helices, β-sheets and unstructured regions, respectively. Once more, despite many glutamine residues being present, few were substrates, with flexible or unstructured regions experiencing the highest reactivity. MTG discriminated notably less against protein-bound lysine as substrates, although those located in disordered regions were indeed more reactive. While this is by no means an exhaustive study of MTG's substrate reactivity with respect to secondary structure, MTG's reactivity towards flexible or unfolded regions for both glutamine and lysine protein substrates is further enforced.

Notwithstanding those advances, searching for superior glutamine recognition sequences that can be grafted onto a desired labeling target (often referred to as a "Q-tag") requires a high-throughput methodology in order to screen varying glutamine-containing sequences in an efficient manner. This had been previously done by phage display [54,55], in which phage-displayed dodecapeptide libraries on the order of 10^{11} members were screened for reactivity toward TG2 and MTG. Regarding MTG, a preference for an aromatic amino acid N-terminal to the glutamine was observed, as well as for an arginine and a hydrophobic amino acid at the +1 or +2 positions. However, no clear preferred amino acid pattern was obvious among the results. Building on this data, sequences determined to be the most reactive were synthesized and tested as penta- and heptapeptide substrates [56]. The pentapeptides' affinity for MTG were as low as Z-QG (in the range of 50 mM); however two heptapeptides, 7M42 (Ac-YELQRPY-NH$_2$) and 7M48 (Ac-WALQRPH-NH$_2$), were found to have a 4.5 and 19-fold decrease in K_m, indicating that the identity of surrounding amino acids affect K_m. Using a complimentary approach, the search for a Q-tag was expanded by recently employing mRNA display as a high-throughput screen [57]. Peptides that served as substrates became covalently bound via MTG reaction with hexa-lysine conjugated beads. Two pentapeptide sequences in particular were reported to have considerably higher reactivity and affinity for MTG (RLQQP and RTQPA), which vary considerably from the results obtained via phage display. In light of these results, valuable insight into the sequence and structural preferences for efficient TGase recognition of glutamine has been obtained. However, they do not yet converge onto a single, high-affinity Q-tag. The identification of a peptide sequence that is highly specific for MTG has also yet to be demonstrated, and so the precise requirements for selective glutamine binding to TGases remain under investigation.

The structural requirement of MTG's amine (lysine) substrate has previously been suggested to be considerably less strict than that of its amide (glutamine) substrate [58–60]. Along the same line of thought, as with the glutamine substrate, a recent study used an *in vivo* Förster resonance energy transfer (FRET) quenching assay in order to screen for highly reactive lysine recognition sequences ("K-tag") in *E. coli* [61]. The sequences screened were limited to pentapeptides with a lysine fixed at the center position. Although there was no repeated or consensus sequence determined by the screen, the pentapeptide KTKTN was found to be of reactivity comparable to a hexa-lysine tag. Synthetic amide and amine substrates were also previously tested for activity in order to determine if MTG could utilize non-natural substrates [62]. This was investigated in greater detail recently by screening amine compounds with increased diversity of chemical substituents and functional groups [63]. Overall, MTG was found to be highly promiscuous for its primary amine substrate, and amines attached to a less hindered carbon as well as amines with a longer hydrocarbon linker exhibited increased reactivity. Aromatic and small, polar amine-bearing compounds were observed to be excellent substrates as well. These studies help broaden the scope for modification of glutamine-containing peptides and proteins by TGases.

4. Assays

Assay development is key to the advancement of medicine, cell biology, and biotechnology. With respect to TGase, some goals for novel or improved assays include: the identification of highly specific substrates or inhibitors, higher sensitivity, cellular visualization in order to better understand the role of TGase in disease, and facilitation of TGase engineering by high-throughput screens. The detection of TGase activity is not immediately obvious due to the fact that none of its reactants or products absorb strongly at a distinctive wavelength, nor are they fluorescent. A standard end-point, colorimetric assay was developed early on (Figure 4A). The assay uses Z-QG as a model glutamine substrate and hydroxylamine as the amine substrate. The addition of TGase catalyzes the formation of an isopeptide bond and a hydroxamate group, and upon the addition of a concentrated ferric chloride solution, results in the development of a yellow color [45]. The hydroxamate assay remains in use to this day in order to determine kinetic constants, but its discontinuous nature and low molar absorptivity limit its applicability. As a result, a number of novel TGase assays have since been developed for use not only *in vitro*, but *in vivo* as well. Some colorimetric and fluorometric examples include sensitive assays involving the enzymatic release of *p*-nitrophenol, 7-hydroxycoumarin, and the production of chromophoric anilide [64–66].

An alternative approach has been to label a protein substrate of interest in a reaction mediated by TG2 with a biotinylated fluorophore and subsequently isolate the newly biotinylated protein with streptavidin beads, allowing for immobilization and separation of the product [67]. The sensitivity of this assay allows for detection of 0.6 mU purified TG2, and can also be applied to crude lysates, making it possible to screen for low transpeptidase activities. However, the sensitivity is less than that of assays using dansylcadaverine to detect product formation, which have been reported to detect as little as 60 μU [68] and 10.8 μU [69] of TG2. This fluorescent alkylamine is commonly used as a substrate for TGases to fluorescently label proteins, and removal of unreacted dansyl cadaverine may reduce background. To address this issue, magnetic dextran coated charcoal has been used to capture and magnetically sediment unreacted dansyl cadaverine, in a method readily adapted to 96-well plate format [69]. The first assay monitoring the change in fluorescence anisotropy has been recently described [70]. A fluorescein-labeled substrate peptide is monitored for an increase in fluorescence anisotropy as it is cross-linked to a significantly larger substrate, bovine serum albumin (BSA). The assay allows for detection of TG2 as low as 300 pM. The assay also detects product formation; however, a large difference in mass between substrates and product is required in order for detection to occur.

Crystal structures of TG2 reveal that the enzyme undergoes a sizeable conformational change upon substrate binding [71]. In the presence of GDP/GTP, TG2 adopts a "closed" conformation that is inactive [72]. When bound to a substrate-mimicking inhibitor, TG2 was found to be in an "open" conformation, suggesting that the open conformation is the catalytically active form of the enzyme [72]. These conformational changes were recently used as a basis for novel activity assays of TG2. In the first assay, TG2 is used as a biosensor that allows for quantitative assessment in live cells using FRET, as measured by fluorescence lifetime imaging microscopy (FLIM) [73] (Figure 4B). This concept was further developed to monitor the real-time, ligand-induced conformational changes of TG2 using kinetic capillary electrophoresis, making this a rapid detection method [74]. As mentioned above, Kim and coworkers recently reported a FRET quenching assay to screen MTG activity in *E. coli* [61]. Each of the two peptide substrates is genetically fused to a fluorescent protein; if the peptide substrates are cross-linked upon exposure to TGase, a FRET quenching results. This approach is highly flexible in that it will allow library screening for either peptide substrate.

Figure 4. Examples of assays used for detection of TGase activity. (**A**) Colorimetric and fluorescent product release activity assays. The hydroxamate assay (top) remains the standard method to determine and compare TGase activity. TG2 activity can also be quantified by the release of *p*-nitrophenol (PNP; λ_{max} = 405 nm), umbelliferone (λ_{em} = 465 nm), or by the formation of an anilide product (λ_{max} = 278 nm) following conjugation with *N,N*-dimethyl-1,4-phenylenediamine (DMPDA); (**B**) Cartoon representation of the TG2 conformational FRET sensor; (**C**) *In vivo* activation of MTG allowing for in-cell assaying.

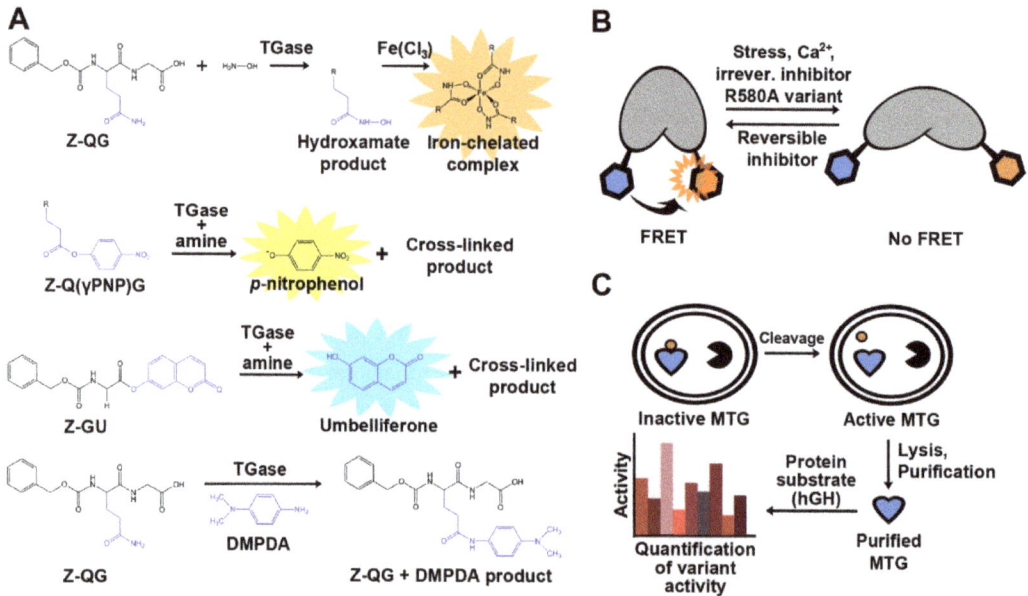

Previously, interest has been expressed to engineer TGases towards novel applications [43,44]. With regard to MTG, its requirement for activation complicates the development of a high-throughput screening assay. In effort to circumvent this obstacle, Zhao and co-workers demonstrated an *in vivo* selection assay for MTG [32] (Figure 4C). MTG was co-expressed with the 3C protease in order to activate the enzyme. The authors performed site-saturation mutagenesis on two different residues, Y62 and Y75, and used the assay to identify a variant that favors the conjugation of PEG to a specific glutamine (Q141) of human growth hormone. Two variants were found to be exclusively specific for Q141, even after 30 h of reaction time. In order to determine activity, a previously established scintillation proximity assay was used [75], complexifying the methodology. A simple, continuous, colorimetric TGase assay was recently adapted in order to easily determine kinetic parameters of

MTG with different substrates. Glutamate dehydrogenase activity was coupled to ammonia release upon deamination of the glutamine substrate for MTG, resulting in a decrease in NADH readily observed at $\lambda_{max} = 340$ nm [56].

5. TGases as Biocatalysts for the Production of Novel Biomaterials

The earliest biocatalytic use of TGases was in the food industry [11,16], which continues on a large scale to this day. Novel biotechnological applications have since been fostered to expand the biocatalytic utility of TGases outside of the food industry. Progress in this field has hastened in conjunction with recognition of their flexibility with respect to the primary amine substrate. This has helped open the door of possibilities with regard to covalently modifying protein- or peptide-bound glutamines with a wide array of compounds. The increasing diversity is welcomed: as previously discussed, a number of polymer-protein conjugates have been prepared with TGase using PEG to tailor the properties of the substrate protein to towards a more favorable therapeutic profile, such as enhanced stability and decreased toxicity. Recently, the polymer repertoire was expanded by synthesizing conjugates using hydroxyethyl starch [76]. It is a biodegradable alternative to PEG for commercial use as a blood plasma volume expander, potentially making it a more suitable polymer for protein conjugation. Taking this concept a step further, protein lipidation was demonstrated using MTG, with the goal of altering the behavior of the conjugated protein by controlling its localization via increased amphiphilicity [77]. Proteins can be regarded as biopolymers themselves, and can thus be assembled into larger biomolecular complexes in order to achieve altered functionality and properties. However, such a complex is only of use if its assembly can be controlled. A supramolecular protein complex, composed of *E. coli* alkaline phosphatase (AP) and streptavidin, was constructed with the aid of MTG [78]. The strong avidin-biotin interaction was exploited to direct the assembly of these two protein building blocks into a larger complex, by having AP site-specifically conjugated with biotin using MTG. The location of biotin conjugation on AP was crucial to create large structures and retain AP activity. Finally, MTG has also been found to be effective at modifying the structure of peptides containing a glutamine and lysine residue by cyclization [79].

Proteins and peptides are not the only biological molecules that have been modified using TGases; MTG has been recently used to site-specifically attach diverse compounds, at multiple positions, onto antibodies [80,81]. Glycosylation normally prevents TGase from effectively modifying antibodies, but the glycosylation pattern was modified such that MTG was able to react at specific locations. The resulting antibody-drug conjugates (ADCs) are of interest as potential therapeutic solutions, and tweaking their pharmokinetic properties by conjugation with different compounds may yield new therapeutic avenues that were previously unfeasible.

6. Protein Labeling

A specific application of TGases that is gaining importance is their use as a tool to site-specifically label proteins with the goal of visualization within complex biological systems, such as in living cells. The typical strategy is to introduce an amide- or amine-containing fluorophore substrate into the system, along with TGase, to form an isopeptide bond with a specific lysine or glutamine, respectively, on the target protein (Figure 5).

Figure 5. General scheme for protein labeling using TGase. The protein of interest (P.O.I.) carries an accessible glutamine residue, for TGase-catalysed reaction with an amine-substituted fluorophore; alternatively, the P.O.I. carries a reactive lysine residue for reaction with a glutamine-modified fluorophore.

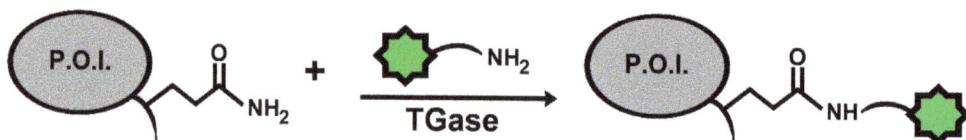

A fluorescent analog of the conventional model glutamine substrate, Z-QG, has been synthesized. Fluorescein-4-isothiocyanate-β-Ala-QG was shown to be an effective glutamine substrate for MTG for reaction with a lysine-containing peptide tag (dubbed as a "K-tag"), genetically encoded at the *N*-terminus of the peptide or protein of interest [82][83]. This K-tag was six amino acids in length, and both the second and fourth residues were lysines (MKHKGS). Mass spectrometry revealed that MTG displayed a high preference for the second lysine. The same group later developed two 13-mer peptidyl loop K-tags, each containing a single lysine, specifically recognized by MTG [84]; no direct comparison of the reactivity of the 6-mer and 13-mer tags was conducted. The 13-mer tags were encoded into bacterial alkaline phosphatase (BAP), which had been selected because MTG does not recognize any of its native glutamine or lysine residues as substrates. High labeling yields (>94%) were obtained when the 13-mer tags were inserted in vicinity of the active site, or at a location distal from the active site (Figure 6A). However, insertion distal from the active site provided higher reactivity. The reactivity of the two 13-mer tags was comparable. Using a different approach, incorporation of a fluorescent substrate was observed by an intramolecular FRET between two fluorescent substrate proteins, allowing an evaluation of transamidation activity of TG2 [85]. With this assay, propargylamine was found to be an excellent substrate for TG2. Following propargylation of a glutamine residue in casein, the resulting alkyne-modified residue was fluorescently labeled through a copper-catalyzed Huigsen cycloaddition with an azido-fluorescein conjugate (click chemistry) [86], thus providing a general route for labeling with a variety of azido-containing compounds. MTG was also found to be capable of using propargylamine as a substrate; additionally, it can use amino azides as substrates, to allow ulterior click chemistry with a variety of alkyne-containing compounds [63]. The techniques above offer high reactivity *in vitro*; however, they have not yet been tested in the context of cellular visualization.

Figure 6. Examples of TGases applied for visualization of biomacromolecules. (**A**) Locations of independently encoded 13-mer peptidyl loop K-tags on bacterial alkaline phosphatase. (**B**) MTG-aided enzymatic detection of nucleic acids. (**C**) The paramagnetic agent is cross-linked to a glutamine, generating the CEST effect. Magnetic resonance saturation is transferred to water following saturation of the amide proton.

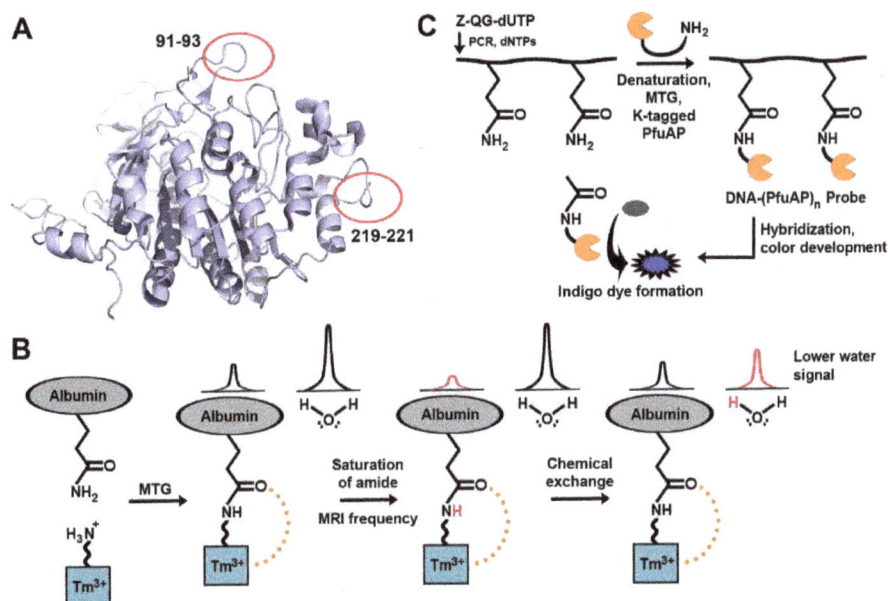

TG2 is associated with tumor growth and drug resistance, but attempts to detect TG2 in tissues can often be plagued by false positives. Magnetic resonance imaging is a powerful diagnostic tool, and TGase may in the future be detected in tumor cells by using a new contrast agent [87] containing a primary amine, designed so that it would serve as a substrate for MTG (Figure 6B). Upon cross-linking the agent onto a tumor, a MRI signal is created. Called chemical exchange saturation transfer (CEST), a particular proton signal associated with the CEST agent is selectively saturated, and the proton remains in exchange with surrounding water molecules. As a result, the MRI signal from the water surrounding the CEST agent is reduced, allowing for its location to be determined. The signal generated before and after cross-linking of the contrast agent differs, allowing for easy differentiation between the two species. Once again, this work remains at the level of *in vitro* experimentation in a model system and has yet to be tested *in vivo*. TGase-mediated labeling has also been further expanded to label biological macromolecules other than proteins, such as DNA and RNA [88,89] (Figure 6C). Nucleic acid hybridization techniques make it possible to detect the expression pattern of a particular gene, which may be indicative of a disease. *In situ* hybridization (ISH) requires binding of a target DNA sequence to a probe, followed by detection with radioisotopes, fluorophores, or antibodies. In a new hybridization procedure dubbed transglutaminase-mediated *in situ* hybridization (TransISH), a Z-QG-labeled DNA-peptide conjugate was synthesized using DNA primers containing Z-QG-dUTP. The labeled DNA can then be denatured and cross-linked to alkaline phosphatase (AP) containing a K-tag in a process mediated by MTG. The DNA-linked AP will then dephosphorylate 5-bromo-4-chloro-3-indolyl phosphate, leading to the development of a blue chromophore. The same concept was also applied to mRNA [90]. As additional detection is not required with TransISH, it simplifies common ISH protocols by bypassing these steps, allowing direct staining after washing the unhybridized probe.

Fluorescent tagging has also been performed using TG2 activity in order to monitor cellular processes as well as the implication of TGases themselves in disease. Click chemistry was employed in a clinical context to monitor native TG2-mediated protein serotonylation (TPS). With little discrimination with regard to its protein substrate, this process involves TG2 cross-linking of serotonin to glutamine residues, and is implicated in necessary biological processes as well as disease [91,92]. A modified analog of serotonin, propargylserotonin, was synthesized so that it could react with azide-functionalized substrates and enhance the understanding of Ras and its role in previously unknown processes [93]. In addition, of clinical relevance, TG2 is known to play a role in fibrosis and vascular calcification. In order to probe this further, mechanism-based fluorescent inhibitors were designed to covalently label TG2, to investigate how its activity may relate to stiffening of arterial tissues [94].

7. Conclusions

Notable progress has been made in both fundamental and applied research of TGases, although many challenges remain. New efforts in engineering their production have been made, with recent biophysical studies supplementing the knowledge base on the enzymes. However, despite recent work with respect to engineering TGase towards new and different capacities, the goals and results remains largely conservative. Better understanding and characterizing the substrate specificity remains a prime interest so that TGase can be effectively applied in existing and for novel applications. The enzymes have also increasingly become a tool to accomplish new feats in biotechnology. New methods have been developed for detecting and quantifying TGase activity, allowing for increased sensitivity and even *in vivo* assessment. TGases' natural ability to use protein and peptide substrates gives them potential to label target proteins or peptides, but is limited by its specificity. Some of the techniques discussed in this review have found ways to work around this limitation, however, many remain at the level of proof-of-concept, leaving room for further development and optimization.

Acknowledgments

The authors would like to acknowledge Alexis Vallée-Bélisle (Université de Montréal) for helpful discussion and comments.

Conflict of Interest

The authors declare no conflict of interest.

References

1. Pattabiraman, V.R.; Bode, J.W. Rethinking amide bond synthesis. *Nature* **2011**, *480*, 471–479.
2. Griffin, M.; Casadio, R.; Bergamini, C.M. Transglutaminases: Nature's biological glues. *Biochem. J.* **2002**, *368*, 377–396.
3. Shleĭkin, A.G.; Danilov, N.P. Evolutionary-biological peculiarities of transglutaminase. Structure, physiological functions, application. *Zh. Evol. Biokhim. Fiziol.* **2011**, *47*, 3–14.
4. Autuori, F.; Farrace, M.G.; Oliverio, S.; Piredda, L.; Piacentini, M. "Tissue" transglutaminase and apoptosis. *Adv. Biochem. Eng. Biotechnol.* **1998**, *62*, 129–136.
5. Abe, S.; Yamashita, K.; Kohno, H.; Ohkubo, Y. Involvement of transglutaminase in the receptor-mediated endocytosis of mouse peritoneal macrophages. *Biol. Pharm. Bull.* **2000**, *23*, 1511–1513.
6. Chen, J.S.; Mehta, K. Tissue transglutaminase: an enzyme with a split personality. *Int. J. Biochem. Cell Biol.* **1999**, *31*, 817–836.
7. Shridas, P.; Sharma, Y.; Balasubramanian, D. Transglutaminase-mediated cross-linking of alpha-crystallin: structural and functional consequences. *FEBS Lett.* **2001**, *499*, 245–250.
8. Shan, L.; Molberg, Ø.; Parrot, I.; Hausch, F.; Filiz, F.; Gray, G.M.; Sollid, L.M.; Khosla, C. Structural basis for gluten intolerance in celiac sprue. *Science* **2002**, *297*, 2275–2279.
9. Schroeder, W.T.; Thacher, S.M.; Stewart-Galetka, S.; Annarella, M.; Chema, D.; Siciliano, M.J.; Davies, P.J.; Tang, H.Y.; Sowa, B.A.; Duvic, M. Type I keratinocyte transglutaminase: expression in human skin and psoriasis. *J. Invest. Dermatol.* **1992**, *99*, 27–34.
10. Ando, H.; Adachi, M.; Umeda, K.; Matsuura, A.; Nonaka, M.; Uchio, R.; Tanaka, H.; Motoki, M. Purification and characteristics of a novel transglutaminase derived from microorganisms. *Agric. Biol. Chem.* **1989**, *53*, 2613–2617.
11. Zhu, Y.; Rinzema, A.; Tramper, J.; Bol, J. Microbial transglutaminase—A review of its production and application in food processing. *Appl. Microbiol. Biotechnol.* **1995**, *44*, 277–282.
12. Suzuki, S.; Izawa, Y.; Kobayashi, K.; Eto, Y.; Yamanaka, S.; Kubota, K.; Yokozeki, K. Purification and characterization of novel transglutaminase from Bacillus subtilis spores. *Biosci. Biotechnol. Biochem.* **2000**, *64*, 2344–2351.
13. Pedersen, L.C.; Yee, V.C.; Bishop, P.D.; Le Trong, I.; Teller, D.C.; Stenkamp, R.E. Transglutaminase factor XIII uses proteinase-like catalytic triad to crosslink macromolecules. *Protein Sci.* **1994**, *3*, 1131–1135.
14. Ikura, K.; Nasu, T.; Yokota, H.; Tsuchiya, Y.; Sasaki, R.; Chiba, H. Amino acid sequence of guinea pig liver transglutaminase from its cDNA sequence. *Biochemistry* **1988**, *27*, 2898–2905.
15. Kashiwagi, T.; Yokoyama, K.-I.; Ishikawa, K.; Ono, K.; Ejima, D.; Matsui, H.; Suzuki, E. Crystal structure of microbial transglutaminase from *Streptoverticillium mobaraense*. *J. Biol. Chem.* **2002**, *277*, 44252–44560.
16. Motoki, M.; Seguro, K. Transglutaminase and its use for food processing. *Trends Food Sci. Technol.* **1998**, *9*, 204–210.

17. Zeugolis, D.I.; Panengad, P.P.; Yew, E.S.Y.; Sheppard, C.; Phan, T.T.; Raghunath, M. An *in situ* and *in vitro* investigation for the transglutaminase potential in tissue engineering. *J. Biomed. Mater. Res. A* **2010**, *92*, 1310–1320.

18. Cortez, J.; Bonner, P.L.; Griffin, M. Application of transglutaminases in the modification of wool textiles. *Enzyme Microb. Technol.* **2004**, *34*, 64–72.

19. Chau, D.Y.S.; Brown, S.V; Mather, M.L.; Hutter, V.; Tint, N.L.; Dua, H.S.; Rose, F.R.A.J.; Ghaemmaghami, A.M. Tissue transglutaminase (TG-2) modified amniotic membrane: a novel scaffold for biomedical applications. *Biomed. Mater.* **2012**, *7*, 045011.

20. Zhu, Y.; Tramper, J. Novel applications for microbial transglutaminase beyond food processing. *Trends Biotechnol.* **2008**, *26*, 559–565.

21. Teixeira, L.S.M.; Feijen, J.; van Blitterswijk, C.A.; Dijkstra, P.J.; Karperien, M. Enzyme-catalyzed crosslinkable hydrogels: emerging strategies for tissue engineering. *Biomaterials* **2012**, *33*, 1281–1290.

22. Gillet, S.M.F.G.; Chica, R.A.; Keillor, J.W.; Pelletier, J.N. Expression and rapid purification of highly active hexahistidine-tagged guinea pig liver transglutaminase. *Protein Expr. Purif.* **2004**, *33*, 256–264.

23. Yokoyama, K.-I.; Nakamura, N.; Seguro, K.; Kubota, K. Overproduction of microbial transglutaminase in *Escherichia coli*, in vitro refolding, and characterization of the refolded form. *Biosci. Biotechnol. Biochem.* **2000**, *64*, 1263–1270.

24. Shi, Q.; Kim, S.-Y.; Blass, J.P.; Cooper, A.J.L. Expression in *Escherichia coli* and purification of hexahistidine-tagged human tissue transglutaminase. *Protein Expr. Purif.* **2002**, *24*, 366–373.

25. Piper, J.L.; Gray, G.M.; Khosla, C. High selectivity of human tissue transglutaminase for immunoactive gliadin peptides: implications for celiac sprue. *Biochemistry* **2002**, *41*, 386–393.

26. Roy, I.; Smith, O.; Clouthier, C.M.; Keillor, J.W. Expression, purification and kinetic characterisation of human tissue transglutaminase. *Protein Expr. Purif.* **2013**, *87*, 41–46.

27. Kobayashi, K.; Hashiguchi, K.; Yokozeki, K.; Yamanaka, S. Molecular clonging of the transglutaminase gene from Bacillus subtilis and its expression in *Escherichia coli*. *Biosci. Biotechnol. Biochem.* **1998**, *62*, 1109–1114.

28. Plácido, D.; Fernandes, C.G.; Isidro, A.; Carrondo, M.A.; Henriques, A.O.; Archer, M. Auto-induction and purification of a Bacillus subtilis transglutaminase (Tgl) and its preliminary crystallographic characterization. *Protein Expr. Purif.* **2008**, *59*, 1–8.

29. Marx, C.K.; Hertel, T.C.; Pietzsch, M. Soluble expression of a pro-transglutaminase from *Streptomyces mobaraensis* in *Escherichia coli*. *Enzyme Microb. Technol.* **2007**, *40*, 1543–1550.

30. Sommer, C.; Volk, N.; Pietzsch, M. Model based optimization of the fed-batch production of a highly active transglutaminase variant in Escherichia coli. *Protein Expr. Purif.* **2011**, *77*, 9–19.

31. Zhang, D.; Zhu, Y.; Chen, J. Microbial transglutaminase production: Understanding the mechanism. *Biotechnol. Genet. Eng. Rev.* **2009**, *26*, 205–222.

32. Zhao, X.; Shaw, A.C.; Wang, J.; Chang, C.-C.; Deng, J.; Su, J. A novel high-throughput screening method for microbial transglutaminases with high specificity toward Gln141 of human growth hormone. *J. Biomol. Screen.* **2010**, *15*, 206–212.

33. Kikuchi, Y.; Date, M.; Yokoyama, K.; Umezawa, Y. Secretion of active-form *Streptoverticillium mobaraense* transglutaminase by *Corynebacterium glutamicum*: processing of the pro-transglutaminase by a cosecreted subtilisin-like protease from *Streptomyces albogriseolus*. *Appl. Environ. Microbiol.* **2003**, *69*, 358–366.

34. Liu, S.; Zhang, D.; Wang, M.; Cui, W.; Chen, K.; Du, G.; Chen, J.; Zhou, Z. The order of expression is a key factor in the production of active transglutaminase in *Escherichia coli* by co-expression with its pro-peptide. *Microb. Cell Fact.* **2011**, *10*, 112.

35. Chen, K.; Liu, S.; Wang, G.; Zhang, D.; Du, G.; Chen, J.; Shi, Z. Enhancement of *Streptomyces* transglutaminase activity and pro-peptide cleavage efficiency by introducing linker peptide in the *C*-terminus of the pro-peptide. *J. Ind. Microbiol. Biotechnol.* **2013**, *40*, 317–325.

36. Yang, M.-T.; Chang, C.-H.; Wang, J.M.; Wu, T.K.; Wang, Y.-K.; Chang, C.-Y.; Li, T.T. Crystal structure and inhibition studies of transglutaminase from *S. mobaraense*. *J. Biol. Chem.* **2011**, *286*, 7301–7307.

37. Eder, J.; Fersht, A.R. Pro-sequence-assisted protein folding. *Mol. Microbiol.* **1995**, *16*, 609–614.

38. Suzuki, M.; Sakurai, K.; Lee, Y.-H.; Ikegami, T.; Yokoyama, K.; Goto, Y. A back hydrogen exchange procedure via the acid-unfolded state for a large protein. *Biochemistry* **2012**, *51*, 5564–5570.

39. Suzuki, M.; Yokoyama, K.; Lee, Y.-H.; Goto, Y. A two-step refolding of acid-denatured microbial transglutaminase escaping from the aggregation-prone intermediate. *Biochemistry* **2011**, *50*, 10390–10398.

40. Savile, C.K.; Janey, J.M.; Mundorff, E.C.; Moore, J.C.; Tam, S.; Jarvis, W.R.; Colbeck, J.C.; Krebber, A.; Fleitz, F.J.; Brands, J.; *et al.* Biocatalytic asymmetric synthesis of chiral amines from ketones applied to sitagliptin manufacture. *Science* **2010**, *329*, 305–309.

41. Clouthier, C.M.; Pelletier, J.N. Expanding the organic toolbox: a guide to integrating biocatalysis in synthesis. *Chem. Soc. Rev.* **2012**, *41*, 1585–1605.

42. Brustad, E.M.; Arnold, F.H. Optimizing non-natural protein function with directed evolution. *Curr. Opin. Chem. Biol.* **2011**, *15*, 201–210.

43. Keillor, J.W.; Chica, R.A.; Chabot, N.; Vinci, V.; Pardin, C.; Fortin, E.; Gillet, S.M.F.G.; Nakano, Y.; Kaartinen, M.T.; Pelletier, J.N.; Lubell, W.D. The bioorganic chemistry of transglutaminase—from mechanism to inhibition and engineering. *Can. J. Chem.* **2008**, *276*, 271–276.

44. Marx, C.K.; Hertel, T.C.; Pietzsch, M. Random mutagenesis of a recombinant microbial transglutaminase for the generation of thermostable and heat-sensitive variants. *J. Biotechnol.* **2008**, *136*, 156–162.

45. Folk, J.; Cole, P. Mechanism of action of guinea pig liver transglutaminase. *J. Biol. Chem.* **1966**, *241*, 5518–5525.

46. Buettner, K.; Hertel, T.C.; Pietzsch, M. Increased thermostability of microbial transglutaminase by combination of several hot spots evolved by random and saturation mutagenesis. *Amino Acids* **2012**, *42*, 987–996.

47. Chen, K.; Liu, S.; Ma, J.; Zhang, D.; Shi, Z.; Du, G.; Chen, J. Deletion combined with saturation mutagenesis of N-terminal residues in transglutaminase from *Streptomyces hygroscopicus* results in enhanced activity and thermostability. *Process Biochem.* **2012**, *47*, 2329–2334.

48. Tagami, U.; Shimba, N.; Nakamura, M.; Yokoyama, K.-I.; Suzuki, E.-I.; Hirokawa, T. Substrate specificity of microbial transglutaminase as revealed by three-dimensional docking simulation and mutagenesis. *Protein Eng. Des. Sel.* **2009**, *22*, 747–752.

49. Coussons, P.J.; Price, N.C.; Kelly, S.M.; Smith, B.; Sawyer, L. Factors that govern the specificity of transglutaminase-catalysed modification of proteins and peptides. *Biochem. J.* **1992**, *282*, 929–930.

50. Hu, B.H.; Messersmith, P.B. Rational design of transglutaminase substrate peptides for rapid enzymatic formation of hydrogels. *J. Am. Chem. Soc.* **2003**, *125*, 14298–14299.

51. Mero, A.; Spolaore, B.; Veronese, F.M.; Fontana, A. Transglutaminase-mediated PEGylation of proteins: direct identification of the sites of protein modification by mass spectrometry using a novel monodisperse PEG. *Bioconjug. Chem.* **2009**, *20*, 384–389.

52. Stachel, I.; Schwarzenbolz, U.; Henle, T.; Meyer, M. Cross-linking of type I collagen with microbial transglutaminase: identification of cross-linking sites. *Biomacromolecules* **2010**, *11*, 698–705.

53. Spolaore, B.; Raboni, S.; Ramos Molina, A.; Satwekar, A.; Damiano, N.; Fontana, A. Local unfolding is required for the site-specific protein modification by transglutaminase. *Biochemistry* **2012**, *51*, 8679–8689.

54. Sugimura, Y.; Hosono, M.; Wada, F.; Yoshimura, T.; Maki, M.; Hitomi, K. Screening for the preferred substrate sequence of transglutaminase using a phage-displayed peptide library: identification of peptide substrates for TGase 2 and Factor XIIIA. *J. Biol. Chem.* **2006**, *281*, 17699–17706.

55. Sugimura, Y.; Yokoyama, K.; Nio, N.; Maki, M.; Hitomi, K. Identification of preferred substrate sequences of microbial transglutaminase from *Streptomyces mobaraensis* using a phage-displayed peptide library. *Arch. Biochem. Biophys.* **2008**, *477*, 379–383.

56. Oteng-Pabi, S.K.; Keillor, J.W. Continuous enzyme-coupled assay for microbial transglutaminase activity. *Anal. Biochem.* **2013**, *441*, 169–173.

57. Lee, J.-H.; Song, C.; Kim, D.-H.; Park, I.-H.; Lee, S.-G.; Lee, Y.-S.; Kim, B.-G. Glutamine (Q)-peptide screening for transglutaminase reaction using mRNA display. *Biotechnol. Bioeng.* **2013**, *110*, 353–362.

58. Ohtsuka, T.; Sawa, a; Kawabata, R.; Nio, N.; Motoki, M. Substrate specificities of microbial transglutaminase for primary amines. *J. Agric. Food Chem.* **2000**, *48*, 6230–6233.

59. Nonaka, M.; Matsuura, Y.; Motoki, M. Incorporation of a lysine- and lysine dipeptides into a_{s1}-Caesin by Ca^{2+} -independent microbial transglutaminase. *Biosci. Biotech. Biochem.* **1996**, *60*, 131–133.

60. Ikura, K.; Sasaki, R.; Motoki, M. Use of transglutaminase in quality-improvement and processing of food proteins. *Agric. Food. Chem.* **1992**, *2*, 389–407.

61. Lee, J.-H.; Song, E.; Lee, S.-G.; Kim, B.-G. High-throughput screening for transglutaminase activities using recombinant fluorescent proteins. *Biotechnol. Bioeng.* **2013**, *110*, 2865–2873.

62. Kulik, C.; Heine, E.; Weichold, O.; Möller, M. Synthetic substrates as amine donors and acceptors in microbial transglutaminase-catalysed reactions. *J. Mol. Catal. B Enzym.* **2009**, *57*, 237–241.

63. Gundersen, M.T.; Keillor, J.W.; Pelletier, J.N. Microbial transglutaminase displays broad acyl-acceptor substrate specificity. *Appl. Microbiol. Biotechnol.* **2013**, doi:10.1007/s00253-013-4886-x.

64. De Macédo, P.; Marrano, C.; Keillor, J.W. A direct continuous spectrophotometric assay for transglutaminase activity. *Anal. Biochem.* **2000**, *285*, 16–20.

65. Leblanc, A.; Gravel, C.; Labelle, J.; Keillor, J.W. Kinetic studies of guinea pig liver transglutaminase reveal a general-base-catalyzed deacylation mechanism. *Biochemistry* **2001**, *40*, 8335–8342.

66. Gillet, S.M.F.G.; Pelletier, J.N.; Keillor, J.W. A direct fluorometric assay for tissue transglutaminase. *Anal. Biochem.* **2005**, *347*, 221–226.

67. Gnaccarini, C.; Ben-Tahar, W.; Lubell, W.D.; Pelletier, J.N.; Keillor, J.W. Fluorometric assay for tissue transglutaminase-mediated transamidation activity. *Bioorg. Med. Chem.* **2009**, *17*, 6354–6359.

68. Jeitner, T.M.; Fuchsbauer, H.; Blass, J.P.; Cooper, A.J.L. A sensitive fluorometric assay for tissue transglutaminase. *Anal. Biochem.* **2001**, *206*, 198–206.

69. Wu, Y.; Tsai, Y. A rapid transglutaminase assay for high-throughput screening applications. *J. Biomol. Screen.* **2006**, *11*, 836–843.

70. Kenniston, J.; Conley, G.P.; Sexton, D.J.; Nixon, A.E. A homogeneous fluorescence anisotropy assay for measuring transglutaminase 2 activity. *Anal. Biochem.* **2013**, *436*, 13–15.

71. Begg, G.E.; Holman, S.R.; Stokes, P.H.; Matthews, J.M.; Graham, R.M.; Iismaa, S.E. Mutation of a critical arginine in the GTP-binding site of transglutaminase 2 disinhibits intracellular cross-linking activity. *J. Biol. Chem.* **2006**, *281*, 12603–12609.

72. Pinkas, D.M.; Strop, P.; Brunger, A.T.; Khosla, C. Transglutaminase 2 undergoes a large conformational change upon activation. *PLoS Biol.* **2007**, *5*, e327.

73. Caron, N.S.; Munsie, L.N.; Keillor, J.W.; Truant, R. Using FLIM-FRET to measure conformational changes of transglutaminase type 2 in live cells. *PLoS One* **2012**, *7*, e44159.

74. Clouthier, C.M.; Mironov, G.G.; Okhonin, V.; Berezovski, M.V; Keillor, J.W. Real-time monitoring of protein conformational dynamics in solution using kinetic capillary electrophoresis. *Angew. Chem. Int. Ed. Engl.* **2012**, *51*, 12464–12468.

75. Mádi, A.; Kárpáti, L.; Kovács, A.; Muszbek, L.; Fésüs, L. High-throughput scintillation proximity assay for transglutaminase activity measurement. *Anal. Biochem.* **2005**, *343*, 256–262.

76. Besheer, A.; Hertel, T.C.; Kressler, J.; Mäder, K.; Pietzsch, M. Enzymatically-catalyzed HESylation using microbial transglutaminase: Proof of feasibility. *J. Pharm. Sci.* **2009**, *98*, 4420–4428.

77. Abe, H.; Goto, M.; Kamiya, N. Protein lipidation catalyzed by microbial transglutaminase. *Chemistry* **2011**, *17*, 14004–14008.

78. Mori, Y.; Wakabayashi, R.; Goto, M.; Kamiya, N. Protein supramolecular complex formation by site-specific avidin-biotin interactions. *Org. Biomol. Chem.* **2013**, *11*, 914–922.

79. Touati, J.; Angelini, A.; Hinner, M.J.; Heinis, C. Enzymatic cyclisation of peptides with a transglutaminase. *Chembiochem* **2011**, *12*, 38–42.

80. Strop, P.; Liu, S.-H.; Dorywalska, M.; Delaria, K.; Dushin, R.G.; Tran, T.-T.; Ho, W.-H.; Farias, S.; Casas, M.G.; Abdiche, Y.; *et al.* Location matters: Site of conjugation modulates stability and pharmacokinetics of antibody drug conjugates. *Chem. Biol.* **2013**, *20*, 161–167.

81. Jeger, S.; Zimmermann, K.; Blanc, A.; Grünberg, J.; Honer, M.; Hunziker, P.; Struthers, H.; Schibli, R. Site-specific and stoichiometric modification of antibodies by bacterial transglutaminase. *Angew. Chem. Int. Ed. Engl.* **2010**, *49*, 9995–9997.

82. Kamiya, N.; Abe, H. New fluorescent substrates of microbial transglutaminase and its application to peptide tag-directed covalent protein labeling. *Bioconjugation Protoc.* **2011**, *751*, 81–94.

83. Kamiya, N.; Abe, H.; Goto, M.; Tsuji, Y.; Jikuya, H. Fluorescent substrates for covalent protein labeling catalyzed by microbial transglutaminase. *Org. Biomol. Chem.* **2009**, *7*, 3407–3412.

84. Mori, Y.; Goto, M.; Kamiya, N. Transglutaminase-mediated internal protein labeling with a designed peptide loop. *Biochem. Biophys. Res. Commun.* **2011**, *410*, 829–833.

85. Gnaccarini, C.; Ben-Tahar, W.; Mulani, A.; Roy, I.; Lubell, W.D.; Pelletier, J.N.; Keillor, J.W. Site-specific protein propargylation using tissue transglutaminase. *Org. Biomol. Chem.* **2012**, *10*, 5258–5265.

86. Kolb, H.C.; Finn, M.G.; Sharpless, K.B. Click chemistry: Diverse chemical function from a few good reactions. *Angew. Chem. Int. Ed. Engl.* **2001**, *40*, 2004–2021.

87. Hingorani, D. V; Randtke, E.A.; Pagel, M.D. A catalyCEST MRI contrast agent that detects the enzyme-catalyzed creation of a covalent bond. *J. Am. Chem. Soc.* **2013**, *135*, 6396–6398.

88. Kitaoka, M.; Tsuruda, Y.; Tanaka, Y.; Goto, M.; Mitsumori, M.; Hayashi, K.; Hiraishi, Y.; Miyawaki, K.; Noji, S.; Kamiya, N. Transglutaminase-mediated synthesis of a DNA-(enzyme)$_n$ probe for highly sensitive DNA detection. *Chemistry* **2011**, *17*, 5387–5392.

89. Takahara, M.; Hayashi, K.; Goto, M.; Kamiya, N. Tailing DNA aptamers with a functional protein by two-step enzymatic reaction. *J. Biosci. Bioeng.* **2013**, doi: 10.1016/j.jbiosc.2013.05.025.

90. Kitaoka, M.; Mitsumori, M.; Hayashi, K.; Hiraishi, Y.; Yoshinaga, H.; Nakano, K.; Miyawaki, K.; Noji, S.; Goto, M.; Kamiya, N. Transglutaminase-mediated *in situ* hybridization (TransISH) system: A new methodology for simplified mRNA detection. *Anal. Chem.* **2012**, *84*, 5885–5891.

91. Watts, S.W.; Priestley, J.R.C.; Thompson, J.M. Serotonylation of vascular proteins important to contraction. *PLoS One* **2009**, *4*, e5682.

92. Walther, D.J.; Stahlberg, S.; Vowinckel, J. Novel roles for biogenic monoamines: From monoamines in transglutaminase-mediated post-translational protein modification to monoaminylation deregulation diseases. *FEBS J.* **2011**, *278*, 4740–4755.

93. Lin, J.C.-Y.; Chou, C.-C.; Gao, S.; Wu, S.-C.; Khoo, K.-H.; Lin, C.-H. An *in vivo* tagging method reveals that Ras undergoes sustained activation upon transglutaminase-mediated protein serotonylation. *Chembiochem* **2013**, *14*, 813–817.

94. Chabot, N.; Moreau, S.; Mulani, A.; Moreau, P.; Keillor, J.W. Fluorescent probes of tissue transglutaminase reveal its association with arterial stiffening. *Chem. Biol.* **2010**, *17*, 1143–1150.

Biophysical Insights into the Inhibitory Mechanism of Non-Nucleoside HIV-1 Reverse Transcriptase Inhibitors

Grant Schauer, Sanford Leuba and Nicolas Sluis-Cremer

Abstract: HIV-1 reverse transcriptase (RT) plays a central role in HIV infection. Current United States Federal Drug Administration (USFDA)-approved antiretroviral therapies can include one of five approved non-nucleoside RT inhibitors (NNRTIs), which are potent inhibitors of RT activity. Despite their crucial clinical role in treating and preventing HIV-1 infection, their mechanism of action remains elusive. In this review, we introduce RT and highlight major advances from experimental and computational biophysical experiments toward an understanding of RT function and the inhibitory mechanism(s) of NNRTIs.

Reprinted from *Biomolecules*. Cite as: G. Schauer, G.; Leuba, S.; Sluis-Cremer, N. Biophysical Insights into the Inhibitory Mechanism of Non-Nucleoside HIV-1 Reverse Transcriptase Inhibitors. *Biomolecules* **2013**, *3*, 889-904.

1. Introduction

HIV-1 reverse transcriptase (RT) is an RNA- or DNA-dependent DNA polymerase and also contains ribonuclease H (RNase H) activity, thereby containing all the necessary enzymatic activity for the multistep conversion of HIV-1 single stranded RNA (ssRNA) into double stranded DNA (dsDNA) for subsequent integration into the human genome. RT thus remains the prime target for new antiretroviral therapies. Non-nucleoside RT inhibitors (NNRTIs) are potent inhibitors of reverse transcription, but despite having been successfully used in the clinic for over 15 years, a comprehensive explanation for their inhibitory mechanism(s) has remained elusive.

2. Structure and Function of HIV-1 RT

2.1. Reverse Transcription

Reverse transcription [1,2] is initiated by RT at the 3'-end of cellular lysyl-tRNA^{Lys,3}, which hybridizes to the primer binding site (PBS) on the HIV-1 genome. During initiation, RNA-primed RT elongates until the 5'-end of the HIV-1 RNA is reached, forming minus-strand strong-stop DNA (Figure 1). Employing the RNase H activity of RT, the remaining HIV-1 genomic RNA is cleaved to allow the nascently synthesized DNA to circularize and hybridize with the repeat sequence (R) at the 3'-end of the HIV-1 ssRNA. After this strand transfer, the nascent DNA strand is further elongated by RT. RT hydrolyzes the remaining RNA, but leaves behind a purine-rich sequence, named the polypurine tract (PPT), which subsequently serves as a primer for the initiation of second strand DNA synthesis. RT then elongates the PPT primer. The RNase H activity of RT removes all remaining RNA, including the transfer-RNA (tRNA) primer and the PPT. Strand transfer takes place by PBS sequence homology. DNA polymerization and strand-displacement followed by further DNA elongation results in an integrase-competent dsDNA, which is flanked by Long Terminal Repeat (LTR) sequences at both ends.

Figure 1. Reverse transcription. Schematic of the multistep process of the conversion of viral RNA (red) into integrase-competent dsDNA (bottom) for insertion into the human genome. PBS, primer binding site.

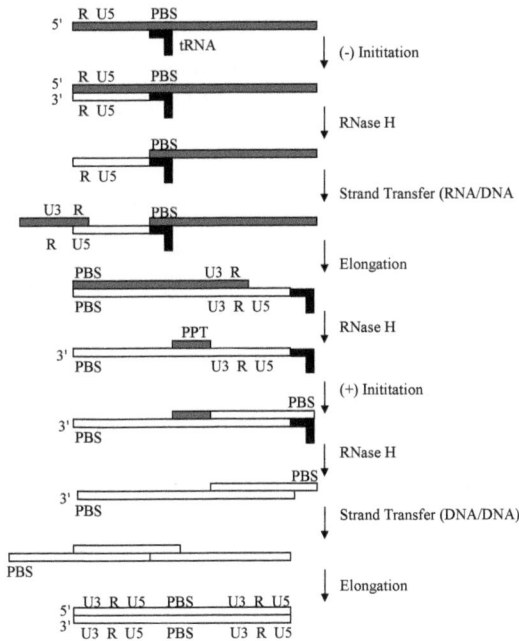

The resulting dsDNA is then a substrate for integrase, which catalyzes the insertion of dsDNA into the human genome [2].

2.2. Structural and Biophysical Studies of RT

With the ability to efficiently catalyze DNA polymerization on both RNA/DNA and DNA/DNA duplexes and also possessing RNase H activity, RT is an astonishingly versatile enzyme, due in large part to its modular structure. RT is a 110 kD heterodimer composed of two subunits: p66 (560 amino acids-long) and p51 (440 amino acids-long) [3]. Both subunits are a product of proteolytic processing of a gag-pol polyprotein by HIV-1 protease. In p51, the RNase-H domain (residues 440–560) has been cleaved, resulting in a structure that shares secondary structural elements with p66. However, since the overall tertiary structure is spatially configured differently than p66, p51 largely plays a scaffolding role for p66, the only subunit in the RT heterodimer to possess polymerase and RNase H activity [4,5].

X-ray crystallography, comprising the majority of biophysical studies on RT, has provided the community with an invaluable mechanistic understanding of RT. Beginning with the first structural elucidation of RT [5], there have since been hundreds of structures of RT solved (at the time of this writing, there were 245 structures of HIV-1 RT deposited in the Protein Database (PDB)). Additionally, a large body of mechanistic information complementary to the structural data has been gleaned from fluorescence-based kinetics studies. Like other DNA polymerases, RT is shaped like a right hand [5] (Figure 2).

Figure 2. Structure of reverse transcriptase (RT). RT is pictured as a solvent-accessible surface area model (taken from PDB ID: 1RTD). The DNA/DNA template/primer is shown as a cartoon. The p51 subdomain is colored in grey, and the p66 subdomain is subdivided into thumb (green), fingers (red), palm (purple), connection (wheat) and RNase H (blue) domains. The polymerase and RNase H active site residues are colored in yellow.

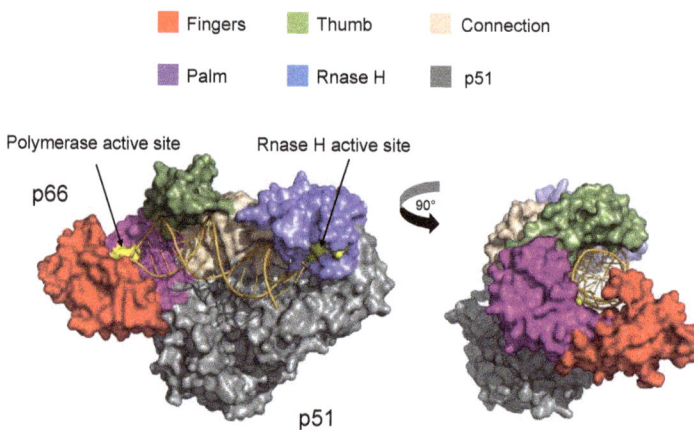

Its subdomains are accordingly named: fingers (residues 1–85 and 118–155), thumb (residues 237–318), palm (residues 86–117 and 156–236) and connection (319–426) subdomains (see Figure 2). In the *apo* structure of RT [6], the thumb and finger domains are nearly in contact, and the thumb resides in the nucleic acid binding cleft; however, to accommodate template/primer (T/P) substrates in the nucleic acid binding cleft, the thumb must extend outward [6,7]. Pre-steady-state kinetic analysis showed that binding to the T/P and deoxynucleotide triphosphate (dNTP) substrates is a two-step process involving initial entry of the T/P into the nucleic acid binding cleft and a slow step dependent on the conformational change of the enzyme to accommodate cognate dNTP, which can increase the overall binding affinity to the T/P substrate [8]. The resultant binary complex contains a T/P substrate simultaneously spanned by polymerase and RNase H active sites, approximately 18 base pairs apart.

2.3. Conformational Dynamics of Reverse Transcription

RT clamps down on the incoming nucleotide with its fingers [9], specifically, via the Lys65, Arg72, Asp113 and Ala114 residues of the β3-β4 loop [10]. Structures of RT complexed with a DNA/DNA template/primer that has been dideoxy terminated at the 3'-end (to create a dead-end complex in the presence of cognate dNTP) identified the binding site of dNTP: Asp113, Tyr115, Phe116 and Gln151 [9]. In agreement from pre-steady-state kinetics data and based on data from other polymerases [11], it was proposed that finger clamping of dNTP is a rate-limiting prerequisite to catalysis [12]. Pre-steady-state kinetic analysis showed that dNTP incorporation rates depend upon the composition of the T/P substrate and suggested that RT can bind T/P substrates in productive or nonproductive complexes in terms of dNTP incorporation and that RT must undergo an isomerization step in order for the RT-T/P complex to be converted into a productive one [13]. The presence of this dead-end complex was later directly visualized with single-pair Förster resonance energy transfer (FRET) via multiparameter fluorescence detection (MFD) [14,15]. It has further been shown, through a combination of stopped-flow fluorescence experiments and a molecular dynamics technique used to extend the timescales of simulations, called directional milestoning [16], that the rate-limiting step of finger bending is on the order of milliseconds and that the conformational change itself governs dNTP specificity [17]. The bending of the finger clamp precisely positions dNTP for incorporation, which is coordinated with the positioning of the growing primer by the "primer grip", composed of the β12-β13 hairpin [4]. Finally, formation of a nascent phosphodiester bond on a growing primer (*i.e.*, DNA polymerization) is coordinated by the catalytic triad in the palm subdomain (D110, D185, D186; part of the conserved YXDD motif, where Y and D stand for Tyrosine and Aspartate, respectively, and X stands for any amino acid), which is a conserved process amongst polymerases and is dependent upon two divalent metals [5]. The process of nucleotide addition ends in the release of pyrophosphate, which is accompanied by finger domain opening. In order for processive replication to continue, the T/P substrate needs to translocate one base pair with respect to RT, a process which is possibly linked to potential energy stored in the YMDD (Tyr-Met-Asp-Asp) loop, akin to a loaded springboard [18,19]. Consistent with this, atomic force microscopy (AFM) experiments demonstrated that finger clamping is likely responsible for generating the motor force necessary for RT translocation [20].

3. NNRTIs and Their Mechanism of Action

3.1. NNRTIs

NNRTIs are amphiphilic compounds that bind to a hydrophobic pocket in HIV-1 RT, called the NNRTI binding pocket (NNRTIBP), that is proximal to, but distinct from, the polymerase active site [21,22]. The NNRTIBP resides close to the p51-p66 interface and does not exist unless an NNRTI is bound [5,21]. NNRTIs typically bind with low nanomolar affinity and are potent inhibitors of reverse transcription [22]. In order of their approval from first to most recent, the five United States Federal Drug Adminstration (USFDA)-approved NNRTIs include nevirapine (NVP), delavirdine (DEL), efavirenz (EFV), etravirine (ETV) and rilpivirine (RIL) (Figure 3).

Figure 3. Chemical structures of USFDA-approved non-nucleoside RT inhibitors (NNRTIs).

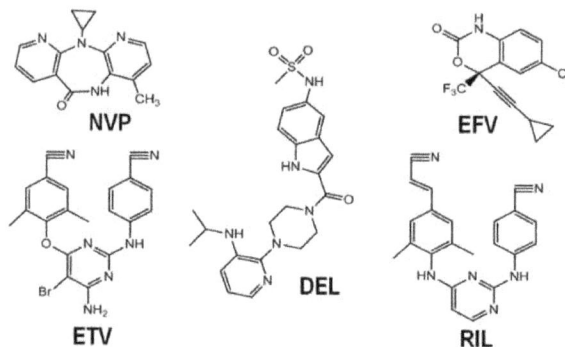

3.2. NNRTI Binding

Binding of NNRTI to RT is accompanied by rearrangements in the residues, Y181 and Y188, as well as in the primer grip motif, thereby forming the cavity of the NNRTIBP [5,6,21]. The fact that this pocket is not observed without the presence of NNRTIs has led some groups to conclude that an induced-fit mechanism [23] is responsible for NNRTI binding [24,25]; however, several other groups have demonstrated that conformational selection likely governs NNRTI binding [26–29]. Fourier transform ion cyclotron resonance mass spectrometry (FT-ICR MS) was originally used to show that p51 or p66 monomers undergo a population shift upon binding to EFV [28], and experiments monitoring EFV binding kinetics via tryptophan fluorescence were subsequently used to show that association of EFV to p51/p66 dimers was extremely slow, consistent with a conformational selection model [29]. Also consistent with this is data from nuclear magnetic resonance (NMR) experiments with RT that was site-specifically spin-labeled, which suggested that the primer grip was much more flexible than previously observed, presumably aiding in NNRTI binding [30]. The dynamic flexibility of the primer grip, comprising part of the NNRTIB, may provide evidence for conformational selection of NNRTIs. The likely important role of conformational selection has been further demonstrated using the Anisotropic Network Model [31] (ANM) combined with principle components analysis (PCA) methodology that both the unbound and NNRTI-bound conformation of RT intrinsically exist, but that NNRTI preferentially binds to conformations of RT within the structural ensemble, which are best predisposed toward NNRTI binding, shifting the population toward the NNRTI-bound form [27].

One obstacle to understanding the inhibitory mechanism of NNRTIs is that NNRTIs are practically insoluble in water at high concentrations (<10 mg/mL), such that traditional techniques for determining the equilibrium dissociation constant, K_d, are made difficult. For instance, traditional K_d determination with isothermal titration calorimetry (ITC), the "gold standard" for measuring reaction thermodynamics, is made difficult, since it typically requires higher concentrations of protein (and, therefore, drug) than attainable for NNRTIs. Most studies therefore use polymerase activity assays to indirectly infer K_d for NNRTIs; however, the disadvantage to this technique is that it only measures dNTP incorporation, such that, e.g., if NNRTIs primarily had an effect on nonproductive binding, it would be difficult to determine an accurate K_d. One alternative is surface plasmon resonance (SPR), which has been used to calculate K_d values for some NNRTIs [26,32,33]. Both SPR and ITC can be limited by extremely slow association and/or dissociation reactions, depending on the experiment [25,29]. One group circumvented the slow association of NNRTI to p51 monomers by extracting the K_d of EFV through the thermodynamic linkage between dimerization and NNRTI binding by combining kinetics from equilibrium dialysis, tryptophan fluorescence and native gel electrophoresis [29]. Another group recently surmounted the solubility barrier to ITC experiments by employing a technique using small, incremental injections of RT at regular intervals into the calorimeter (the Multiple Injection Method, or MIM [34]) containing fixed concentrations of NNRTI, demonstrating that, contrary to most reports, rather than acting on RT-DNA complexes, NNRTIs preferentially bind to free RT. This study showed that NNRTI-bound RT can then associate with DNA and form either a DNA-RT-NNRTI complex that exists in either a polymerase-competent incompetent configuration, both of which dNTP is unable to bind to [35].

3.3. Putative Mechanisms of Inhibition by NNRTIs

Interestingly, binding of NNRTIs does not appear to affect the ability of RT to bind incoming dNTPs [36,37]. Since the NNRTIBP is ~1 nm away from the polymerase active site and since binding of NNRTIs is noncompetitive with dNTP or template/primer binding [38], NNRTIs are considered classic allosteric inhibitors of HIV-1 RT DNA polymerization [21,39]. Despite their widespread use and remarkable efficacy, the precise mechanism(s) behind inhibition of reverse transcription by NNRTIs remains unclear [2,40–42], but proposed mechanisms have included restriction of thumb flexibility [5], distortion of the catalytic triad [43], primer grip repositioning [44], repositioning of the primer [45], enhancement of RNase H activity [46,47] and loosening of the thumb/finger clamp on template/primer substrates [48].

3.4. Molecular Arthritis

One persistent observation from the solved crystal structures of RT in the presence of NNRTIs has been the hyperextension of the thumb domain and a further opening of the finger domain accompanied by a marked decrease in flexibility, also known as "molecular arthritis [5]" (see Figure 4). Using hydrogen exchange mass spectrometry (HXMS), it was demonstrated that binding of EFV is allosterically coupled to regions of RT that are up to 6 nm away from the NRTIBP, primarily acting to stabilize the dynamics of these regions [39]. Elastic network models [31] and multicopy molecular dynamics simulations have shown that molecular arthritis appears to be closely related to the existence of a hinge region between the p51 and p66 subdomains [49,50]. Evaluating the slowest ANM modes, it was also shown that the presence of NNRTI changes the direction of finger and thumb motions, while the actual restriction of mobility was primarily seen in the presence of EFV, but not NVP [51]. Recently, however, one group using molecular dynamics simulations suggested that thumb mobility is not constrained as much as previously reported [52]. Notwithstanding, restriction of thumb flexibility has long been considered a key element in the inhibition mechanism [5], but whether molecular arthritis is directly and functionally tied to inhibition of polymerization is unclear.

Figure 4. Molecular arthritis. The structures of *apo* wild-type (WT) RT (left; PDB ID: 1DLO) and WT RT bound to efavirenz (right; PDB ID: 1FK9). Structures are represented by solvent-accessible surface area. The p51 subunit is colored in grey, and the p66 subunit is colored according to crystallographic B-factors, with blue being the least mobile and red the most mobile residues. EFV, efavirenz; NNRTIBP, NNRTI binding pocket.

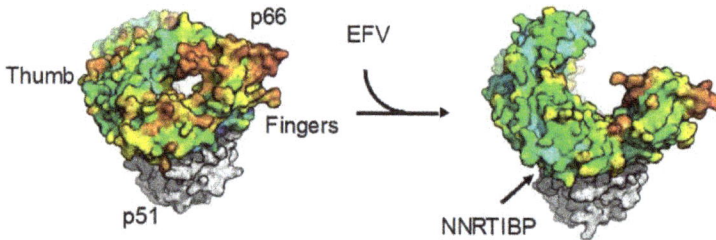

One possible effect of NNRTI-induced molecular arthritis is distortion of the catalytic triad [43]. In addition to the observation from crystal structures, repositioning of the catalytic triad into a polymerase incompetent configuration was directly observed in large, multicopy simulations of *apo* and NNRTI-bound RT [50]. Possibly linked to thumb hyperextension or simply to local rearrangements resulting from NNRTI binding, distortion of the precise constellation residues in the YXDD motif is presumed to be deleterious to polymerization activity. In a similar, but distinct, mechanism, it has also been postulated that NNRTI-induced molecular arthritis is responsible for repositioning the primer grip, eliminating the coordination of primer to the catalytic triad [44]. Furthermore, observation from crystal structures suggested that molecular arthritis is linked to the opening up of the RNase H domain, thereby providing access to degradation of DNA/RNA duplexes [53]. Consistent with this, EFV was shown to enhance RNase H activity [54].

3.5. Effect of NNRTIs on RT Dimerization

NNRTIs have been shown to enhance or stabilize the rate of RT heterodimerization, depending on the NNRTI studied, suggesting diversity in binding modes depending on chemical structure [55]. Perhaps counterintuitively, it has been demonstrated that some NNRTIs, such as EFV, act as potent chemical enhancers of HIV-1 RT heterodimerization [56,57]. To date, efavirenz was found to be the most potent enhancer of RT heterodimerization, whereas nevirapine has a weak effect, and delavirdine has no effect at all [56]. While some studies have demonstrated the effects of some potent NNRTIs, (e.g., efavirenz, dapivirine and etravirine) on the late stages of HIV replication [58,59], results from pre-steady-state kinetics experiments indicated that there does not appear to be a correlation between the impact of NNRTI-mediated enhancement of RT heterodimerization and the defects in RT polymerase function [60].

3.6. NNRTI Resistance Mutations

Due to the error-prone nature of RT, resistance mutations in and around the NNRTIBP arise during treatment regimens involving NNRTI therapy and are associated with virologic failure [61].

Because NNRTI resistance mutations are necessarily linked to RT function and to the mechanism of susceptibility of RT to NNRTIs, it is instructive to study them in order to better understand NNRTI mechanism [61]. It is generally understood that NNRTI resistance mutations can affect inhibitor binding by either altering one or more favorable interactions between the inhibitor and NNRTIBP (e.g., the Y181C mutation eliminates π-stacking interactions between this residue and the aromatic ring of the NNRTI [62]), by introducing steric barriers to NNRTI binding (e.g., G190E introduces a bulky side-chain, which may sterically interfere with NNRTI binding [63,64]) or by eliminating or altering the inter-residue network of the NNRTI-binding pocket, interfering with the ability of other residues in the pocket to envelop the NNRTI [21].

3.6.1. K103N

Although a discussion of all resistance mutations is beyond the scope of this review, particularly in light of the accessibility of growing RT crystals for structural determination, resulting in an abundance of solved structures of RT with various resistance mutations, we will discuss K103N as a prime example of an NNRTI-resistance mutation, since it is the most commonly reported clinical mutation [65]. K103N confers high level resistance to a wide range of NNRTIs, notably efavirenz (EFV) and nevirapine (NVP) (approximately 20-fold reduction in susceptibility) [66]. Despite its devastating effects on susceptibility to first-generation NNRTIs, the mechanism of resistance by K103N remains unclear. Observations from the first structures of K103N RT [62,67] indicated that neither K103 nor the mutant N103 residue make any contacts with EFV or NVP (although K103 can H-bond with delavirdine (DEL)) [65]. It was initially proposed that the K103N mutation was responsible for adding an extra H-bond with Y188 in the NNRTIBP, stabilizing the *apo* form of RT [67]; however, the energy of an H-bond is relatively weak compared to that of NNRTI binding, and surface plasmon resonance (SPR) studies showed that K103N actually facilitates entry and exit into the NNRTIBP [38]. It was later inferred from a K103N/Y181C double mutant that the extra H-bond was possibly mediated by a Na^+ ion and water molecules in the NNRTIBP [68]. Unlike first generation NNRTIs, the next generation diarylpyrimidine NNRTIs, etravirine (ETR) and rilpivirine (RIL), are effective against K103N RT [69–73]. At the moment, however, it is unclear what advantage these inhibitors have over first generation NNRTIs, although the crystal structures of K103N/Y181C RT and K103N/L101I RT suggest that the flexibility of ETR and RIL may allow the NNRTIBP to conform to these drugs, even in the presence of resistance mutations in the NNRTIBP [71]. It is also possible that the strengthened H-bond network conferred by K103N is broken by this new class of NNRTIs through a binding mode with extra favorable interactions [73]. Alternately, the diarylpyrimidine NNRTIs may be able to overcome K103N in a yet-to-be determined mechanism.

3.7. Structures of NNRTI-Bound RT-T/P Complexes

Until recently, there only existed structures of RT complexed with dsDNA template/primer (T/P) mimic substrates (mostly DNA/DNA, DNA/PPT) or structures of RT complexed with NNRTIs; however, there was no structure of a ternary RT-T/P-NNRTI complex. Recently, however, a structure of RT crosslinked to a DNA/DNA T/P substrate and bound to nevirapine (NVP) was elucidated [45], wherein the authors observed a distortion of the primer grip accompanied by thumb hyperextension and a 5.5 Å shift of the 3'-end primer away from the active site, dNTP binding site distortion and a reduction in RT-T/P contacts. By restricting the mobility of RT, it is possible that crosslinking of RT to the T/P substrate could lead to experimental artifacts. Soon after, structures of RT bound to several DNA/RNA T/P substrates in the presence of NVP and EFV were solved without the use of crosslinking agents [47]. The structure showed that NNRTIs pushed RT toward a degradative/RNase H-competent mode (as opposed to a polymerase competent mode) in the context of a hybrid substrate, which is consistent with the findings that EFV accelerates RNA degradation [54].

3.8. Insights into RT Dynamics from Time-Resolved Single-Molecule Experiments

Given the heterogeneity and complexity of the processes involved in reverse transcription and the suspected dynamic nature of RT-T/P interactions, there is great interest in observing single kinetic processes of reverse transcription. Due to the brief amount of time spent in the observation volume (~1 ms), single-molecule methods based on confocal fluorescence microscopy provide instantaneous, albeit detailed, structural information from FRET signals [14,15,74]. In contrast, time-resolved single-molecule techniques, relying on surface-tethering schemes, offer a glimpse into a broad range of dynamic processes for up to several minutes. One method to visualize RT dynamics on nucleic acid substrates is through direct visualization of the lengthening of flow-stretched, bead-tethered ssDNA [75] by RT as it completes primer extension [76]. Using this technique, different rates of primer extension and strand displacement were observed, and it was shown that RT dynamically switches between these modes, depending on the composition of the substrate [77]. Crucially, single-pair FRET experiments using total internal reflection fluorescence microscopy (TIRFM) [78] revealed that RT slides on nucleic acid substrates in a highly dynamic manner [48]. While cognate dNTP stabilized the polymerase competent configuration, NNRTI destabilized this configuration, enhancing the sliding dynamics of RT on the T/P. Remarkably, RT was shown to flip on template/primer substrates and can reside in different relative orientations based on the composition of the template/primer alone. It was further shown that RT bound T/P substrates in opposite orientations depending on whether it contains a DNA or RNA primer [77]. The relative orientation was a direct predictor of enzymatic activity; *i.e.*, when assayed for activity, the orientations were shown to be either polymerase-competent or RNase H-competent. When bound to a T/P with a PPT primer, RT could flip between these orientations, and the rate of flipping could be slowed by dNTP (directing RT toward a polymerase-competent configuration) or enhanced by NNRTIs (directing it toward an RNA-degradative orientation) [77]. Taken together, these results indicated that modulation of the grip on the T/P substrate itself by NNRTIs may alter RT-T/P dynamics, disfavoring the polymerase mode, suggesting that NNRTI-induced molecular arthritis affects the grip on the template/primer substrate. Intriguingly, it was recently demonstrated that the binding of the various dimeric isoforms of RT could be distinguished using a single-molecule fluorescence method, called Protein-Induced Fluorescence Enhancement (PIFE) [79], where the authors were able to monitor the binding of RT via the fluorescence intensity enhancement of a Cy3-labeled T/P resulting from the proximity of RT to Cy3 [80].

4. Conclusions and Future Directions

Combining results from many interdisciplinary biophysical experiments, a comprehensive picture of the mechanism(s) of action of NNRTIs is emerging, but is far from complete. Clearly, molecular arthritis plays a role in the inhibitory mechanism of NNRTI, but the exact link between modulation of structural dynamics as it relates to the attenuation of RT function remains unclear. Exciting new means of obtaining the crystal structures of T/P-bound RT in the presence of NNRTIs have emerged, and novel structures of T/P-bound, NNRTI-resistant RT mutants complexed to their relative NNRTIs are likely soon to follow. In X-ray crystallographic studies, crystal packing can lead to underestimation of flexibility, as shown for RT with Hydrogen-Deuterium Exchange Mass Spectrometry (HXMS) [81] and NMR [30], highlighting the necessity of using molecular dynamics simulations to probe the conformational dynamics of solved structures. Advances in sampling techniques for molecular simulations combined with the continually increasing computational power afforded by Moore's Law [82] will help bring these structures to life, providing unprecedented knowledge of the conformational dynamics of reverse transcription and its inhibition by NNRTIs. Advances in the techniques used to quantify the thermodynamics of NNRTI binding may help in understanding the evolutionary rationale for certain NNRTI resistance mutations. Novel spin-label probes for NMR experiments will permit measurement of the dynamics of new regions of RT in the presence or absence of NNRTIs. Although traditional biophysical experiments have afforded crucial insight into the mechanisms of reverse transcription and its inhibition by NNRTIs, single-molecule biophysical experiments offer many strategic advantages over bulk experiments when it comes to understanding the kinetic mechanisms of a dynamic enzyme like RT. For instance, since traditional bulk fluorescence spectroscopy experiments represent an ensemble average of many unsynchronized kinetic processes occurring simultaneously (not all of which are related to the observable of interest), data from these techniques may be difficult to interpret [83]. Furthermore, crystallographic structures represent an ensemble average of structural states at equilibrium, but cannot provide information on the transitional intermediates between these states. Eliminating bulk averaging and enabling the visualization of rare events not associated with low-energy structures, single-molecule techniques will likely be increasingly used to resolve signals from individual RT complexes without the need for synchronization [83]. It will be interesting to see whether the techniques involving the multiplexed observation of flow-stretched DNA molecules will be put to use to probe NNRTI function. Completely new types of information have been made available from single-pair FRET, and these experiments are likely to continue. Although experiments cannot provide the detailed structural and/or orientation information, it is nonetheless an extensible technique that will likely see more use in the near future. Since PIFE does not require exogenous labeling of RT, it does not require structural perturbation and also may be more accessible to some laboratories than FRET. Furthermore, through observation of signals from T/P in the presence of unlabeled RT, single-molecule protein induced fluorescence enhancement (PIFE) experiments [80] allow the observation of physiologically relevant RT concentrations by providing a workaround to the "concentration problem" [83] seen in single-molecule FRET experiments, which are limited to the use of low nanomolar concentrations of labeled protein. Biophysical studies of RT structure, function and inhibition by NNRTI are all interrelated; e.g., the results from time-resolved single-molecule experiments must be informed by the structural data, the interpretation of which is, in turn, aided by new advances in computational simulation and biophysical techniques to measure protein dynamics. Combining these powerful methodologies, a great wave of enlightening structural information about HIV-1 RT is imminent, hopefully providing new strategies for rational drug design against this highly elusive target.

Acknowledgments

Our work on NNRTIs has been funded by grants AI081571, GM068406 and T32GM088119 from the National Institutes of Health (USA).

Conflicts of Interest

The authors declare no conflict of interest.

References

1. Hu, W.-S.; Hughes, S.H. HIV-1 reverse transcription. *Cold Spring Harb. Perspect. Med.* **2012**, *2*, doi:10.1101/cshperspect.a006882.
2. Sluis-Cremer, N.; Tachedjian, G. Mechanisms of inhibition of HIV replication by non-nucleoside reverse transcriptase inhibitors. *Virus Res.* **2008**, *134*, 147–156.
3. Divita, G.; Restle, T.; Goody, R.S. Characterization of the dimerization process of HIV-1 reverse transcriptase heterodimer using intrinsic protein fluorescence. *FEBS Lett.* **1993**, *324*, 153–158.
4. Jacobo-Molina, A.; Ding, J.; Nanni, R.G.; Clark, A.D.; Lu, X.; Tantillo, C.; Williams, R.L.; Kamer, G.; Ferris, A.L.; Clark, P. Crystal structure of human immunodeficiency virus type 1 reverse transcriptase complexed with double-stranded DNA at 3.0 A resolution shows bent DNA. *Proc. Natl. Acad. Sci. USA* **1993**, *90*, 6320–6324.
5. Kohlstaedt, L.A.; Wang, J.; Friedman, J.M.; Rice, P.A.; Steitz, T.A. Crystal structure at 3.5 Å resolution of HIV-1 reverse transcriptase complexed with an inhibitor. *Science* **1992**, *256*, 1783–1790.
6. Rodgers, D.W.; Gamblin, S.J.; Harris, B.A.; Ray, S.; Culp, J.S.; Hellmig, B.; Woolf, D.J.; Debouck, C.; Harrison, S.C. The structure of unliganded reverse transcriptase from the human immunodeficiency virus type 1. *Proc. Natl. Acad. Sci. USA* **1995**, *92*, 1222–1226.
7. Esnouf, R.; Ren, J.; Ross, C.; Jones, Y.; Stammers, D.; Stuart, D. Mechanism of inhibition of HIV-1 reverse transcriptase by non-nucleoside inhibitors. *Nat. Struct. Mol. Biol.* **1995**, *2*, 303–308.
8. KruhØfter, M.; Urbanke, C.; Grosse, F. Two step binding of HIV-1 reverse transcriptase to nucleic acid substrates. *Nucleic Acids Res.* **1993**, *21*, 3943–3949.
9. Huang, H.; Chopra, R.; Verdine, G.L.; Harrison, S.C. Structure of a covalently trapped catalytic complex of HIV-1 reverse transcriptase: Implications for drug resistance. *Science* **1998**, *282*, 1669–1675.
10. Grice, S.F.J.L. Human immunodeficiency virus reverse transcriptase: 25 Years of research, drug discovery, and promise. *J. Biol. Chem.* **2012**, *287*, 40850–40857.

11. Kati, W.M.; Johnson, K.A.; Jerva, L.F.; Anderson, K.S. Mechanism and fidelity of HIV reverse transcriptase. *J. Biol. Chem.* **1992**, *267*, 25988–25997.

12. Sarafianos, S.G.; Das, K.; Ding, J.; Boyer, P.L.; Hughes, S.H.; Arnold, E. Touching the heart of HIV-1 drug resistance: The fingers close down on the dNTP at the polymerase active site. *Chem. Biol.* **1999**, *6*, R137–R146.

13. Wöhrl, B.M.; Krebs, R.; Goody, R.S.; Restle, T. Refined model for primer/template binding by HIV-1 reverse transcriptase: Pre-steady-state kinetic analyses of primer/template binding and nucleotide incorporation events distinguish between different binding modes depending on the nature of the nucleic acid substrate. *J. Mol. Biol.* **1999**, *292*, 333–344.

14. Rothwell, P.J.; Berger, S.; Kensch, O.; Felekyan, S.; Antonik, M.; Wöhrl, B.M.; Restle, T.; Goody, R.S.; Seidel, C.A.M. Multiparameter single-molecule fluorescence spectroscopy reveals heterogeneity of HIV-1 reverse transcriptase:primer/template complexes. *Proc. Natl. Acad. Sci. USA* **2003**, *100*, 1655–1660.

15. Sisamakis, E.; Valeri, A.; Kalinin, S.; Rothwell, P.J.; Seidel, C.A.M. Accurate single-molecule FRET studies using multiparameter fluorescence detection. *Methods Enzymol.* **2010**, *475*, 455–514.

16. Faradjian, A.K.; Elber, R. Computing time scales from reaction coordinates by milestoning. *J. Chem. Phys.* **2004**, *120*, 10880–10889.

17. Kirmizialtin, S.; Nguyen, V.; Johnson, K.A.; Elber, R. How conformational dynamics of DNA polymerase select correct substrates: Experiments and simulations. *Structure* **2012**, *20*, 618–627.

18. Götte, M.; Rausch, J.W.; Marchand, B.; Sarafianos, S.; le Grice, S.F.J. Reverse transcriptase in motion: Conformational dynamics of enzyme-substrate interactions. *Biochim. Biophys. Acta* **2010**, *1804*, 1202–1212.

19. Sarafianos, S.G.; Clark, A.D.; Das, K.; Tuske, S.; Birktoft, J.J.; Ilankumaran, P.; Ramesha, A.R.; Sayer, J.M.; Jerina, D.M.; Boyer, P.L.; *et al.* Structures of HIV-1 reverse transcriptase with pre- and post-translocation AZTMP-terminated DNA. *EMBO J.* **2002**, *21*, 6614–6624.

20. Lu, H.; Macosko, J.; Habel-Rodriguez, D.; Keller, R.W.; Brozik, J.A.; Keller, D.J. Closing of the fingers domain generates motor forces in the HIV reverse transcriptase. *J. Biol. Chem.* **2004**, *279*, 54529–54532.

21. Sluis-Cremer, N.; Temiz, N.A.; Bahar, I. Conformational changes in HIV-1 reverse transcriptase induced by nonnucleoside reverse transcriptase inhibitor binding. *Curr. HIV Res.* **2004**, *2*, 323–332.

22. De Béthune, M.-P. Non-nucleoside reverse transcriptase inhibitors (NNRTIs), their discovery, development, and use in the treatment of HIV-1 infection: A review of the last 20 years (1989–2009). *Antiviral Res.* **2010**, *85*, 75–90.

23. Zhou, H.-X. From induced fit to conformational selection: A continuum of binding mechanism controlled by the timescale of conformational transitions. *Biophys. J.* **2010**, *98*, L15–L17.

24. Basavapathruni, A.; Anderson, K.S. Reverse transcription of the HIV-1 pandemic. *FASEB J.* **2007**, *21*, 3795–3808.

25. Elinder, M.; Selhorst, P.; Vanham, G.; Oberg, B.; Vrang, L.; Danielson, U.H. Inhibition of HIV-1 by non-nucleoside reverse transcriptase inhibitors via an induced fit mechanism-importance of slow dissociation and relaxation rates for antiviral efficacy. *Biochem. Pharmacol.* **2010**, *80*, 1133–1140.

26. Geitmann, M.; Unge, T.; Danielson, U.H. Biosensor-based kinetic characterization of the interaction between HIV-1 reverse transcriptase and non-nucleoside inhibitors. *J. Med. Chem.* **2006**, *49*, 2367–2374.

27. Bakan, A.; Bahar, I. The intrinsic dynamics of enzymes plays a dominant role in determining the structural changes induced upon inhibitor binding. *Proc. Natl. Acad. Sci. USA* **2009**, *106*, 14349–14354.

28. Braz, V.A.; Barkley, M.D.; Jockusch, R.A.; Wintrode, P.L. Efavirenz binding site in HIV-1 reverse transcriptase monomers. *Biochemistry* **2010**, *49*, 10565–10573.

29. Braz, V.A.; Holladay, L.A.; Barkley, M.D. Efavirenz binding to HIV-1 reverse transcriptase monomers and dimers. *Biochemistry* **2010**, *49*, 601–610.

30. Zheng, X.; Mueller, G.A.; DeRose, E.F.; London, R.E. Solution characterization of [methyl-13C]methionine HIV-1 reverse transcriptase by NMR spectroscopy. *Antiviral Res.* **2009**, *84*, 205–214.

31. Chennubhotla, C.; Rader, A.J.; Yang, L.-W.; Bahar, I. Elastic network models for understanding biomolecular machinery: From enzymes to supramolecular assemblies. *Phys. Biol.* **2005**, *2*, S173–S180.

32. Radi, M.; Maga, G.; Alongi, M.; Angeli, L.; Samuele, A.; Zanoli, S.; Bellucci, L.; Tafi, A.; Casaluce, G.; Giorgi, G.; *et al.* Discovery of chiral cyclopropyl dihydro-alkylthio-benzyl-oxopyrimidine (S-DABO) derivatives as potent HIV-1 reverse transcriptase inhibitors with high activity against clinically relevant mutants. *J. Med. Chem.* **2009**, *52*, 840–851.

33. Geitmann, M.; Unge, T.; Danielson, U.H. Interaction kinetic characterization of HIV-1 reverse transcriptase non-nucleoside inhibitor resistance. *J. Med. Chem.* **2006**, *49*, 2375–2387.

34. Burnouf, D.; Ennifar, E.; Guedich, S.; Puffer, B.; Hoffmann, G.; Bec, G.; Disdier, F.; Baltzinger, M.; Dumas, P. kinITC: A new method for obtaining joint thermodynamic and kinetic data by isothermal titration calorimetry. *J. Am. Chem. Soc.* **2012**, *134*, 559–565.

35. Bec, G.; Meyer, B.; Gerard, M.-A.; Steger, J.; Fauster, K.; Wolff, P.; Burnouf, D.Y.; Micura, R.; Dumas, P.; Ennifar, E. Thermodynamics of HIV-1 reverse transcriptase in action elucidates the mechanism of action of non-nucleoside inhibitors. *J. Am. Chem. Soc.* **2013**, *135*, 9743–9752.

36. Rittinger, K.; Divita, G.; Goody, R.S. Human immunodeficiency virus reverse transcriptase substrate-induced conformational changes and the mechanism of inhibition by nonnucleoside inhibitors. *Proc. Natl. Acad. Sci. USA* **1995**, *92*, 8046–8049.

37. Spence, R.; Kati, W.; Anderson, K.; Johnson, K. Mechanism of inhibition of HIV-1 reverse transcriptase by nonnucleoside inhibitors. *Science* **1995**, *267*, 988–993.

38. Divita, G.; Mueller, B.; Immendoerfer, U.; Gautel, M.; Rittinger, K.; Restle, T.; Goody, R.S. Kinetics of interaction of HIV reverse transcriptase with primer/template. *Biochemistry* **1993**, *32*, 7966–7971.

39. Seckler, J.M.; Barkley, M.D.; Wintrode, P.L. Allosteric suppression of HIV-1 reverse transcriptase structural dynamics upon inhibitor binding. *Biophys. J.* **2011**, *100*, 144–153.

40. Esposito, F.; Corona, A.; Tramontano, E. HIV-1 reverse transcriptase still remains a new drug target: Structure, function, classical inhibitors, and new inhibitors with innovative mechanisms of actions. *Mol. Biol. Int.* **2012**, *2012*, 1–23.

41. Sarafianos, S.G.; Marchand, B.; Das, K.; Himmel, D.M.; Parniak, M.A.; Hughes, S.H.; Arnold, E. Structure and function of HIV-1 reverse transcriptase: Molecular mechanisms of polymerization and inhibition. *J. Mol. Biol.* **2009**, *385*, 693–713.

42. Ren, J.; Nichols, C.E.; Stamp, A.; Chamberlain, P.P.; Ferris, R.; Weaver, K.L.; Short, S.A.; Stammers, D.K. Structural insights into mechanisms of non-nucleoside drug resistance for HIV-1 reverse transcriptases mutated at codons 101 or 138. *FEBS J.* **2006**, *273*, 3850–3860.

43. Ren, J.; Esnouf, R.; Garman, E.; Somers, D.; Ross, C.; Kirby, I.; Keeling, J.; Darby, G.; Jones, Y.; Stuart, D. High resolution structures of HIV-1 RT from four RT-inhibitor complexes. *Nat. Struct. Biol.* **1995**, *2*, 293–302.

44. Das, K.; Ding, J.; Hsiou, Y.; Clark, A.D., Jr.; Moereels, H.; Koymans, L.; Andries, K.; Pauwels, R.; Janssen, P.A.; Boyer, P.L.; *et al.* Crystal structures of 8-Cl and 9-Cl TIBO complexed with wild-type HIV-1 RT and 8-Cl TIBO complexed with the Tyr181Cys HIV-1 RT drug-resistant mutant. *J. Mol. Biol.* **1996**, *264*, 1085–1100.

45. Das, K.; Martinez, S.E.; Bauman, J.D.; Arnold, E. HIV-1 reverse transcriptase complex with DNA and nevirapine reveals non-nucleoside inhibition mechanism. *Nat. Struct. Mol. Biol.* **2012**, *19*, 253–259.

46. Delviks-Frankenberry, K.A.; Nikolenko, G.N.; Pathak, V.K. The "connection" between HIV drug resistance and RNase H. *Viruses* **2010**, *2*, 1476–1503.

47. Lapkouski, M.; Tian, L.; Miller, J.T.; Le Grice, S.F.J.; Yang, W. Complexes of HIV-1 RT, NNRTI and RNA/DNA hybrid reveal a structure compatible with RNA degradation. *Nat. Struct. Mol. Biol.* **2013**, *20*, 230–236.

48. Liu, S.; Abbondanzieri, E.A.; Rausch, J.W.; Grice, S.F.J.L.; Zhuang, X. Slide into action: Dynamic shuttling of HIV reverse transcriptase on nucleic acid substrates. *Science* **2008**, *322*, 1092–1097.

49. Bahar, I.; Erman, B.; Jernigan, R.L.; Atilgan, A.R.; Covell, D.G. Collective motions in HIV-1 reverse transcriptase: Examination of flexibility and enzyme function. *J. Mol. Biol.* **1999**, *285*, 1023–1037.

50. Ivetac, A.; McCammon, J.A. Elucidating the inhibition mechanism of HIV-1 non-nucleoside reverse transcriptase inhibitors through multicopy molecular dynamics simulations. *J. Mol. Biol.* **2009**, *388*, 644–658.

51. Temiz, N.A.; Bahar, I. Inhibitor binding alters the directions of domain motions in HIV-1 reverse transcriptase. *Proteins Struct. Funct. Genet.* **2002**, *49*, 61–70.

52. Wright, D.W.; Sadiq, S.K.; de Fabritiis, G.; Coveney, P.V. Thumbs down for HIV: Domain level rearrangements do occur in the NNRTI-bound HIV-1 reverse transcriptase. *J. Am. Chem. Soc.* **2012**, *134*, 12885–12888.

53. Shaw-Reid, C.A.; Feuston, B.; Munshi, V.; Getty, K.; Krueger, J.; Hazuda, D.J.; Parniak, M.A.; Miller, M.D.; Lewis, D. Dissecting the effects of DNA polymerase and ribonuclease H inhibitor combinations on HIV-1 reverse-transcriptase activities. *Biochemistry* **2005**, *44*, 1595–1606.

54. Radzio, J.; Sluis-Cremer, N. Efavirenz accelerates HIV-1 reverse transcriptase ribonuclease H cleavage, leading to diminished zidovudine excision. *Mol. Pharmacol.* **2008**, *73*, 601–606.

55. Tachedjian, G.; Goff, S.P. The effect of NNRTIs on HIV reverse transcriptase dimerization. *Curr. Opin. Investig. Drugs* **2003**, *4*, 966–973.

56. Tachedjian, G.; Orlova, M.; Sarafianos, S.G.; Arnold, E.; Goff, S.P. Nonnucleoside reverse transcriptase inhibitors are chemical enhancers of dimerization of the HIV type 1 reverse transcriptase. *Proc. Natl. Acad. Sci. USA* **2001**, *98*, 7188–7193.

57. Venezia, C.F.; Howard, K.J.; Ignatov, M.E.; Holladay, L.A.; Barkley, M.D. Effects of efavirenz binding on the subunit equilibria of HIV-1 reverse transcriptase. *Biochemistry* **2006**, *45*, 2779–2789.

58. Tachedjian, G.; Moore, K.L.; Goff, S.P.; Sluis-Cremer, N. Efavirenz enhances the proteolytic processing of an HIV-1 pol polyprotein precursor and reverse transcriptase homodimer formation. *FEBS Lett.* **2005**, *579*, 379–384.

59. Figueiredo, A.; Moore, K.L.; Mak, J.; Sluis-Cremer, N.; de Bethune, M.-P.; Tachedjian, G. Potent nonnucleoside reverse transcriptase inhibitors target HIV-1 Gag-Pol. *PLoS Pathog.* **2006**, *2*, e119.

60. Xia, Q.; Radzio, J.; Anderson, K.S.; Sluis-Cremer, N. Probing nonnucleoside inhibitor-induced active-site distortion in HIV-1 reverse transcriptase by transient kinetic analyses. *Protein Sci.* **2007**, *16*, 1728–1737.

61. Menéndez-Arias, L. Molecular basis of human immunodeficiency virus type 1 drug resistance: Overview and recent developments. *Antiviral Res.* **2013**, *98*, 93–120.

62. Ren, J.; Nichols, C.; Bird, L.; Chamberlain, P.; Weaver, K.; Short, S.; Stuart, D.I.; Stammers, D.K. Structural mechanisms of drug resistance for mutations at codons 181 and 188 in HIV-1 reverse transcriptase and the improved resilience of second generation non-nucleoside inhibitors. *J. Mol. Biol.* **2001**, *312*, 795–805.

63. Huang, W.; Gamarnik, A.; Limoli, K.; Petropoulos, C.J.; Whitcomb, J.M. Amino acid substitutions at position 190 of human immunodeficiency virus type 1 reverse transcriptase increase susceptibility to delavirdine and impair virus replication. *J. Virol.* **2003**, *77*, 1512–1523.

64. Yap, S.-H.; Sheen, C.-W.; Fahey, J.; Zanin, M.; Tyssen, D.; Lima, V.D.; Wynhoven, B.; Kuiper, M.; Sluis-Cremer, N.; Harrigan, P.R.; *et al.* N348I in the connection domain of HIV-1 reverse transcriptase confers zidovudine and nevirapine resistance. *PLoS Med.* **2007**, *4*, e335.

65. Ren, J.; Stammers, D.K. Structural basis for drug resistance mechanisms for non-nucleoside inhibitors of HIV reverse transcriptase. *Virus Res.* **2008**, *134*, 157–170.

66. Clotet, B. Efavirenz: Resistance and cross-resistance. *Int. J. Clin. Pract. Suppl.* **1999**, *103*, 21–25.

67. Hsiou, Y.; Ding, J.; Das, K.; Clark, A.D., Jr.; Boyer, P.L.; Lewi, P.; Janssen, P.A.; Kleim, J.-P.; Rösner, M.; Hughes, S.H.; *et al.* The Lys103Asn mutation of HIV-1 RT: A novel mechanism of drug resistance. *J. Mol. Biol.* **2001**, *309*, 437–445.

68. Das, K.; Sarafianos, S.G.; Clark, A.D., Jr.; Boyer, P.L.; Hughes, S.H.; Arnold, E. Crystal structures of clinically relevant Lys103Asn/Tyr181Cys double mutant HIV-1 reverse transcriptase in complexes with ATP and non-nucleoside inhibitor HBY 097. *J. Mol. Biol.* **2007**, *365*, 77–89.

69. Andries, K.; Azijn, H.; Thielemans, T.; Ludovici, D.; Kukla, M.; Heeres, J.; Janssen, P.; de Corte, B.; Vingerhoets, J.; Pauwels, R.; *et al.* TMC125, a novel next-generation nonnucleoside reverse transcriptase inhibitor active against nonnucleoside reverse transcriptase inhibitor-resistant human immunodeficiency virus type 1. *Antimicrob. Agents Chemother.* **2004**, *48*, 4680–4686.

70. Das, K.; Bauman, J.D.; Clark, A.D.; Frenkel, Y.V.; Lewi, P.J.; Shatkin, A.J.; Hughes, S.H.; Arnold, E. High-resolution structures of HIV-1 reverse transcriptase/TMC278 complexes: Strategic flexibility explains potency against resistance mutations. *Proc. Natl. Acad. Sci. USA* **2008**, *105*, 1466–1471.

71. Azijn, H.; Tirry, I.; Vingerhoets, J.; de Béthune, M.-P.; Kraus, G.; Boven, K.; Jochmans, D.; van Craenenbroeck, E.; Picchio, G.; Rimsky, L.T. TMC278, a next-generation nonnucleoside reverse transcriptase inhibitor (NNRTI), active against wild-type and NNRTI-resistant HIV-1. *Antimicrob. Agents Chemother.* **2010**, *54*, 718–727.

72. Lansdon, E.B.; Brendza, K.M.; Hung, M.; Wang, R.; Mukund, S.; Jin, D.; Birkus, G.; Kutty, N.; Liu, X. Crystal structures of HIV-1 reverse transcriptase with etravirine (TMC125) and rilpivirine (TMC278): Implications for drug design. *J. Med. Chem.* **2010**, *53*, 4295–4299.

73. Rawal, R.K.; Murugesan, V.; Katti, S.B. Structure-activity relationship studies on clinically relevant HIV-1 NNRTIs. *Curr. Med. Chem.* **2012**, *19*, 5364–5380.

74. Kalinin, S.; Peulen, T.; Sindbert, S.; Rothwell, P.J.; Berger, S.; Restle, T.; Goody, R.S.; Gohlke, H.; Seidel, C.A.M. A toolkit and benchmark study for FRET-restrained high-precision structural modeling. *Nat. Methods* **2012**, *9*, 1218–1225.

75. Kim, S.; Blainey, P.C.; Schroeder, C.M.; Xie, X.S. Multiplexed single-molecule assay for enzymatic activity on flow-stretched DNA. *Nat. Methods* **2007**, *4*, 397–399.

76. Kim, S.; Schroeder, C.M.; Xie, X.S. Single-molecule study of DNA polymerization activity of HIV-1 reverse transcriptase on DNA templates. *J. Mol. Biol.* **2010**, *395*, 995–1006.

77. Abbondanzieri, E.A.; Bokinsky, G.; Rausch, J.W.; Zhang, J.X.; Le Grice, S.F.J.; Zhuang, X. Dynamic binding orientations direct activity of HIV reverse transcriptase. *Nature* **2008**, *453*, 184–189.

78. Fagerburg, M.V.; Leuba, S.H. Optimal practices for surface-tethered single molecule total internal reflection fluorescence resonance energy transfer analysis. *Methods Mol. Biol.* **2011**, *749*, 273–289.

79. Hwang, H.; Kim, H.; Myong, S. Protein induced fluorescence enhancement as a single molecule assay with short distance sensitivity. *Proc. Natl. Acad. Sci. USA* **2011**, *108*, 7414–7418.

80. Marko, R.A.; Liu, H.-W.; Ablenas, C.J.; Ehteshami, M.; Götte, M.; Cosa, G. Binding kinetics and affinities of heterodimeric *versus* homodimeric HIV-1 reverse transcriptase on DNA—DNA substrates at the single-molecule level. *J. Phys. Chem. B* **2013**, *117*, 4560–4567.

81. Seckler, J.M.; Howard, K.J.; Barkley, M.D.; Wintrode, P.L. Solution structural dynamics of HIV-1 reverse transcriptase heterodimer. *Biochemistry* **2009**, *48*, 7646–7655.
82. Moore, G.E. *Cramming More Components onto Integrated Circuits*; McGraw-Hill: New York, NY, USA, 1965.
83. Van Oijen, A.M. Single-molecule approaches to characterizing kinetics of biomolecular interactions. *Curr. Opin. Biotechnol.* **2011**, *22*, 75–80.

Research Applications of Proteolytic Enzymes in Molecular Biology

János András Mótyán, Ferenc Tóth and József Tőzsér

Abstract: Proteolytic enzymes (also termed peptidases, proteases and proteinases) are capable of hydrolyzing peptide bonds in proteins. They can be found in all living organisms, from viruses to animals and humans. Proteolytic enzymes have great medical and pharmaceutical importance due to their key role in biological processes and in the life-cycle of many pathogens. Proteases are extensively applied enzymes in several sectors of industry and biotechnology, furthermore, numerous research applications require their use, including production of Klenow fragments, peptide synthesis, digestion of unwanted proteins during nucleic acid purification, cell culturing and tissue dissociation, preparation of recombinant antibody fragments for research, diagnostics and therapy, exploration of the structure-function relationships by structural studies, removal of affinity tags from fusion proteins in recombinant protein techniques, peptide sequencing and proteolytic digestion of proteins in proteomics. The aim of this paper is to review the molecular biological aspects of proteolytic enzymes and summarize their applications in the life sciences.

Reprinted from *Biomolecules*. Cite as: Mótyán, J.A.; Tóth, F.; Tőzsér, J. Research Applications of Proteolytic Enzymes in Molecular Biology. *Biomolecules* **2013**, *3*, 923-942.

1. Scope of the Review

Proteolytic enzymes are capable of hydrolyzing peptide bonds and are also referred to as peptidases, proteases or proteinases [1].

The physiological function of proteases is necessary for all living organisms, from viruses to humans, and proteolytic enzymes can be classified based on their origin: microbial (bacterial, fungal and viral), plant, animal and human enzymes can be distinguished.

Proteolytic enzymes belong to the hydrolase class of enzymes (EC 3) and are grouped into the subclass of the peptide hydrolases or peptidases (EC 3.4). Depending on the site of enzyme action the proteases can also be subdivided into exopeptidases or endopeptidases. Exopeptidases catalyze the hydrolysis of the peptide bonds near the *N*- or *C*-terminal ends of the substrate. Aminopeptidases (Figure 1) can liberate single amino acids (EC 3.4.11), dipeptides (dipeptidyl peptidases, EC 3.4.14) or tripeptides (tripeptidyl peptidases EC 3.4.14) from the N-terminal end of their substrates. Single amino acids can be released from dipeptide substrates by dipeptidases (EC 3.4.13) or from polypeptides by carboxypeptidases (EC 3.4.16-3.4.18) (Figure 1), while peptidyl dipeptidases (EC 3.4.15) liberate dipeptides from the *C*-terminal end of a polypeptide chain. Endopeptidases (Figure 1) cleave peptide bonds within and distant from the ends of a polypeptide chain [2].

Figure 1. Action of aminopeptidases and carboxypeptidases removing the terminal amino acid residues as well as endopeptidases on a polypeptide substrate (having n residues). Red arrows show the peptide bonds to be cleaved.

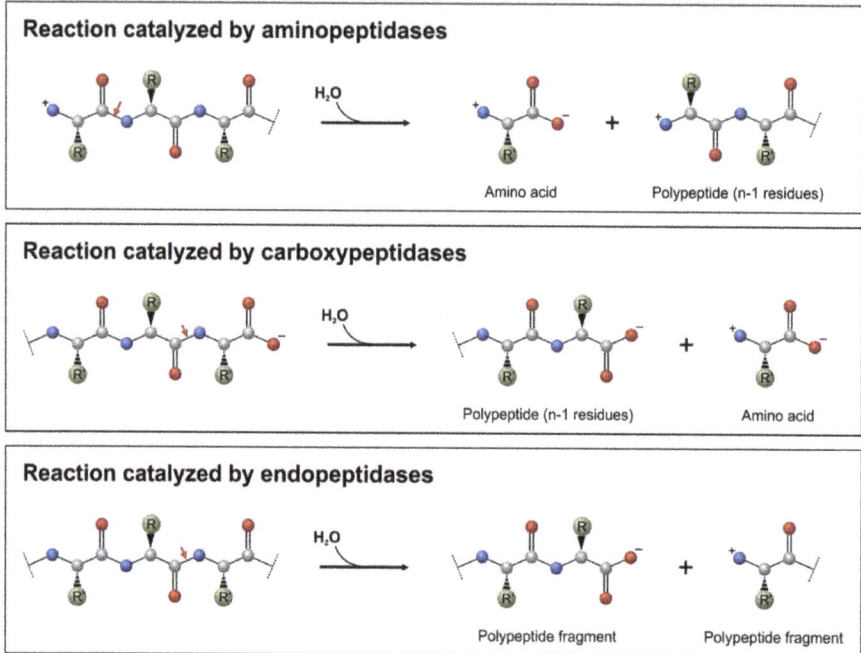

Based on the catalytic mechanism and the presence of amino acid residue(s) at the active site the proteases can be grouped as aspartic proteases, cysteine proteases, glutamic proteases, metalloproteases, asparagine proteases, serine proteases, threonine proteases, and proteases with mixed or unknown catalytic mechanism [3].

The current classification system further classifies the proteases into families based on sequence similarities, furthermore, homologous families are grouped into clans using a structure-based classification [3,4]. Classification and nomenclature of proteolytic enzymes as well as a detailed description of individual proteases is available in the MEROPS database [3].

Action of the proteolytic enzymes is essential in several physiological processes, e.g., in digestion of food proteins, protein turnover, cell division, blood-clotting cascade, signal transduction, processing of polypeptide hormones, apoptosis and the life-cycle of several disease-causing organisms including the replication of retroviruses [5,6]. Due to their key role in the life-cycle of many hosts and pathogens they have great medical, pharmaceutical, and academic importance [7–9].

It was estimated previously that about 2% of the human genes encode proteolytic enzymes [8] and due to their necessity in many biological processes proteases have become important therapeutic targets [8]. They are intensively studied to explore their structure-function relationships, to investigate their interactions with the substrates and inhibitors, to develop therapeutic agents for antiviral therapies [9] or to improve their thermostability, efficiency and to change their specificity by protein engineering for industrial or therapeutic purposes [7]. Studying proteolytic enzymes is highly justified by their key role in several fields of industry [2,10–12], as well. The worldwide market of industrial enzymes was estimated to reach \$3.3 billion value in 2010 and the largest segment of this market is related to proteases [13].

Proteases are extensively applied enzymes in several sectors of industry and biotechnology, furthermore, numerous research applications require the use of them, including the production of Klenow fragments, peptide synthesis, digestion of unwanted proteins during nucleic acid purification, use of proteases in cell culture experiments and in tissue dissociation, preparation of recombinant antibody fragments for research, diagnostics and therapy, exploration of the structure-function relationships by structural studies, removal of affinity tags from fusion proteins in recombinant protein techniques, peptide sequencing, and proteolytic digestion of proteins in proteomics.

This review focuses on the application of proteolytic enzymes in life sciences, especially in the field of molecular biology. The summary table of proteases discussed in this review (Table 1) contains the substrate specificities of the enzymes which are grouped based on their catalytic mechanisms.

2. Molecular Biology Research Applications

2.1. Klenow Fragment Production

The Klenow fragment is the large fragment of the *E. coli* DNA polymerase I enzyme. While the holoenzyme has 5'→3' polymerase, 3'→5' and 5'→3' exonuclease activities, the Klenow fragment has only the polymerase and the 3'→5' exonuclease activities. The Klenow fragment has several applications in the recombinant DNA technology, including the labeling, sequencing, and site-specific mutagenesis of DNA.

The enzymatic method to release the large protein fragment from the DNA polymerase I holoenzyme by proteolysis was published in 1970 [14]. Subtilisin-catalyzed proteolytic cleavage was used to produce Klenow fragment leading to the retention of the polymerase and the 3'→5' exonuclease activities and to the loss of 5'→3' exonuclease activity of the intact polymerase [6].

Nowadays, commercially available Klenow fragment is produced in recombinant ways in *E. coli* strains which carry the gene of large fragment of DNA polymerase I, therefore, the proteolytic production of Klenow fragment has mainly historical significance.

2.2. Enzymatic Peptide Synthesis

While enzymatic peptide synthesis has been frequently used to synthesize peptides for pharmaceutical and nutritional purposes (Table 2), this method is also essential for several research applications. The enzymatic method has several advantages compared to chemical methods, such as stereo specificity with side-chain protection, and the non-toxic nature of solvents coupled with the possibility of recycling the reagents used for synthesis. Enzymes have been selected considering their specificity for amino acid residues (Table 2), but this type of application is limited by the possibility of the hydrolysis of the peptide bond. The types of the enzymatic synthesis and its requirements have been reviewed [15–17]. Enzymatic peptide synthesis can be made by equilibrium- or kinetically-controlled methods.

Table 1. Substrate specificity of some proteolytic enzymes used in molecular biology research. Proteases are classified based on their catalytic mechanisms, furthermore, the main sources and enzyme specificities are indicated. The arrows indicate the sites of cleavages.

Enzyme	Main Source	Cleavage Site
Endopeptidases		
Serine proteases		
Trypsin	bovine	-Arg or Lys↓nonspecific-
Chymotrypsin	bovine	-Trp (or Phe, Leu, Tyr)↓nonspecific-
Enterokinase	bovine	Asp-Asp-Asp-Lys↓nonspecific-
Endoproteinase Arg-C	microbial	-Arg↓nonspecific-
Endoproteinase Glu-C	microbial	-Glu (or Asp)↓nonspecific-
Endoproteinase Lys-C	microbial	-Lys↓nonspecific-
Elastase	porcine	-Ala (or Gly or Val)↓nonspecific-
Subtilisin	microbial	-Trp (or Tyr, Phe, Leu)↓nonspecific-
Proteinase K	fungal	-aromatic, aliphatic or hydrophobic ↓nonspecific-
Thrombin	bovine	-Arg (or Lys)↓nonspecific- specific for -Leu-Val-Pro-Arg-↓Gly-Ser-
Factor Xa	bovine	-Arg (or Lys)↓nonspecific- specific for -Leu-Val-Pro-Arg-↓Gly-Ser-
WNV protease	*E. coli*	-Lys (or Arg)-Arg↓Gly-Ser-
Cysteine proteases		
Bromelain	plant	-nonspecific↓nonspecific-
Papain	plant	-Arg (or Lys)↓nonspecific-
Ficin (ficain)	plant	-nonspecific↓nonspecific-
Rhinovirus 3C	*E. coli*	Gly-Pro dipeptide after the scissile bond highly specific for -Leu-Glu-Val-Leu-Phe-Gln↓Gly-Pro-
TEV protease	*E. coli*	specific for -Gln-Asn-Leu-Tyr-Phe-Gln↓Gly-
TVMV protease	*E. coli*	specific for -Glu-Thr-Val-Arg-Phe-Gln↓Ser-
Metalloproteases		
Endoproteinase Asp-N	microbial	-nonspecific↓Asp-
Thermolysin	microbial	-Leu (or Phe)↓Leu (or Phe, Val, Met, Ala, Ile)-
Collagenase	microbial	-Pro-neutral↓Gly-Pro-
Dispase	microbial	-nonspecific↓non-polar-
Aspartic proteases		
Pepsin	porcine	-Phe (or Tyr, Leu, Trp)↓Trp (or Phe, Tyr, Leu)-
Cathepsin D	bovine	-Phe (or Leu)↓nonspecific (not Val, Ala)-
Exopeptidases		
Serine proteases		
Carboxypeptidase Y	yeast	-nonspecific↓nonspecific
Cysteine proteases		
Cathepsin C	bovine	removes N-terminal dipeptide
DAPase	porcine	removes N-terminal dipeptide
Metalloproteases		
Carboxypeptidase A	bovine	-nonspecific↓aromatic or branched preferred
Carboxypeptidase B	porcine	specific for C-terminal Arg or Lys

Table 2. Examples of peptides synthesized by proteases.

Peptide	Sequence	Enzyme(s)	Reference
Aspartame	Asp-Phe	Thermolysin	[18]
Nutritional peptide	Tyr-Trp-Val	α-Chymotrypsin, papain	[19]
Somatostatin	Ala-Gly-Cys-Lys-Phe-Phe-Trp-Lys-Thr-Phe-Thr-Ser-Cys	Thermolysin, chymotrypsin	[20]
Vasopressin	Tyr-Phe-Phe-Gln	Thermolysin, chymotrypsin	[21]
Oxytocin	Cys-Tyr Tyr-Ile Pro-Leu Leu-Gly	Papain, thermolysin, chymotrypsin	[21]
mouse EGF (21–31)	His-Ile-Glu-Ser-Leu-Asp-SerTyr-Thr-Cys	Papain, trypsin	[22]

2.2.1. Kinetically Controlled Peptide Synthesis

The scheme for chymotrypsin-catalyzed kinetically-controlled Z-D-Leu-L-Leu-NH$_2$ synthesis [23] is illustrated in Figure 2. The acyl donor Z-D-Leu that is activated by carbamoylmethyl (Cam) ester and chymotrypsin (E) form the enzyme-substrate complex first and after that the covalently linked Z-D-Leu-E intermediate with the loss of the carbamoylmethyl ester. If this intermediate is attacked by water, hydrolysis occurs, which results in the Z-D-Leu-OH fragment. However if a more powerful nucleophile (e.g., alcohol or thiol) is present in the media, the enzyme produces a peptide bond instead of the cleavage [15] and the Z-D-Leu-L-Leu-NH$_2$ dipeptide may be formed in the presence of H-L-Leu-NH$_2$ nucleophile (Figure 2). The product yield depends on the kinetics of the two nucleophilic reactions, however, the reaction is faster and requires lower substrate enzyme ratios compared to the equilibrium-controlled synthesis, due to the activated acyl donor.

The acyl donor activating agent must not only be an ester, but an amide or a nitrile as well. Only serine or cysteine proteases can be used to perform the kinetically controlled peptide synthesis, as these enzymes can act as transferase and hence are able to catalyze the transfer of an acyl group from the acyl donor to the nucleophile through the formation of a covalent acyl enzyme intermediate. Papain, thermolysin, trypsin and α-chymotrypsin are mostly used for kinetically-controlled peptide synthesis [24]. The yield of peptide product will depend on the apparent ratio of transferase to hydrolase rate constants $(K_T/K_H)_{app}$ and the rate at which the peptide product is hydrolyzed. The $(K_T/K_H)_{app}$ values of proteases used for kinetically-controlled synthesis are in the range of 10^2–10^4 [17].

2.2.2. Equilibrium-Controlled Synthesis

In the case of the equilibrium-controlled synthesis the process is the reverse of hydrolysis. Important problems of this enzymatic method of peptide synthesis are the low reaction rates and the need of increased yield because proteases do not alter the equilibrium of the reaction. A high amount of the enzyme is often required together with the precise reaction conditions to drive the equilibrium towards synthesis [15]. A higher rate of peptide bond formation can be reached by the appropriate pH of the reaction medium (changing the equilibrium of ionization) but there are several other ways to increase the yield of the reaction:

(a) Precipitation of the product is the classical method. When certain soluble carboxyl amine components are used as reactants the products will precipitate and the reduced concentration of soluble products will drive the equilibrium towards synthesis. In this case the yield of the product depends on the concentration of the starting materials and can be determined by the solubility of the product [17].

(b) In a biphasic system the enzyme acts in an aqueous environment that is surrounded by a water immiscible medium; the water content of the system is around 2%–5%. The reactants (dissolved in high concentrations) can diffuse from the organic phase into the water until the equilibrium is reached; the enzyme-catalyzed synthesis is followed by the diffusion of the products back into the organic phase. The organic phase reduces the dielectric constant of the medium and thus the acidity of the carboxyl group of the acyl donor as well, which in turn promotes the synthesis of the peptide bond instead of hydrolysis [24]. This method is applicable only for the synthesis of water insoluble products.

(c) The dissolved state system can be used for the synthesis of water-soluble products (short peptides, high molecular weight peptides and proteins). In this environment forcing the reaction towards peptide synthesis requires the mass action, the addition of a water-miscible organic co-solvent in high concentration or the excess of one reactant. In serine protease-catalyzed reaction in water, the rate determining feature is the acylation of the enzyme while the product yield at equilibrium depends on the partition coefficient and the ratio of the aqueous and organic volumes [17]. The chymotrypsin- and subtilisin-catalyzed synthesis of N-Bz-L-Tyr-L-Leu-NH$_2$ is more efficient in hydrophobic organic solvents; adding water in sub-saturating concentration increases the yield of the chymotrypsin-catalyzed peptide synthesis [25].

Figure 2. Kinetically-controlled synthesis of Z-D-Leu-L-Leu-NH$_2$ dipeptide. After the formation of enzyme-substrate complex (K$_1$) a covalent enzyme-substrate intermediate is formed (K$_2$). The intermediate is subjected to the attack from H$_2$O or other nucleophiles (Nu). K$_H$ is the equilibrium constant of hydrolysis, K$_T$ is the equilibrium constant of the transferase reaction.

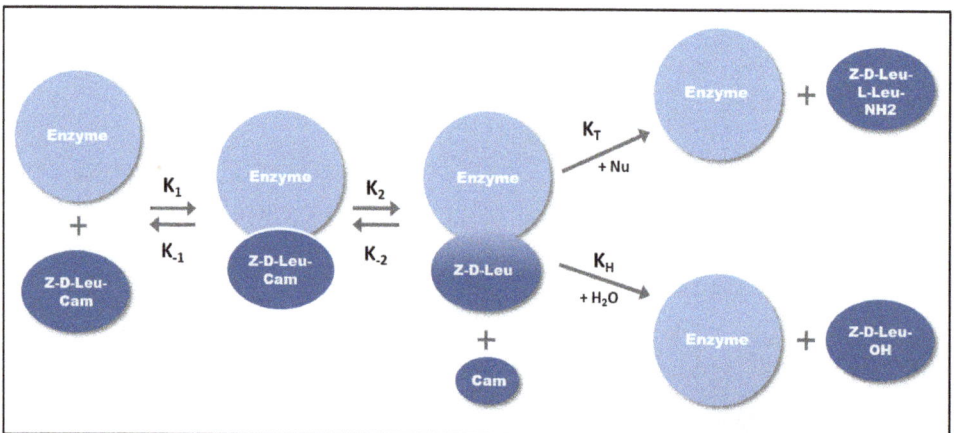

2.2.3. Strategies Used in Enzymatic Synthesis

The *use of enzymes in organic solvents* have several advantages compared to aqueous solvents which have led to their widespread application: the thermodynamic equilibrium can be shifted towards synthesis, the undesirable side reactions can be reduced, the nonpolar substrates are more soluble in organic solvents, the separation process and enzyme recovery is more effective in a low water-containing environment [26–29]. Many proteases, such as thermolysin, subtilisin and α-chymotrypsin [26,29] can maintain their active conformation in organic solvents and show good functionality in the synthesis of aspartame and demorphin derivatives.

However, the use of enzymes in organic solvent has also disadvantages such as the unfavorable effects of the organic solvents on enzyme activity and stability. The *modification of biocatalysts* by protein engineering [30,31] and/or chemical modification or the use of naturally solvent-tolerant proteases [32] for peptide synthesis is a developing field. The driving force of this field is the aim of making biocatalysts with proper features to suit them for the reactions under specific synthesis conditions. Site-directed mutagenesis is a very effective tool and can be used by protein engineers to screen mutants with enhanced stability, activity or specificity, furthermore, this method can be used to explore structure-function relationships (rational design).

Subtilisin has been extensively studied and engineered via site-directed mutagenesis to make it more capable of peptide bond formation in aqueous solution [33]. Single and multiple mutations have been introduced into subtilisin to increase its stability and make it more resistant against oxidizing agents, thermal denaturations and inactivation effects of polar solvents [28].

Thermolysin has a higher synthesis rate compared to the solvent stable PST-01 protease from *Pseudomonas aeruginosa*. Considering the high structural similarity of these enzymes, the synthetic activity of PST-01 protease was increased by the Y114F mutation [31], moreover, the Y114R and Y114S mutations resulted in better activity enhancement.

Chemical modification is also an efficient method to modify the properties of enzymes used for peptide synthesis. Thiol-subtilisin, in which the serine residue has been chemically changed to cysteine at the active site, shows an enhanced aminolysis to hydrolysis ratio in aqueous solution and in dimethyl sulphoxide. The stability of proteases can also be increased by chemical modification e.g., a hydrophilic carbohydrate-polyacrylate polymer coat can make the enzymes highly active and stable in polar solvents and more resistant against thermal inactivation [28].

Immobilization of proteases is the most frequently applied method for the recovery of products without great loss of the catalysts, which greatly decreases the cost of the synthesis. This approach also ensures better operational stability of biocatalysts and control of the reaction. Enzyme immobilization techniques can be divided into five groups: (a) covalent attachment to solid support; (b) absorption on solid support; (c) entrapment in polymeric gel; (d) crosslinking with bifunctional reagents and (e) encapsulation [17,34].

Substrate engineering means the manipulation of the leaving group and is a powerful tool to increase the specificity of the proper enzyme and/or increase the rate and the yield of the reaction [24].

Protease-catalyzed synthesis of stereochemically modified peptides is also a preferable application compared to chemical synthesis due to stereospecificity of the proteases.

Proteases can bind not only natural substrates, but also specifically designed substrate mimetics, which are also very useful tools to increase the yield of peptide synthesis. Substrate mimetics can bind to the active site of the enzyme and in this way proteases can be used for the synthesis of products containing non-specific amino acids. The undesired cleavage of the newly synthesized peptide bonds can be avoided using this method and it is not required to change the properties of the medium or the enzyme [17].

The production of peptides with amides at their C-termini is a great challenge for enzymatic peptide synthesis, but amidation may be required to retain biological activity.

2.3. Nucleic Acid Isolation

Generally, the first step of nucleic acid isolation protocols is the lysis of the biological material containing the DNA or RNA of interest. Before the purification and concentration of nucleic acids the contaminating proteins and other macromolecules have to be removed from the sample. Undamaged nucleic acids can be isolated when the degradation of the DNA and RNA present in the sample is avoided by the inhibition and removal of DNases and RNases. The nucleases can be inhibited by the addition of chelators (e.g., EDTA) which bind the ions essential for their action. Besides the inactivation of nucleases, proteolytic enzymes are applied during the nucleic acid isolation to remove total protein content of the sample.

The most widely used proteolytic enzyme in nucleic acid purification is the Proteinase K, which was described in 1974 [35]. Proteinase K is a non-specific serine endopeptidase which can catalyze the cleavage of peptide bonds at the carboxylic side of aromatic, aliphatic, or hydrophobic amino acid residues. Besides the digestion of unwanted proteins, Proteinase K also quickly inactivates the nucleases which might degrade the nucleic acids present in the sample [36]. This proteolytic digestion decreases the level of contaminants in the nucleic acid extract and prevents nucleic acids from degradation leading to a higher yield of the DNA or RNA to be isolated.

2.4. Cell Isolation and Tissue Dissociation

Cell biology studies frequently require the dissociation of primary tissues and the isolation of viable cells for tissue culturing. The most common method for cell isolation is the enzymatic digestion of the junctions connecting the cells and the components of the surrounding extracellular matrix, by which the cells can be released from a wide variety of tissues. Several enzymes are available in the market for the detachment of cultured cells, cell dissociation and cell component or membrane-associated protein isolation [37,38]. Besides the polysaccharidases, nucleases and lipases, the proteases are the most important enzymes used widely to dissociate cells from tissues.

The experimental conditions of cell isolation are functions of several parameters, including the type of the tissue and the source of its origin. Cells with high viability can be isolated in high yield using a suitable enzyme or the optimal combination of enzymes. As proteases differ in their specificities, different enzymes are recommended to be used use for most effective tissue disruption, depending on the origin and type of the tissue. We describe below the enzymes most commonly used for cell isolation.

The matrix metalloproteinase collagenase was first isolated in 1953 [39]. This endopeptidase can digest the collagenous extracellular matrix in a zinc-dependent manner. Collagenase cleaves the peptide bonds within the triple helices of native collagen, between a neutral amino acid and Gly within the Pro-X-Gly-Pro sequence. This sequence can be found most frequently in the collagen; therefore collagenases digest other proteins less efficiently. A commercially available collagenase (clostridiopeptidase A) is produced by *Clostridium histolyticum*, and it is capable of digesting collagen fibers very effectively. Solutions supplied for tissue dissociation contain collagenase and other additional proteinases which can digest the components of the extracellular matrix [38,40]. The serine protease elastase is a unique enzyme which can cleave the peptide bonds in elastin, therefore, it is generally used to dissociate tissues containing a high amount of elastin connective fibers. Elastase cleaves peptide bonds next to smaller neutral amino acids and besides its protease activity it also has esterase and amidase activities. Papain is a cysteine peptidase of *Carica papaya* latex. Papain, similarly to elastase, also has amidase and esterase activities and has a broad specificity. Papain has less damaging effects on tissues and therefore it is typically applied for cell dissociation of neuronal tissues. Besides cell dissociation, papain is also widely used for integral membrane protein solubilization and for digestion of proteoglycans. The serine protease trypsin is a very specific proteinase cleaving the peptide bonds at the *C*-terminal end of positively charged Lys and Arg side chains. Due to the high specificity of trypsin the digestion of tissue proteins is less effective and it is generally used for tissue dissociation together with other proteolytic enzymes. Serine protease chymotrypsin cleaves peptide bonds preferentially at the carboxyl side of aromatic Tyr, Trp and Phe residues. Chymotrypsin is less widely used for tissue dissociation; the use of other additional proteases is required for efficient digestion. The Zn-metalloprotease dispase is also a neutral protease. This non-specific protease cleaves the peptide bonds of proteins at the amino side of non-polar amino acid residues.

2.5. Cell Culturing

Cells isolated from a tissue can be cultured separately from the organism in cell culture flasks using appropriate growth medium. Adherent cells grown in a cell culture flask are attached to the surface by protein bridges which have to be disrupted during passaging. The cells can be released from the cell flask surface mechanically using a cell scraper or can be detached by a protease treatment using trypsin solution.

Trypsinization means the process used for the detachment of adherent cells using trypsin solution to digest the adhesion molecules by which the cells are attached to the surface of the culture flask. Trypsin solutions generally contain EDTA to reduce the concentration of metal ions that might inhibit trypsin.

Although trypsinization is the most commonly used method to detach adherent cells from cell culture flasks, the effects of this protease treatment were only recently studied in detail. It was found that trypsinization can affect the extracellular matrix surrounding the cells [41] and has physiological effects on cells grown in cell cultures [42]. Trypsin treatment can lead to cleavage of membrane proteins and receptors, which can cause significant changes in the expression level of different proteins: level of growth- and metabolism-related protein expressions were found to be down-regulated after trypsinization, while up-regulation of apoptosis-related protein expressions was seen after the protease treatment [42,43]. This effect should be taken into account when trypsinization is involved in experimental design.

2.6. Antibody Fragment Production

Antibody molecules are produced by the immune system against foreign substances and are classified into the immunoglobulin superfamily of the proteins (Figure 3A). They consist of four polypeptide chains, two identical heavy chains (H) and two identical light chains (L) which are connected by disulfide bridges. Both the H and the L chains contain variable (V_H and V_L) and constant (C_H1, C_H2, C_H3 and C_L) regions, respectively. The V_H and V_L chains, containing hypervariable regions, are responsible for the antigen-antibody interactions and determine the antigen specificity [6].

Fragments of the monoclonal antibodies are widely used in diagnostics, therapeutics and in biopharmaceutical research [44–46] having beneficial properties compared to the whole immunoglobulin molecules due to their smaller size and lower immunogenicity [44]. Fragments of whole immunoglobulin molecules can be produced using recombinant DNA technology or can be generated by enzymatic digestion. Here we discuss the proteolytic antibody fragmentation method.

Generally, the papain, pepsin and ficin proteases are used for the specific digestion of IgG molecules. Digestion of an antibody by the cysteine protease papain results in three fragments due to the cleavage of peptide bonds in the hinge region between C_H1 and C_H2 domains: one Fc (crystallizable) and two identical Fab (antigen binding) fragments are released (Figure 3B). While both released Fab fragments carry one antigen-binding site, the Fc fragment does not have antigen-binding ability. The aspartic acid protease pepsin cleaves the peptide bonds of the antibody near the disulfide bonds connecting the H chains (Figure 3C). This digestion results in the release of the peptides of the Fc region and one F(ab')$_2$ fragment containing both antigen binding sites. The cysteine protease ficin can release both F(ab')$_2$ or Fab fragments (Figure 3D), depending on the cysteine concentration [44].

The *in vivo* applications of the large, pentameric IgM immunoglobulines could be restricted because of their large size. Proteolytic fragmentation of IgM moleucles is also a useful method to produce smaller, active Fab, Fab', F(ab')$_2$ or "IgG-like" fragments which have beneficial properties compared to the whole IgM molecules. Trypsin and pepsin are useful enzymes for IgM fragmentation, pepsin can generate Fab and F(ab')$_2$ fragments, while trypsin can generate "IgG-like" fragments, as well. Papain cannot be used for IgM fragmentation because of the production of heterogeneous fragments.

Digestion of monoclonal antibodies by papain or pepsin is still used to produce Fab or F(ab')$_2$ fragments [44]. There are several products available on the market obtained by proteolytic cleavage of antibodies, furthermore, several companies supply fragmentation kits for antibody fragment preparation. In some cases it could be preferable to produce the Fab fragments in high quality by recombinant expression in cell lines and obtain the fragment in sufficient quantity. For example, the Fab fragments produced by recombinant expression were found to be more preferable for the crystallization experiments because of the higher quality of the protein sample [47].

Figure 3. Structure of IgG antibody molecules (**A**) and fragments released after proteolytic digestion using papain (**B**), pepsin (**C**) or ficin (**D**).

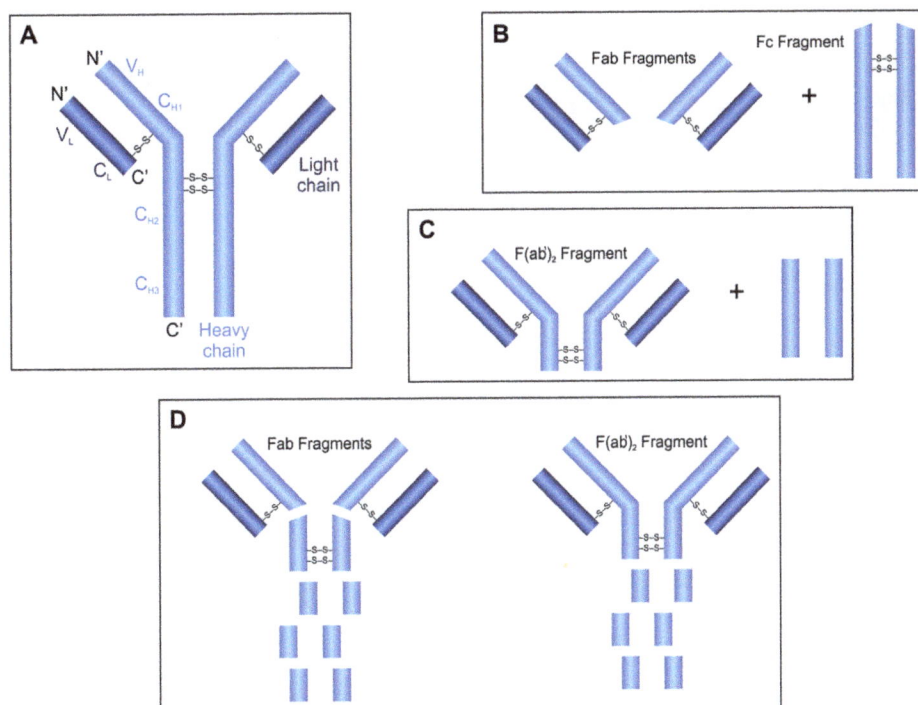

Antibody fragments have several beneficial properties for *in vivo* applications compared to whole antibody molecules. Due to their smaller size they have higher mobility and can penetrate tissues or permeate cell membranes more easily. As antigen-binding fragments lack the Fc fragments, they have lower immunogenicity, as they contain only their antigen-binding domain sites (Fab, Fab' or F(ab')₂ fragments) and do not carry the regions responsible for antibody effector functions, furthermore, they do not form large immunocomplexes.

The antigen-binding fragments of antibodies have great importance from the viewpoint of clinical and therapeutic applications. Antibody fragments could be administered to prevent the development of a disease (e.g., restenosis), could be applied during the diagnosis (e.g., metastatic breast and colon cancer) or for the treatment of some diseases (e.g., macular degeneration) or to detect toxins or neutralize snake venoms [44,45]. The current number of antibody-based therapeutics approved by the FDA is 35, while several other antibodies are in clinical trials. The relevance of antibody fragments in structural studies is discussed in detail in the following paragraph. Further important biotechnological applications of antibody fragments, e.g., as immunodetection, immunopurification and detoxification, have been reviewed in the recent past [46].

2.7. Structural Studies

Crystallographers have great challenges in the structure determination of transmembrane proteins. It is difficult to crystallize these proteins due to their high molecular flexibility, hydrophobic surfaces and low solubility. Antibody fragments are very useful tools for solving these problems. Specific binding of antibody fragments can increase the overall hydrophilicity of proteins and the solubility of the transmembrane proteins, furthermore, they can decrease the flexibility and stabilize the conformation of the molecule [48]. The structures of the membrane proteins co-crystallized with antibody fragments can be determined at higher resolution because these crystals have a higher diffraction quality [49–51].

The proteases have great indirect significance in structure determination, because the antibody fragments produced by proteolytic cleavage of whole immunoglobulins can be used to improve the crystallization properties [52–54].

The proteases are not only tools for crystallographers but are also important target molecules for structural biologists and have great relevance in antiviral therapies, drug and therapeutics development from the viewpoint of structural biology. Besides interest in proteases with unknown structure, the results of structural studies can help researchers evaluate the structure-function relationships more efficiently; increasing knowledge on the structural organization of viral proteases can help to explore their action, perform comparative studies by which we can better understand the structure-function and evolutionary relationships and recognize general or specific features [55–57]. One of the main driving forces of structure determination of proteases is the need for the development of efficient drugs for antiviral therapies [7,9,58–60]. Both structural and enzymatic inhibition studies are required for the structure-based drug development of protease inhibitors [61]. Structural data can also help protein engineers to alter the specificity and to improve the enzymatic properties of proteases by structure-guided mutagenesis [62–64] for several purposes.

2.8. Fusion Tag Removal

The proteins produced by recombinant techniques are typically linked with a fusion partner termed a fusion tag. The introduction of a fusion tag means the fusion of an additional protein or peptide to the recombinant protein. These fusion tags are extensively used from basic research to high-throughput structural biology owing to the several advantages they provide in the expression of different recombinant proteins [65,66]. The tags largely aid the detection and purification of proteins; moreover they also could have a favorable effect on protein yield and/or solubility. Tags can prevent proteins from proteolytic digestion, can protect antigenicity or facilitate the folding of the fusion protein. On the other hand, they can also negatively alter solubility, structural integrity and biological activity [47,67,68] or may cause a disadvantage for further application of the protein, so the removal of a tag can be crucial [66].

Commonly used affinity tags and fusion protein partners are the hexahistidine-tag (His_6), FLAG-tag, maltose binding protein (MBP), glutathione S-transferase (GST), thioredoxin (TRX), small ubiquitin-like modifier (SUMO), ubiquitin (Ub) and green fluorescent protein (GFP) [69].

In some cases the tag can be removed by a chemical treatment but those methods are rather unspecific compared to enzymatic cleavages and may lead to protein denaturation and/or side chain modifications of amino acids in the target protein. The specificity and detergent sensitivity of common proteases used for tag removal have been examined and reviewed previously [70–73]. Both endo- and exo-proteases could be suitable for fusion tag removal.

2.8.1. Endoproteases

Serine proteases such as enterokinase (also referred to as enteropeptidase), factor Xa and thrombin have been widely used for many years to remove *N*-terminal tags, but several cases have been reported in which they cleaved not only at the desired cleavage site but also in the protein of interest. These incidents led to the extensive application of viral proteases like human rhinovirus (HRV) 3C protease and tobacco etch virus (TEV) protease. While sequences recognized by a cellular serine protease and the viral proteases could be similar, the viral proteases cleave the protein substrates at the undesired sites less efficiently due to their high specificity and low catalytic rate, moreover, recombinant viral proteases can be produced in high quantities in *E. coli* [73]. These findings and the limited activity of the generally used serine proteases in some detergents, which are needed to study the membrane proteins, inspired the search for other viral proteases for tag removal, such as Tobacco Vein Mottling Virus (TVMV) protease [74], West Nile Virus (WNV) protease [75] and some alphaviral proteases: Venezuelan Equine Encephalitis Virus (VEEV) protease, Semliki Forest Virus (SFV) and Sindbis Virus (SIN) protease [76].

2.8.2. Exopeptidases

Aminopeptidases and carboxypeptidases are not as widely used as endopeptidases, as they frequently leave amino acid residues on the target protein, while it is easier to design cleavage sites with endopeptidases not to leave extra residues after the cleavage. However, if is still desired to add a tag onto the C-terminal of the target protein a carboxypeptidase may be used for its removal. Among metallocarboxypeptidases, type A carboxypeptidases remove mostly aromatic or branched aliphatic side chain containing amino acids, while type B carboxypeptidases prefer basic amino acids. Carboxypeptidases can be utilized to remove a His$_6$ tag from the *C*-terminal end of a protein [77]. Dipeptidyl aminopeptidase (DAPase) is a useful enzyme for the removal of *N*-terminal dipeptides.

2.9. Proteomic Applications

Proteomic studies are made with the aim to identify, characterize, and quantify the required samples and typically involve mass spectrometric (MS) analysis. Besides determination of the composition of protein complexes, chemical properties, post-translational modifications and structural properties of proteins can also be revealed by MS.

MS is a powerful analytical method to measure the mass of proteins or peptides by the analysis of mass-to-charge ratio (*m/z*) ratio. Generally, the samples to be analyzed contain a mixture of various proteins and/or polypeptides that have to be separated and digested into smaller fragments before the MS analysis. Protein separation can be performed efficiently by polyacrylamide gel electrophoresis.

The separated proteins can be digested after the electrophoresis by chemical cleavage or by enzyme-catalyzed digestion of peptide bonds. The process in which the bands or spots are cut out from the gel followed by the addition of protease(s) to the gel containing the protein(s) of interest is called in-gel digestion [78]. Proteolysis of whole proteins leads to the release of smaller peptides with different molecular masses which are suitable for MS analysis (Figure 4).

Figure 4. Steps of proteomic analysis using mass-spectrometry after separation and in-gel digestion of proteins of interest.

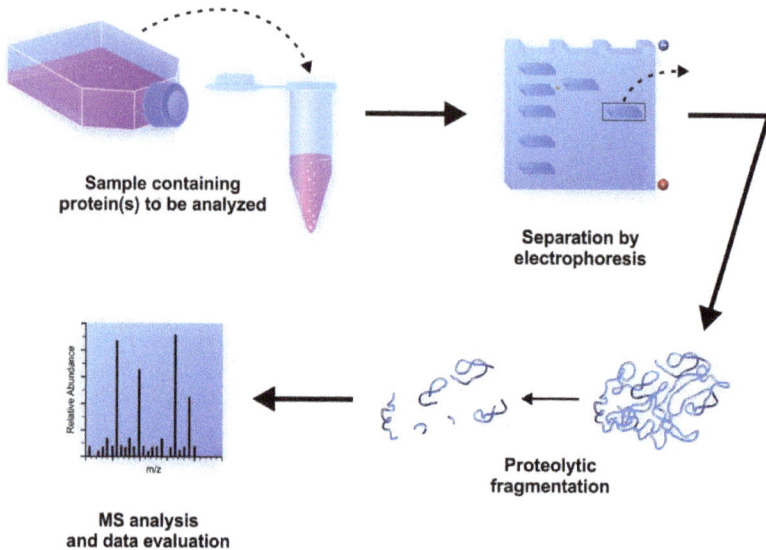

Sample containing protein(s) to be analyzed

Separation by electrophoresis

Proteolytic fragmentation

MS analysis and data evaluation

Trypsin is the most widely used proteolytic enzyme for protein digestion in MS analysis. Due to its high specificity it is easy to predict the cleavage sites and to compare the results of experimental enzymatic and theoretical *in-silico* digestion. The Asp-N, Lys-C, Arg-C and Glu-C enyzmes are also highly sequence-specific endoproteases but they are less active [78]. Chymotrypsin, pepsin, papain, elastase, subtilisin, proteinase K, thrombin, factor Xa and some other proteases are also suitable enzymes for fragmentation in MS analysis [79].

Several proteases are available for this fragmentation of which specificities are well established [79,80]. The number and length of released peptide fragments depends on the protease(s) applied for selective proteolysis of the targeted protein. Applications developed for *in silico* protein fragmentation are useful to predict the proteolytic fragments and to choose the most proper enzyme for the most effective digestion based on the enzyme specificities (http://prospector.ucsf.edu).

Generally, highly sequence-specific proteases are preferred for protein fragmentation instead of less specific enzymes, as the latter ones produce a very complex mixture of fragments. In the case of the efficient fragmentation the peptide, the fragments have a proper length and are released in high yield, and the complete sequence of the whole protein can be covered by the analysis of the proteolytic fragments.

3. Summary

Besides extended application for nutritional and pharmaceutical purposes, proteases from natural sources are also widely used tools in molecular biology practice. Their degradative properties make them useful for general protein digestion in tissue dissociation, cell isolation, and cell culturing. The specificity and the predictability of cleavages by proteases enables their use for more specific tasks such as antibody fragment production, the removal of affinity tags from recombinant proteins and specific protein digestion in the proteomics field mainly for protein sequencing. Moreover, the already mentioned specificity makes proteases—in a water restricted environment—able to synthesize the peptide bonds instead of hydrolyzing them. This property combined with their enantioselectivity has also promoted their use in peptide synthesis.

The expansion of knowledge has assisted the increase of applications of proteolytic enzymes for several purposes, and the application fields are widening with the help of protein engineering techniques and by chemical modification of the enzymes [7,62]. Studies made with the aim to better understand the structure and function of existing proteolytic enzymes and to obtain new, engineered proteases with altered properties for therapeutic, industrial or research fields require the use of the applications discussed in this paper.

Acknowledgments

This work was supported by the TÁMOP 4.2.2.A-11/1/KONV-2012-0023 "VÉD-ELEM" and by the Hungarian Science and Research Fund (OTKA 101591) implemented through the New Hungary Development Plan co-financed by the European Social Fund and the European Regional Development Fund.

Conflicts of Interest

The authors declare no conflict of interest.

References

1. Barrett, A.J.; McDonald, J.K. Nomenclature: Protease, proteinase and peptidase. *Biochem. J.* **1986**, *237*, 935.
2. Rao, M.B.; Tanksale, A.M.; Ghatge, M.S.; Deshpande, V.V. Molecular and biotechnological aspects of microbial proteases. *Microbiol. Mol. Biol. Rev.* **1998**, *62*, 597–635.
3. Rawlings, N.D.; Barrett, A.J.; Bateman, A. MEROPS: The database of proteolytic enzymes, their substrates and inhibitors. *Nucleic Acids Res.* **2012**, *40*, D343–D350.
4. Rawlings, N.D.; Barrett, A.J. Evolutionary families of peptidases. *Biochem. J.* **1993**, *290*, 205–218.
5. Neurath, H.; Walsh, K.A. Role of proteolytic enzymes in biological regulation (a review). *Proc. Natl. Acad. Sci. USA* **1976**, *73*, 3825–3832.
6. Devlin, T.M. *Textbook of Biochemistry with Clinical Correlations*, 5th ed.; Wiley & Sons: New York, NY, USA, 2002.

7. Li, Q.; Yi, L.; Marek, P.; Iverson, B.L. Commercial proteases: Present and future. *FEBS Lett.* **2013**, *587*, 1155–1163.

8. Craik, C.S.; Page, M.J.; Madison, E.L. Proteases as therapeutics. *Biochem. J.* **2011**, *435*, 1–16.

9. Antonelli, G.; Turriziani, O. Antiviral therapy: Old and current issues. *Int. J. Antimicrob. Agents* **2012**, *40*, 95–102.

10. Kirk, O.; Borchert, T.V.; Fuglsang, C.C. Industrial enzyme applications. *Curr. Opin. Biotechnol.* **2002**, *13*, 345–351.

11. Rani, K.; Rana, R.; Datt, S. Review on latest overview of proteases. *Int. J. Curr. Life Sci.* **2012**, *2*, 12–18.

12. Ray, A. Protease enzyme- potential industrial scope. *Int. J. Technol.* **2012**, *2*, 1–4.

13. Sarrouh, B.; Santos, T.M.; Miyoshi, A.; Dias, R.; Azevedo, V. Up-to-date insight on industrial enzymes applications and global market. *J. Bioprocess. Biotech.* **2012**, S4:002

14. Klenow, H.; Henningsen, I. Selective elimination of the exonuclease activity of the deoxyribonucleic acid polymerase from Escherichia coli B by limited proteolysis. *Proc. Natl. Acad. Sci. USA* **1970**, *65*, 168–175.

15. Morihara, K. Using proteases in peptide synthesis. *Trends Biotechnol.* **1987**, *5*, 164–170.

16. Bhalla, T.C.; Kumar, D.; Gajju, H.; Agrawal, H.O. Thermophilic bacterial proteases. *J. Punjab Acad. Sci.* **1999**, *1*, 77–91

17. Kumar, D.; Bhalla, T.C. Microbial proteases in peptide synthesis: Approaches and applications. *Appl. Microbiol. Biotechnol.* **2005**, *68*, 726–736.

18. Kühn, D.; Dürrschmidt, P.; Mansfeld, J.; Ulbrich-Hofmann, R. Biolysin and thermolysin in dipeptide synthesis: A comparative study. *Biotechnol. Appl. Biochem.* **2002**, *36*, 71–76.

19. Kimura, Y.; Muraya, K.; Araki, Y.; Matsuoka, H.; Nakanishi, K.; Matsuno, R. Synthesis peptides consisting of essential amino acids by a reactor system using three proteinases and an organic solvent. *Agric. Biol. Chem.* **1990**, *54*, 3331–3333.

20. Bille, V.; Ripak, C.; van Aasche, I.; Forni, I.; Degelaen, L.; Searso, A. A Semi-Enzymatic Synthesis of Somatostatin. In Proceedings of 21st European Peptide Symposium. ESCOM, Leiden, The Netherlands, 1991; Giralt, E., Andreu, D., Eds.; pp. 253–254.

21. Rizo, J.; Gierarch, L.M. Constrained peptides: Models of bioactive peptides and protein structures. *Ann. Rev. Biochem.* **1992**, *61*, 387–418.

22. Widmer, F.; Bayne, S.; Houen, G.; Rigby, R.B.; Whittaker, R.G.; Johansen, J.T. Use of Proteolytic Enzymes for the Synthesis of Fragments of Mouse Epidermal Growth Factor. In Proceedings of Peptides 1984, Almquist, Stockholm, 1985; Ragnurrson, U., Ed.; pp. 193–196.

23. Salam, S.M.; Kagawa, K.; Kawashiro, K. Alpha-chymotrypsin-catalyzed peptide synthesis using *N*-protected D-amino acid carbamoylmethyl esters as acyl donors. *Biotechnol. Lett.* **2005**, *27*, 1199–1203.

24. Guzmán, F.; Barberis, S.; Illanes, A. Peptide synthesis: Chemical or enzymatic. *Electron. J. Biotechnol.* **2007**, *10*, 279–314.

25. Sergeeva, M.V.; Paradkar, V.M.; Dordick, J.S. Peptide synthesis using proteases dissolved in organic solvents. *Enzyme Microb. Technol.* **1997**, *20*, 623–628.

26. Dordick, J.S. Enzymatic catalysis in monophasic organic solvents. *Enzyme Microb. Technol.* **1989**, *11*, 194–211.
27. Khemlnitski, Y.L.; Levashov, A.V.; Klyachko, N.L.; Martinek, K. Engineering biocatalytic systems in organic media with low water content. *Enzyme Microb. Technol.* **1988**, *10*, 710–724.
28. Gill, I.; Fandino, R.L.; Jobra, X.; Vulfson, E.N. Biologically active peptides and enzymatic approaches to their production. *Enzyme Microb. Technol.* **1996**, *18*, 162–183.
29. Shen, H.Y.; Tian, G.L.; Ye, Y.H. Synthesis of demorphin (1–4) derivatives catalysed by proteases in organic solvents. *J. Pept. Res.* **2004**, *65*, 143–148.
30. Wells, J.A.; Estell, D.A. Subtilisin: An enzyme designed to be engineered. *Trends Biochem. Sci.* **1988**, *13*, 291–297.
31. Ogino, H.; Tsuchiyama, S.; Yasuda, M.; Doukyu, N. Enhancement of the aspartame precursor synthetic activity of an organic solvent-stable protease. *Protein Eng. Des. Sel.* **2010**, *23*, 147–152.
32. Xu, J.X.; Jiang, M.; Sun, H.L.; He, B.F. An organic solvent-stable protease from organic solvent-tolerant Bacillus cereus WQ9–2: Purification, biochemical properties, and potential application in peptide synthesis. *Bioresour. Technol.* **2010**, *101*, 7991–7994.
33. Abrahmsén, L.; Tom, J.; Burnier, J.; Butcher, K.A.; Kossiakoff, A.; Wells, J.A. Engineering subtilisin and its substrates for efficient ligation of peptide bonds in aqueous solution. *Biochemistry* **1991**, *30*, 4151–4159.
34. Adamczak, M.; Krishna, S.H. Enzyme for efficient biocatalysis. *Food Technol. Biotechnol.* **2004**, *42*, 251–264.
35. Ebeling, W.; Hennrich, N.; Klockow, M.; Metz, H.; Orth, H.D.; Lang, H. Proteinase K from Tritirachium album Limber. *Eur. J. Biochem.* **1974**, *47*, 91–97.
36. Carpi, F.M.; di Pietro, F.; Vincenzetti, S.; Mignini, F.; Napolioni, V. Human DNA extraction methods: Patents and applications. *Recent Pat. DNA Gene Seq.* **2011**, *5*, 1–7.
37. Sigma-Aldrich Corporation. Enzymes for cell dissociation and lysis. *Biofiles Life Sci. Res.* **2006**, Avaiable online: http://www.sigmaaldrich.com/ etc/medialib/docs/Sigma/ General_Information/2/biofiles_issue2.Par.0001.File.tmp/biofiles_issue2.pdf (accessed on 20 July 2013).
38. Santangelo, C. Worthington biochemical online tissue dissociation guide. *Worthington Biochem. Corp.* **2011**. Avaiable online: http://www.worthington-biochem.com/ tissuedissociation/ default.html (accessed on 20 July 2013).
39. Mandl, I.; Maclennan, J.D.; Howes, E.L. Isolation and characterization of proteinase and collagenase from Cl. histolyticum. *J. Clin. Investig.* **1953**, *32*, 1323–1329.
40. Kin, T.; Johnson, P.R.; Shapiro, A.M.; Lakey, J.R. Factors influencing the collagenase digestion phase of human islet isolation. *Transplantation* **2007**, *83*, 7–12.
41. Canavan, H.E.; Cheng, X.; Graham, D.J.; Ratner, B.D.; Castner, D.G. Cell sheet detachment affects the extracellular matrix: A surface science study comparing thermal liftoff, enzymatic, and mechanical methods. *J. Biomed. Mater. Res. A* **2005**, *75*, 1–13.

42. Huang, H.L.; Hsing, H.W.; Lai, T.C.; Chen, Y.W.; Lee, T.R.; Chan, H.T.; Lyu, P.C.; Wu, C.L.; Lu, Y.C.; Lin, S.T.; *et al.* Trypsin-induced proteome alteration during cell subculture in mammalian cells. *J. Biomed. Sci.* **2012**, *17*, doi:10.1186/1423-0127-17-36.

43. Danhier, P.; Copetti, T.; de Preter, G.; Leveque, P.; Feron, O.; Jordan, B.F.; Sonveaux, P.; Gallez, B. Influence of cell detachment on the respiration rate of tumor and endothelial cells. *PLoS One* **2013**, *8*, e53324.

44. Rader, C. Overview on concepts and applications of Fab antibody fragments. *Curr. Protoc. Protein Sci.* **2009**, *55*, 6.9.1–6.9.14.

45. Flanagan, R.J.; Jones, A.L. Fab antibody fragments: Some applications in clinical toxicology. *Drug Saf.* **2004**, *27*, 1115–1133.

46. De Marco, A. Biotechnological applications of recombinant single-domain antibody fragments. *Microb. Cell Fact.* **2011**, *10*, doi:10.1186/1475-2859-10-44.

47. Zhao, Y.; Gutshall, L.; Jiang, H.; Baker, A.; Beil, E.; Obmolova, G.; Carton, J.; Taudte, S.; Amegadzie, B. Two routes for production and purification of Fab fragments in biopharmaceutical discovery research: Papain digestion of mAb and transient expression in mammalian cells. *Protein Expr. Purif.* **2009**, *67*, 182–189.

48. Hunte, C.; Michel, H. Crystallisation of membrane proteins mediated by antibody fragments. *Curr. Opin. Struct. Biol.* **2002**, *12*, 503–508.

49. Kovari, L.C.; Momany, C.; Rossmann, M.G. The use of antibody fragments for crystallization and structure determinations. *Structure* **1995**, *3*, 1291–1293.

50. Caffrey, M. Membrane protein crystallization. *J. Struct. Biol.* **2003**, *42*, 108–132.

51. Bill, R.M.; Henderson, P.J.; Iwata, S.; Kunji, E.R.; Michel, H.; Neutze, R.; Newstead, S.; Poolman, B.; Tate, C.G.; Vogel, H. Overcoming barriers to membrane protein structure determination. *Nat. Biotechnol.* **2011**, *29*, 335–340.

52. Zhou, Y.; Morais-Cabral, J.H.; Kaufman, A.; MacKinnon, R. Chemistry of ion coordination and hydration revealed by a K+ channel-Fab complex at 2.0 A resolution. *Nature* **2001**, *414*, 43–48.

53. Rasmussen, S.G.F.; Choi, H.J.; Rosenbaum, D.M.; Kobilka, T.S.; Thian, F.S.; Edwards, P.C.; Burghammer, M.; Ratnala, V.R.; Sanishvili, R.; Fischetti, R.F.; *et al.* Crystal structure of the human beta2 adrenergic G-protein-coupled receptor. *Nature* **2007**, *450*, 383–387.

54. Kwong, P.D.; Wyatt, R.; Robinson, J.; Sweet, R.W.; Sodroski, J.; Hendrickson, W.A. Structure of an HIV gp120 envelope glycoprotein in complex with the CD4 receptor and a neutralizing human antibody. *Nature* **1998**, *393*, 648–659.

55. Bagossi, P.; Sperka, T.; Fehér, A.; Kádas, J.; Zahuczky, G.; Miklóssy, G.; Boross, P.; Tőzsér, J. Amino acid preferences for a critical substrate binding subsite of retroviral proteases in type 1 cleavage sites. *J. Virol.* **2005**, *79*, 4213–4218.

56. Eizert, H.; Bander, P.; Bagossi, P.; Sperka, T.; Miklóssy, G.; Boross, P.; Weber, I.T.; Tőzsér, J. Amino acid preferences of retroviral proteases for amino-terminal positions in a type 1 cleavage site. *J. Virol.* **2008**, *82*, 10111–10117.

57. Tőzsér, J. Comparative studies on retroviral proteases: Substrate specificity. *Viruses* **2010**, *2*, 147–165.

58. Patick, A.K.; Potts, K.E. Protease inhibitors as antiviral agents. *Clin. Microbiol. Rev.* **1998**, *11*, 614–627.

59. Wlodawer, A.; Gustchina, A. Structural and biochemical studies of retroviral proteases. *Biochim. Biophys. Acta* **2000**, *1477*, 16–34.

60. De Clercq, E. Strategies in the design of antiviral drugs. *Nat. Rev. Drug Discov.* **2000**, *1*, 13–25.

61. Wlodawer, A. Structure-based design of AIDS drugs and the development of resistance. *Vox Sang.* **2002**, *83* (Suppl. 1), 23–26.

62. Pogson, M.; Georgiou, G.; Iverson, B.L. Engineering next generation proteases. *Curr. Opin. Biotechnol.* **2009**, *20*, 390–397.

63. Lim, E.J.; Sampath, S.; Coll-Rodriguez, J.; Schmidt, J.; Ray, K.; Rodgers, D.W. Swapping the substrate specificities of the neuropeptidases neurolysin and thimet oligopeptidase. *J. Biol. Chem.* **2007**, *282*, 9722–9732.

64. Villa, J.P.; Bertenshaw, G.P.; Bond, J.S. Critical amino acids in the active site of meprin metalloproteinases for substrate and peptide bond specificity. *J. Biol. Chem.* **2003**, *278*, 42545–42550.

65. Derewenda, Z.S. The use of recombinant methods and molecular engineering in protein crystallization. *Methods* **2004**, *34*, 354–363.

66. Waugh, D.S. Making the most of affinity tags. *Trends Biotechnol.* **2005**, *23*, 316–320.

67. Renzi, F.; Panetta, G.; Vallone, B.; Brunori, M.; Arceci, M.; Bozzoni, I.; Laneve, P.; Caffarelli, E. Large-scale purification and crystallization of the endoribonuclease XendoU: Troubleshooting with His-tagged proteins. *Acta Crystallogr. Sect. F Struct. Biol. Cryst. Commun.* **2006**, *62*, 298–301.

68. Horchani, H.; Ouertani, S.; Gargouri, Y.; Sayari, A. The *N*-terminal His-tag and the recombination process affect the biochemical properties of Staphylococcus aureus lipase produced in Escherichia coli. *J. Mol. Catal. B Enzym.* **2009**, *61*, 194–201.

69. Terpe, K. Overview of tag protein fusions: From molecular and biochemical fundamentals to commercial systems. *Appl. Microbiol. Biotechnol.* **2003**, *60*, 523–533.

70. Jenny, R.J.; Mann, K.G.; Lundblad, R.L. A critical review of the methods for cleavage of fusion proteins with thrombin and factor Xa. *Protein Expr. Purif.* **2003**, *31*, 1–11.

71. Arnau, J.; Lauritzen, C.; Petersen, G.E.; Pedersen, J. Current strategies for the use of affinity tags and tag removal for the purification of recombinant proteins. *Protein Expr. Purif.* **2005**, *48*, 1–13.

72. Vergis, J.M.; Wiener, M.C. The variable detergent sensitivity of proteases that are utilized for recombinant protein affinity tag removal. *Protein Expr. Purif.* **2011**, *78*, 139–142.

73. Waugh, D.S. An overview of enzymatic reagents for the removal of affinity tags. *Protein Expr. Purif.* **2011**, *80*, 283–293.

74. Nallamsetty, S.; Kapust, R.B.; Tözsér, J.; Cherry, S.; Tropea, J.E.; Copeland, T.D.; Waugh, D.S. Efficient site-specific processing of fusion proteins by tobacco vein mottling virus protease *in vivo* and *in vitro*. *Protein Expr. Purif.* **2004**, *38*, 108–115.

75. Huang, Q.; Li, Q.; Chen, A.S.; Kang, C. West Nile virus protease activity in detergent solutions and application for affinity tag removal. *Anal. Biochem.* **2013**, *435*, 44–46.

76. Zhang, D.; Tőzsér, J.; Waugh, D.S. Molecular cloning, overproduction, purification and biochemical characterization of the p39 nsp2 protease domains encoded by three alphaviruses. *Protein Expr. Purif.* **2009**, *64*, 89–97.

77. Austin, B.P.; Tőzsér, J.; Bagossi, P.; Tropea, J.E.; Waugh, D.S. The substrate specificity of Metarhizium anisopliae and Bos taurus carboxypeptidases A: Insights into their use as tools for the removal of affinity tags. *Protein Expr. Purif.* **2011**, *77*, 53–61.

78. Steen, H.; Mann, M. The ABC's (and XYZ's) of peptide sequencing. *Nat. Rev. Mol. Cell Biol.* **2004**, *5*, 699–711.

79. Granvogl, B.; Plöscher, M.; Eichacker, L.A. Sample preparation by in-gel digestion for mass spectrometry-based proteomics. *Anal. Bioanal. Chem.* **2007**, *389*, 991–1002.

80. Meyers, A.; Trauger, S.; Webb, W.; Reisdorph, N.; Wranik, C.; Peters, E.; Siuzdak, G. Protein identification and profiling with mass spectrometry. *Spectroscopy* **2003**, *17*, 1–15.

Microbial Enzymes: Tools for Biotechnological Processes

Jose L. Adrio and Arnold L. Demain

Abstract: Microbial enzymes are of great importance in the development of industrial bioprocesses. Current applications are focused on many different markets including pulp and paper, leather, detergents and textiles, pharmaceuticals, chemical, food and beverages, biofuels, animal feed and personal care, among others. Today there is a need for new, improved or/and more versatile enzymes in order to develop more novel, sustainable and economically competitive production processes. Microbial diversity and modern molecular techniques, such as metagenomics and genomics, are being used to discover new microbial enzymes whose catalytic properties can be improved/modified by different strategies based on rational, semi-rational and random directed evolution. Most industrial enzymes are recombinant forms produced in bacteria and fungi.

Reprinted from *Biomolecules*. Cite as: Adrio, J.L.; Demain, A.L. Microbial Enzymes: Tools for Biotechnological Processes. *Biomolecules* **2014**, *4*, 117-139.

1. Introduction

Microbial enzymes are known to play a crucial role as metabolic catalysts, leading to their use in various industries and applications. The end use market for industrial enzymes is extremely wide-spread with numerous industrial commercial applications [1]. Over 500 industrial products are being made using enzymes [2,3]. The demand for industrial enzymes is on a continuous rise driven by a growing need for sustainable solutions. Microbes have served and continue to serve as one of the largest and useful sources of many enzymes [4]. Many industrial processes, including chemical synthesis for production of chemicals and pharmaceuticals, have several disadvantages: low catalytic efficiency, lack of enantiomeric specificity for chiral synthesis, need for high temperature, low pH and high pressure. Also, the use of organic solvents leads to organic waste and pollutants. Enzymes are more useful for these applications as they work under mild reaction conditions (e.g., temperature, pH, atmospheric conditions), do not need protection of substrate functional groups, have a long half-life, a high stereo-selectivity yielding stereo- and regio-chemically-defined reaction products at an acceleration of 10^5 to 10^8-fold, and, in addition, they work on unnatural substrates [5]. Furthermore, enzymes can be selected genetically and chemically-modified to enhance their key properties: stability, substrate specificity and specific activity. There are drawbacks however, to the use of enzymes, e.g., certain enzymes require co-factors. However, various approaches such as cofactor recycling and use of whole cells can solve this problem. About 150 industrial processes use enzymes or whole microbial cell catalysts.

The global industrial enzymes market is very competitive with Novozymes being the largest player in the industry, followed by DSM, and DuPont (after it acquired a majority stake in Danisco and its Genencor division), among others. The companies mainly compete on the basis of product quality, performance, use of intellectual property rights, and the ability to innovate, among other such factors. North America and Europe are the largest consumers of industrial enzymes although the Asia Pacific region will undergo a rapid increase in enzyme demand in China, Japan and India, reflecting the size and strength of these country's economies.

2. Discovering Enzymes

Nature provides a vast amount of microbial enzyme resources. Our ability to tap into such immense biodiversity depends on the tools available to expand the search for new enzymes by (i) metagenome screening [6–10]); (ii) genome mining in more than 2000 sequenced microbial genomes [11–14]; and (iii) exploring the diversity of extremophiles [15,16]).

2.1. Metagenomic Screening

Although numerous microbes inhabit the biosphere, less than 1% can be cultivated through standard laboratory techniques. Metagenomics has appeared as an alternative strategy to conventional microbe screening by preparing a genomic library from environmental DNA and systematically screening such a library for the open reading frames potentially encoding putative novel enzymes [10,17].

Metagenomic screening is mostly based on either function or sequence approaches [8,10]. Function-based screening is a straightforward way to isolate genes that show the desired function by direct phenotypical detection, heterologous complementation, and induced gene expression [18]. On the other hand, sequence-based screening is performed using either the polymerase chain reaction (PCR) or hybridization procedures. Usually, the common procedure is to use a set of degenerated primers that have been designed based on consensus amino acid sequences.

Studies from different habitats such as volcanic vents, arctic tundra, cow rumen [19], marine environments [20], and termite guts [21] have yielded microbial enzymes with potential for biocatalytic applications, such as lipase [22,23], oxidoreductase [24], amidase [25], amylase [26], nitrilase [27], beta-glucosidase [28,29]), decarboxylase [30], and epoxide hydrolase [31].

Function-based screening of metagenomic libraries is somehow problematic mainly due to insufficient, biased expression of foreign genes in *Escherichia coli* as this bacterium is usually used as surogate host [8]. To overcome such hurdles, alternative bacterial host and expression systems are currently being examined including *Streptomyces lividans*, *Pseudomonas putida* and *Rhizobium leguminosarum*, among others [32,33].

Hit rate (probability of identifying a certain gene) also depends on other factors such as size of the target gene and the assay method. Enzyme activities are usually assayed on agar plates supplemented with different substrates Sensitivity of agar plate-based screening can be improved by using cell lysates [34], screening for genes giving resistance to toxic compounds [35,36], or linking the target activity to the expression of a reporter gene such as green fluorescent protein (GFP) [37] or β-galactosidase [38]. Also, development of flow cytometry based screens as SIGEX are leading the way as they enable more rapid screening of large metagenomic libraries [39]. Genes obtained through sequence-based screening are limited to those having homology to the sequences used as probes.

2.2. Microbial Genomes

Recent success of genome sequencing programs has resulted in an explosion of information available from sequence databases, thus creating an opportunity to explore the possibility of finding new natural products (including enzymes) by database mining [40]. The next generation sequencing platforms (454 from Roche, Solexa from Illumina or SoLiD from ABI), hold promise to reduce time and cost of genome sequencing. Using these platforms, as well as cutting edge approaches such as resequencing, helps to complete multiple whole genomes in less than two weeks. So far, more than 2000 genome sequences and draft assemblies are available in the NCBI database [41].

Two approaches are being followed to discover new enzymes [42]. On one hand, genome hunting is based on searching for open reading frames in the genome of a certain microorganism. Sequences that are annotated as putative enzymes are subjected to subsequent cloning, over-expression and activity screening. Another approach, called data mining, is based on homology alignment among all sequences deposited in databases. Using different bioinformatics tools (e.g., BLAST), a search for conserved regions between sequences yields homologous protein sequences that are identified as possible candidates for further characterization.

2.3. Extremophiles

Over 30 articles on extremophiles have been published in a special issue [43]. Due to their capability to survive under environments of extreme conditions, both physical as temperature (−2 to 12 °C, 60–110 °C), pressure or radiation, and geochemical such as salinity (2–5 NaCl) and pH (<2, >9), extremophiles are a very interesting source of enzymes with extreme stability under conditions regarded as incompatible with biological materials. Recent studies show that the diversity of organisms in these extreme environments could be even greater than was initially thought [16,44]. However, because the majority of these microorganisms have not yet been isolated in pure culture, useful characterization of their enzymes still remains quite difficult.

Thermophilic proteases, lipases as well as cellulases and amylases are being used in many different industrial applications [16,45]. Extreme thermophiles (growing at 60–80 °C) are widely distributed among several bacterial genera such as *Clostridium*, *Thermus*, *Thermotoga*, and *Bacillus*, whereas most of hyperthermophiles belong to Archaea such as *Pyrococcus*, *Thermococcus* or *Methanopyrus*, among others. The Taq DNA polymerase, isolated from the thermophilic *Thermus aquaticus*, had 2009 sales of $500 million [46].

Also, enzymes from psychrophiles have become quite interesting for many industrial applications, partly because of the ongoing efforts to reduce energy consumption. Therefore, enzymes like proteases, amylases or lipases have great commercial potential for development of detergents to reduce wear and tear of textile fibers. Polymer-degrading activities (e.g., cellulases, xylanases,) are quite interesting for the pulp and paper industry, as well as for saccharification of pre-treated lignocellulosic biomass for the production of second generation biofuels [47]. These cold-active enzymes also have potential for many other applications [16,48], such as extraction and clarification of fruit juices, improvement of bakery products, polishing and stone-washing of textiles, and bioremediation of waters contaminated with oils or hydrocarbons [49].

Enzymes from halophites have to cope with very high concentrations of salts (e.g., sodium or potassium chloride). Such proteins have adapted to these environments by acquiring a large number of negatively-charged amino acid residues of their surfaces to prevent precipitation. Such a property has been taken advantage of by use of non-aqueous media [50]. Xylanases, amylases, proteases and lipases from *Halobacterium*, *Halobacillus* and *Halothermothrix* have been produced and their potential has been reviewed [51,52]).

Microorganisms that can survive under extreme pH values could be good sources of thermoalkaliphilic enzymes, like proteases and lipases, particularly useful for applications as additives in laundry and dishwashing detergents [16,53].

3. Strategies to Improve Properties of Microbial Enzymes

The continuously expanding application of enzymes is creating a growing demand for biocatalysts that exhibit improved or new properties [46]. Although enzymes have favorable turnover numbers, they do not necessary fulfill all process requirements and need further fine tuning to achieve industrial scale production. Among those hurdles are: substrate/product inhibition, stability, narrow substrate specificity or enantioselectivity [54]. Genetic modification is very important and recombinant DNA techniques have increased production by 100-fold [55]. Development of new/improved biocatalysts is a challenging and complex task (Figure 1). There are two major ways in which enzymes can be modified to adapt their functions to applied ends: (i) rational redesign of existing biocatalysts and (ii) combinatorial methods which search for the desired functionality in libraries generated at random.

Figure 1. Discovery and development of biocatalysts.

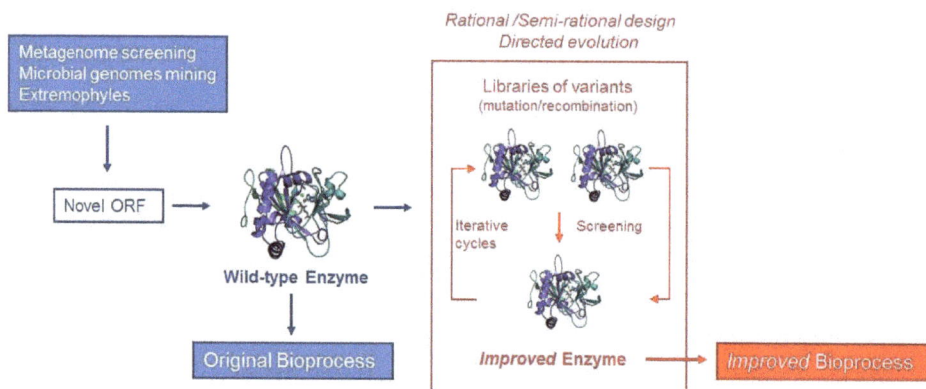

3.1. Rational Design

This approach includes site-directed mutagenesis to target amino acid substitutions, thus requiring knowledge of detailed information about the 3-dimensional structure and chemical mechanism of the enzymatic reaction, some of which may not be available. However, the increasing growth of databases containing protein structures and sequences is helping to overcome this lack of information.

Comparison of the sequence of a new biocatalyst identified in a screening program with the thousands deposited in the databases can identify related proteins whose functions or/and structures are already known. Because new enzymes have evolved in nature by relatively minor modification of active-site structures, the goals of homology-driven experiments include engineering binding sites to fit different substrates as well as construction of new catalytic residues to modify functions and mechanisms [56]. A small number of variants are produced which are then screened. Although in many cases, results are poor compared to natural enzymes, there have been successes [57,58].

Computational protein design starts with the coordinates of a protein main chain and uses a force field to identify sequences and geometries of amino acids that are optimal for stabilizing the backbone geometry [59]. Because of the amazing number of possible sequences generated, the combination of predictive force fields and search algorithms is now being applied to functional protein design [60].

3.2. Directed Evolution

Combinatorial methods such as directed evolution create a large number of variants for screening for enantioselectivity, catalytic efficiency, catalytic rate, solubility, specificity and enzyme stability, but do not require extensive knowledge about the enzyme. Directed evolution is a fast and inexpensive way of finding variants of existing enzymes that work better than naturally occurring enzymes under specific conditions [3,61–63]. Directed evolution includes an entire range of molecular biological techniques that allow the achievement of genetic diversity mimicking mechanisms of evolution occurring in nature. It involves random mutagenesis of the protein-encoding gene by different techniques including the error-prone polymerase chain reaction (PCR) [64], repeated oligonucleotide directed mutagenesis [65], or chemical agents [66], among others. Error prone PCR accomplishes introduction of random point mutations in a population of enzymes. Such molecular breeding techniques (DNA shuffling, Molecular Breeding^{TM}) allow *in vitro* random homologous recombination, typically between parent genes with homology higher than 70% [67]. After cloning and expression, a large collection of enzyme variants (10^4–10^6) is typically generated and is subjected to screening or selection.

All the approaches mentioned above are not mutually exclusive as the fields of rational, semi-rational and random redesign of enzymes are moving closer. Thus, directed evolution techniques make use, where possible, of smaller enzyme variant libraries designed by rational or semi-rational methods to reduce the screening effort but without compromising the likelihood of finding better variants [61,63]. One option is to target the active site residues (about 10–15 amino acids) and those closest to it (another 20–30 amino acids) as mutations closer to these regions seem to be more beneficial [68]. Another strategy, called CASTing, is based on a combinatorial active site testing [69], in which libraries are generated from groups of two or three residues made from the active site residues. Hits obtained from these initial libraries are combined and new libraries are generated and screened in an iterative way. By changing the nucleotide components during PCR, the amino acid alphabet can be reduced yielding new proteins composed by only 12 amino acids [70]. Screening of such libraries can lead to remarkable improvements in activity by using saturation mutagenesis at homologous enzyme positions [71].

As the fitness of a gene will increase more rapidly in a breeding population with high genetic variability that is under the influence of selection, DNA Family Shuffling, an improvement in the breeding technique based on recombination of several homologous sequences, yielded an improvement in activity of about 30 to 80 times higher than when each gene was shuffled independently [72]. Further techniques can create shuffle exons or domains [73], loop regions [74], random truncations [75] or insertions and deletions of codons [76].

Random redesign techniques are being currently used to generate enzymes with improved properties, such as: activity and stability at different pH values and temperatures [77], increased or modified enantioselectivity [78], altered substrate specificity [79], stability in organic solvents [80], novel substrate specificity and activity [81] and increased biological activity of protein pharmaceuticals and biological molecules [82,83]. Directed evolution increased the activity of glyphosate-N-acetyltransferase by 10,000-fold and at the same time, its thermostability increased 5-fold [84]. Proteins from directed evolution work were already on the market in 2000 [85,86]. These were GFP of Clontech and Novo Nordisk's LipoPrime® lipase.

4. Production of Recombinant Proteins in Microbial Hosts

In 2005, there were 4200 biotechnology companies worldwide. Total revenue amounted to $63 billion. Recombinant DNA technology has been remarkably advanced by their development of efficient and scale-up expression systems to produce enzymes from industrially-unknown microorganisms and other living organisms using industrial organisms such as *E. coli*, *Bacillus subtilis* and other species of *Bacillus*, *Ralstonia eutropha*, *Pseudomonas fluorescens*, *Saccharomyce cerevisiae*, *Pichia pastoris*, *Hansenula polymorpha*, and species of *Aspergillus and Trichoderma* [87]. Approximately 90% of industrial enzymes are recombinant versions.

E. coli has been extensively used as a recombinant host for many reasons including (i) ease of quickly and precisely modifying the genome; (ii) rapid growth to high cell densities; (iii) ease of culture in cheap media; and (iv) ease of reduction of protease activity. *E. coli* can accumulate heterologous proteins up to 50% of its dry cell weight [88]. However, it has several drawbacks, such as: inability for post-translational modifications, presence of toxic cell wall pyrogens or, sometimes, formation of inclusion bodies containing inactive, aggregated and insoluble heterologous protein. Despite this, high level production and excretion has been obtained with the following heterologous proteins: alkaline phosphatase (PhoA) at 5.2 g/L into the periplasm, and levan fructotransferase LFT at 4 g/L into the medium. In 1993, recombinant processes in *E. coli* were responsible for almost $5 billion worth of products (87). *R. eutropha* produced organophosphohydrolase at 10 g/L [89]. The *P. fluorescens* culture of the Pfenex company is capable of producing 20 g/L of protein [90].

S. cerevisiae offers certain advantages over bacteria as a cloning host [91]. This yeast can be grown rapidly in simple media and to a high cell density, can secrete heterologous proteins into the extracellular broth, and its genetics are more advanced than any other eukaryote. Glucose oxidase from *Aspergillus niger* has been produced at 9 g/L by this yeast (87). Despite these advantages, *S. cerevisiae* is sometimes regarded as a less than optimal host for large-scale production of mammalian proteins because of drawbacks such as hyperglycosylation, presence of α-1, 3-linked mannose residues that could cause an antigenic response in patients, and absence of strong and tightly-regulated promoters.

P. pastoris has become one of the most extensively used expression systems [87,92]. Over 700 proteins have been produced by this yeast [93]. Production of recombinant proteins reached 22 g/L for intracellular proteins [94] and 14.8 g/L for secreted proteins [95]. Claims have been made that *P. pastoris* can produce up to 30 g/L of recombinant proteins [96]. Among the advantages of this methylotrophic yeast over *S. cerevisiae* are (i) an efficient and tightly-regulated methanol promoter (AOX1) which yields alcohol oxidase at 30% of soluble protein; (ii) less extensive glycosylation, due to shorter chain lengths of *N*-linked high-mannose oligosaccharides, usually up to 20 residues lacking the terminal α-1,3-mannose linkages [97]; (iii) integration of multicopies of foreign DNA into chromosomal DNA yielding stable transformants; (iv) ability to secrete high levels of foreign proteins; and (v) high-density growth and straight-forward scale-up [98].

Heterologous gene expression in the methylotropic yeast *H. polymorpha* is similar to that of *P. pastoris*. The promoter of the methanol oxidase gene is used to express foreign genes. As with AOX1 in *P. pastoris*, the MOX gene in *H. polymorpha* is highly expressed and tightly-regulated, giving enzyme levels up to 37% of total cell protein [99]. One major difference is that expression of the MOX gene is significantly derepressed in the absence of glucose or during glucose limitation [100] and therefore tight regulation of the MOX promoter is lost in the high glucose conditions usually used for high-biomass fermentations. *H. polymorpha* can produce 1.4 g/L of secreted glucoamylase and 13.5 g/L of phytase.

The development of molecular techniques for production of recombinant heterologous proteins in filamentous fungi has been laborious and contrasts markedly with the success achieved in yeasts. The ability to introduce or delete genes remains difficult, although some advances in transformation have been reported, e.g., restriction enzyme-mediated integration [101] and *Agrobacterium tumefaciens*-Ti plasmid-mediated transformation [102]. Levels of production of non-fungal proteins have been low compared to those of homologous proteins. Different strategies have been developed to overcome these problems, including the construction of protease-deficient strains [103], introduction of a large number of gene copies [104], use of strong fungal promoters, efficient secretion signals [104,105], and gene fusions with a gene which encodes part of or an entire well-secreted protein [105]. Little research has been carried out on glycosylation in molds although hyper-glycosylation does not seem to occur and low-mannose side chains are formed. *Aspergillus awamori* produces 4.6 g/L of glucoamylase from *A. niger*. *Aspergillus oryzae* yields 3.3 g/L of *Mucor* rennin. *Acremonium chrysogenum* produces 4 g/L of *Fusarium* alkaline protease. *Trichoderma reesei* produces 35 g/L of recombinantproteins.A recent entry into the field is *Chrysosporium lucknowense*, which produces high levels of proteins (50–80 g/L), and from which low-viscosity and low-protease mutants have been obtained [106,107].

5. Enzymatic Biocatalysis

Biocatalysts have been widely applied in the brewing and food industries for a long time but ar finding new applications in many fields including industrial chemistry [108]. Biocatalysis involves the application of whole microbial cells, cell extracts, purified enzymes, immobilized cells, or immobilized enzymes as catalysts for any of the above mentioned processes [109,110]. As mentioned in the previous sections, its rapid development was due to the recent advances in large-scale genome sequencing, directed evolution, protein expression, metabolic engineering, high throughput screening, and structural biology [111,112].

5.1. Technical Applications

Enzymes are very important for processes of industrial, pharmaceutical and biotechnological significance [113]. The total market for industrial enzymes reached $3.3 billion in 2010 and it is estimated to reach a value of 4.4 billion by 2015 [114]. Of these, technical enzymes are typically used as bulk enzymes in the detergent, textile, pulp and paper industries, and in the biofuels industry, among others. Usage for leather and bioethanol is responsible for the highest sales figures. Technical enzymes had revenues of nearly $1.2 billion in 2011 which is expected to reach $1.5 billion in 2015 and $1.7 billion in 2016. The highest sales are expected to be in the biofuels (bioethanol) market [115]. Use of enzymes for foods and beverages is expected to reach $1.3 billion by 2015.

The use of enzymes as detergent additives represents a major application of industrial enzymes. Proteases, lipases, amylases, oxidases, peroxidases and cellulases are added to detergents where they catalyze the breakdown of chemical bonds on the addition of water. To be suitable, they must be active under thermophilic (60 °C) and alkalophilic (pH 9–11) conditions, as well as in the presence of the various components of washing powders.

Proteases constitute over 60% of the global market for enzymes. They are used to produce pharmaceuticals, foods, detergents, leather, silk and agrochemical products. In laundry detergents, they account for approximately 25% of the total worldwide sales of enzymes. The first detergent containing a bacterial protease ("Biotex") was introduced by Novo Industry A/S (now Novozymes) in 1956. It contained an alcalase produced by *Bacillus licheniformis*. In 1994, Novo Nordisk introduced Lipolase™, the first commercial recombinant lipase for use in a detergent, by cloning the *Humicola lanuginose* lipase into the *A. oryzae* genome. In 1995, Genencor International introduced two bacterial lipases, one from *Pseudomonas mendocina* (Lumafast™), and another from *Pseudomonas alcaligenes* (Lipomax™). An enzyme added recently to detergents is Mannaway™, a *Bacillus* mannanase which removes food stains containing guar gum [116].

In the textile industry, enzymes are also increasingly being used to develop cleaner processes and reduce the use of raw materials and production of waste. The application of cellulases for denim finishing and laccases for decolorization of textile effluents and textile bleaching are the most recent commercial advances [117]. An alternative enzymatic process in the manufacturing of cotton has been recently developed based on a pectate lyase [118]. The process is performed at much lower temperatures and uses less water than the classical method.

Another application of enzymes with increasing importance is the use of lipases, xylanases and laccases in removing pitch (hydrophobic components of wood, mainly triglycerides and waxes) in the pulp industry [119]. A lipase from *Candida rugosa* is used by Nippon Paper Industries to remove up to 90% of these compounds [120]. The use of enzymes as alternatives to chemicals in leather processing has proved successful in improving leather quality and in reducing environmental pollution. Alkaline lipases from *Bacillus* strains, which grow under highly alkaline conditions, in

435

combination with other alkaline or neutral proteases, are currently being used in this industry. Laccases oxidize phenolic and non-phenolic lignin-related compounds as well as environmental pollutants [121]. They are used to detoxify industrial effluents from the paper and pulp, textile, and petrochemical industries, as a medical diagnostic tool, for bioremediation of herbicides, pesticides, and explosives in soil, as a cleaning agent for water purification systems, as a catalyst in drug manufacture and as cosmetic ingredients.

Although cellulases have been widely used in textile applications for many years, these enzymes are gaining additional consideration in the enzyme market owing to their ability in the degradation of lignocellulosic feedstocks. The cost of cellulases is a key issue in achieving a low price conversion of lignocellulosic biomass into biofuels and other products [122–124]. Filamentous fungi can produce native cellulases at levels greater than 100 g/L [87]. Enzymes needed to hydrolyze cellulose include (1) endoglucanases, which break down cellulose chains in a random manner; (2) cellobiohydrolases, which liberate glucose dimers from both ends of cellulose chains; and (3) beta-glucosidases, which produce glucose from oligomer chains. *Hypocrea jecorina (Trichoderma reesei)* is the main industrial source of cellulases and hemicellulases used to depolymerize plant biomass to simple sugars [125–127]. The overall action of *T. reesei* on cellulosic biomass is limited by its low content of beta-glucosidase. The result is accumulation of cellobiose which limits further breakdown. The expression of the beta-glucosidase gene from *Pericona* sp in *T. reesei* resulted in an increased level of beta-glucosidase, thus increasing overall cellulase activity and action on biomass residues [128]. Cellulases are formed adaptively, and several positive (XYR1, ACE2, HAP2/3/5) and negative (ACE1, CRE1) components involved in this regulation are now known [127]. In addition, its complete genome sequence has been published [129], thus making the organism susceptible to targeted improvement by metabolic engineering. It has recently been reported that the extreme thermophilic bacterium *Caldicelluloseruptor bescil* produces a cellulase/hemicellulase system twice as active as that from *T. reesei* [130].

5.2. Enzymes in the Feed Industry

The global market for feed enzymes is a promising segment in the enzyme industry and is expected to reach about $730 million in 2015 [131]. Feed enzymes can increase the digestibility of nutrients, leading to greater efficiency in feed utilization. Also, they can degrade unacceptable components in feed, which are otherwise harmful or of little or no value [132]. Currently, feed enzymes commercially available are phytases, proteases, α-galactosidases, glucanases, xylanases, α-amylases, and polygalacturonases, mainly used for swine and poultry [133]. Developments of heat-stable enzymes, improved specific activity, some new non-starch polysaccharide-degrading enzymes, and rapid, economical and reliable assays for measuring enzyme activity have always been the focus and have been intensified recently. The use of enzymes as feed additives is restricted in many countries by local regulatory authorities [134] and applications may therefore vary from country to country.

5.3. Enzymes in Food Processing

Food and beverage enzymes constitute the largest segment of industrial enzymes with revenues of nearly $1.2 billion in 2011 which is expected to grow to $1.8 billion by 2016, at a composed annual growth rate of 10.4% [115].

Lipases are commonly used in the production of a variety of products, ranging from fruit juices, baked foods, and vegetable fermentations to dairy enrichment. Fats, oils and related compounds are the main targets of lipases in food technology. Accurate control of lipase concentration, pH, temperature and emulsion content is required to maximize the production of flavor and fragrance. The lipase mediation of carbohydrate esters of fatty acids offers a potential market for use as emulsifiers in foods, pharmaceuticals and cosmetics. There are three recombinant fungal lipases currently used in the food industry, one from *Rhizomucor miehi*, one from *Thermomyces lanuginosus* and another from *Fusarium oxysporum*; all being produced in *A. oryzae* [135,136].

The major application of proteases in the dairy industry is for the manufacture of cheese. Calf rennin had been preferred in cheese making due to its high specificity, but microbial proteases produced by GRAS microorganisms like *Mucor miehei*, *Bacillus subtilis*, *Mucor pusillus Lindt* and *Endothia parasitica* are gradually replacing it. The primary function of these enzymes in cheese making is to hydrolyze the specific peptide bond (Phe105-Met106) that generates para-k-casein and macropeptides [137]. Production of calf rennin (chymosin) in recombinant *A. niger var awamori* amounted to about 1 g/L after nitrosoguanidine mutagenesis and selection for 2-deoxyglucose resistance [138]. Further improvement was done by parasexual recombination resulting in a strain producing 1.5 g/L from parents producing 1.2 g/L [139]. Four recombinant proteases have been approved by FDA for cheese production [140,141].

Bacterial glucose isomerase, fungal α-amylase and glucoamylase are currently used to produce "high fructose corn syrup" from starch in a $1 billion business. Other enzymes useful in the food industry include invertase from *Kluyveromyces fragilis*, *Saccharomyces carlsbergensis* and *S. cerevisiae* for candy and jam manufacture, β-galactosidase (lactase) from *Kluyveromyces lactis*, *K. fragilis* or *Candida pseudotropicalis* for hydrolysis of lactose from milk or whey, and galactosidase from *S. carlsbergensis* for crystallization of beet sugar. "Fructose syrup", produced by xxylose isomerase on glucose is at a production level of 15 million tons per year [142].

In terms of government regulation, enzymes used in food can be divided into food additives and processing aids. Most food enzymes are considered as processing aids, with only a few used as additives, such as lysozyme and invertase [143]. The processing aids are used during the manufacturing process of foodstuffs, and do not have a technological function in the final food. All these materials are expected to be safe, under the guidance of good manufacturing practice (GMP). The key issue in evaluating safety of enzyme preparations is the safety assessment of the production strain. Only about nine recombinant microorganisms are considered "Generally Recognized As Safe" (GRAS) based on FDA regulations. These are from a relatively small number of bacterial and fungal species primarily *A. oryzae*, *A. niger*, *B. subtilis* and *B. licheniformis*. Olempska-Beer [144] has reviewed the microbial strains engineered for food enzyme production from a security point of view.

5.4. Enzymes in Chemical and Pharmaceutical Processes

Successful application of enzymatic processes in the chemical industry depends mainly on cost competitiveness with the existing and well-established chemical methods [145]. Lower energy demand, increased product titer, increased catalyst efficiency, less catalyst waste and byproducts, as well as lower volumes of wastewater streams, are the main advantages that biotechnological processes have as compared to well-established chemical processes. There are estimated to be only around 150 biocatalytic processes currently applied in industry [146]. However, new scientific developments in genomics, as well as in protein engineering, facilitate the tailoring of enzyme properties to increase that number significantly [147,148].

An enzymatic conversion was devised to produce the amino acid L-tyrosine [149]. Phenol, pyruvate, pyridoxal phosphate and ammonium chloride are converted to L-tyrosine using a thermostable and chemostable tyrosine phenol lyase obtained from *Symbiobacterium toebii*. The titer produced was 130 g/L after 30 h with continuous feeding of substrate.

Industrial scale biocatalysis is focused primarily on hydrolases, a few ketoreductases (KREDs), cofactor regeneration and protein stability in organic solvents. The numerous biocatalytic routes scaled up for pharmaceutical manufacturing have been recently reviewed by Bornscheuer *et al.* [112], showing the competitiveness of enzymes versus traditional chemical processes.

Enzymes are useful for preparing beta-lactam antibiotics such as semi-synthetic penicillins and cephalosporins [150]. Beta-lactams constitute 60%–65% of the total antibiotic market.

Preparation of chiral medicines, *i.e.*, the synthesis of complex chiral pharmaceutical intermediates efficiently and economically, is one of the most important applications in biocatalysis. Esterases, lipases, proteases and KREDs (ketoreductases) are widely applied in the preparation of chiral alcohols, carboxylic acids, amines or epoxides, among others [116,151,152].

The inherent inefficiency of kinetic resolution (maximum 50% yield) can be overcome by novel asymmetric reactions catalyzed by improved microbial enzymes which can provide a 100% yield [153]. Asymmetric reduction of tetrahydrothiophene-3-one with a wild-type reductase gave the desired alcohol ((R)-tetrahydrothiophene-3-ol), a key component in sulopenem, a potent antibacterial developed by Pfizer, but only in 80%–90% ee (enantiomeric excess). A combination of random mutagenesis, gene shuffling and ProSAR analysis was used to improve the enantio-selectivity of a ketoreductase towards tetrahydrothiophene-3-one. The best variant increased enantio-selectivity from 63% ee to 99% ee [154].

Atorvastatin, the active ingredient of Lipitor, a cholesterol-lowering drug that had global sales of US$12 billion in 2010, can be produced enzymatically. The process is based on three enzymatic activities: a ketone reductase, a glucose dehydrogenase and a halohydryn dehalogenase. Several iterative rounds of DNA shuffling for these three enzymes, with screening in the presence of iteratively higher concentrations of product, led to a 14-fold reduction in reaction time, a 7-fold increase in substrate loading, a 25-fold reduction in enzyme use, and a 50% improvement in isolated yield [155].

Kinetic resolution of racemic amines is a common method used in the synthesis of chiral amines. Acylation of a primary amine moiety by a lipase is used by BASF for the resolution of chiral primary amines in a multi-thousand ton scale [156]. Recently, asymmetric synthesis from the corresponding chiral ketones, using transaminases, is gaining attention [152]. Some (R)-selective transaminases have been recently discovered using *in silico* strategies for a sequence-based prediction of substrate specificity and enantio-preference [157]. Optically pure (S)-amines were obtained using a recombinant ω-transaminase with 99% ee and 97% yield [158]. These enantiopure amines may find use as inhibitors of monoamine oxidase in the treatment of diverse neurological disorders such as Parkinson's and Alzheimer's diseases.

An effective enzymatic process using enzyme evolution was developed by the biotechnology company Codexis, in cooperation with Pfizer, to produce 2-methyl pentanol, an important intermediate for manufacture of pharmaceuticals and liquid crystals [159]. Quite recently, protein engineering expanded the substrate range of transaminases to ketones. In an impressive piece of work developed by Merck and Codexis, the chemical manufacture of sitagliptin, the active ingredient in Januvia which is a leading drug for type 2 diabetes, was replaced by a new biocatalytic process. Several rounds of directed evolution were applied to create an engineered amine transaminase with a 40,000-fold increase in activity [160]. Such a process not only reduced total waste (by 19%), but also increased overall yield (by 13%) and productivity (by 53%). Codexis scientists also developed enzymatic processes for the production of montelukast (Singulair) and silopenem [161]. They also developed an improved LovD enzyme (an acyltransferase) for improved conversion of the cholesterol-lowering agent, lovastatin, to simvastatin [162].

Optically active carboxylic acids have been usually synthesized through different enzymatic routes catalyzed by lipases, nitrilases or hydroxynitrile lyases. Recent advances have improved the efficiency of such procedures. The synthesis of 2-arylpropanoic acids (e.g., ketoprofen, ibuprofen and naproxen) is mainly achieved through the kinetic resolution of racemic substrates by lipases from *Candida antarctica* or *Pseudomonas* sp. A process using a novel substrate, (R,S)-N-profenylazoles, instead of their correspondent esters, proved to be more efficient.

(R)-o-chloromandelic acid is a key intermediate for manufacture of Clopidogrel, a platelet aggregation inhibitor, with global sales of $10 billion per year. The asymmetric reduction of methyl o-chlorobenzoylformate with a versatile recombinant carbonyl reductase from *S. cerevisiae* expressed in *E. coli* yielded (R)-o-chloromandelate at a concentration of 178 g/L and 99% ee [163].

Application of enzymes in several industrial bioconversions has been broadened by the use of organic solvents replacing water [45,50], an important development in enzyme engineering. Many chemicals and polymers are insoluble in water and its presence leads to undesirable by-products and degradation of common organic reagents. Although switching from water to an organic solvent as the reaction medium might suggest that the enzyme would be denatured, many crystalline or lyophilized enzymes are actually stable and retain their activities in such anhydrous environments. Yeast lipases have been used to catalyze butanolysis in anhydrous solvents to obtain enantiopure 2-chloro- and 2-bromo-propionic acids that are used for the synthesis of herbicides and pharmaceuticals [151]. Another lipase is used in a stereoselective step, carried out in acetonitrile, for the acetylation of a symmetrical diol during the synthesis of an antifungal agent [164].

From a biotechnological perspective, there are many advantages of employing enzymes in organic, as opposed to aqueous, media [165], including higher substrate solubility, reversal of hydrolytic reactions, and modified enzyme specificity, which result in new enzyme activities. On the other hand, enzymes usually show lower catalytic activities in organic than in aqueous solution.

6. Conclusion and Future Perspectives

Microorganisms provide an impressive amount of catalysts with a wide range of applications across several industries such as household care, food, animal feed, technical industries, fine chemicals and pharma. The unique properties of enzymes such as high specificity, fast action and biodegradability allow enzyme-assisted processes in industry to run under milder reaction conditions, with improved yields and reduce waste generation.

However, naturally occurring enzymes are often not suitable for such biocatalytic processes without further tailoring or redesign of the enzyme itself in order to fine-tune substrate specificity activity or other key catalytic properties.

Recent advances in genomics, metagenomics, proteomics, efficient expression systems and emerging recombinant DNA techniques have facilitated the discovery of new microbial enzymes from nature (through genome and metagenome) or by creating (or evolving) enzymes with improved catalytic properties.

The ongoing progress and interest in enzymes provide further success in areas of industrial biocatalysis. The next years should see a lot of exciting developments in the area of biotransformations. There are many factors influencing the growing interest in biocatalysis which include enzyme promiscuity, robust computational methods combined with directed evolution and screening technologies to improve enzyme properties to meet process prospects, the application of one-pot multistep reactions using multifunctional catalysts and the *de novo* design and selection of catalytic proteins catalyzing any desired chemical reaction.

Many future investigations will use combinations of engineered and *de novo* designed enzymes coupled with chemistry to generate more (and most likely new) chemicals and materials from cheaper (and renewable) resources, which will consequently contribute to establishing a bio-based economy and achieving low carbon green growth.

Conflicts of Interest

The authors declare no conflict of interest.

References

1.   Adrio, J.L.; Demain, A.L. Microbial Cells and Enzymes—A Century of Progress. In *Methods in Biotechnology. Microbial Enzymes and Biotransformations*; Barredo, J.L., Ed.; Humana Press: Totowa, NJ, USA, 2005; Volume 17, pp. 1–27.
2.   Johannes, T.W.; Zhao, H. Directed evolution of enzymes and biosynthetic pathways. *Curr. Opin. Microbiol.* **2006**, *9*, 261–267.
3.   Kumar, A.; Singh, S. Directed evolution: Tailoring biocatalysis for industrial application. *Crit. Rev. Biotechnol.* **2013**, *33*, 365–378.

4. Demain, A.L.; Adrio, J.L. Contributions of microorganisms to industrial biology. *Mol. Biotechnol.* **2008**, *38*, 41–45.

5. Johnson, E.A. Biotechnology of non-*Saccharomyces* yeasts- the ascomycetes. *Appl. Microbiol. Biotechnol.* **2013**, *97*, 503–517.

6. Rondon, M.R.; Goodman, R.M.; Handelsman, J. The Earth's bounty: Assessing and accessing soil microbial diversity. *Trends Biotechnol.* **1999**, *17*, 403–409.

7. Verenium, A Pioneer of 21st Century Bioscience, is Working to Transform Industries. Available online: http://www.diversa.com (access on 1 July 2013).

8. Uchiyama, T.; Miyazaki, K. Functional metagenomics for enzyme discovery: Challenges to efficient screening. *Curr. Opin. Biotechnol.* **2009**, *20*, 616–622.

9. Ferrer, M.; Beloqui, A.; Timmis, K.M.; Golyshin, P.N. Metagenomics for mining new genetic resources of microbial communities. *J. Mol. Microbiol. Biotechnol.* **2009**, *16*, 109–123.

10. Gilbert, J.A.; Dupont, C.L. Microbial metagenomics: Beyond the genome. *Annu. Rev. Mar. Sci.* **2011**, *3*, 347–371.

11. The Institute for Genomic Research (TIGR)-JCVI. http://cmr.jcvi.org/tigr (accessed on 1 July 2013).

12. The National Center for Biotechnology Information. Available online: http://www.ncbi.nlm.nih.gov (accessed on 1 July 2013).

13. Ahmed, N. A flood of microbial genomes—Do we need more? *PLoS One* **2009**, *4*, 1–5.

14. Kaul, P.; Asano, Y. Strategies for discovery and improvement of enzyme function: State of the art and opportunities. *Microbiol. Biotechnol.* **2012**, *5*, 18–33.

15. Schiraldini, C.; de Rosa, M. The production of biocatalysts and biomolecules from extremophiles. *Trends Biotechnol.* **2002**. *20*, 515–521.

16. Kumar, L.; Awasthi, G.; Singh, B. Extremophiles: A novel source of industrially important enzymes. *Biotechnology* **2011**, *10*, 1–15.

17. Steele, H.L.; Jaeger, K.E.; Daniel, R.; Streit, W.R. Advances in recovery of novel biocatalysts from metagenomes. *J. Mol. Microbiol. Biotechnol.* **2009**, *16*, 25–37.

18. Li, S.; Yang, X.; Yang, S.; Zhu, M.; Wang, X. Technology prospecting on enzymes: Application, marketing and engineering. *Comput. Struct. Biotechnol. J.* **2012**, *2*, 1–11.

19. Hess, M.; Sczyrba, A.; Egan, R.; Kim, T.W.; Chokhawala, H.; Schroth, G.; Luo, S.; Clark, D.S.; Chen, F.; Zhang, T.; *et al.* Metagenomic discovery of biomass-degrading genes and genomes from cow rumen. *Science* **2011**, *331*, 463–467.

20. Kennedy, J.; Marchesi, J.R.; Dobson, A.D. Marine metagenomics: Strategies for the discovery of novel enzymes with biotechnological applications from marine environments. *Microb. Cell Fact.* **2008**, *7*, 27–37.

21. Warnecke, F.; Luginbühl, P.; Ivanova, N.; Ghassemian, M.; Richardson, T.H.; Stege, J.T.; Cayouette, M.; McHardy, A.C.; Djordjevic, G.; Aboushadi, N.; *et al.* Metagenomic and functional analysis of hindgut microbiota of a wood-feeding higher termite. *Nature* **2007**, *450*, 560–565.

22. Jeon, J.H.; Kim, J.T.; Kim, Y.J.; Kim, H.K.; Lee, H.S.; Kang, S.G.; Kim, S.J.; Lee, J.H. Cloning and characterization of a new-cold active lipase from a deep-se sediment metagenome. *Appl. Microbiol. Biotechnol.* **2009**, *81*, 865–874.

23. Fernández-Álvaro, E.; Kourist, R.; Winter, J.; Böttcher, D.; Liebeton, K.; Naumer, C. Enantioselective kinetic resolution of phenylalkyl carboxylic acids using metagenome-derived esterases. *Microb. Biotechnol.* **2010**, *3*, 59–64.

24. Knietsch, A.; Waschkowitz, T.; Bowien, S.; Henne, A.; Daniel, R. Construction and screening of metagenomic libraries derived from enrichment cultures: Generation of a gene bank for genes conferring alcohol oxidoreductase activity on *Escherichia coli*. *Appl. Environ. Microbiol.* **2003**, *69*, 1408–1416.

25. Gabor, E.M.; de Vries, E.J.; Janssen, D.B. Construction, characterization, and use of small-insert gene banks of DNA isolated from soil and enrichment cultures for the recovery of novel amidases. *Environ. Microbiol.* **2004**, *6*, 948–958.

26. Rondon, M.R.; August, P.R.; Betterman, A.D.; Brady, S.F.; Grossman, T.H.; Liles, M.R. Cloning the soil metagenome: A strategy for accesing the genetic and functional diversity of uncultured microorganisms. *Appl. Environ. Microbiol.* **2000**, *66*, 2541–2547.

27. Bayer, S.; Birkemeyer, C.; Ballschmiter, M. A nitrilase from ametagenomic library acts regioselectively on aliphatic dinitriles. *Appl. Microbiol. Biotechnol.* **2011**, *89*, 91–98.

28. Wang, K.; Li, G.; Yu, S.Q.; Zhang, C.T.; Liu, Y.H. A novel metegenome-derived β-galactosidase: Gene cloning, overexpression, purification and characterization. *Appl. Microbiol. Biotechnol.* **2010**, *88*, 155–165.

29. Jiang, C.; Li, S.X.; Luo, F.F.; Jin, K.; Wang, Q.; Hao, Z.Y. Biochemical characterization of two novel β-glucosidase genes by metagenome expression cloning. *Bioresour. Technol.* **2011**, *102*, 3272–3278.

30. Jiang, C.; Shen, P.; Yan, B.; Wua, B. Biochemical characterization of a metagenome-derived decarboxylase. *Enzyme Microb. Technol.* **2009**, *45*, 58–63.

31. Kotik, M.; Stepanek, V.; Grulich, M.; Kyslik, P.; Archelas, A. Access to enantiopure aromatic epoxides and diols using epoxide hydrolases derived from total biofilter DNA. *J. Mol. Catal. B Enzym.* **2010**, *65*, 41–48.

32. Martínez, A.; Kolvek, S.J.; Yip, C.L.T.; Hopke, J.; Brown, K.A.; MacNeil, I.A.; Osburne, M.S. Genetically modified bacterial strains and novel bacterial artificial chromosome shuttle vectors for constructing environmental libraries and detecting heterologous naturals products in multiple expression hosts. *Appl. Environ. Microbiol.* **2004**, *70*, 2452–2463.

33. Wexler, M.; Bond, P.L.; Richardson, D.J.; Johnston, A.W. A wide host-range metagenomic library from a waste water treatment plants yields a novel alcohol/aldehyde dehydrogenase. *Environ. Microbiol.* **2005**, *7*, 1917–1926.

34. Suenaga, H.; Ohnuki, T.; Miyazaki, K. Functional screening of a metagenomic library for genes involved in microbial degradation of aromatic compounds. *Environ. Microbiol.* **2007**, *9*, 2289–2297.

442

35. Mirete, S.; de Figueras, C.G.; González-Pastor, J.E. Novel nickel resistance genes from the rhizosphere metagenome of plants adapted to acid mine drainage. *Appl. Environ. Microbiol.* **2007**, *73*, 6001–6011.

36. Mori, T.; Mizuta, S.; Suenaga, H.; Miyazaki, K. Metagenomic screening for bleomycin resistance genes. *Appl. Environ. Microbiol.* **2008**, *74*, 6803–6805.

37. Uchiyama, T.; Abe, T.; Ikemura, T.; Watanabe, K. Substrate-induced gene-expression screening of environmental metagenome libraries for isolation of catabolic genes. *Nat. Biotechnol.* **2005**, *23*, 88–93.

38. Schipper, C.; Hornung, C.; Bijtenhoorn, P.; Quistchau, M.; Grond, S.; Streit, W.R. Metagenome-derived clones encoding two novel lactonase family proteins involved in biofilm inhibition in *Pseudomonas aeruginosa*. *Appl. Environ. Microbiol.* **2009**, *75*, 224–233.

39. Uchiyama, T.; Watanabe, K. Substrate-induced gene expression (SIGEX) screening of metagenome libraries. *Nat. Protoc.* **2008**, *3*, 1202–1212.

40. Van Lanen, S.; Shen, B. Microbial genomics for the improvement of natural product discovery. *Curr. Opin. Microbiol.* **2006**, *9*, 252–260.

41. NCBI Microbial Genomes. Available online: http://www.ncbi.nlm.nhi.gov/genomes/microbial (accessed on 10 July 2013).

42. Luo, X.J.; Yu, H.L.; Xu, J.H. Genomic data mining: An efficient way to find new and better enzymes. *Enzyme Eng.* **2012**, *1*, 104–108.

43. Cavicchioli, R.; Amils, R.; Wagner, D.; McGenity, T. Life and applications of extremophiles. *Environ. Microbiol.* **2011**, *13*, 1903–1907.

44. Pikuta, E.V.; Hoover, R.B.; Tang, J. Microbial Extremophiles at the limit of life. *Crit. Rev. Microbiol.* **2007**, *33*, 183–209.

45. Atomi, H.; Sato, T.; Kanai, T. Application of hyperthermophiles and their enzymes. *Curr. Opin. Biotechnol.* **2011**, *22*, 618–626.

46. De Carvalho, C.C. Enzymatic and whole cell catalysis: Finding new strategies for old processes. *Biotechnol. Adv.* **2011**, *29*, 75–83.

47. Hess, M. Thermoacidophilic proteins for biofuels production. *Trends Microbiol.* **2008**, *16*, 414–419.

48. Chen, Z.W.; Liu, Y.Y.; Wu, J.F.; She, Q.; Jiang, C.Y.; Liu, S.J. Novel bacterial sulphur oxygenase reductases from bioreactors treating gold-bearing concentrates. *Appl. Microbiol. Biotechnol.* **2007**, *74*, 688–698.

49. Margesin, R.; Feller, G.; Gerday, C.; Rusell, N. Cold-Adapted Microorganisms: Adaptation Strategies and Biotechnological Potential. In *The Encyclopedia of Environmental Microbiology*; Bitton, G., Ed.; John Wiley and Sons: New York, NY, USA, 2002; pp. 871–885.

50. Klibanov, A.M. Improving enzymes by using them in organic solvents. *Nature* **2001**, *409*, 241–246.

51. Gomes, I.; Gomes, J.; Steiner, W. Highly thermostable amylase and pullulanase of the extreme thermophilic eubacterium *Rhodothermus marinus*: Production and partialcharacterization. *Bioresour. Technol.* **2003**, *90*, 207–214.

52. Van den Burg, B. Extremophiles as a source for novel enzymes. *Curr. Opin. Microbiol.* **2003**, *6*, 213–218.

53. Shukla, A.; Rana, A.; Kumar, L.; Singh, B.; Ghosh, D. Assessment of detergent activity of *Streptococcus* sp. AS02 protease isolated from soil of Sahastradhara, Doon Valley, Uttarakhand. *Asian J. Microbiol. Biotechnol. Environ. Sci.* **2009**, *11*, 587–591.

54. Marrs, B.; Delagrave, S.; Murphy, D. Novel approaches for discovering industrial enzymes. *Curr. Opin. Microbiol.* **1999**, *2*, 241–245.

55. Singhania, R.R.; Patel, A.K.; Pandy, A. *Industrial Biotechnology: Sustainable Growth and Economic Success*; Soetaert, W., Vandamme, E.J., Eds.; Wiley VCH Verlag GmbH: Weinheim, Germany, 2010; pp. 207–226.

56. Cedrone, F.; Menez, A.; Quemeneur, E. Tailoring new enzyme functions by rational redesign. *Curr. Opin. Struct. Biol.* **2000**, *10*, 405–410.

57. Beppu, T. Modification of milk-clotting aspartic proteinases by recombinant DNA techniques. *Ann. N. Y. Acad. Sci.* **1990**, *613*, 14–25.

58. Van den Burg, B.; de Kreij, A.; van der Veek, P.; Mansfeld, J.; Venema, G. Engineering an enzyme to resist boiling. *Proc. Natl. Acad. Sci. USA* **1998**, *95*, 2056–2060.

59. Bolon, D.N.; Voigt, C.A.; Mayo, S.L. *De novo* design of biocatalysts. *Curr. Opin. Struct. Biol.* **2002**, *6*, 125–129.

60. Shimaoka, M.; Shiftman, J.M.; Jing, H.; Tagaki, J.; Mayo, S.L.; Springer, T.A. Computational design of an integrin I domain stabilized in the open high affinity conformation. *Nat. Struct. Biol.* **2000**, *7*, 674–678.

61. Turner, N.J. Directed evolution drives the next generation of biocatalysts. *Nat. Chem. Biol.* **2009**, *5*, 567–573.

62. Schmidt, M.; Boettcher, D.; Bornscheuer, U.T. *Industrial Biotechnology: Sustainable Growth and Economic Success*; Soetaert, W., Vandamme, E.J., Eds.; Wiley VCH Verlag GmbH: Weinheim, Germany, 2010; pp. 155–187.

63. Dalby, P.A. Strategy and success for the directed evolution of enzymes. *Curr. Opin. Struct. Biol.* **2011**, *21*, 473–480.

64. Leung, D.W.; Chen, E.; Goeddel, D.V. A method for random mutagenesis of a defined DNA segment using a modified polymerase chain reaction. *Technique* **1989**, *1*, 11–15.

65. Reidhaar-Olson, J.; Bowie, J.; Breyer, R.M.; Hu, J.C.; Knight, K.L.; Lim, W.A.; Mossing, M.C.; Parsell, D.A.; Shoemaker, K.R.; Sauer, R.T. Random mutagenesis of protein sequences using oligonucleotide cassettes. *Methods Enzymol.* **1991**, *208*, 564–586.

66. Taguchi, S.; Ozaki, A.; Momose, H. Engineering of a cold-adapted protease by sequential random mutagenesis and a screening system. *Appl. Environ. Microbiol.* **1998**, *64*, 492–495.

67. Ness, J.E.; del Cardayre, S.B.; Minshull, J.; Stemmer, W.P. Molecular breeding: The natural approach to protein design. *Adv. Protein Chem.* **2000**, *55*, 261–292.

68. Morley, K.L.; Kazlauskas, R.J. Improving enzyme properties: When are closer mutations better? *Trends Biotechnol.* **2005**, *3*, 231–237.

69. Reetz, M.T.; Kahakeaw, D.; Lohmer, R. Addressing the numbers problem in directed evolution. *ChemBioChem* **2008**, *9*, 1797–1804.

70. Muñoz, E.; Deem, M.W. Amino acid alphabet size in protein evolution experiments: Better to search a small library thoroughly or a large library sparsely? *Protein Eng. Des. Sel.* **2008**, *1*, 311–317.

71. Reetz, M.T.; Wu, S. Greatly reduced amino acid alphabets in directed evolution: Making the right choice for saturation mutagenesis at homologous enzyme positions. *Chem. Commun.* **2008**, 5499–5501, doi:10.1039/b813388c.

72. Crameri, A.; Raillard, S.A.; Bermudez, E.; Stemmer, W.P. DNA shuffling of a family of genes from diverse species acelerates directed evolution. *Nature* **1998**, *391*, 288–291.

73. Kolkman, J.A.; Stemmer, W.P. Directed evolution of proteins by exon shuffling. *Nat. Biotechnol.* **2001**, *19*, 423–428.

74. Hackel, B.J.; Kapila, A.; Wittrup, K.D. Picomolar affinity fibronectin domain engineering utilizing loop length diversity, recursive mutagenesis, and loop shuffling. *J. Mol. Biol.* **2008**, *381*, 1238–1252.

75. Ostermeier, M.; Nixon, A.E.; Shim, J.H.; Benkovic, S.J. Combinatorial protein engineering by incremental truncation. *Proc. Natl. Acad. Sci. USA* **1999**, *96*, 3562–3567.

76. Fujii, R.; Kitakoa, M.; Hayashi, K. RAISE: A simple and novel method of generating random insertion and deletion mutations. *Nucleic Acid Res.* **2006**, *34*, e30.

77. Ness, J.E.; Welch, M.; Giver, L.; Bueno, M.; Cherry, J.R.; Borchert, T.V.; Stemmer, W.P.; Minshull, J. DNA shuffling of subgenomic sequences of subtilisin. *Nat. Biotechnol.* **1999**, *17*, 893–896.

78. Jaeger, K.E.; Reetz, M.T. Directed evolution of enantioselective enzymes for organic chemistry. *Curr. Opin. Chem. Biol.* **2000**, *4*, 68–73.

79. Suenaga, H.; Mitsokua, M.; Ura, Y.; Watanabe, T.; Furukawa, K. Directed evolution of biphenyl dioxygenase: Emergence of enhanced degradation capacity for benzene, toluene, and alkylbenzenes. *J. Bacteriol.* **2001**, *183*, 5441–5444.

80. Song, J.K.; Rhee, J.S. Enhancement of stability and activity of phospholipase A(1) in organic solvents by directed evolution. *Biochim. Biophys. Acta* **2001**, *1547*, 370–378.

81. Raillard, S.; Krebber, A.; Chen, Y.; Ness, J.E.; Bermudez, E.; Trinidad, R.; Fullem, R.; Davis, C.; Welch, M.; Seffernick, J.; *et al.* Novel enzyme activities and functional plasticity revealed by recombining highly homologous enzymes. *Chem. Biol.* **2001**, *8*, 891–898.

82. Kurtzman, A.L.; Govindarajan, S.; Vahle, K.; Jones, J.T.; Heinrichs, V.; Patten, P.A. Advances in directed protein evolution by recursive genetic recombination: Applications to therapeutic proteins. *Curr. Opin. Biotechnol.* **2001**, *12*, 361–370.

83. Patten, P.A.; Howard, R.J.; Stemmer, W.P. Applications of DNA shuffling to pharmaceuticals and vaccines. *Curr. Opin. Biotechnol.* **1997**, *8*, 724–733.

84. Siehl, D.L.; Castle, L.A.; Gorton, R.; Chen, Y.H.; Bertain, S.; Cho, H.J.; Keenan, R.; Liu, D.; Lassner, M.W. Evolution of a microbial acetyl transferase for modification of glyphosate: A novel tolerance strategy. *Pest Manag. Sci.* **2005**, *61*, 235–240.

85. Tobin, M.B.; Gustafsson, C.; Huisman, G.W. Directed evolution: The "rational" basis for "irrational" design. *Curr. Opin. Struct. Biol.* **2000**, *10*, 421–427.

86. Cherry, J.R.; Fidanstel, A.L. Directed evolution of industrial enzymes: An update. *Curr. Opin. Biotechnol.* **2003**, *14*, 438–443.

87. Demain, A.L.; Vaishnav, P. Production of recombinant proteins by microbes and higher organisms. *Biotechnol. Adv.* **2009**, *27*, 297–306.

88. Swartz, J.R. *Escherichia coli* Recombinant DNA Technology. In *Escherichia coli and Salmonella: Cellular and Molecular Biology*, 2nd ed.; Neidhardt, F.C., Ed.; American Society of Microbiology Press: Washington, DC, USA, 1996; pp. 1693–1771.

89. Barnard, G.C.; Henderson, G.E.; Srinivasan, S.; Gerngross, T.U. High level recombinant protein expression in *Ralstonia eutropha* using T7 RNA polymerase based amplification. *Protein Expr. Purif.* **2004**, *38*, 264–271.

90. Squires, C.H.; Lucy, P. Vendor voice: A new paradigm for bacterial strain engineering. *BioProcess Int.* **2008**, *6*, 22–27.

91. Romanos, M.A.; Scorer, C.A.; Clare, J.J. Foreign gene expression in yeast: A review. *Yeast* **1992**, *8*, 423–488.

92. Higgins, D.R.; Cregg, J.M. Introduction to *Pichia pastoris*. In *Pichia Protocols*; Higgins, D.R., Cregg, J.M., Eds.; Humana Press: Totowa, NJ, USA, 1998; pp. 1–15.

93. Zhang, A.L.; Luo, X.J.; Zhang, T.Y.; Pan, Y.N. Recent advances on the GAP promoter-derived expression system of *Pichia pastoris*. *Mol. Biol. Rep.* **2009**, *36*, 1611–1619.

94. Hasslacher, M.; Schall, M.; Hayn, M.; Bora, R.; Rumbold, K.; Luecki, J.; Grieng, H.; Kohlwein, S.D.; Schwab, H. High-level intracellular expression of hydroxynitrile lyase from the tropical rubber tree *Hevea brassiliensis* in microbial hosts. *Protein Expr. Purif.* **1997**, *11*, 61–71.

95. Werton, M.W.T.; van den Bosch, T.J.; Wind, R.D.; Mooibroek, H.; de Wolf, F.A. High-yield secretion of recombinant gelatins by *Pichia pastoris*. *Yeast* **1999**, *15*, 1087–1096.

96. Morrow, K.J. Improving protein production processes. *Gen. Eng. Biotechnol. News* **2007**, *27*, 50–54.

97. Bretthauer, R.K.; Castellino, F.J. Glycosylation of *Pichia pastoris*-derived proteins. *Biotechnol. Appl. Biochem.* **1999**, *30*, 193–200.

98. Romanos, M.A. Advances in the use of *Pichia pastoris* for high-level expression. *Curr. Opin. Biotechnol.* **1995**, *6*, 527–533.

99. Giuseppin, M.; van Eijk, H.M.; Bes, B.C. Molecular regulation of methanol oxidase activity in continuous cultures of *Hansenula polymorpha*. *Biotechnol. Bioeng.* **1988**, *32*, 577–583.

100. Egli, T.; van Dijken, J.P.; Veenhuis, M.; Harder, W.; Feichter, A. Methanol metabolism in yeasts: Regulation of the synthesis of catabolite enzymes. *Arch. Microbiol.* **1980**, *124*, 115–121.

101. Shuster, J.R.; Connelley, M.B. Promoter-tagged restriction enzyme-mediated insertion mutagenesis in *Aspergillus niger*. *Mol. Gen. Genet.* **1999**, *262*, 27–34.

102. Gouka, R.J.; Gerk, C.; Hooykaas, P.J.J.; Bundock, P.; Musters, W.; Verrips, C.T.; de Groot, M.J.A. Transformation of *Aspergillus awamori* by *Agrobacterium tumefaciens*-mediated homologous recombination. *Nat. Biotechnol.* **1999**, *6*, 598–601.

103. Van der Hombergh, J.P.; van de Vondervoort, P.J.; van der Heijden, N.C.; Visser, J. New protease mutants in *Aspergillus niger* result in strongly reduced *in vitro* degradation of target proteins; genetical and biochemical characterization of seven complementation groups. *Curr. Genet.* **1997**, *28*, 299–308.

104. Gouka, R.J.; Punt, P.J.; van den Hondel, C.A.M.J.J. Efficient production of secreted proteins by *Aspergillus*: Progress, limitations and prospects. *Appl. Microbiol. Biotechnol.* **1997**, *47*, 1–11.

105. Moralejo, F.J.; Cardoza, R.E.; Gutierrez, S.; Martín, J.F. Thaumatin production in *Aspergillus awamori* by use of expression cassettes with strong fungal promoters and high gene dosage. *Appl. Environ. Microbiol.* **1999**, *65*, 1168–1174.

106. Gusakov, A.V.; Salanovich, T.N.; Antonov, A.I.; Ustinov, B.B.; Okunev, O.N.; Burlingame, R.; Emalfarb, M.; Baez, M.; Sinitsyn, A.P. Design of highly efficient cellulase mixtures for enzymatic hydrolysis of cellulose. *Biotechnol. Bioeng.* **2007**, *97*, 1028–1038.

107. Verdoes, J.C.; Punt, P.J.; Burlingame, R.; Bartels, J.; van Dijk, R.; Slump, E.; Meens, M.; Joosten, R.; Emalfarb, M. A dedicated vector for efficient library construction and high throughput screening in the hyphal fungus *Chrysosporium lucknowense*. *Ind. Biotechnol.* **2007**, *3*, 48–57.

108. Wohlgemuth, R. Biocatalysis—Key to sustainable industrial chemistry. *Curr. Opin. Biotechnol.* **2010**, *21*, 713–724.

109. Gong, J.S.; Lu, Z.M.; Li, H.; Shi, J.S.; Zhou, Z.M.; Xu, Z.H. Nitrilases in nitrile biocatalysis: Recent progress and forthcoming research. *Microb. Cell Fact.* **2012**, *11*, 142–160.

110. Schmid, A.; Dordick, J.S.; Hauer, B.; Kiener, A.; Wubbolts, M.; Witholt, B. Industrial biocatalysis today and tomorrow. *Nature* **2001**, *409*, 258–268.

111. Ran, N.; Zhao, L.; Chen, Z.; Tao, J. Recent applications of biocatalysis in developing green chemistry for chemical synthesis at the industrial scale. *Green Chem.* **2008**, *10*, 361–372.

112. Bornscheuer, U.T.; Huisman, G.W.; Kazlauskas, R.J.; Lutz, S.; Moore, J.C.; Robins, K. Engineering the third wave of biocatalysis. *Nature* **2012**, *485*, 185–194.

113. Sanchez, S.; Demain, A.L. Enzymes and bioconversions of industrial, pharmaceutical, and biotechnological significance. *Org. Process Res. Dev.* **2011**, *15*, 224–230.

114. BBC Research. *Report BIO030 F Enzymes in Industrial Applications: Global Markets*; BBC Research: Wellesley, MA, USA, 2011.

115. World Enzymes. Freedonia Group: Cleveland, OH, USA, **2011**.

116. Kirk, O.; Borchert, T.V.; Fuglsang, C.C. Industrial enzyme applications. *Curr. Opin. Biotechnol.* **2002**, *13*, 345–351.

117. Araujo, R.; Casal, M.; Cavaco-Paulo, A. Application of enzymes for textiles fibers processing. *Biocatal. Biotechnol.* **2008**, *26*, 332–349.

118. Tzanov, T.; Calafell, M.; Guebitz, G.M.; Cavaco-Paulo, A. Bio-preparation of cotton fabrics. *Enzyme Microb. Technol.* **2001**, *29*, 357–362.

119. Gutiérrez, A.; del Río, J.C.; Martínez, A.T. Microbial and enzymatic control of pitch in the pulp and paper industry. *Appl. Microbiol. Biotechnol.* **2009**, *82*, 1005–1018.

120. Farrell, R.L.; Hata, K.; Wall, M.B. Solving pitch problems in pulp and paper processes by the use of enzymes or fungi. *Adv. Biochem. Eng. Biotechnol.* **1997**, *57*, 197–212.

121. Rodriguez-Couto, S.; Toca-Herrera, J.L. Industrial and biotechnological applications of laccases: A review. *Biotechnol. Adv.* **2006**, *24*, 500–513.

122. Rubin, E.M. Genomics of cellulosic biofuels. *Nature* **2008**, *454*, 841–845.

123. Wilson, B.D. Cellulases and biofuels. *Curr. Opin. Biotechnol.* **2009**, *20*, 295–299.

124. Zhang, Y.H.P. What is vital (and not vital) to advance economically-competitive biofuels production. *Process Biochem.* **2011**, *46*, 2091–2110.

125. Zhang, Y.H.P.; Himmmel, M.E.; Mielenz, J.R. Outlook for cellulose improvement: Screening and selection strategies. *Biotechnol. Adv.* **2006**, *24*, 452–481.

126. Kumar, R.; Singh, S.; Singh, O.V. Bioconversion of lignocellulosic biomass: Biochemical and molecular perspectives. *J. Ind. Microbiol. Biotechnol.* **2008**, *35*, 377–391.

127. Kubicek, C.P.; Mikus, M.; Schuster, A.; Schmoll, M.; Seiboth, B. Metabolic engineering strategies for the improvement of cellulase production by *Hypocrea jecorina. Biotechnol. Biofuels* **2009**, *2*, 19–31.

128. Dashtban, M.; Qin, W. Overexpression of an exotic thermotolerant β-glucosidase in *Trichoderma reesei* and its significant increase in cellulolytic activity and saccharification of barley straw. *Microb. Cell Fact.* **2012**, *11*, 63–78.

129. Martinez, D.; Berka, R.M.; Henrissat, B.; Saloheimo, M.; Arvas, M.; Baker, S.E.; Chapman, J.; Chertkov, O.; Coutinho, P.M.; Cullen, D.; *et al.* Genome sequence analysis of the cellulolytic fungus *Trichoderma reesei* (syn. *Hypocrea jecorina*) reveals a surprisingly limited inventory of carbohydrate active enzymes. *Nat. Biotechnol.* **2008**, *26*, 553–560.

130. Kanafusa-Shinkai, S.; Wakayama, J.; Tsukamoto, K.; Hayashi, N.; Miyazaki, Y.; Ohmori, H.; Tajima, K.; Yokoyama, H. Degradation of microcrystalline cellulose and non-pretreated plant biomass by a cell-free extracellular cellulose/hemicellulase system from the extreme thermophilic bacterium *Caldicellulosiruptor bescii. J. Biosci. Bioeng.* **2013**, *115*, 64–70.

131. *Feed Enzymes: The Global Scenario*; Frost & Sullivan: London, UK, 2007.

132. Choct, M. Enzymes for the feed industry: Past, present and future. *World Poult. Sci.* **2006**, *62*, 5–15.

133. Selle, P.H.; Ravindran, V. Microbial phytase in poultry nutrition. *Anim. Feed Sci. Technol.* **2007**, *135*, 1–41.

134. Pariza, M.W.; Cook, M. Determining the safety of enzymes used in animal feed. *Regul. Toxicol. Pharmcol.* **2010**, *56*, 332–342.

135. Mendez, C.; Salas, J.A. Altering the glycosylation pattern of bioactive compounds. *Trends Biotechnol.* **2001**, *19*, 449–456.

136. Okanishi, M.; Suzuki, N.; Furita, T. Variety of hybrid characters among recombinants obtained by interspecific protoplast fusion in streptomycetes. *Biosci. Biotechnol. Biochem.* **1996**, *6*, 1233–1238.

137. Rao, M.B.; Tanksale, A.M.; Ghatge, M.S.; Deshpande, V.V. Molecular and biotechnological aspects of microbial proteases. *Microbiol. Mol. Biol. Rev.* **1998**, *62*, 597–635.

138. Dunn-Coleman, N.S.; Bloebaum, P.; Berka, R.; Bodie, E.; Robinson, N.; Armstrong, G.; Ward, M.; Przetak, M.; Carter, G.L.; LaCost, R.; *et al.* Commercial levels of chymosin production by *Aspergillus. Biotechnology* **1991**, *9*, 976–981.

448

139. Bodie, E.A.; Armstrong, G.L.; Dunn-Coleman, N.S. Strain improvement of chymosin-producing strains of *Aspergillus niger var awamori* using parasexual recombination. *Enzyme Microb. Technol.* **1994**, *16*, 376–382.

140. Pariza, M.W.; Johnson, E.A. Evaluating the safety of microbial enzyme preparations used in food processing: Update for a new century. *Regul. Toxicol. Pharmacol.* **2001**, *33*, 173–186.

141. US FDA. Center for Food Safety and Applied Nutrition. http://vm.cfsan.fda.gov (accessed on 1 July 2013).

142. Vandamme, E.J.; Cerdobbel, A.; Soetaert, W. Biocatalysis on the rise. Part 1. Principles. *Chem. Today* **2005**, *23*, 57–61.

143. *Collection of Information on Enzymes*; Austrian Federal Evironment Agency: Vienna, Austria, 2002.

144. Olempska-Beer, Z.S.; Merker, R.I.; Ditto, M.D.; DiNovi, M.J. Food-processing enzymes from recombinant microorganisms—A review. *Regul. Toxicol. Pharmcol.* **2006**, *45*, 144–158.

145. Tufvesson, P.; Lima-Ramos, J.; Nordblad, M.; Woodley, J.M. Guidelines and cost analysis for catalyst production in biocatalytic processes. *Org. Process Res. Dev.* **2011**, *15*, 266–274.

146. Panke, S.; Wubbolts, M. Advances in biocatalytic synthesis of pharmaceutical intermediates. *Curr. Opin. Chem. Biol.* **2005**, *9*, 188–194.

147. Jäckel, C.; Hilvert, D. Biocatalysts by evolution. *Curr. Opin. Biotechnol.* **2010**, *21*, 753–759.

148. Lutz, S. Reengineering enzymes. *Science* **2010**, *329*, 285–287.

149. Kim, D.Y.; Rha, E.; Choi, S.-L.; Song, J.J.; Hong, S.-P.; Sung, M.-H.; Lee, S.-G. Development of bioreactor system for L-tyrosine synthesis using thermostable tyrosine phenol-lyase. *J. Microb. Biotechnol.* **2007**, *17*, 116–122.

150. Volpato, G.; Rodrigues, R.C.; Fernandez-Lafuente, R. Use of enzymes in the production of semi-synthetic penicillins and cephalosporins: Drawbacks and perspectives. *Curr. Med. Chem.* **2010**, *17*, 3855–3873.

151. Kirchner, G.; Scollar, M.P.; Klibanov, A. Resolution of racemic mixtures via lipase catalysis in organic solvents. *J. Am. Chem. Soc.* **1995**, *107*, 7072–7076.

152. Zheng, G.W.; Xu, J.H. New opportunities for biocatalysis: Driving the synthesis of chiral chemicals. *Curr. Opin. Biotechnol.* **2011**, *22*, 784–792.

153. Wohlgemuth, R. Asymmetric biocatalysis with microbial enzymes and cells. *Curr. Opin. Microbiol.* **2010**, *13*, 283–292.

154. Liang, J.; Mundorff, E.; Voladri, R.; Jenne, S.; Gilson, L.; Conway, A.; Krebber, A.; Wong, J.; Huisman, G.; Truesdell, S.; *et al.* Highly Enantioselective Reduction of a small heterocyclic ketone: Biocatalytic reduction of tetrahydrothiophene-3-one to the corresponding (*R*)-alcohol. *Org. Process Res. Dev.* **2010**, *14*, 185–192.

155. Ma, S.K.; Gruber, J.; Davis, C.; Newman, L.; Gray, D.; Wang, A.; Grate, J.; Huisman, G.W.; Sheldon, R.A. A green-by-design biocatalytic process for atorvastatin intermediate. *Green Chem.* **2010**, *12*, 81–86.

156. Sheldom, R.A. E factors, green chemistry and catalysis: An odyssey. *Chem. Commun.* **2008**, 3352–3365, doi:10.1039/b803584a.

157. Höhne, M.; Schätzle, S.; Jochens, H.; Robins, K.; Bornscheuer, U.T. Rational assignment of key motifs for function guides in silico enzyme identification. *Nat. Chem. Biol.* **2010**, *6*, 807–813.

158. Koszelewski, D.; Göritzer, M.; Clay, D.; Seisser, B.; Kroutil, W. Synthesis of optically active amines employing recombinant ω-transaminases in *E. coli* cells. *ChemCatChem* **2010**, *2*, 73–77.

159. Gooding, O.; Voladri, R.; Bautista, A.; Hopkins, T.; Huisman, G.; Jenne, S.; Ma, S.; Mundorff, E.C.; Savile, M.M.; Truesdell, S.J. Development of a practical biocatalytic process for (R)-2-methylpentanol. *Org. Process Res. Dev.* **2010**, *14*, 119–126.

160. Savile, C.K.; Janey, J.M.; Mundorff, E.C.; Moore, J.C.; Tam, S.; Jarvis, W.R.; Colbeck, J.C.; Krebber, A.; Fleits, F.J.; Brands, J.; *et al.* Biocatalytic asymmetric synthesis of chiral amines from ketones applied to sitagliptin manufacture. *Science* **2010**, *329*, 305–309.

161. Liang, J.; Lalonde, J.; Borup, B.; Mitchell, V.; Mundorff, E.; Trinh, N.; Kochreckar, D.A.; Cherat, R.N.; Ganesh, P.G. Development of a biocatalytic process as an alternative to the (-)-DIP-Cl-mediated asymmetric reduction of a key intermediate of Montelukast. *Org. Process Res. Dev.* **2010**, *14*, 193–198.

162. Ritter, S. Green chemistry awards. Honors: Presidential challenge highlights innovations that promote sustainability. *Chem. Eng. News* **2012**, *90*, 11.

163. Ema, T.; Sayaka, I.; Nobuyasu, O.; Sakai, T. Highly efficient chemoenzymatic synthesis of methyl (R)-*o*-chloromandelate, a key intermediate for clopidogrel, *via* asymmetric reduction with recombinant *Escherichia coli*. *Adv. Synth. Catal.* **2008**, *350*, 2039–2044.

164. Zaks, A.; Dodds, D.R. Application of biocatalysis and biotransformations to the synthesis of pharmaceuticals. *Drug Discov. Today* **1997**, *2*, 513–531.

165. Lee, M.Y.; Dordick, J.S. Enzyme activation for nonaqueous media. *Curr. Opin. Biotechnol.* **2002**, *13*, 376–384.

MDPI AG
Klybeckstrasse 64
4057 Basel, Switzerland
Tel. +41 61 683 77 34
Fax +41 61 302 89 18
http://www.mdpi.com/

Biomolecules Editorial Office
E-mail: biomolecules@mdpi.com
http://www.mdpi.com/journal/biomolecules

www.ingramcontent.com/pod-product-compliance
Lightning Source LLC
Chambersburg PA
CBHW050345230326
41458CB00102B/6418